Student CONSULT Built with inkling | E books

Any screen. Any time. Anywhere.

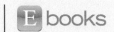

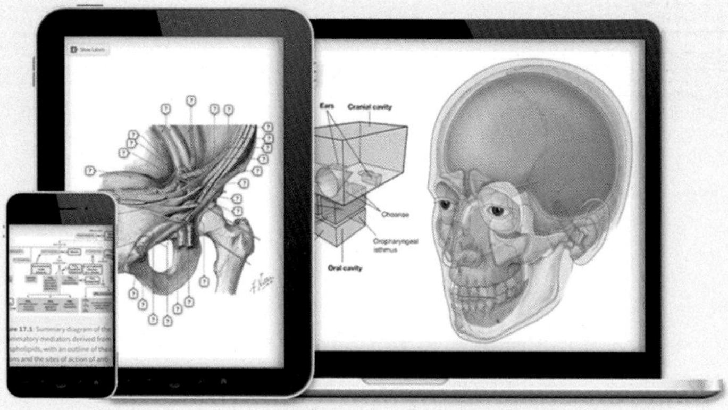

Activate the eBook version of this title at no additional charge.

Student Consult eBooks give you the power to browse and find content, view enhanced images, share notes and highlights—both online and offline.

Unlock your eBook today.

1. Visit studentconsult.inkling.com/redeem
2. Scratch off your code
3. Type code into "Enter Code" box
4. Click "Redeem"
5. Log in or Sign up
6. Go to "My Library"

It's that easy!

Scan this QR code to redeem your eBook through your mobile device:

Place Peel Off Sticker Here

For technical assistance:
email studentconsult.help@elsevier.com
call 1-800-401-9962 (inside the US)
call +1-314-447-8200 (outside the US)

ELSEVIER

HUTCHISON'S CLINICAL METHODS

Executive Content Strategist: Laurence Hunter
Content Development Specialist: Carole McMurray
Project Manager: Louisa Talbott
Designer: Christian Bilbow
Illustration Manager: Amy Faith Heyden
Illustrator: Sara Jarret, CMI; Amanda Williams

24th Edition

HUTCHISON'S CLINICAL METHODS

An integrated approach to clinical practice

Edited by

Michael Glynn MA MD FRCP FHEA

Consultant Physician, Gastroenterologist and Hepatologist
Barts Health NHS Trust;
Honorary Senior Lecturer
Barts and the London School of Medicine and Dentistry;
Former National Clinical Director for GI and Liver Diseases
NHS England

William M. Drake DM FRCP

Professor of Clinical Endocrinology
St Bartholomew's Hospital
London, UK

ELSEVIER

Edinburgh London New York Oxford Philadelphia St Louis Sydney Toronto 2018

ELSEVIER

First edition 1897
Twenty-fourth edition 2018

ISBN 978-0-7020-6739-6
International ISBN 978-0-7020-6740-2

Notices
Knowledge and best practice in this field are constantly changing. As new research and experience broaden our understanding, changes in research methods, professional practices or medical treatment may become necessary.

Practitioners and researchers must always rely on their own experience and knowledge in evaluating and using any information, methods, compounds or experiments described herein. In using such information or methods they should be mindful of their own safety and the safety of others, including parties for whom they have a professional responsibility.

With respect to any drug or pharmaceutical products identified, readers are advised to check the most current information provided (i) on procedures featured or (ii) by the manufacturer of each product to be administered to verify the recommended dose or formula, the method and duration of administration and contraindications. It is the responsibility of practitioners, relying on their own experience and knowledge of their patients, to make diagnoses, to determine dosages and the best treatment for each individual patient, and to take all appropriate safety precautions.

To the fullest extent of the law, neither the Publisher nor the authors, contributors, or editors assume any liability for any injury and/or damage to persons or property as a matter of products liability, negligence or otherwise, or from any use or operation of any methods, products, instructions or ideas contained in the material herein.

Printed in China

Last digit is the print number: 9 8 7 6 5 4 3 2 1

Preface to the Twenty-fourth Edition

Hutchison's Clinical Methods is a book for students of all ages and all degrees of experience. Although the scope, complexity and technology of clinical medicine continues to evolve with great speed, the aim of this text is exactly as it was when Robert Hutchison published the very first edition in 1897: to provide insight into the acquisition of the traditional clinical skills of history taking and physical examination leading to the formulation of a differential diagnosis and management plan. This approach remains as essential as ever to providing good patient care; indeed, as the array of potential investigations expands (and the overall cost continues to rise), it is imperative that such technological advances are integrated with traditional methods. Even though many patients now have easy access, via the Internet, to information about disease and diagnosis, it is the editors' experience that patients appreciate just as much as ever time spent listening to their symptoms, careful physical examination and simple human compassion. Although the circumstances of clinical practice of the readers will vary hugely across the world (with different structures and levels of funding of healthcare), a sound clinical method is indispensable. The organisation of this edition adheres to Hutchison's original approach, with sections on the overall patient assessment, assessment in particular situations, the core body systems and key clinical specialties. Overall, this forms a logical sequence if read straight through but also allows study of each section separately.

As in previous editions, new contributors have joined the book. Some have written entirely new chapters and others have modified the work of their predecessors (including the work of Alan Naftalin, Consultant Gynaecologist, who has sadly died since the last edition was published). All the contributors are accustomed to working closely together and the book reflects these professional relationships. It is the editors' responsibility to mould the chapters into a single text with a logical narrative, but the expertise lies with the contributing authors, whose time and dedication is gratefully acknowledged, as are the extensive contributions of previous experts.

Some of the changes to the previous edition have been made as a result of formally gathered feedback from the newly formed International Advisory Board. In addition a reader survey elicited a range of positive suggestions for improvements to the book. Constructive readers' comments direct to the editors are always welcome.

Michael Glynn and Will Drake
Royal London and St Batholomew's Hospitals

Sir Robert Hutchison MD FRCP

(1871-1960)

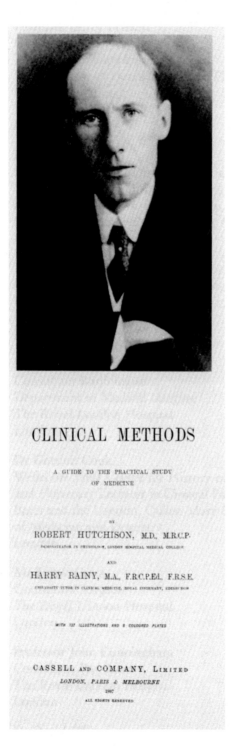

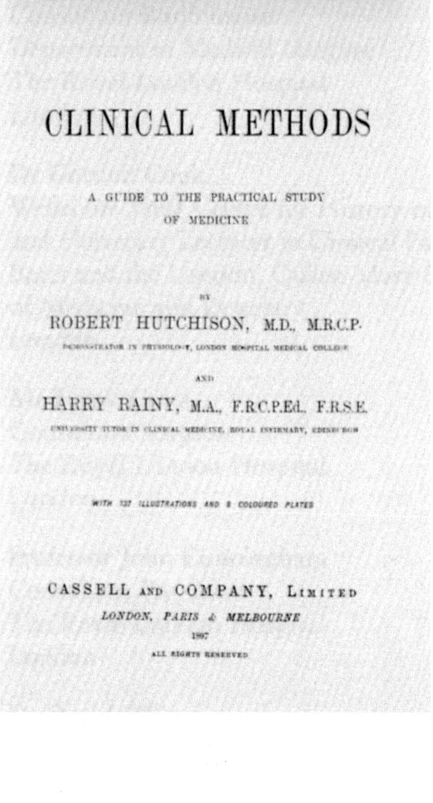

CLINICAL METHODS

A GUIDE TO THE PRACTICAL STUDY OF MEDICINE

BY

ROBERT HUTCHISON, M.D., M.R.C.P.

DEMONSTRATOR IN PHYSIOLOGY, LONDON HOSPITAL MEDICAL COLLEGE

AND

HARRY RAINY, M.A., F.R.C.P.Ed., F.R.S.E.

UNIVERSITY TUTOR IN CLINICAL MEDICINE, ROYAL INFIRMARY, EDINBURGH

WITH 137 ILLUSTRATIONS AND 8 COLOURED PLATES

CASSELL AND COMPANY, LIMITED

LONDON, PARIS & MELBOURNE

1897

ALL RIGHTS RESERVED

Clinical Methods began in 1897, three years after Robert Hutchison was appointed Assistant Physician to The London Hospital (named the Royal London Hospital since its 250th anniversary in 1990). He was appointed full physician to The London and to the Hospital for Sick Children, Great Ormond Street in 1900. He steered *Clinical Methods* through no less than 13 editions, at first with the assistance of Dr H. Rainy and then, from the 9th edition, published in 1929, with the help of Dr Donald Hunter. Although Hutchison retired from hospital practice in 1934, he continued to direct new editions of the book with Donald Hunter, and from 1949 with the assistance also of Dr Richard Bomford. The 13th edition, the first produced without Hutchison's guiding hand, was published in 1956 under the direction of Donald Hunter and Richard Bomford. Dr A. Stuart Mason and Dr Michael Swash joined Richard Bomford on Donald Hunter's retirement to produce the 16th edition, published in 1975, and following Richard Bomford's retirement prepared the 17th, 18th and 19th editions. Dr Swash edited the 20th and 21st editions himself and was joined by Dr Michael Glynn for the 22nd edition. On Dr Swash's retirement Prof William Drake joined Dr Glynn as a co-editor on the 23rd and now this 24th edition. In keeping with the tradition that lies behind the book, each of these editions has been revised with the help of colleagues at The Royal London Hospital, and the other hospitals which now form Barts Health NHS Trust, namely St Bartholomew's Hospital, Whipps Cross University Hospital and Newham University Hospital.

Sir Robert Hutchison died in 1960 in his 90th year. It is evident from the memoirs of his contemporaries that he had a remarkable personality. Many of his clinical sayings became, in their day, aphorisms to be remembered and passed on to future generations of students. Of these, the best known is his petition, written in 1953, his 82nd year:

'From inability to let well alone;
from too much zeal for the new
and contempt for what is old;
from putting knowledge before wisdom, science before art, and cleverness before common sense;
from treating patients as cases;
and from making the cure of the disease more grievous than the endurance of the same, Good Lord, deliver us.'

Michael Glynn and Will Drake
Royal London Hospital

Contributors

Rino Cerio BSc FRCP(Lon) FRCP(Edin) FRCPath DipRCPath ICDPath
Consultant Dermatologist and Professor of Dermatopathology
Department of Cutaneous Medicine and Surgery
Barts Health NHS Trust
London, UK

Tahseen A. Chowdhury MD FRCP
Consultant Physician
Department of Diabetes and Metabolism
Barts Health NHS Trust
London, UK

Andrew Coombes BSc MBBS FRCOphth
Consultant Eye Surgeon and Lead Clinician for Ophthalmology
Barts Health NHS Trust;
Honorary Senior Lecturer
Barts and the London School of Medicine and Dentistry
London, UK

Ceri Davies MD FRCP
Consultant Cardiologist
Barts Health NHS Trust
London, UK

William M. Drake DM FRCP
Professor of Clinical Endocrinology
St Bartholomew's Hospital
London, UK

Adam Feather FRCP
Consultant Acute Physician
Barts Health NHS Trust
London, UK

Michael Glynn MA MD FRCP FHEA
Consultant Physician, Gastroenterologist and Hepatologist
Barts and the London NHS Trust;
Honorary Senior Lecturer
Barts and the London School of Medicine and Dentistry;
Regional Adviser, Royal College of Physicians (London)

James Green LLM FRCS(Urol)
Consultant Urological Surgeon
Department of Urology
Whipps Cross University Hospital
Barts Health NHS Trust;
Visiting Professor
London South Bank University
London, UK

Lina Hijazi
Consultant Physician
Associate Foundation Programme Director
Whipps Cross University Hospital
Barts Health NHS Trust
London, UK

Ali Jawad MBChB MSc(Lond) DCH FRCP(Lond) FRCP(Edin) DMedRehab
Consultant Rheumatologist
Barts Health NHS Trust
London, UK

Stephen Kelly MB ChB MRCP
Consultant Rheumatologist
Barts Health NHS Trust
London, UK

Rehan Khan MRCOG DipIPM
Consultant Obstetrician and Gynaecologist
St Bartholomew's and Royal London Hospitals
Barts and the London NHS Trust
London, UK

Richard Langford MB BS
Consultant in Anaesthesia and Pain Medicine
Barts Health NHS Trust
London, UK

Geraint Morris BMedSc MB BS FRCP DCH FRCEM
Consultant in Emergency Medicine
Homerton University Hospital Foundation NHS Trust
London, UK

John Peters FRCS
Consultant Urologist
Whipps Cross University Hospital
Barts Health NHS Trust
London, UK

Shankar Ramaswamy MBBS MD FRCA FFPMRCA EDRA
Locum Consultant in Anaesthesia and Pain Medicine
Barts and the London NHS Trust
London, UK

Anna Riddell BSc MBBS MRCPCH
Consultant Paediatrician
The Royal London Children's Hospital
Barts Health NHS Trust
London, UK

Andrew Rochford MSc FRCP
Consultant Gastroenterologist
Barts Health NHS Trust
London, UK

Caryn Rosmarin MBBCh DTM&H FCPath(SA) FRCPath(UK)
Consultant Microbiologist
Division of Infection
Barts and the London School of Medicine and Dentistry
Barts and the London NHS Trust
London, UK

Trevor Turner
Honorary Consultant Psychiatrist
East London Foundation Trust;
Former Vice-President of the Royal College of Psychiatrists
London, UK

Rodney W.H. Walker MA BM PhD FRCP
Consultant Neurologist
Barts Health NHS Trust
London, UK

Michael P. Wareing MBBS BSc FRCS(ORL-HNS)
Consultant Otolaryngologist, Head and Neck Surgeon
Barts Health NHS Trust
London, UK

Veronica L.C. White
Consultant Respiratory Physician
Barts and the London NHS Trust
London, UK

International Advisory Board

Professor M.D. Selvam
Professor of Medicine, Sri Muthukumaran Medical College Hospital and Research Institute, Chennai; Former Professor of Medicine, Stanley Medical College and Government Stanley Hospital, Chennai, India

Professor I. Uthman
Professor of Clinical Medicine, Head, Division of Rheumatology, Department of Internal Medicine, American University of Beirut Medical Center, Beirut, Lebanon

Acknowledgements

The Editors would like to acknowledge the contribution of all past authors to this textbook. Each new edition builds on the expertise of the many writers whose work has shaped this book over more than a century. In particular we would like to acknowledge the following who stepped down after the last edition to allow new authors to take their place: Runa Ali; Andrew Archbold; David D'Cruz; Jayne Gallagher; Robert Ghosh; Beng Goh; John Monson; John Moore-Gillon; the late Alan Naftalin; Serge Nikolic; Ruth Taylor; Adam Timmis; and Raj Thuraisingham.

The Editors and Publishers would like to thank all the students and doctors who have provided valuable feedback on this textbook and whose comments have helped shape this new edition. We hope we have listed all those who have contributed and apologise if any names have been accidentally omitted.

As part of the publishers' review, students from numerous medical schools supplied many innovative ideas on how to enhance the book. We are indebted to the following for their enthusiastic support: Emir Abadi; Suhel Abbas; Shaik Kariuddin Abdullah; Santosh Acharya; Mamun David Ebne Ahamed; Salsabil Alfadly; Nouman Safdar Ali; Hemant Atri; Keerthi Ananthula; Noah Anvesh; Sumant Arora; Mohan Babu; Pirmal Bachani; Suranjana Banik; Ankit Bansal; Siddhartha Barnawal; Suranjana Basak; Manognya Bethapudi; Sunil Bhardwaj; Ifrah Binyamin; Sagnik Biswas; Sugandh Chadha; Subhankar Chatterjee; Prajwal Dahal; Amrutha Denduluri; Ugur Demirpek; Mansi Dhingra; Shubham Dixit; Arpan Dutta; Mohammed Omar Farooq; Samreen Fathima; Neil Dominic Fernanes; Priya Gala; Vikash Gautam; Apeksha Ghai; Spandita Ghosh; Akanksha Grover; Prakriti Gupta; Nishedh Gyawali; Riffat Humayun; Mobin Imtiaz; Vibhu Jain; Ruwandika Jayawickrama; Govind Jha; Tushar Jha; Kaushal Raj Kafle; Sowmyashree Mayur Kaku; Pavan Kamble; Kiran Kanchankoti; Vivekanand Kattimani; Abhishek Kaushik; Muneeb Khalid; Sharoj Khan; Zahila Khan; Supreet Khare; Balaram Krishna; Anita Kum; Akshay Kumar; Amit Kumar; Deepak Kumar; Manish Kumar; Praveen Kumar; Vivek Kumar; Dhairya Lakhani; Mirza Umm E Laila; Manikho Lawrence; Jin Xiang Lui; Mohd Luqman; Surjeet Kumar Malakar; Aaron Mascarenhas; Abhishek Mittal; Patel Mrugank; Abhishek Mittal; Sudeb Mukherjee; Vineet Nair; Naren Srinath Nallapeta; Dilip Neupane; Patel Nida; Avinash Pallav; Anup Pandeya; Ambikapathi Panneerselvam; Sabin Parajuli; Ashwin Singh Parihar; Kishor Pokharel; Arun Prasad; Nikhil Prasad; Varun Venkat Raghavan MS; Vishal Raj; Pradhum Ram; Jai Ranjan; Piyush Ranjan; Amuda Regmi; Sudeep Regmi; Sudip Regmi; Peter Richards; Arpit Rustagi; Simrina Kaur Sabharwal; Sujit Kumar Sah; Shreyas Samaga; Bipin Sapkota; Priyanka Satish; Somya Saxena; Deeksha Seth; Sakhi Shah; Syed Mohammad Usman Shah; Anmol Sharma; Anurag Sharma; Bhanu Sharma; Dhan Bahadur Shrestha; Jeevan Shrestha; Suhana Shrestha; Veena Shriram; Amber Tahir Siddiqui; Ankita Singh; Arashdeep Singh; Avinainder Singh; Bishnu Singh; Jeevika Singh; Nidhi Singh; Chopperla SK SK Dattatreya Sitaram; Sakar Raj Sitaula; Soundarya Soundararajan; Amit Srivastava; Shashank K. Srivastava; Sepuri Bala Ravi Teja; Priyesh Thakurathi; Akhilesh Tripathi; Subhrajyoti Tripathy; Mohammad Yousuf Ul Islam; Rajiv Vasusumi; Ashwin P Vinod; Farhan Khan Virk; Waiz A. Wasey; Rajat Kumar Yadav; Saroj Yadav; and Vikrant Yadav.

Contents

SECTION 1

General patient assessment

Doctor and patient: General principles of history taking

1

Michael Glynn

Introduction

If asked why they entered medicine, most doctors would say that they wish to relieve human suffering and disease. In order to achieve this aim for every patient, it is essential to understand what has gone wrong with normal human physiology in that individual and how the patient's personality, beliefs and environment are interacting with the disease process. History taking and clinical examination are initial but crucial steps to achieving this understanding, even in an era in which the availability of sophisticated investigations might suggest to a lay person that a blood test or scan will give all the answers. In addition, even though many diseases are now curable, the relief of symptoms is usually what the patient expects from the medical process.

The phrase 'Clinical Methods' is used less than it used to be. It can be defined as the set of skills doctors use to diagnose and treat disease and the manner in which doctors approach clinical problems and relate to patients. The skills that make up Clinical Methods are acquired during a lifetime of medical work, and they evolve and change as new techniques and new concepts arise and as the experience and maturity of the doctor develop. Clinical methods are acquired by a combination of study and experience, and there is always something new to learn.

The aims of any first consultation are to understand patients' own perceptions of their problems and to start or complete the process of diagnosis. This double aim requires knowledge of disease and its patterns of presentation, together with an ability to interpret a patient's symptoms (what the patient reports/complains of, e.g. cough or headache) and the findings on observation or physical examination (called physical signs or, often, simply 'signs'). Appropriate skills are needed to elicit the symptoms from the patient's description and conversation and the signs by observation and by physical examination. This requires not only experience and considerable knowledge of people in general, but also the skill to strike up a relationship, in a short space of time, with a range of very different individuals.

There are two main steps to making a diagnosis:

1. To establish the clinical features by history and examination – this represents the clinical database.
2. To interpret the clinical database in terms of disordered function and potential causative pathologies, whether physical, mental, social or a combination of these.

This book is about this process. This first chapter introduces the basic principles of history taking and examination, while more detail about the history and examination of each system (cardiovascular, respiratory, etc.) is set out in individual succeeding chapters. Throughout the book, the patient is referred to as 'he', the editors preferring this to 'he/she' or 'they' (except in specific scenarios involving female patients).

Setting the scene

Most medical encounters or consultations do not occur in hospital wards or Emergency Departments but in primary care or outpatient settings. Whatever the setting, a certain familiarity to the context of the consultation, including the consulting room itself, the waiting area and all the associated staff, makes the process of clinical diagnosis easier. Patients are less often assessed in their own home than previously, and many doctors now find this a strange concept.

Meeting the patient in the waiting room allows the doctor to make an early assessment of his demeanour, hearing, walking and any accompanying persons. It is good to offer a greeting and careful introduction and to observe the response unobtrusively but with care. It is important to remember that patients are easily confused by medical titles and hierarchies. All of the following questions should be quickly assessed:

- Does the patient appear relaxed and smiling or furtive and anxious?
- Does the patient make good eye contact?
- Is he frightened or depressed?

- Are posture and stance normal?
- Is he short of breath or wheezing?

In some conditions (e.g. congestive heart failure, acute asthma, Parkinson's disease, stroke, jaundice), the general nature of the problem is immediately obvious. It is very important to identify the patient correctly, particularly if he has a name that is very common in the local community. Carefully check the full name, date of birth and address and any numerical identifier used by the local health system (in the UK, the hospital registration number or the NHS number)

Pleasant surroundings are very important. It is essential that both patient and doctor feel at ease, and especially that neither feels threatened by the encounter. Avoid having patients full-face across a desk. Note taking is important during consultations while being able to see the patient and establish eye contact and to show sympathy and awareness of his needs during the discussion of symptoms, much of which may be distressing or even embarrassing. If the doctor is right-handed and the patient sits on the doctor's left, at an angle to the desk, the situation is less formal, and clues such as agitated foot and hand movements are more evident. If other people are present, arrange the seating to make it clear that it is the patient who is the centre of attention rather than any others present. Increasingly doctors are entering information directly into a computer, rather than writing, and this affects positioning.

Emergency presentations

If the patient is being seen as an emergency, the whole process of history taking is altered according to the surroundings and the degree of illness. No history may be obtainable from a severely ill or unconscious patient, but collateral history from bystanders, relatives or emergency medical personnel should not be ignored. In retrospect this information can be hard to get later on in the patient's illness and can be crucial to diagnosis (e.g. was the patient seen to have a grand mal seizure, or did he complain of sudden pain, before a collapse).

History taking

Having overcome the strangeness of meeting and talking to a wide variety of people that he might not ordinarily meet, the new medical student usually feels that history taking ought to be fairly simple but that physical examination is full of pitfalls such as unrecognized heart murmurs and confusing parts of the neurological examination. However, the experienced doctor comes to realize that history taking is immensely skilled, and that the extent to which this skill goes on increasing with experience is probably greater than for clinical examination.

Beginning the history

The process of gathering information about a patient often begins by reading any referral documentation and with the immediate introduction of doctor and patient. However, once the social introductions are achieved, the doctor will usually begin with a single opening question. Broadly, there are two ways to do this.

A single open-ended question along the lines of 'Tell me about what has led up to you coming here today' gives the opportunity for the patient to begin with what he feels to be most important to him and avoids any prejudgement of issues or exclusion of what at first hearing may seem less important. However, at this stage the patient may be very anxious and nervous and still making his own assessment of how he will react to the doctor as a person. A beginning which focuses on issues which may be more factual and less emotive can be more rewarding and lead to a more satisfactory consultation. Box 1.1 lists some of the areas of questioning that can be usefully included at the beginning of the history. It is important to inform the patient that this is going to be the order of things so that he does not feel that his pressing problems are being ignored. A statement along the lines of 'Before we discuss why you have come today, I want to ask you some background questions' should inform the patient satisfactorily.

There is a particular logic in taking the past medical history at this stage. For many conditions, the distinction as to what is a current problem and what is past history is unclear and arbitrary in the patient's mind. A patient presenting with an acute exacerbation of chronic obstructive pulmonary disease may have a history of respiratory problems going back many years. Therefore, taking the history along a 'timeline' will often build up a much better picture of all of the patient's problems, how they have developed and how they now interact with life and work.

Once these preliminaries have been completed, the doctor should use a simple and open-ended question to encourage the patient to give a full and free account of the current issues. Say something along the lines of 'Tell me about what has led up to you coming here today'. This wording leaves as open as possible any question about the cause of the

Box 1.1 Areas of questioning that can be covered at the beginning of history taking

- Confirm date of birth and age
- Occupation and occupational history
- Past medical history
- Smoking
- Alcohol consumption
- Drug and treatment history
- Family history

patient's problems and why he is seeing a doctor, and could give rise to an initial answer beginning with such varied phrases as 'I have this pain …', 'I feel depressed …', 'I am extremely worried about …', 'I don't know but my family doctor thought …', 'My wife insisted …' or even 'I thought you would already know from the letter my family doctor wrote to you'. All of these answers are perfectly valid but each gives a different clue as to what are the real issues for the patient, and how to develop the history-taking process further for that individual.

This part of history taking is probably the most important and the most dependent on the skill of the doctor. It is always tempting to interrupt too early and, once interrupted, the patient rarely completes what he was intending to say. Even when he appears to have finished giving his reasons for the consultation, always ask if there are any more broad areas that will need discussion before beginning to discuss each in more detail.

Developing themes

This stage of the history is likely to see the patient talking much more than the doctor, but it remains vital for the doctor to steer and mould the process so that the information gathered is complete, coherent and, if possible, logical. Some patients will present a clear, concise and chronologically perfect history with little prompting, although they are in the minority. For most patients, the doctor will need to do a substantial amount of clarifying and summarizing with statements such as 'You mean that …', 'Can I go back to when …', Can I check I have understood …', So up to that point you …', 'I am afraid I am not at all clear about …' and 'I really do not understand, can we go over that again?' If a patient clearly indicates that he does not wish to discuss particular aspects of the history, then this wish must be respected and the diagnosis based on what information is available, although it is also important to explain to the patient the limitations that may be imposed by this lack of information.

Non-verbal communication

Within any consultation, the non-verbal communication is as important as what the patient says. There may be contradictions such as a patient who does not admit to any worries or anxieties but who clearly looks as if he has many. Particular gestures during the description of pain symptoms can give vital clinical clues (Box 1.2). While concentrating on the conversation with the patient, the doctor should keep a wide awareness of all other clues that can be gleaned from the consultation. These include the patient's demeanour, dress and appearance, any walking aids, the interaction between the patient and any accompanying people and the way that the patient reacts to the developing consultation.

Box 1.2 Particular gestures useful in analysing specific pain symptoms

- A squeezing gesture to describe cardiac pain
- Hand position to describe renal colic
- Rubbing the sternum to describe heartburn
- Rubbing the buttock and thigh to describe sciatica
- Arms clenched around the abdomen to describe mid-gut colic

Box 1.3 Words and phrases that need clarification

Ordinary English words

- Diarrhoea
- Constipation
- Wind
- Indigestion
- Being sick
- Dizziness
- Headache
- Double vision
- Pins and needles
- Rash
- Blister

Medical terms that may be used imprecisely by patients

- Arthritis
- Sciatica
- Migraine
- Fits
- Stroke
- Palpitation
- Angina
- Heart attack
- Diarrhoea
- Constipation
- Nausea
- Piles/haemorrhoids
- Anaemia
- Pleurisy
- Eczema
- Urticaria
- Warts
- Cystitis

Vocabulary

It is very important to use vocabulary that the patient will understand and use appropriately. This understanding needs to be on two levels: he must understand the basic words used, and his interpretation of those words must be understood and clarified by the doctor. Box 1.3 lists words and phrases that may be used in the consultation that the doctor needs to be very careful to clarify with the patient. If the patient uses one of the ordinary English words listed, its meaning must be clarified. A patient who says he is dizzy could be describing actual vertigo, but could just mean light-headedness or a feeling that he is going to faint. A patient who says that he has diarrhoea could mean liquid stools passed hourly throughout the day and night or could mean a couple of urgent soft stools passed first thing in the morning only. Therefore, the doctor needs to use words that are almost certainly going to be clearly understood by the patient, and the doctor must clarify any word or phrase that the patient uses to avoid any possibility of ambiguity.

Indirect and direct questions

Broadly, questions asked by the doctor can be divided into indirect or open-ended and direct or closed. Indirect or open-ended questions can be regarded as an invitation for the patient to talk about the general area that the doctor indicates to be of interest. These questions will often start with phrases like 'Tell me more about …', 'What do you think about …', 'How does that make you feel …', 'What happened next …' or 'Is there anything else you would like to tell me?' They inform the patient that the agenda is very much with him, that he can talk about whatever is important and that the doctor has not prejudged any issues. If skilfully used, and if the doctor is sensitive to the clues presented in the answers, a series of such questions should allow the doctor to understand the issues that are most important from the patient's point of view. The patient will also be allowed to describe things in his own words.

Many patients are in awe of doctors and have some conscious or subconscious need to please them and go along with what they say. If the doctor prejudges the patient's problems and tends to 'railroad' the conversation to fit their assumed diagnosis too early in the process, then the patient can easily go along with this and give simple answers that do not fully describe his situation. Box 1.4 illustrates this extremely simple, common and important pitfall of history taking.

Disease-centred versus patient-centred

An interview that uses lots of direct questions is often 'disease centred', whereas a 'patient centred' interview will contain enough open-ended questions for patients to talk about all of their problems and be given enough time to do so. This will also help to avoid the situation in which the doctor and the patient have different agendas. There can often appear to be a conflict if the patient complains of symptoms that are probably not medically serious, such as tension headache, while the doctor is focusing on some potentially serious but relatively asymptomatic condition, such as anaemia or hypertension. In this situation, a patient-centred approach will allow the patient to air all of his problems and will allow a skilled doctor to educate the patient as to why the other issues are also important and must not be ignored. A GP may rightly refuse a demand for antibiotics for a sore

Box 1.4 Example of a history that leads to a poor conclusion

A GP is seeing a 58-year-old man who is known to be hypertensive and a smoker. The receptionist has already documented that he is coming in with a problem of chest pain. The GP makes an automatic assumption that the pain is most likely to be angina pectoris, because that is probably the most serious cause and the one that the patient is likely to be most worried about, and therefore starts taking the history with the specific purpose of confirming or refuting that diagnosis.

GP: I gather you've had some chest pain?

Patient: Yes, it's been quite bad.

GP: Is it in the middle of your chest?

Patient: Yes.

GP: And does it travel to your left arm?

Patient: Yes – and to my shoulder.

GP: Does it come on when you walk?

Patient: Yes.

GP: And is it relieved by rest?

Patient: Yes – usually.

GP: I'm afraid I think this is angina and I will need to refer you to a heart specialist.

The GP has only asked very direct and closed questions. Each answer has begun with 'Yes'. The patient has already been quite firmly tagged with a 'label' of angina, and anxiety has been raised by the specialist referral.

Alternatively, the GP keeps an open mind and starts as follows:

GP: Tell me why you have come to see me today.

Patient: Well – I have been having some chest pain.

GP: Tell me more about what it's like.

Patient: It's in the centre of my chest and tends to go to my left arm. Sometimes it comes on when I've been walking.

GP: Tell me more about that.

Patient: Sometimes it comes when I am walking and sometimes when I'm sitting down at home after a long walk.

GP: If the pain comes on when you are walking, what do you do?

Patient: I usually slow down, but if I'm in a hurry I can walk on with the pain.

GP: I am a little worried that this might be angina but some things suggest it might not be, so I am going to refer you to a heart specialist to make sure it isn't angina.

The GP has asked questions which are either completely open-ended or leave the patient free to describe exactly what happens within a directed area of interest. Clarifying questions have been used. While being reassuring, the GP expresses some concern about angina and is clear about the exact reason for the specialist referral (for clarification).

throat that is likely to be viral but should use the opportunity to educate and inform the patient about the true place of antibiotic treatment and the risks of excess and inappropriate use. The doctor needs to grasp the difference between the disease framework (what the diagnosis is) and the illness framework (what are the patient's experiences, ideas, expectations and feelings) and to be able to apply both frameworks to a clinical situation, varying the degree of each, according to the differing demands.

Judging the severity of symptoms

Many symptoms are subjective and the degree of severity expressed by the patient will depend on his own personal reaction and also on how the symptoms interact with his life. A tiny alteration in the neurological function of the hands and fingers will make a huge impression on a professional musician, whereas most others might hardly notice the same dysfunction. A mild skin complaint might be devastating for a professional model but cause little worry in others.

Trying to assess how the symptoms interact with the patient's life is an important skill of history taking. A simple question such as 'How much does this bother you?' might suffice. It may be helpful to ask specific questions about how the patient's daily life is affected, with comparison to events that many patients will experience. Box 1.5 illustrates some of the relevant areas.

Medical symptomatology often involves pain, which is more subjective than almost anything else. Many patients are stoical and bear severe pain uncomplainingly whereas others seem to complain much more about apparently less severe pain. A simple pain scale can be very helpful in assessing the severity of pain. The patient is asked to rate his pain on a scale from 1 to 10, with 1 being a pain that is barely noticeable and 10 the worst pain he can imagine or the worst pain he has ever experienced. It is also useful to clarify what the reference point is for '10', which for many women will be the pain of labour. The pain scale assessment is useful in diagnosis and in monitoring disease, treatment and analgesia. Assessing a patient with pain is discussed in more detail in Chapter 11.

Which issues are important?

A problem for those doctors wishing to take the history in chronological order – 'Start at the beginning and tell me all about it' – is that people usually start with the part of the problem that they regard as the most important. This is, of course, entirely valid from the patient's viewpoint, and it is also important to the doctor, since the issue that most bothers the patient is then brought to attention. Curing disease may not always be possible, so it is important to be aware of the important symptoms since, for example, pain may be relieved even though the underlying cause of the pain is still present. It is very common for the doctor to be pleased that one condition has been solved, but the patient still complains of the main symptom that he originally came with.

A schematic history

A suggested schematic history is detailed in Box 1.6. There will be many clinical situations in which it will be clear that a different scheme should be followed. An important part of learning about history taking is that each doctor develops his own personal scheme that works for him in the situations that he generally comes across. Nevertheless, it is useful to start with a basic outline in mind.

Direct questions about bodily systems

Within the variety of disease processes that may present to doctors, many have features that occur in many of the bodily systems which at first may not seem to be related to the patient's main complaint. A patient presenting with back pain may have had

Box 1.5 Areas of everyday life that can be used as a reference for the severity, importance or clarification of symptoms

Exercise tolerance: 'How far can you walk on the flat going at your own speed?', 'Can you climb one flight of stairs slowly without stopping?', 'Can you still do simple housework such as vacuum cleaning or making a bed?'

Work: 'Has this problem kept you off work?', 'Why exactly have you not been able to work?'

Sport: 'Do you play regular sport and has this been affected?'

Eating: 'Has this affected your eating?', 'Do any particular foods cause trouble?'

Social life: 'What do you do in your spare time and has this been restricted in any way?', 'Has your sex life been affected?'

Box 1.6 Suggested scheme for basic history taking

- Name, age, occupation, country of birth, other clarification of identity
- Main presenting problem
- Past medical history – 'Before we talk about why you have come, I need to ask you to tell me about any serious medical problems that you have had in the whole of your life'
- Specific past medical history – e.g. diabetes, jaundice, TB, heart disease, high blood pressure, rheumatic fever, epilepsy
- History of main presenting complaint
- Family history
- Occupational history
- Smoking, alcohol, allergies
- Drug and other treatment history
- Direct questions about bodily systems not covered by the presenting complaint

some haematuria from a renal cell carcinoma that has spread and is the cause of the presenting symptom. For this reason, any thorough assessment of a patient must include questions about all the bodily systems and not just areas that the patient perceives as problematic. This area of questioning should be introduced with a statement such as 'I am now going to ask you about other possible symptoms that could be important and relevant to your problem'. A list of such question areas is given in Box 1.7.

In addition, during any medical consultation, however brief, it is the duty of the doctor to be alert to all aspects of the patient's health and not just the area or problem that he has presented with. For example, a GP would not ignore a high blood pressure reading in a patient presenting with a rash, even though the two are probably not connected. This function of any consultation can be regarded as 'screening' the patient. In health economic terms, a true screening programme for a particular disease across a whole population (such as for cervical cancer) has to be evaluated as being useful, economic and with no negative effects. However, once the patient with a complaint has attended a doctor, a simple screening process can be incorporated into the consultation with little extra time or effort. The direct questions (and full routine examination) encompass this screening function as well as contributing to solving the patient's presenting problems.

Clarifying detail

One of the basic principles of history taking is not to take what the patient says at face value but to clarify it as much as possible. Almost all of the history will involve clarification but there are specific areas where this is particularly important.

Pain

Whenever a patient complains of pain, there should follow a series of clarifying questions as listed in Box 1.8. Of all symptoms, pain is perhaps the most subjective and the hardest for the doctor to truly comprehend. A simple pain scale has been described above. The other characteristics are vital in analysing what might be the cause of pain. Some painful conditions have classic sites for the pain and the radiation (myocardial ischaemia is classically felt in the centre of the chest radiating to the left arm). Pain from a hollow organ is classically colicky (such as biliary or renal colic). The pain of a subarachnoid haemorrhage is classically very sudden, 'like a hammer blow to the head'. Some pains have clear aggravating or relieving factors (peptic ulcer pain is classically worse when hungry and better after food). Colicky right upper quadrant abdominal pain accompanied by jaundice suggests a gallstone obstructing the bile duct, and a headache accompanied by preceding flashing lights suggests migraine. It is always worth making sure that any symptom of pain has been clarified in this way,

Box 1.7 Bodily systems and questions relevant to taking a full history from most patients. If the specific questions have been covered by the history of the presenting complaint, they do not need to be included again. If the answers are positive, the characteristics of each must be clarified

Cardiorespiratory

- Chest pain
- Intermittent claudication
- Palpitation
- Ankle swelling
- Orthopnoea
- Nocturnal dyspnoea
- Shortness of breath
- Cough with or without sputum
- Haemoptysis

Gastrointestinal

- Abdominal pain
- Dyspepsia
- Dysphagia
- Nausea and/or vomiting
- Degree of appetite
- Weight loss or gain
- Bowel pattern and any change
- Rectal bleeding
- Jaundice

Genitourinary

- Haematuria
- Nocturia
- Frequency
- Dysuria
- Menstrual irregularity – women
- Urethral discharge – men

Locomotor

- Joint pain
- Change in mobility

Neurological

- Seizures
- Collapses
- Dizziness
- Eyesight
- Hearing
- Transient loss of function (vision, speech, sight)
- Paraesthesia

Box 1.8 List of clarifications for a complaint of pain

- Site
- Radiation
- Character
- Severity
- Time course
- Aggravating factors
- Relieving factors
- Associated symptoms

Box 1.9 Clarifying questions in the drug history

- Can you tell me all the drugs or medicines that you take?
- Have any been prescribed from another clinic, doctor or dentist?
- Do you buy any yourself from a pharmacy?
- Are you sure you have told me about all tablets, capsules and liquid medicines?
- What about inhalers, skin creams or patches, suppositories or tablets to suck?
- Were you taking any medicines a little while ago but stopped recently?
- Do you ever take any medicines prescribed for other people such as your spouse?
- Do you use herbal or other complementary medicines?

Box 1.10 Detail of the family history

Are there any illnesses that run in your family?

Occasionally this will reveal major genetic trends such as haemophilia. More often there will be an answer such as 'They all have heart trouble'.

Basic family tree of first-degree relatives

This should be plotted on a diagram for most patients, including major illnesses and cause and age of any deaths.

Specific questions about occurrence of problems similar to the patient's

Ask the patient about items in the developing differential diagnosis, for example 'Does any one in your family have gallstones/epilepsy/high blood pressure?' if these seem a likely diagnosis for the patient under consideration.

and while some of the points will come out in the open-ended part of the history taking, others will need specific questions.

Drug history

At first glance, asking a patient what drugs he is taking would seem to be one of the simplest and most reliable parts of taking a history. In practice, this could not be further from the truth, and there are many pitfalls for the inexperienced. This is partly because many patients are not very knowledgeable about their own medications and also because patients often misinterpret the question, giving a very narrow answer when the doctor wants to know about medications in the widest sense. The need for clarification in the drug history is given in Box 1.9. The drug history, almost more than any other, benefits from being repeated at another time and in a slightly different way. For example, in trying to define a possible drug reaction as a cause of liver dysfunction, it is not unusual to find that the patient has taken a few relevant tablets (such as over-the-counter non-steroidal anti-inflammatory drugs) just before the onset of the problem and only remembered or realized it was important to say so when asked repeatedly and in great detail.

Family history

Like the drug history, the family history would seem at first glance to be simple and reliably quoted. In general this is true, but it can be dissected into sections that will uncover more information. These are set out in Box 1.10.

Occupational history

It is always useful to know the patient's occupation if he has one, as it is such an important part of life and one with which any illness is bound to interact. In some situations, a patient's occupation will be directly relevant to the diagnostic process. The classic industrial illnesses, such as lead poisoning and other toxic exposures, are now extremely rare in developed industrial countries, but accidental exposure continues to occur. Other problems, such as asbestosis or silicosis, produce effects many years after exposure, and a careful chronological occupational history may be required to elucidate the exposure. For patients with non-organic problems, the work environment can often be the trigger for the development of the problem.

Alcohol history

The detrimental effects of alcohol on health cause a variety of problems, and the frequency of excess alcohol use means that up to 10% of adult hospital inpatients have a problem related to alcohol. To make an accurate estimate of alcohol consumption and any possible dependency, it is essential to enquire carefully and not to take what the patient says at face value but to probe the history in different ways (Box 1.11). For documentation, the reported amount should then be converted into units of alcohol per week (Box 1.12). If the reported amount seems at all excessive then an assessment should be made of possible dependency for which the CAGE questions are very useful (Box 1.13).

Retrospective history

The concept of retrospective history taking is a refinement of taking the past medical history and develops the theme of never taking what the patient says at face value. Many patients will clearly say that they have had certain illnesses or previous symptoms using medical terminology. This information may not be accurate either because the patient has misinterpreted it or because they were given the wrong information or diagnosis in the first place. This area becomes particularly important if any new diagnosis is going to rely on this type of information. For instance, in assessing a patient presenting with chest pain at rest, a past history of angina of effort will be considered a risk factor for acute myocardial infarction

Box 1.11 Probing the alcohol history

Doctor: Do you drink any alcoholic drinks?

Patient: Oh yes, but not much – just socially.

Doctor: Do you drink some every day?

Patient: Yes.

Doctor: Tell me what you drink.

Patient: I usually have two pints of beer at lunchtime and two or three on my way home from work.

Doctor: And at the weekend?

Patient: I usually go out Saturday nights and have four or five pints.

Doctor: Do you drink anything other than beer?

Patient: On Saturdays I have a double whisky with each pint.

The first answer does not suggest a problem, but based on the figures in Box 1.12, the actual amount adds up to 70 units per week which clearly confers considerable health risks to this patient.

Box 1.12 Units of alcohol (1 unit contains 10 g of pure alcohol)

The units of alcohol can be determined by multiplying the volume of the drink (in ml) by its % alcohol by volume (abv) and dividing this by 1000. For example, 1 pint (568 ml) of beer at 3.5% abv contains: $(568 \times 3.5) / 1000 = 1.988$ units.

It is important to bear in mind that alcohol strength varies widely within each category of drink, but here is a guide to the most common alcoholic drinks:

- Standard-strength beer (3.5% abv): 1 pint = 2 units
- Very strong lagers (6% abv): 1 pint = 3.5 units
- Spirits (whisky, gin, etc., 40% abv): 1 UK pub measure (about 25 ml) = 1 unit
- Wine (12%): 1 standard glass (175 ml) = 2 units

The UK Government now recommends that to minimize alcohol-related health effects, both men and women should keep to less than 14 units of alcohol per week.

Box 1.13 The CAGE assessment for alcohol dependency

- C – Have you ever felt the need to Cut down your alcohol consumption?
- A – Have you ever felt Angry at others criticizing your drinking?
- G – Do you ever feel Guilty about excess drinking?
- E – Do you ever drink in the mornings (Eye-opener)?

Two or more positive answers could indicate a problem of dependency.

and will increase the likelihood of that as the current diagnosis. However, on closer questioning, it might become clear that what the patient was told was angina (perhaps by a relative and not even a doctor) was in fact a vague chest ache coming on after a period of heavy work and not a clear central chest pain coming on during exertion.

Clearly the possibility of retaking the history for everything the patient says about his medical past may not be practical in the time available, but the possibility and value of doing this should always be borne in mind and can completely alter the developing differential diagnosis.

Particular situations

It is true to say that while there are many themes, patterns and common areas to history taking and some areas of history taking might seem routine, the process of history taking for different patients will never be identical. There are some particular and often challenging situations that deserve some further description.

Garrulous patients

A new medical student will soon meet a patient who says a huge amount without really revealing any of the information that goes towards a useful medical history. This will be in marked contrast to some other patients who, from the first introductory question (e.g. 'Tell me about what has led up to you coming here today'), will reveal a perfect history with virtually no prompting. A fictitious but typical history from the former type of patient is given in Box 1.14. When faced with such a patient, the doctor will need to significantly alter the balance of open-ended and direct questions. Open-ended questions will tend to lead to such a patient giving a long recitation but with little useful content. The doctor will have to use many more clear, direct questions which may just have yes/no answers. The overall history will inevitably be less satisfactory but it is not possible to get the 'perfect' history in every patient.

Angry patients

Only a few patients are overtly angry when they see a doctor, but anger expressed during a clinical consultation may be an important diagnostic clue while at the same time get in the way of a smooth diagnostic process. Some patients will be angry with the immediate circumstances such as a late-running outpatient clinic. Others will have longer-term anger against the surgery, department or institution which will be more difficult to address. It is always important to acknowledge anger and to try to tease out what underlies it. Even if it is not the doctor's immediate fault that the clinic is running late or there have been other problems, it is always worth apologizing on behalf of the unit or institution.

For some patients, anger may be part of the symptomatology or expressed as a reaction to the diagnosis or treatment. This will be particularly true in patients with a non-organic diagnosis who insist that there is 'something wrong' and that the doctor must do something. Many types of presentation will fall into

Box 1.14 A typical 'garrulous' history

Doctor: Tell me about what has led up to you coming here today.

Patient: Well doctor, you see, it was like this. I woke up one day last week – I am not quite sure which day it was – it might have been Tuesday – or, no, I remember it was Monday because my son came round later to visit – he always comes on a Monday because that's his day off college – he's studying law – I'm so pleased that he's settled down to that – he was so wild when he was younger – do you know what he did once ...?

Doctor (interrupting): Can you tell me what did happen when you woke up last Monday?

Patient: Oh yes – it was like this – I am not sure what woke me up – it may have been the pain – no, more likely it was the dustmen collecting the rubbish – they do come so early and make such a noise – that day it was even worse because their usual dustcart must have been broken and they came with this really old noisy one ...

Doctor (interrupting): So you had some pain when you woke up then?

Patient: Yes – I think it must have been there when I woke up because I lay in bed wondering where on earth there might be some indigestion remedy – I knew I had some but I am one of those people who can never remember where things are – do you know what I managed to lose last year ...?

Doctor (interrupting): Was the pain burning or crushing?

Patient: Well, that depends on what you mean by ...

Doctor (interrupting): Yes, but did you have any crushing pain?

The doctor gradually changes from very open-ended to very closed questions in order to try to get some information that is useful to building up the diagnostic picture – eventually a question is asked that just has a yes/no answer.

this group, including tension headache, irritable bowel and back pain. There may be obvious secondary gain for the patient (such as staying off work and claiming benefits) and challenging this pattern of behaviour may provoke anger.

It is the duty of a doctor to attempt to work with and help a wide variety of patients, and those who are angry are no exception. However, occasionally it may be best to acknowledge that the doctor–patient relationship has broken down and that facilitating a change to another doctor may be in the best interests of the patient.

The well-informed patient

In the last century, doctors often looked after patients for a long time without really explaining their illness to them, and patients were reasonably happy taking the attitude that 'the doctor knows best'. This approach is no longer acceptable and it is the duty of a doctor to give the patient as much information about his illness as possible, particularly so that he is able to make informed choices about treatments. This change of approach has led to many patients seeking out information about their problems from many other sources, particularly the Internet. It is not unusual for a patient to come into the first consultation with a new doctor, armed with printouts from various websites that he feels are relevant or information on their smart phone.

The doctor must take all this in their stride, go through the information with the patient and help him by showing what is relevant and what is not. Many medical websites are created by individuals or groups without proper information for a sound basis of knowledge, but it can be difficult for the patient to make a judgement about this. Being able to inform patients of a few relevant and reliable websites can be very helpful. In general, it is easy and more rewarding to look after well-informed patients, provided they do not fall into the very small group that have such fixed and erroneous ideas about their problems that the diagnostic and treatment process is impeded.

Accompanying persons

Some people come to consultations alone and others with one or more friends or family members. Always spend time during the initial exchange of greetings identifying who is present and getting some idea of the group dynamics. If the patient appears to be alone, ask whether there is someone waiting outside. There is always a reason people come accompanied, but if there appear to be too many people present or if the presence of others might threaten the relationship with the patient at any time in the consultation, it is appropriate to consider asking the others to leave, even if only briefly. It is reasonable, if in doubt, to ascertain why others wish to be present, and certainly whether this is also the patient's wish. It is very important to be certain that the patient is happy for any others to be present and to be as certain as possible that the patient does not wish to object but feels unable to do so. This is particularly difficult if the doctor does not speak the patient's language but can speak to those accompanying. Consider whether specific questions about the history should be asked of those accompanying, either with the patient or separately, with specific consent.

Beware of a situation in which the accompanying people answer all the questions, even if there is not a language difficulty. Many clues to diagnosis may be masked if direct communication with the patient is not possible (using an interpreter/advocate for patients who do not speak the same language as the doctor is discussed below). There may be many reasons that the patient does not speak for himself. These may include embarrassment in front of those accompanying (such as a teenager with his parents). In such circumstances, it may be necessary to leave parts of the history until those accompanying can reasonably be asked to leave, such as during the examination. Occasionally it is clear that the patient will not talk for himself, in which case the history from those accompanying will have to be the working information.

Using interpreters/advocates

Particularly in the inner cities of Western countries, there will often be a large immigrant population who do not speak the first language of the country, even if they have been resident for some years, and it is impractical for each patient to be looked after by health professionals who speak their language. In these circumstances, the medical consultation has to be undertaken with an interpreter. The most immediate solution may be to use a family member, but if the issues are private or embarrassing, this often does not work well. It is also unethical to use an underage family member as an interpreter (under 16).

The best solution is to have available an independent interpreter/advocate for the consultation, although in areas where many patients are not native speakers, many interpreters will be needed for a range of languages. Another solution for infrequently encountered languages is a telephone interpreting service.

When taking a history via an interpreter/advocate, the overall style usually has to change. The breadth of history and the clinical clues that can be obtained from a good initial open-ended question may well be lost in the double translation, and the doctor often changes to a much more direct style of questioning for which the answers will be unambiguous even when going through the double translation. It is also not unusual for the interpreter/advocate and the patient to have a few minutes of conversation following an apparently simple question from the doctor, but then a very short answer is returned to the doctor. This leaves the doctor bemused as to what is really going on with the patient. Finally, history taking via an interpreter/advocate usually takes much longer than when the doctor and the patient speak the same language.

Analysing symptoms

The objective of the history and examination is to begin identifying the disturbance of function and structure responsible for the patient's symptoms. This is done by analysis of the symptoms and signs leading to a differential diagnosis (a list of possible diagnoses that will account for the symptoms and signs, usually set out in descending order of likelihood). This list of possibilities is then often refined by the use of special investigations, but in up to 80% of patients the likely diagnosis is reasonably clear after the initial history. The process of analysis can be likened to detective work, in which the symptoms and signs are the evidence. When a medical student is first faced with the myriad data gleaned on taking a history, he is often baffled as to how to start the analysis, but inevitably the process becomes easier as more medical knowledge is acquired. An analysis of symptoms from a medical student is more based on facts learned from textbooks, whereas an experienced doctor will tend to base the analysis more on patterns of disease presentation that they have encountered many times. While the analytical process is largely acquired through this type of experience, some principles can be described. This topic is discussed further in Chapter 3.

'Hard and soft' symptoms

A detective analysing evidence of a crime will put a lot of weight on fingerprint or DNA evidence and less weight on identification evidence. The same principles apply to analysing symptoms. A 'hard' symptom can be thought of as one which, if clearly present, adds a lot of weight to a particular diagnosis. A 'soft' symptom may be thought of as one which is either reported by patients so variably that its true presence is often in doubt, or one which is present in such a variety of conditions as to not be useful in confirming or refuting a diagnosis. Examples of these two groupings are given in Box 1.15.

Time course

A simple epithet states that the character of the symptom suggests the 'anatomy' of the problem and the time course the 'pathology' of it. For instance, a vascular event such as a myocardial infarct, stroke or subarachnoid haemorrhage usually has a sudden onset, whereas something that gradually progresses or for

Box 1.15 'Hard' and 'soft' symptoms

'Hard' symptoms

- Pneumaturia: almost always due to a colovesical fistula
- Fortification spectra: if associated with unilateral headache, strongly suggests classical migraine
- Rigors: strongly suggests bacteraemia, viraemia or malaria
- A bitten tongue: if associated with a seizure, strongly suggests a grand mal fit
- A sudden severe headache 'like a hammer blow': strongly suggests a subarachnoid haemorrhage
- Pleuritic chest pain: strongly suggests pleural irritation due to infection or a pulmonary embolus
- Itching: if associated with jaundice, indicates intra- or extrahepatic cholestasis

'Soft' symptoms

- Dizziness
- Light-headedness
- Tiredness
- Back pain
- Headache
- Wind

which the onset cannot be exactly dated by the patient, such as weight loss or dysphagia, may be a malignant process. There are some pitfalls in this type of analysis which must be borne in mind to avoid confusion.

Disease processes that gradually progress may start off by being asymptomatic and the patient may only notice symptoms when they start to interfere with his lifestyle and activities. For example, exertional breathlessness in a largely sedentary patient may develop late in a cardiorespiratory disease process, whereas a patient who actively exercises is likely to notice symptoms much earlier. This phenomenon is also seen where the relevant bodily organ or system has a lot of reserve and the symptom may show itself only when the reserve is used up. This could be true for a relatively chronic liver disease such as primary biliary cirrhosis apparently presenting acutely. The proverb of the 'straw that broke the camel's back' is a good analogy of this sort of situation (a camel is steadily loaded up with straw until suddenly it appears that a single piece of straw is sufficient to make the camel collapse). In addition, the disease process may have a step-wise worsening rather than a linear decline, such as in a situation of multiple small strokes when the patient may not present until a single small stroke makes a big difference to his functional ability.

Pattern recognition versus logical analysis

It is important to realize that in some clinical situations the diagnosis may be clear based on previous experience, and in others the diagnosis has to be built up through a process of logical analysis of symptoms, signs and special investigations. The fact that the process of gaining information from symptoms, signs and special investigations is never completely exact must also be borne in mind so that the patient with an atypical presentation is not assigned the wrong diagnosis. The area of medicine that probably most often uses pattern recognition is dermatology, but recently skin biopsies are used much more to clarify diagnoses that were previously assumed. A patient presenting with chest pain and signs of underperfusion may easily be thought to be having a myocardial infarction but a brief history of the character of the pain (tearing and going through to the back) may prompt a search for a dissecting aortic aneurysm.

Negative data

An experienced history taker will begin the analysis from the outset of the clinical encounter. This means that during the initial process and without the need for so much later review, questions can be asked for which a negative answer is as important as a positive one. These questions are usually very specific and direct, often with a yes/no answer. A patient whose presenting complaint is exertional chest pain can immediately be asked if the pain is worse on increased exertion and how long a period of rest is needed to relieve it. Pain that is not predictably produced by exertion and is not reliably relieved by rest may well not be angina pectoris. However, it remains very important that interjected questions of this type do not spoil the flow of the patient's story.

Box 1.16 General reasons that patients come to see doctors (other than for a severe or acute problem)

- Cannot tolerate ongoing symptoms and wants to be rid of them
- Someone else noticing specific problems (e.g. jaundice)
- Another doctor noticing specific problems (e.g. high blood pressure)
- Worry about underlying diagnosis (often induced by relatives, friends, books, media or Internet)
- Spouse or relative worried about patient
- Cannot work with symptoms
- Colleagues/bosses complaining about patient's work or time off
- Requirement of others (insurance, employment benefit, litigation)

What does the patient actually want?

If a patient comes to a doctor with a long history, it is always worth trying to find out why he has come for medical help and what he actually wants from the consultation. There may be various scenarios as listed in Box 1.16. It is always worth trying to find out which might apply to the individual patient, because it sets the scene for giving advice and treatment, particularly if an exact diagnosis or a complete treatment cannot be provided. It is often much easier to reassure a patient that there is nothing seriously wrong than to give him an exact diagnosis or fully relieve his symptoms.

Retaking the history

It is clear that history taking is an inexact process, heavily influenced by the doctor and by the patient. The logical conclusion of this is that no two histories taken from the same patient about the same set of symptoms will be identical, even if the same doctor repeats the process. Given two slightly or significantly different histories, it may be hard to know on which one to base the diagnosis, or whether to regard history taking for that patient as so unreliable as to be useless. The main message is that a single attempt at the history may not suffice and repeated histories taken at different times by different people and in different ways may provide just as much extra information on which to base a diagnosis as more and more detailed special investigations. When a patient is seen for a second or alternative opinion, the doctor usually spends more time on retaking the history than on repeating the examination.

Note taking

When making notes, it is important to keep eye contact with the patient. Notes should not be made only at times that might suggest to the patient what items of information are regarded as important. It is better to listen carefully and just record enough to help remember the important points later. A fuller account can be written up afterwards or dictated for typing later. In this, the exact history, the weight placed on various items and, most importantly, what the patient actually said can be recorded. What patients say, word for word, is often as important as any later reconstruction of the history. Increasingly doctors are entering information directly into computers, rather than writing, during a consultation. If an experienced doctor starts this for the first time, it can feel intrusive, but can soon be mastered so as to become second nature. Patients will generally accept the presence of the computer as being part of the fabric of modern life.

Conclusion

History taking is the cornerstone of medical practice. It combines considerable interpersonal skill and diversity with the need for logical thought based on a wealth of medical knowledge and represents the beginning of treating and caring for patients in the widest sense. Almost all the attributes of good medical practice as set out by the UK General Medical Council (Box 1.17) are encompassed in good history taking. Taking a detailed history while getting to know a patient and arriving at a likely diagnosis is as rewarding in itself as performing a technical procedure for a patient or seeing him get better in the end.

Box 1.17 Duties of doctors registered with the UK General Medical Council (2013)

Knowledge, skills and performance

- Make the care of your patient your first concern
- Keep your professional knowledge and skills up to date
- Recognize and work within the limits of your competence

Safety and quality

- Take prompt action if you think that patient safety, dignity or comfort is being compromised.

Communication, partnership and teamwork

- Protect and promote the health of patients and the public
- Treat patients politely and considerately
- Respect patients' right to confidentiality
- Listen to, and respond to, patients' concerns and preferences
- Give patients the information they want or need in a way they can understand
- Respect patients' right to reach decisions with you about their treatment and care
- Support patients in caring for themselves to improve and maintain their health

Maintaining trust

- Be honest and open and act with integrity
- Never discriminate unfairly against patients or colleagues
- Never abuse your patients' trust in you or the public's trust in the medical profession
- You are personally accountable for your professional practice and must always be prepared to justify your decisions and actions

General patient examination and differential diagnosis

2

William M. Drake and Tahseen A. Chowdhury

Introduction

The separation of the history from the examination is artificial as the latter starts with the first greeting and ends when the patient departs. There may be physical findings that prompt further questioning; do not be concerned that your history taking was inadequate, but revisit these areas at the conclusion of the examination or during it. From the outset, the clinician is assimilating potentially relevant information from the patient's posture, appearance, speech, demeanour and response to questions. Who is this patient? What kind of person is he? What are his anxieties? What is the reason for consulting a doctor at this time? In the outpatient setting, note the patient's grooming and appropriateness of dress. If the patient is in hospital, are there outward signs of social support, such as get-well cards or indicators of a religious faith?

General examination of a patient

Many patients are apprehensive about being examined; the environment is unfamiliar, they may feel exposed and are likely to have anxieties about the findings. Be open about your status as a medical student or junior doctor. Reassure the patient that the extra length of time you take to complete your examination compared to someone more senior is because you are less experienced and that it does not necessarily imply the findings are worrying. Many students, early in their training, are anxious about touching and examining patients. Persevere, as with practice and experience, confidence will quickly come.

The examination should be conducted in a warm, private, quiet area. Daylight is preferable to artificial light, which may make the recognition of subtle changes in skin colour (e.g. mild jaundice) difficult. A cold room increases anxiety levels and shivering muscle generates strange noises on auscultation of the chest. In hospital, you may need to ask neighbouring patients to turn down the volume on their television or radio.

A thorough examination requires the patient to be adequately exposed. Patients should be asked to undress completely or at least to their underclothes and then to cover themselves with a sheet or an examination gown. If the patient keeps his underclothes on, do not forget to examine the covered areas (buttocks, breasts, genitalia, perineum). Ideally a chaperone should be present when a male doctor examines a female patient and is essential for intimate examinations such as rectal, vaginal and breast examinations. This is to reassure the patient and to protect the doctor from subsequent accusations of impropriety. Although the patient's attendance at a consultation suggests he is happy to be examined, this may not be the case and it is always courteous to ask permission. Check he is able to prepare for the examination by disrobing and mounting the couch unaided. Do not embarrass him by waiting for him to fail and ask for help.

For most patients, start the examination on the right of the bed/couch with the patient semi-recumbent (approximately 45°). Do not dent the confidence of an already anxious patient with heart failure or peritonitis by moving him unnecessarily from the position he finds most comfortable. From the right-hand side of the patient, it is easier to examine the jugular veins, apex beat and abdominal viscera, although left-handed students will take longer to master this approach. Try to expose only the area you are examining at the time. With practice, you will become adept at using the gown or drape to cover the body part just examined as you proceed to the next. Regular attention to the patient's comfort, such as adjustment/replacement of pillows, helps strengthen the professional bond and reassures him that you are concerned about his welfare.

Quickly make a global assessment of the severity of the patient's illness. Ask yourself: 'Does this person look well, mildly ill or severely ill?' If the patient is severely ill then it is appropriate to postpone a detailed examination until the acute situation has been attended to. Do not put severely ill patients to inconvenience or distress that is not essential at that moment.

Posture and gait

In the outpatient or primary care setting, observe your patient from the moment you meet him in the waiting area. Does he rise easily from a chair? Does he walk freely, stiffly or with a limp; confidently or apparently fearful of falling; aided or unaided? In the hospital setting, note the patient's posture in bed. Healthy people adjust their position at will, without difficulty. In disease, this ability is lost to variable degrees, and severely ill patients may be sufficiently helpless that they adopt positions that are very uncomfortable. Patients with left heart failure typically find that lying horizontally worsens their sense of breathlessness (orthopnoea). The pain of peritonitis typically compels patients to lie supine, sometimes with the legs drawn up, still and quiet, with shallow breathing movements in order to minimise the pain that movement induces. This contrasts with the restlessness of renal colic, in which the patient often rolls around in a futile attempt to find a position free from pain. With acute inflammatory or infective joint disease, the affected limbs often lie motionless. In severe cases of meningitis, the neck may bend backwards and appear to burrow into the pillow.

Speech and interaction

Much information comes out of the first interaction. The face, particularly the eyes, indicate real feelings better than words. Did your patient smile when you introduced yourself? Was it symmetrical or was there obvious facial weakness? Did he make eye contact? Was the face animated or expressionless as in Parkinson's disease? Was the voice hoarse due to laryngeal disease, recurrent laryngeal nerve palsy or myxoedema? Was the speech pressured, as in thyrotoxicosis or mania or monotonous and expressionless as in severe depression? Was it slurred from cerebellar disease or a previous stroke?

Physique and nutrition

The nutritional state of a patient may provide an important indicator of disease, and prompt correction of a deficient nutritional state may improve recovery. The more detailed methodologies available for nutritional assessment and management in the context of complex gastrointestinal disease are covered in Chapter 14. In the general survey, note if the patient is cachectic, slim, plump or obese (Box 2.1). If obese, is it generalized or centrally distributed? Wasting of the temporalis muscle leads to a gaunt appearance, and recent weight loss may result in prominence of the ribs. Other clues to poor nutrition include cracked skin, loss of scalp and body hair and poor wound healing. Malnutrition together with acute or chronic illness results in blood albumin being low, leading to oedema and making overall body weight an unreliable marker of malnutrition. A smooth, often sore tongue without papillae (atrophic glossitis, Fig. 2.1) suggests important vitamin B deficiencies. Angular stomatitis (cheilosis, a softening of the skin at the angles of the mouth followed by cracking) may occur with a severe deficiency of iron or B vitamins. Niacin deficiency, if profound, may cause the typical skin changes of pellagra (Fig. 2.2).

Box 2.1 Body mass index

BMI = weight (kg)/height (m)^2

In Europeans:

- Normal BMI: 20-25
- Overweight: 25.1-30
- Obese: 30.1-35
- Grossly obese: >35.1

In Asians:

- Normal BMI: 18-23
- Overweight: 23.1-28
- Obese: 28.1-33
- Grossly obese: >33.1

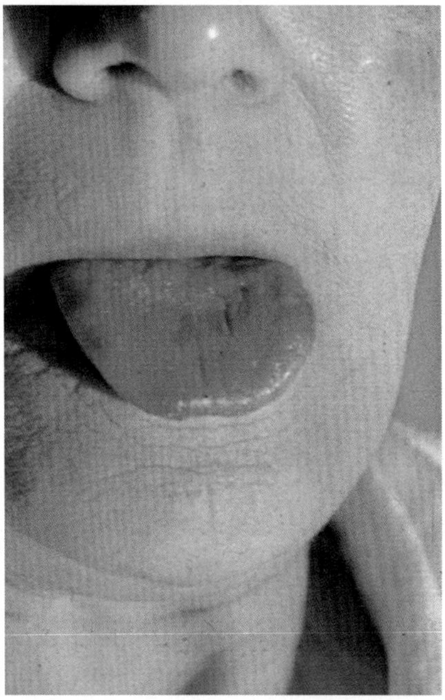

Figure 2.1 Atrophic glossitis in a patient with severe vitamin B12 deficiency. There is also angular stomatitis from severe iron deficiency. (From Forbes and Jackson 2002 Color Atlas and Text of Clinical Medicine, 3rd edn, Mosby, Edinburgh. Reproduced by kind permission.)

Temperature

Body temperature may be recorded in the mouth, axilla, ear or rectum. A 'normal' mouth temperature is 35.8-37°C. Those in the ear and rectum are 0.5°C higher and in the axilla 0.5°C lower. There is a diurnal

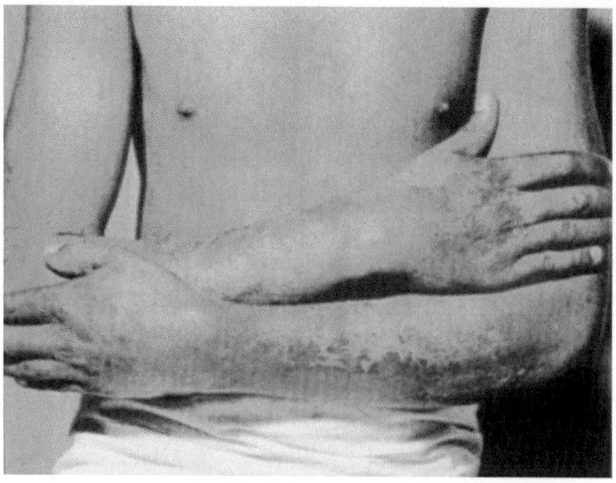

Figure 2.2 Pellagra as a result of niacin deficiency. (From Forbes and Jackson 2002 Color Atlas and Text of Clinical Medicine, 3rd edn, Mosby, Edinburgh. Reproduced by kind permission.)

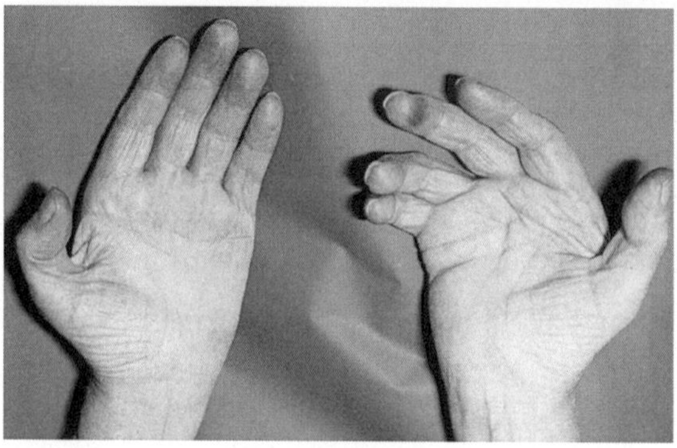

Figure 2.3 Dupuytren's contracture. (From Forbes and Jackson 2002 Color Atlas and Text of Clinical Medicine, 3rd edn, Mosby, Edinburgh. Reproduced by kind permission.)

variation in temperature; the lowest values are recorded in the early morning with a maximum between 6 and 10 pm. In women, ovulation is associated with a 0.5°C rise in temperature. In hospitalized patients, regular temperature measurements may identify certain characteristic patterns of disturbance. A persistent fever is one that does not fluctuate by more than 1°C during 24 hours; a remittent fever oscillates by 2°C during the course of a day; and an intermittent or spiking fever is present for only several hours at a time before returning to normal. None has great sensitivity or specificity for any particular diagnosis, but changes may provide useful information about the course of a disease.

Hands

Examine the hands carefully as diagnostic information from a variety of pathologies may be evident. The strength of the patient's handshake may be informative with regard to underlying neurological or musculoskeletal disorders. Characteristic patterns of muscular wasting may accompany various neuropathies and radiculopathies (see Ch. 16). Make note of any tremor, taking care to distinguish the fine tremor of thyrotoxicosis or recent beta-adrenergic therapy from the rhythmical 'pill rolling' tremor of Parkinsonism (see Ch. 16) and from the coarse jerky tremor of hepatic or uraemic failure (sufficiently slow to be referred to as a metabolic 'flap') or the intention tremor of cerebellar disease.

Feel for Dupuytren's contracture in both hands, the first sign of which is usually a thickening of tissue over the flexor tendon of the ring finger at the level of the distal palmar crease. With time, puckering of the skin in this area develops, together with a thick fibrous cord, leading to flexion contracture of the metacarpophalangeal and proximal interphalangeal joints. Flexion contracture of the other fingers may follow (Fig. 2.3).

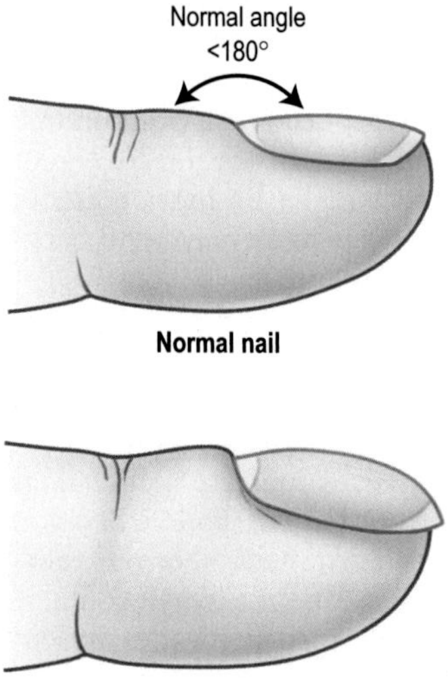

Figure 2.4 Lovibond's angle refers to the angulation between the nail plate and the skin below the nail, when viewed laterally. Normally it is less than 180°. When clubbing is present, the angle is at least 180°, or more.

Check for clubbing of the fingers. Normally, the angle of the fingernail and the nail base (Lovibond's angle) is approximately 180° and the base feels firm to palpation (Fig. 2.4). As clubbing develops, the tissues at the base of the nail are thickened and Lovibond's angle is lost. Subsequently, the nail becomes more convex both transversely and longitudinally and seems to 'float' in a softened nailbed. In normal nails, when both thumbnails are apposed, a diamond-shaped gap is created, called Schamroth's window. With clubbing, a combination of the thickened nail bed and the loss of Lovibond's angle dictates that this window is reduced or even obliterated. In gross cases (usually due to severe cyanotic heart disease, bronchiectasis or empyema), the volume of the finger pulp increases (Fig. 2.5) and becomes bulbous like the end of a drumstick. The toes may also be affected. Lesser degrees of clubbing may be seen in bronchial carcinoma, fibrosing alveolitis,

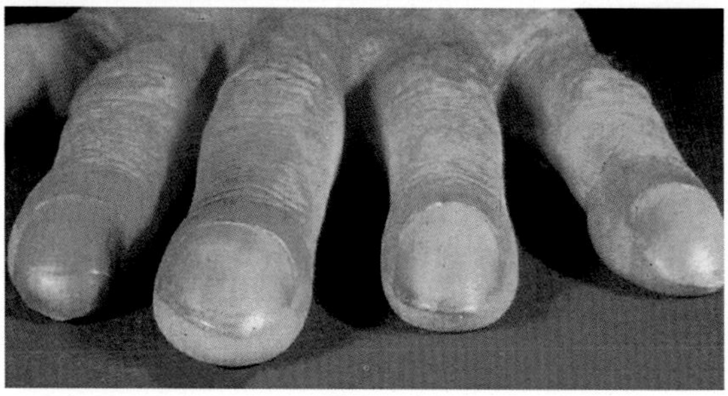

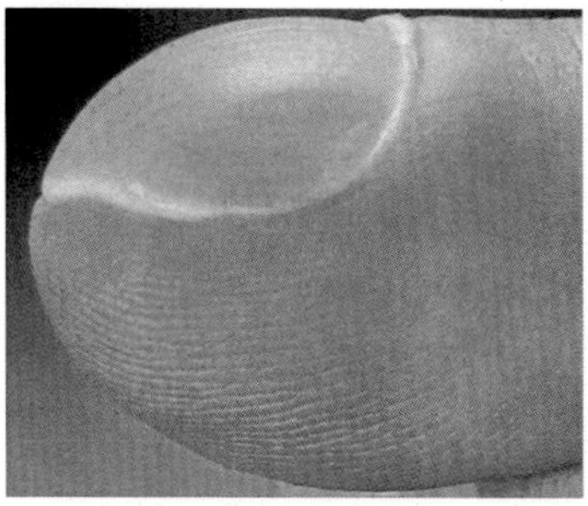

Figure 2.5 Clubbing of the fingers. This case is very marked. (From Forbes and Jackson 2002 Color Atlas and Text of Clinical Medicine, 3rd edn, Mosby, Edinburgh. Reproduced by kind permission.)

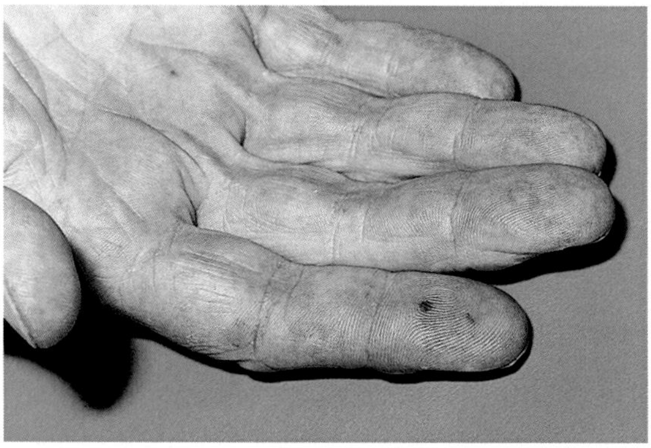

Figure 2.6 Small dermal infarcts in infective endocarditis. (From Forbes and Jackson 2002 Color Atlas and Text of Clinical Medicine, 3rd edn, Mosby, Edinburgh. Reproduced by kind permission.)

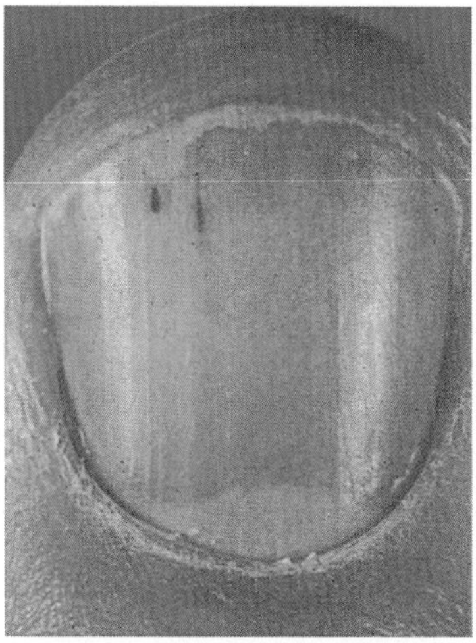

Figure 2.7 Splinter haemorrhages. (From Forbes and Jackson 2002 Color Atlas and Text of Clinical Medicine, 3rd edn, Mosby, Edinburgh. Reproduced by kind permission.)

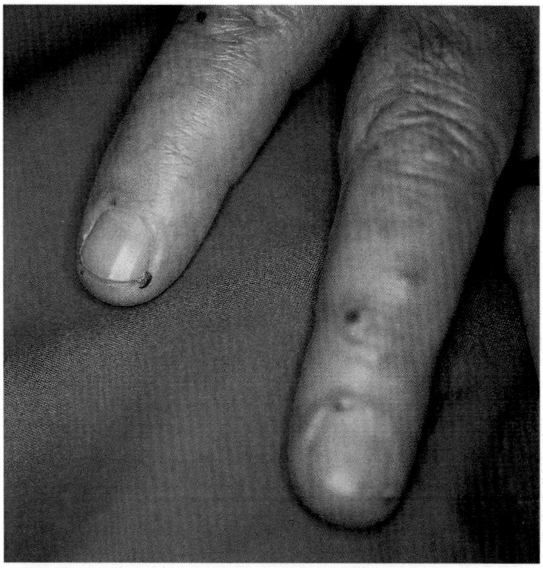

Figure 2.8 Nail-fold infarction. (From Forbes and Jackson 2002 Color Atlas and Text of Clinical Medicine, 3rd edn, Mosby, Edinburgh. Reproduced by kind permission.)

inflammatory bowel disease and infective endocarditis. The last of these may also be associated with Osler's nodes – transient, tender swellings due to dermal infarcts from septic cardiac vegetations (Fig. 2.6). Splinter haemorrhages (Fig. 2.7) and nail-fold infarctions (Fig. 2.8) may be signs of a vasculitic process but may also be the result of trauma in normal individuals and are therefore rather non-specific.

Trophic changes may be evident in the skin in certain neurological diseases and in peripheral circulatory disorders such as Raynaud's syndrome, in which vasospasm of the digital arterioles causes the fingers to become white and numb, followed by blue/purple cyanosis and then redness due to arteriolar dilatation and reactive hyperaemia (Fig. 2.9).

In koilonychia the nails are soft, thin and brittle and the normal convexity replaced by a spoon-shaped concavity (Fig. 2.10). It is a rare feature of longstanding iron-deficiency. Leuconychia (opaque white nails) may occur in chronic liver disease and other conditions associated with hypoalbuminaemia (Fig. 2.11) but are not particularly useful for making a clinical diagnosis of chronic liver disease.

Beau's lines are horizontal (transverse) depressions in the nail that may result from any disease process, illness, chemotherapy or malnutrition that constitutes a sufficient insult to affect the growth plate of the

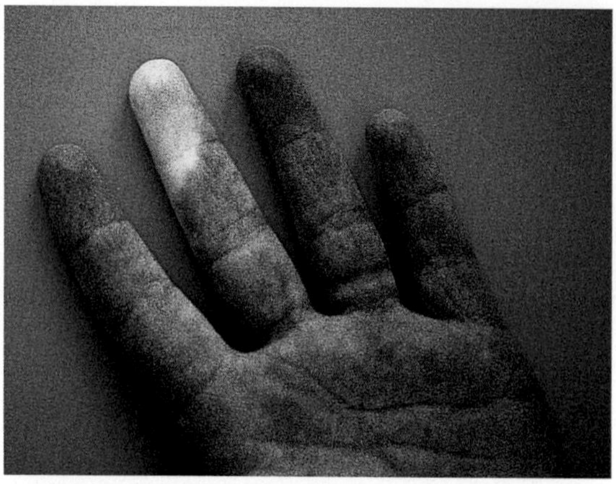

Figure 2.9 Raynaud's syndrome in the acute phase with severe blanching of the tip of one finger. (From Forbes and Jackson 2002 Color Atlas and Text of Clinical Medicine, 3rd edn, Mosby, Edinburgh. Reproduced by kind permission.)

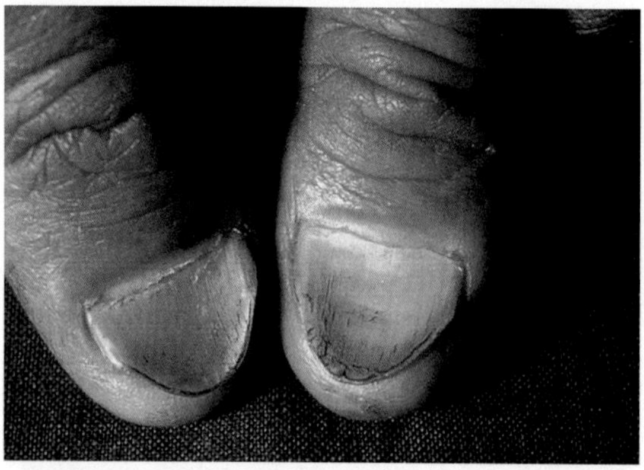

Figure 2.10 Koilonychia. (Reproduced with permission from Mir 2003 Atlas of Clinical Diagnosis, 2nd edn, Saunders, Edinburgh.)

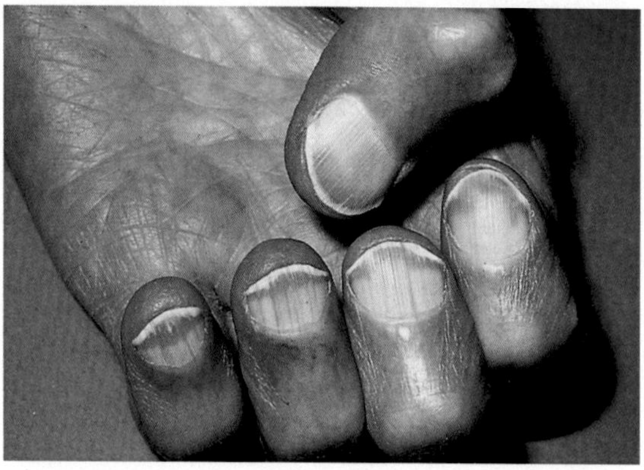

Figure 2.11 Leuconychia in a patient with chronic liver disease. (From Forbes and Jackson 2002 Color Atlas and Text of Clinical Medicine, 3rd edn, Mosby, Edinburgh. Reproduced by kind permission.)

nail. Fingernails grow at a rate of 1 mm per day, so the timing of the disease onset can be estimated by measuring the distance from the Beau's line to the nail bed. They disappear over several months as the nail grows out.

Odours

Certain odours may provide diagnostic clues. The odour of alcohol on the patient's breath is easily recognizable, but do not assume that an alcoholic foetor implies alcoholism or that all the patient's current symptoms and signs are related to alcohol intoxication. Patients with alcohol dependence may have reversible problems such as hypoglycaemia or a subdural haematoma. The odour of diabetic ketoacidosis resembles acetone ('pear drops' or nail varnish remover) and those of hepatic failure and uraemia have been described as 'ammonia-like' or 'mousy', respectively, but such terms are rather subjective and their use is limited. Halitosis (bad breath) is common in patients with suppurative lung diseases and those with gingivitis due to poor dental hygiene. As with all smells, they are difficult to describe but can be characteristic when previously experienced and learnt.

Face and neck

In addition to important expressions and features of mood and attitude noted above, important diagnostic clues may be easily apparent on inspection of the face. Examination of the cranial nerves is covered in Chapter 16, but palsies of the III (Fig. 16.5) and VII (Fig. 2.12) nerves may be obvious simply on inspection. Parotid swellings are usually easily apparent; the tender bilateral parotid swelling of mumps or the unilateral swelling with reddening of the skin from acute parotitis can be contrasted with the non-tender bilateral enlargement that sometimes accompanies chronic alcohol use (and possibly accompanying liver disease). Some patients with mitral stenosis have a bright, circumscribed flush over the malar bones, and in some patients with systemic lupus erythematosus there is a red raised eruption on the bridge of the nose extending onto the cheeks in a 'butterfly' distribution (Fig. 2.13). Telangiectases, minute capillary tortuosities, may be seen on the face in liver disease and rarely, as a hereditary disorder (Fig. 2.14). In systemic sclerosis, there may be radial puckering (furrows) around the mouth (Fig. 2.15) that, as the skin becomes tighter, limits the extent to which the mouth may be opened (Fig. 2.16).

The neck should be inspected and palpated. Examination of the jugular venous pulse (JVP) is described in detail in Chapter 13 but is an important part of the examination in all patients, not just those with suspected cardiovascular disease. It may contribute useful information regarding the severity of lung disease, and its careful assessment is particularly important in patients with suspected disturbance of fluid and electrolyte balance.

Neck swellings are usually best felt from behind the patient. The general principles of lymph node palpation are described below, and the details of examination of the thyroid are covered in Chapter 18.

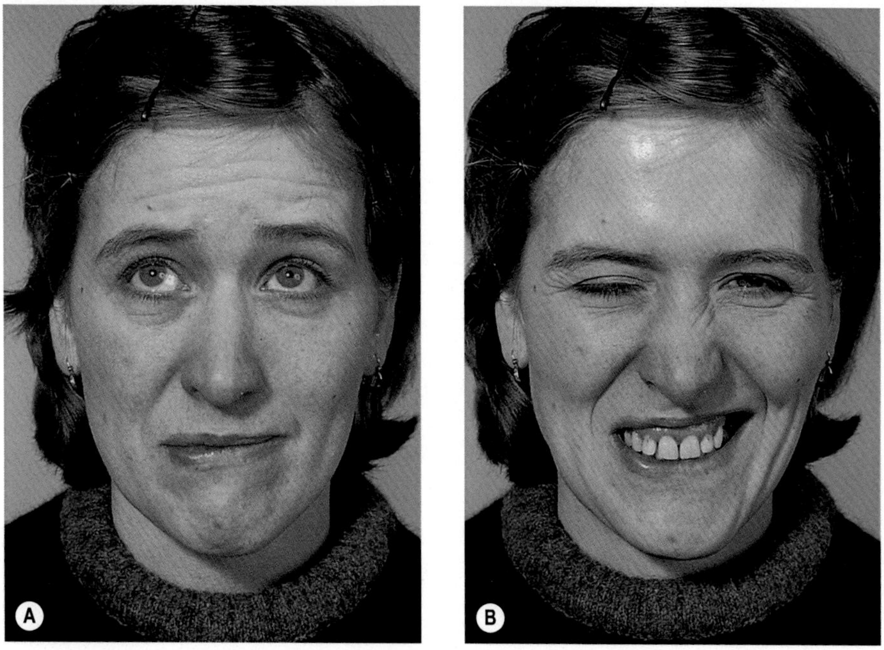

Figure 2.12 A,B Lower motor neuron palsy of the right facial nerve (Bell's palsy).

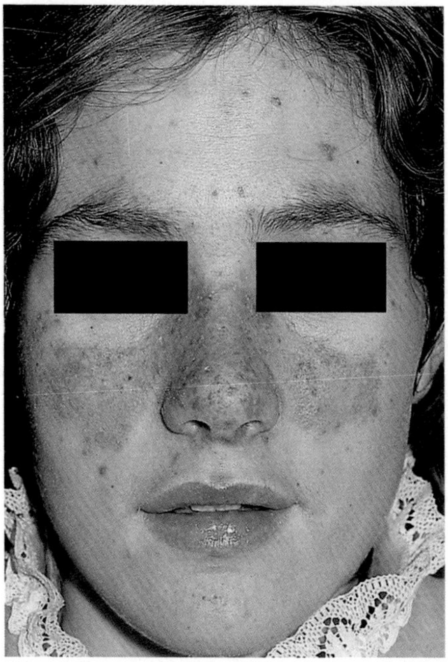

Figure 2.13 Classic butterfly wing rash in a young patient with systemic lupus erythematosus.

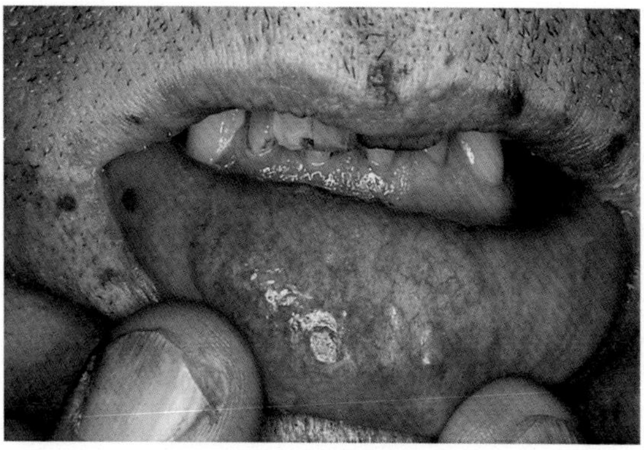

Figure 2.14 Hereditary telangiectasia. The telangiectasia can be seen at the margin of the lips and on the lower lip.

Lymph glands and lymphadenopathy

Details pertaining to the examination of specific lymph node groups may be found in the relevant chapters (e.g. Ch. 21 for cervical lymphadenopathy). Here, the principles of palpating for lymphadenopathy will be covered. Lymph nodes are interposed along the course of lymphatic channels, and their enlargement should always be noted. Lymph from the arm drains into the axillary nodes. These should be routinely examined but particularly in conjunction with examination of the breast (see below). Lymph from the lower limbs drains via deep and superficial inguinal nodes, although only the latter can be palpated and, in turn, comprise a vertical and horizontal group. The vertical inguinal nodes lie close to the upper part of the long saphenous vein and drain the leg. The horizontal group lies above the inguinal ligament and drains the lower abdominal skin, anal canal, external genitalia (excluding the testes), buttocks and lower vagina.

Examination of lymph nodes involves inspection and palpation. Inflammation of the overlying skin and associated pain usually implies an infective aetiology, whereas malignant lymphadenopathy is

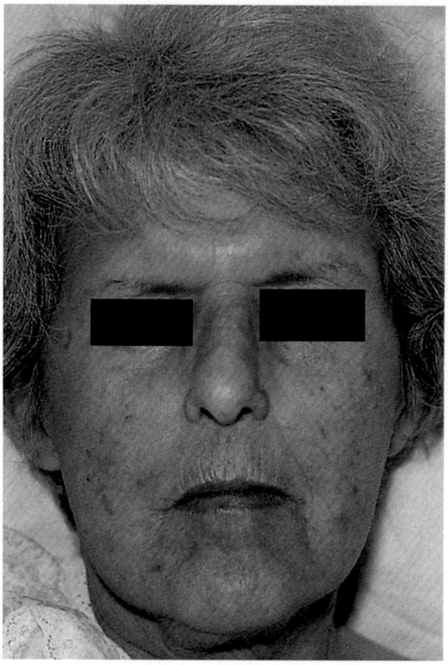

Figure 2.15 Radial puckering (furrows) around the mouth in systemic sclerosis.

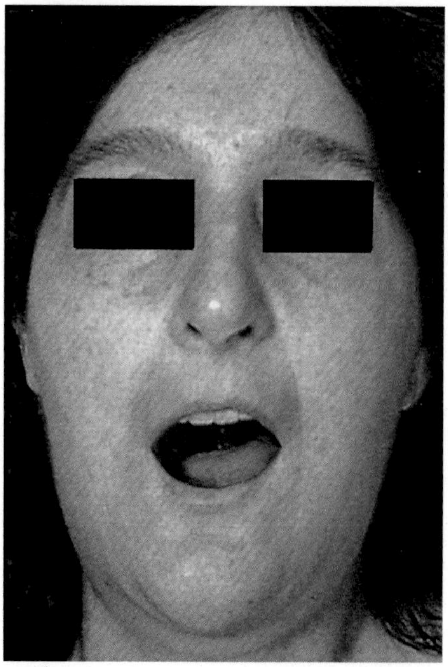

Figure 2.16 Limited mouth opening in systemic sclerosis.

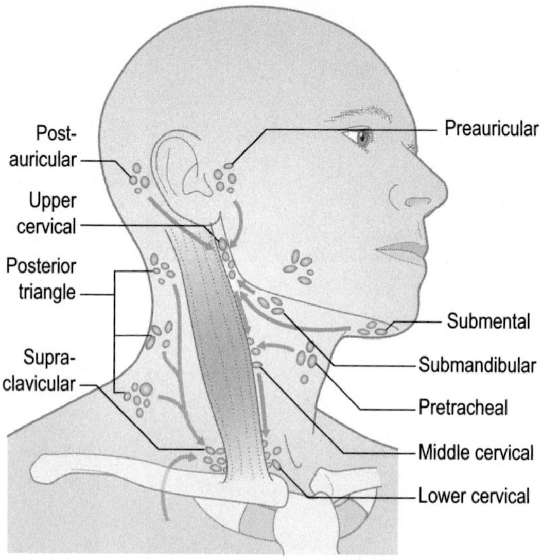

Figure 2.17 The cervical lymph node groups.

usually non-tender. To palpate for lymphadenopathy, use the pulps of your fingers (usually the index and middle but, for large nodes, the ring as well) to move the skin overlying the potentially enlarged node(s). Determine the size, position, shape, consistency, mobility, tenderness and whether it is an isolated lymph node or whether several coalesce. For the head and neck nodes, it is often helpful to tilt the head slightly towards the side of examination in order to relax the overlying muscles. Feel for each of the groups shown in Fig. 2.17 in whatever order you find most efficient and reliable. Muscles and arteries in the neck and groin may be mistaken for lymph nodes. If in doubt, try to move the structure in question in two directions (laterally and superior to inferior). It should be possible to move a lymph node in two directions but not an artery or muscle.

Determining whether a lymph node is pathological can be difficult and requires practice and experience. In general, small, mobile, discrete lymph nodes are frequently found in normal individuals, particularly those who are slim and have little overlying adipose tissue. The finding of an enlarged lymph node should prompt the question 'Is this consequent upon local pathology, for example infection or malignancy, or is it part of a more generalized abnormality of the reticuloendothelial system (including other lymph node groups, liver and spleen)?' (Fig. 2.18).

Axillae

Most information from examination of the axillae comes from palpation for possible lymphadenopathy (Fig. 2.19), but inspection may reveal an absence/paucity of secondary sexual hair in either gender (most commonly in association with chronic liver disease but also in certain endocrinopathies), abnormal skin colouring, such as the dark velvety appearance of acanthosis nigricans (characteristic of insulin resistance and occasionally gastric cancer, Fig. 2.20), or (very rarely and almost always in the presence of café au lait spots elsewhere) the characteristic freckling of von Recklinghausen's disease (Fig. 2.21).

Support the weight of the patient's arm by holding his arm at the elbow with your non-examining hand so that the patient's pectoral muscles are relaxed.

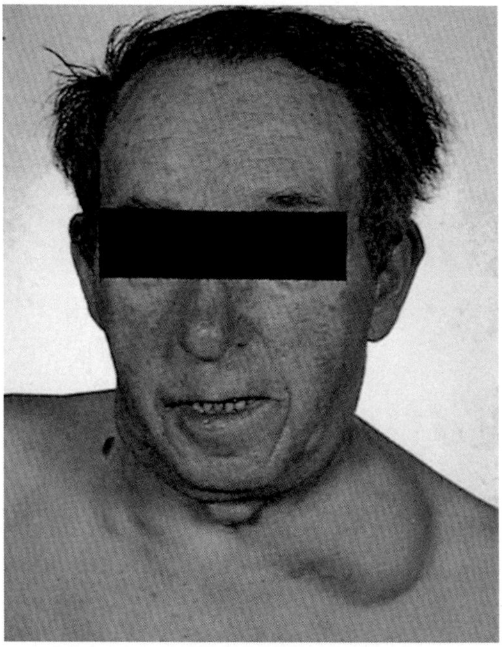

Figure 2.18 Gross enlargement of supraclavicular and cervical lymph nodes. (From Forbes and Jackson 2002 Color Atlas and Text of Clinical Medicine, 3rd edn, Mosby, Edinburgh. Reproduced by kind permission.)

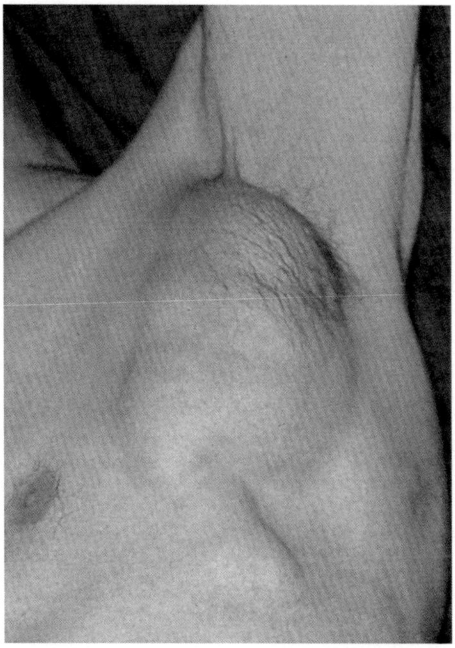

Figure 2.19 Gross (in this case, painless) axillary lymph node enlargement. (From Forbes and Jackson 2002 Color Atlas and Text of Clinical Medicine, 3rd edn, Mosby, Edinburgh. Reproduced by kind permission.)

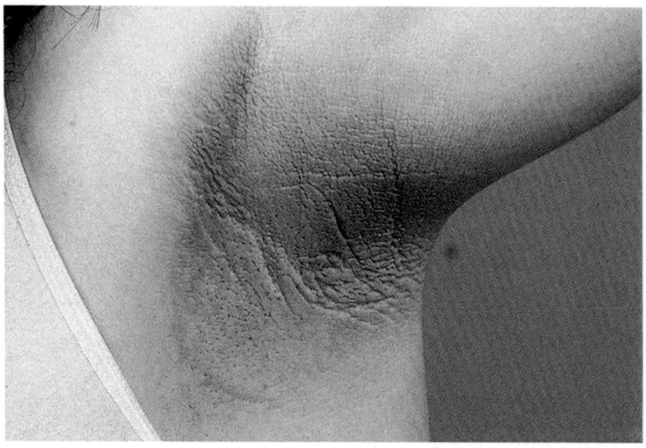

Figure 2.20 Acanthosis nigricans (sometimes seen in insulin resistance and gastric cancer) visible in the axilla.

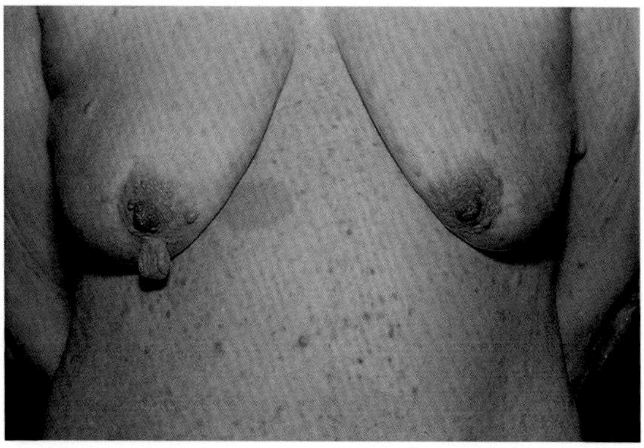

Figure 2.21 Freckling and neurofibromas in von Recklinghausen's disease.

With the fingers of your right hand cupped together, probe the apex of the left axilla, then slide them downwards against the chest wall to feel for lymphadenopathy. Next, 'sweep' your fingers along the inside of the anterior and posterior axillary folds, feeling for enlargement of the pectoral and subscapular lymph nodes respectively. Use your left hand in the same way to examine the right axilla.

Skin

Examination of the skin with respect to specific dermatological diagnoses is covered in Chapter 19. In the context of the general examination, the most important features relate to temperature, hydration, pallor, colour/pigmentation and cyanosis. Use the back of your fingers to assess the temperature of the skin. This complements rather than replaces the formal measurement with a thermometer. There may be generalized warmth in febrile illness or thyrotoxicosis or localized warmth if there is regional inflammation. Cold skin may be localized, such as when a limb is deprived of its blood supply, or generalized in states of circulatory failure, when the skin feels clammy and sweaty.

Lift a fold of skin and make note of its thickness, mobility and how easily it returns to its original position (turgor). The skin on the back of the hand is often thin and fragile in elderly patients, may show decreased mobility in scleroderma (Fig. 2.22) or in oedematous states and have reduced turgor in the

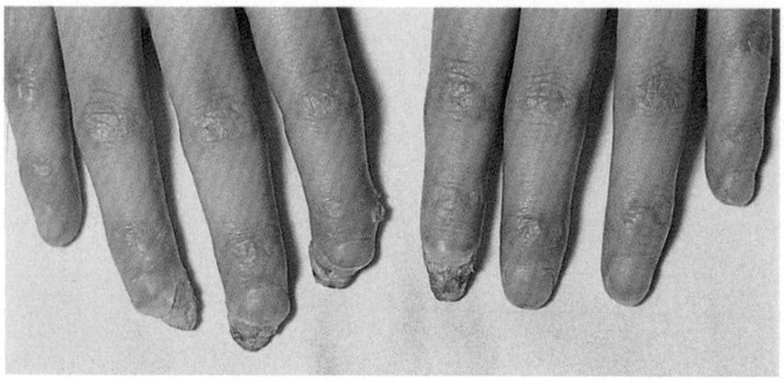

Figure 2.22 Advanced scleroderma. (From Forbes and Jackson 2002 Color Atlas and Text of Clinical Medicine, 3rd edn, Mosby, Edinburgh. Reproduced by kind permission.)

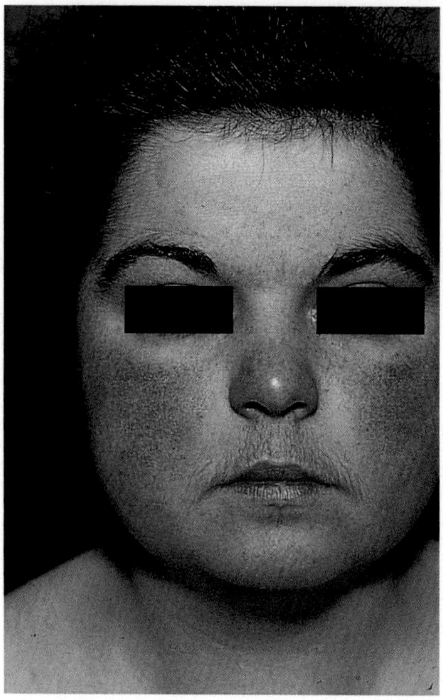

Figure 2.23 The characteristic plethoric appearance of a patient with Cushing's syndrome. (From Forbes and Jackson 2002 Color Atlas and Text of Clinical Medicine, 3rd edn, Mosby, Edinburgh. Reproduced by kind permission.)

presence of dehydration. The skin of acromegalic patients is typically thick and greasy.

Make note of the colour of the skin (the following description is less relevant to people with dark skin). Normal skin colour varies considerably; some people have a fresh complexion and others, although completely healthy, a pale one. Pallor may be seen temporarily in haemorrhage, shock and in intense emotion. Anaemic patients are often pale, but not all pale people are anaemic. The colour of the mucous membrane of the eyelids and mouth is a better indication of anaemia than the colour of the skin.

Yellowness of the skin is usually due to jaundice. A pale lemon-yellow tinge is characteristic of haemolytic jaundice, whereas in obstructive jaundice there is a dark yellow or orange tint, sometimes accompanied by scratch marks from itching caused by bile salts. Lemon tinge may also be associated with uraemia, which may occasionally also cause a 'frosting' of the lips or forehead – so-called 'uraemic frost'.

An important determinant of skin colour is the relative amount of oxyhaemoglobin and deoxyhaemoglobin. Oxyhaemoglobin is a bright red pigment. An increase in its flow beneath thinned facial skin causes the characteristic plethora of Cushing's syndrome (Fig. 2.23), whereas a decrease in flow causes pallor. As blood passes through the capillary bed, oxygen is given up to metabolizing tissues to produce deoxyhaemoglobin. This has a darker, less red, more bluish pigment, and its presence in peripheral blood vessels in increased amounts causes the clinical sign of cyanosis. There are two physiological types of cyanosis: peripheral and central. Peripheral cyanosis is associated with increased extraction of oxygen from capillaries when peripheral blood flow is slowed, often due to vasospasm caused by cold, heart failure or anxiety. The cyanosed extremity is usually cold and the tongue is unaffected. Any condition causing slowing of the peripheral circulation may lead to peripheral cyanosis as there is more time for oxygen extraction. Central cyanosis is caused by inadequate oxygenation of blood, in turn due to heart failure, serious respiratory disease or mixing of venous and arterial blood across a right to left cardiac shunt. In the latter situation, blood passes directly from the right to the left side of the heart, without passing through the pulmonary circulation, thereby failing to become oxygenated. Central cyanosis is generalized and the peripheries are often warm. At least 5 g/dl of reduced haemoglobin is necessary to produce central cyanosis, and it is therefore less marked in anaemic patients. The cyanosis of heart failure is often due to both peripheral and central causes. The presence of central cyanosis is best appreciated at the lips, mucous membranes and conjunctivae, where the keratinized skin is thinnest (Fig. 2.24).

Pulses

Arterial pulses are detected by compressing the relevant vessel against a firm underlying structure, usually a bone. Details of the characteristic pulse abnormalities that help in the diagnosis of various cardiac disorders are described in Chapter 13, but palpation of all the peripheral pulses should form part of the general examination of all patients. Some may be difficult to feel and you may need to vary the degree of pressure in order to pick up the relevant pulsation. On occasion, you may confuse the patient's pulse with your own. Feel your own pulse on the side of your forehead with your other hand and compare it with the patient's, as they will usually be different.

The radial pulse is palpated by gentle pressure of the artery against the distal shaft of the radius, using

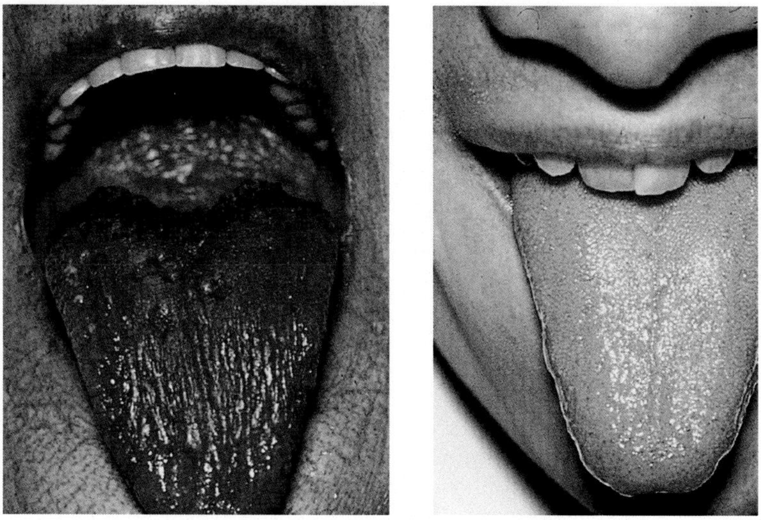

Figure 2.24 Central cyanosis in a patient with severe respiratory disease (left) compared to the tongue of a normal person. (From Forbes and Jackson 2002 Color Atlas and Text of Clinical Medicine, 3rd edn, Mosby, Edinburgh. Reproduced by kind permission.)

the tips of the index and middle fingers. It provides information about rate and rhythm, although significant abnormalities in character may also be detected. If the rhythm is regular, it is safe to count the number of beats for 15 seconds and multiply by 4 for the rate. Irregular and very slow pulses require palpation for a full minute. Palpating both radial pulses simultaneously can give useful information in selected patients. Atheromatous narrowing of the axillary artery may cause reduced strength of one radial pulse compared to the other, as may aortic dissection.

To palpate the femoral pulse, press deeply below the inguinal ligament, midway between the anterior superior iliac spine and the symphysis pubis. The pulse is usually easily felt against the underlying femur. In obese patients it may be useful to use two hands, one on top of the other. Occasionally, such as in young patients with hypertension, it may be appropriate to examine for radio-femoral delay. Here, the radial and femoral pulses on one side of the body are palpated at the same time. The pulsation should occur simultaneously; any delay may suggest coarctation of the aorta, in which the aorta is constricted just beyond the subclavian artery. Blood flow to the arms is good, but to the legs is poor such that the pulse is weak and delayed.

The popliteal pulse is the most difficult to palpate. Flex the knee to approximately 120° and, with your thumbs on the patella, place your fingers in the popliteal fossa such that they meet in the midline. Occasionally, it may be necessary to have the patient lie prone with the knee flexed to 90° and the leg resting against the shoulder or upper arm; press the thumbs deep into the popliteal fossa.

The dorsalis pedis (DP) pulse is palpated by pressing against the tarsal bones just lateral to the extensor tendon of the great toe, although in some patients it may be necessary to explore the dorsum of the foot more widely. In general, it is most convenient to use the right hand to examine the left DP pulse; the right pulse is often best felt with the right hand from the left side of the patient.

To feel the posterior tibial (PT) pulse, with the patient's foot relaxed between plantar- and dorsiflexion, press your curved fingers against the distal part of the tibia, approximately 1 cm behind and below the medial malleolus. The PT pulse may be difficult to feel and require extra patience and pressure in obese or oedematous patients.

Blood pressure

The physiology of blood pressure measurement (including a description of the Korotkoff sounds) is given in Chapter 13. Many doctors and medical students neglect to measure the blood pressure routinely in the belief that it is somehow a 'nursing' observation. This is a poor habit to adopt, not least because, once the technique has been mastered, it can be easily combined with simultaneous, unobtrusive observations of the patient that may provide useful diagnostic information without his feeling self-conscious. Although not necessary or appropriate to perform routinely, assessment for postural (orthostatic) hypotension is frequently informative in older patients, particularly those with symptoms of unsteadiness, syncope or presyncope, or those taking medication for hypertension. It is defined as a drop in blood pressure of >20/10 mmHg within 3 minutes of changing from a supine to an upright position. Various 'protocols' are adopted; the authors favour measurement of blood pressure supine after a period of calm rest and then every minute for 3 minutes after moving to a vertical position. Together with assessment of the JVP, it can provide important information about volume status in the evaluation of patients with fluid and electrolyte abnormalities, such as those with recent gastrointestinal bleeding.

Legs and feet

Examination of the legs requires adequate exposure from the groins and buttocks to the toes. Note the colour and texture of the skin. Peripheral vascular disease often makes the skin shiny and hair does not grow on ischaemic legs or feet (Fig. 2.25). Pressure on the toes of ischaemic feet will cause blanching of the characteristic purple colour with subsequent slow return. Passive elevation of an ischaemic leg leads to marked pallor of the foot as perfusion against gravity falls. Painless trophic lesions, often with deep ulceration, may be seen in diabetic peripheral neuropathy. The posterior aspect of the heels is a particularly important area to inspect in elderly, emaciated or neurologically impaired patients, all of whom are vulnerable to pressure ulcers caused by obliteration of arteriolar and capillary blood flow to the skin.

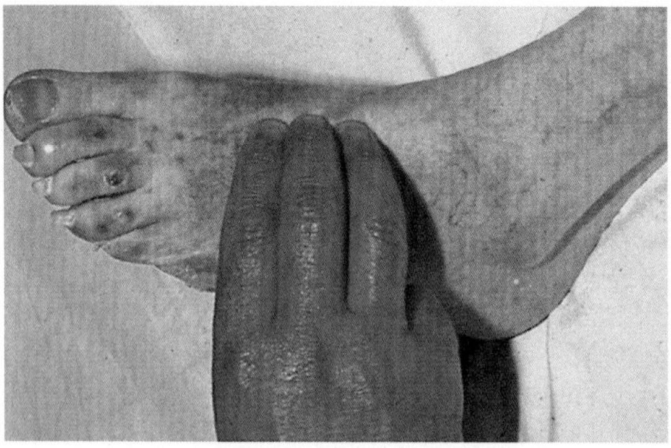

Figure 2.25 Peripheral vascular disease. There is pallor, loss of hair and early ulceration on the dorsum of three toes. (From Forbes and Jackson 2002 Color Atlas and Text of Clinical Medicine, 3rd edn, Mosby, Edinburgh. Reproduced by kind permission.)

Inspect the legs for easily seen oedema (fluid in the subcutaneous tissue that appears as swelling) and examine for pitting oedema. Press firmly but gently behind the medial malleolus, over the dorsum of the foot and on the shin. If oedema is present, a depression/concavity will form and persist for some time (Fig. 2.26). The skin over oedematous feet and shins has a pallid, glossy appearance and a characteristic doughy feel. The best place to look for mild degrees of oedema in cardiac disease is behind the malleoli in patients who are ambulant and over the sacrum in those who are confined to bed. Usually, 5-10 seconds of finger pressure is sufficient to produce the typical shallow pit but it may be necessary to press for 20-30 seconds to avoid overlooking mild degrees of oedema. Some doctors grade oedema on a 4-point scale (slight and short-lived after relief of pressure to very marked and long lasting), although the system is poorly standardized. Oedema due to cardiac disease or to conditions associated with a low plasma protein level is bilateral. In local venous obstruction the oedema is confined to the parts from which the return of blood is impeded. Thus, oedema of an arm occurs when malignant lymph nodes constrict the axillary vein, and unilateral leg oedema will develop if the ileofemoral vein is occluded. The oedema of lymphatic obstruction does not pit on pressure.

Varicose veins should be looked for with the patient standing (Fig. 2.27). Superficial varicosities are generally obvious in this position, whereas the efficiency of the valves of the long saphenous vein should be assessed by Trendelenburg's test. With the patient lying, the saphenous vein is emptied by elevating the

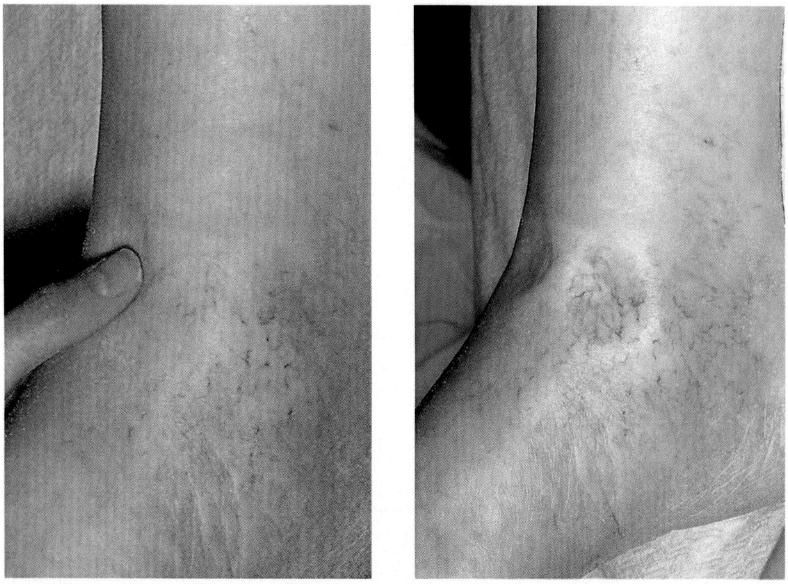

Figure 2.26 Pitting oedema in a patient with cardiac failure. A depression remains in the oedema for several minutes after firm fingertip pressure is applied. (From Forbes and Jackson 2002 Color Atlas and Text of Clinical Medicine, 3rd edn, Mosby, Edinburgh. Reproduced by kind permission.)

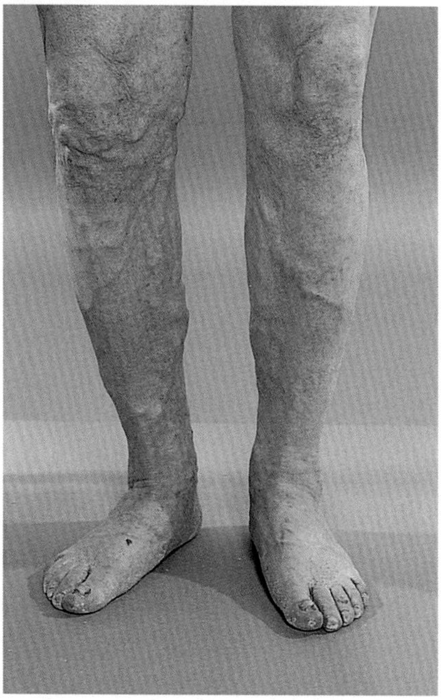

Figure 2.27 Varicose veins. (From Forbes and Jackson 2002 Color Atlas and Text of Clinical Medicine, 3rd edn, Mosby, Edinburgh. Reproduced by kind permission.)

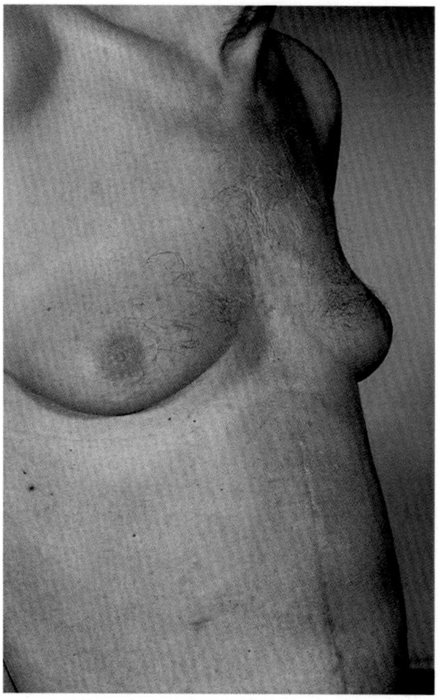

Figure 2.28 Gynaecomastia in a male patient. (From Forbes and Jackson 2002 Color Atlas and Text of Clinical Medicine, 3rd edn, Mosby, Edinburgh. Reproduced by kind permission.)

leg. Occlude the upper end of the vein by finger pressure on the saphenous vein opening (alternatively use a tourniquet) and ask the patient to stand while maintaining this pressure. If the valves are incompetent, the veins will rapidly fill from above when the pressure is released.

Venous thrombosis is rare in healthy mobile subjects but frequently complicates enforced bed rest, particularly after surgery. The affected limb will be swollen. The circumference of the calf should be measured and compared with the unaffected leg at the same distance below the tibial tuberosity. A discrepancy of more than 1 cm is significant. The affected leg is also tender and warmer than normal, with dilated superficial veins which do not collapse when the leg is elevated. Forceful dorsiflexion of the foot may cause pain in the calf (Homan's sign). Sometimes a deep vein thrombosis may extend up the thigh leading to a tender, hard, palpable femoral vein.

Breasts

Examination of the breasts should form part of the routine clinical assessment, usually at the time of examination of the chest. It requires tact and sensitivity and should be conducted with a chaperone. With the patient disrobed to the waist, the arms should be in a relaxed position by the sides. By inspection, make note of the size, symmetry, contour (e.g. any dimpling) and colour of the breasts. Inflammatory breast cancer with oedema of the overlying skin may produce a characteristic look and texture termed peau d'orange (orange peel skin). Note any asymmetry or inversion of the nipples. Simple longstanding inversion is often a normal phenomenon, but associated retraction of the areola or recent nipple inversion are more sinister. Ask the patient to raise her arms above her head. This manoeuvre allows inspection of the inframammary fold and may expose subtle contour abnormalities. Now, with the patient supine, ask the patient to rest one arm above her head. This helps spread the breast tissue more evenly across the chest and makes palpation of any nodules easier. For ease of annotation, the breast is usually divided into four quadrants, with the upper outer quadrant extending into an axillary tail. Use the pads of your middle three fingers to palpate the breast, using rotatory movements gently to compress the tissue against the chest wall. Proceed systematically to examine all quadrants, the tail and areola. Sometimes it is useful to support the breast with the other hand in order to aid examination, especially when the breasts are large.

Breast tissue is variable between patients, ranging from smooth to granular, and may change in a given individual with the menstrual cycle. For any nodule, note its size, shape, consistency, tenderness, mobility and the presence of any tethering or skin ulceration. Ask the patient to press her hands against her hips. If the lump becomes less mobile, it is likely to be attached to the pectoral muscles. Fixation to skin may be assessed by moving the skin overlying the lump independently. If this is not possible then skin involvement is likely.

Swelling of male breast tissue is usually easily apparent (Fig. 2.28). Distinguishing true glandular enlargement from pectoral fat may be facilitated with the patient's arms above his head. At some stage of puberty, most boys will have a palpable disc of tissue.

Putting it all together

The information given in this and subsequent chapters describes techniques of physical examination that *may* be helpful in elucidating the cause of a patient's symptoms. It is not implicit that *all* of these examinations should be performed in *all* patients. For example, it is not appropriate to make a detailed assessment of the neurological system in someone in severe respiratory distress due to pulmonary oedema or in abdominal pain from peritonitis. Initially, both alone and during teaching, you will probably practise examining individual systems (e.g. the cardiovascular system). Soon, however, you will be ready to conduct a complete examination. The following is a suggested order for the student to practise, and doctor to perform, in all hospitalized patients who are not acutely ill, in order to exclude any major abnormality in the various bodily systems.

General

- Overall appearance (well, unwell, severely ill; neglected or well-cared for).
- Posture and gait.
- Nutrition, obesity, oedema.
- Skin colour, cyanosis, jaundice, anaemia.
- Skin lesions (spider naevi, vitiligo, purpura, petechiae).
- Body hair (distribution, quantity).
- Vital signs (temperature, pulse, respiration rate).
- Obvious features of endocrine disease (e.g. Cushing's, acromegaly, hyperlipidaemia).

Mouth and pharynx

- Odours, lips, tongue (ask to protrude), teeth, gums, buccal mucous membrane, tonsils.

Hands

- Clubbing, tremor, wasting, arthropathy, metabolic flap, Dupuytren's contracture, splinter haemorrhages, nail-fold infarcts, koilonychia, leuconychia, nicotine stains.

Cardiovascular and respiratory (anterior, patient semi-recumbent)

- Radial pulse: rate, rhythm, character.
- Blood pressure, lying and standing.
- Jugular venous pulse.
- Carotid pulses, separately, both sides.
- Inspection for symmetry, scars, dilated vessels, breasts, nipples.
- Praecordial palpation: apex beat, thrills, heaves.
- Auscultate the heart sounds.
- Palpate tracheal position.
- Chest expansion.
- Tactile vocal fremitus.
- Percuss the lungs.
- Auscultate the breath sounds.
- Vocal resonance.

Cardiovascular and respiratory (posterior, sitting forward)

- Inspect for symmetry of movement, scars.
- Chest expansion.
- Tactile vocal fremitus.
- Percuss the lungs.
- Auscultate the breath sounds.
- Vocal resonance.
- Inspect for sacral oedema.

Neck (while sitting forward)

- Thyroid palpation.
- Cervical, submandibular lymphadenopathy.

Abdomen

- Inspection: size, distension, asymmetry, scars, abdominal wall movements, dilated vessels, visible peristalsis, pulsations, pubic hair, spider naevi.
- Palpation: tenderness, rigidity, hyperaesthesia, masses, organomegaly, hernial orifices, inguinal lymphadenopathy, genitalia, digital rectal (where relevant).
- Percussion: organomegaly, masses.
- Auscultation: bowel sounds, bruits.

Upper limbs

- Inspection: fasciculations, wasting, trophic changes.
- Test for tone, power, reflexes, coordination and cutaneous sensation.
- Test joints for swelling, pain and movement, if relevant.

Lower limbs

- Inspection: fasciculations, wasting, trophic changes, ulceration, varicose veins, oedema.
- Test for tone, power, reflexes, coordination and cutaneous sensation.
- Test joints for swelling, pain and movement, if relevant.
- Peripheral pulses.

Cranial nerves

- Visual acuity, pupillary responses, visual fields, extraocular movements, nystagmus fundoscopy.
- Facial movements and sensation.
- Rinne and Weber test.
- Palatal elevation, tongue appearance and protrusion.

Documentation and communication

An accurate, concise record of a clinical episode is crucial for effective care. It serves as a tool for ordering the doctor's thoughts as he reviews the findings before constructing a provisional differential diagnosis. It may identify errors or missing data (did I examine the reflexes?). It serves as a reminder of those thought processes at future consultations as the results of investigations become available and/or the condition evolves, and it allows colleagues to pick up the 'thread' of a case in the event of the initial assessing doctor being unavailable. Furthermore, as rising expectations and increasing availability of medical information via the Internet embolden more patients to question the quality of their care, accurate documentation is vital in order to provide the evidence for the quality of the decision making and assessment in the event of a disagreement between patient and doctor. All medical note entries should be dated, timed and signed and each page should have the patient's name and hospital record number clearly written.

The style and extent of note-taking will vary according to circumstance. For example, a postoperative visit to a surgical outpatient clinic after a routine repair of a hernia is likely to focus exclusively on issues relating to pain and scar healing, with brief documentation. In contrast, the initial consultation at a falls clinic will involve the expert in elderly medicine gathering potentially relevant information about past medical history, current medication, social support and the history of the current problem, and will certainly require a comprehensive physical examination. A GP is likely already to know the details of the patient's family, social, past medical and drug histories, so in the limited time available will focus on the current problem. In all of these situations, however, the clinician should avoid being constantly engaged in writing notes or, increasingly, looking at a computer screen. Maintain eye contact as the patient talks about his problems. The following suggestions refer to a new patient consultation in the outpatient clinic or a non-acutely ill hospitalized patient. The goal is to write a complete yet concise record of the patient's problem that can easily be followed as a logical narrative by the next doctor to see that patient.

Start with the routine social data: name, address, marital status, occupation, dependent family members and children. The order in which the family, past medical and presenting complaint histories are documented is not rigidly set. For those patients who have enjoyed good health to the point of the current illness, the presenting complaint and history of the current problem fall naturally out of the context of the above background information. Medical notes for such a patient with (for example) a spontaneous pneumothorax might read as follows:

Mr JW, aged 32, manual labourer, married, 2 children.

Generally in excellent health and symptom free. Keen sportsman.

No relevant past medical history.

PC: Breathlessness.

HPC:

- Sudden-onset right-sided chest pain.
- Worse on inspiration.
- Associated severe breathlessness; unable to get comfortable.
- No cough or sputum or haemoptysis.
- No injury or trauma to chest.
- No previous similar episodes.
- No recent periods of immobility.
- No leg swelling or pain.

PMH:

- Appendectomy age 6.
- Varicocoele found and surgically corrected age 25 following assessment for primary infertility.

An important differential diagnosis in a patient with pneumothorax is pulmonary embolism, sometimes with prior deep venous thrombosis. The 'negative' features of the history (no leg symptoms, no recent immobility) 'steer' the narrative and any subsequent reader of the history away from this diagnosis but serve as a focus for its consideration. If a rigid system were recommended of documenting all *potentially* relevant past medical and family history prior to the presenting problem, the same history might read:

Mr JW, age 32, manual labourer, married, 2 children.

Generally in excellent health and symptom free. Keen sportsman.

No family history of deep vein thrombosis or pulmonary embolism. No family history of tall stature, lens dislocation, valvular heart disease (all features of Marfan's syndrome, an important association with pneumothorax in young patients). Varicocoele surgery age 25 with no history of postoperative deep vein thrombosis or pulmonary embolism.

PC: Breathlessness.

HPC:

- Sudden-onset right-sided chest pain.
- Worse on inspiration.
- Associated severe breathlessness; unable to get comfortable.
- No cough or sputum or haemoptysis.
- No injury or trauma to chest.
- No previous similar episodes.
- No recent periods of immobility.
- No leg swelling or pain.

Although used as an extreme example, such a style of documentation could 'obstruct access' to the presenting complaint. For many patients, however, it *is* appropriate to detail a pertinent family history and/or past medical history prior to the current problem or as an 'introduction/context' to it. Good examples of this would include a middle-aged man with rectal bleeding and a strong family history of carcinoma of the colon, or a young person, breathless on exertion, who underwent corrective surgery for congenital heart disease as a child. For other patients,

Box 2.2 Example of a cardiovascular system statement

- Pulse 76 regular, peripheral pulses normal
- Neck veins not distended. No peripheral oedema
- BP 130/80
- Apex beat not displaced
- Heart sounds I and II heard in all areas
- No murmurs, lungs clear

the current problem is the latest development of a long-standing illness, such as cough and breathlessness in a patient with chronic obstructive pulmonary disease. This skill of interweaving the past/family history with the current problem will develop with experience, so do not be disheartened if your notes initially seem disjointed.

Many patients have had medical and surgical episodes in their history that are essentially 'closed events', for example cataract removal, hernia repair or tonsillectomy as a child. Although they may seem irrelevant to the current problem, they may subsequently provide important useful information and it is important to document them meticulously. For example, knowing that a bilateral oophorectomy was performed at the time of a hysterectomy is helpful information in the assessment of a woman with ascites. The past medical history (if accurate) makes a diagnosis of carcinoma of the ovary highly improbable. Documentation of any surgical procedures, however minor, can provide reassuring or helpful anticipatory information in patients likely to undergo general anaesthesia. Recording of the history concludes with the full list of drugs, dosages and dosing intervals, any adverse reactions to previously prescribed medicines and documentation of the review of systems (see Ch. 1).

Details of the physical examination should be documented in a clear, structured framework. Start with a general, non-judgemental comment about the patient's overall appearance, such as 'well man with moderate generalized adiposity' or 'drawn, anxious woman, breathless on undressing'. Record important positive and negative features on general examination, for example jaundice, clubbing, rash, fever, lymphadenopathy. The remainder of the examination should be documented under bodily systems: cardiovascular, respiratory, gastrointestinal (often referred to as abdominal), nervous system, skin, limbs and joints. Negative findings are often as pertinent as positive ones. Simple line drawings are often particularly effective. A concise summary of the findings in the cardiovascular system might read as in Box 2.2.

The case notes should conclude with a brief summary of the history and the major abnormalities found on examination, which leads to the differential diagnosis and management plan (Boxes 2.3 and 2.4).

Box 2.3 Framework of pathological processes informing a differential diagnosis

- Congenital
- Degenerative
- Infective/inflammatory
- Metabolic
- Neoplastic
- Nutritional
- Toxic
- Traumatic
- Vascular

Box 2.4 Order of tasks to follow when constructing a provisional management plan

1. List the monitoring/nursing recommendations that are imperative to the patient's immediate comfort, well being and safety
2. List the investigations that need to be done immediately (e.g. blood cultures and malaria film in a patient returning from overseas with a fever of unknown origin)
3. Document the medications you propose to prescribe, including the dosages and frequency of administration (this includes intravenous fluid therapy)
4. List the investigations that may need to be done at some stage in order to provide further diagnostic information

Presenting a case

It is very valuable to your learning to practice making short summaries of your findings, emphasizing both important positive findings and relevant negative ones. The summary should begin with the name, age, sex and occupation of the patient and end with a brief statement of the problem. Another important skill to acquire is that of oral presentations of the cases you see to colleagues; the ultimate test is the ability to communicate a difficult problem to a senior colleague on the telephone. The history and findings on examination should be communicated in temporal, coherent order, making an interesting and easily grasped narrative.

Summary

Ultimately, the goal is for the clinician to use a combination of experience, knowledge and appreciation of the accuracy and limitations of history taking and examination to try to come to a correct diagnosis, or diagnoses, and facilitate the best treatment with the least discomfort and anxiety for the patient. As with everything described in this chapter, there is no substitute for practice and an open-ended willingness to learn from both success and error.

The next steps: Differential diagnosis and initial management

3

Michael Glynn

Introduction

The term 'Differential Diagnosis' used to be very widely used by doctors, but it now seems to be used less and is less well understood. It might be better termed as 'Differential Diagnoses', because the process of preparing it is to formulate a list of possible diagnoses that cover the clinical situation that presents itself, usually written in the descending order of likelihood. It is a very important part of the overall management of a patient from initial presentation, particularly in the emergency situation. The doctor clerking a patient may write a thorough history and complete a detailed examination and may write a good plan of management, but the intermediate step of preparing the differential diagnosis is often missed or replaced by something which is entitled 'Impression' and this may only consider one possibility. Box 3.1 gives three illustrations of situations in which the 'Impression' is too restrictive, whereas a full differential diagnosis would allow the treating doctors to consider the full range of possibilities, including those that are quite rare but nevertheless vitally important for the patient.

One of the most common reasons for attendance at an emergency department with chest pain is because the patient himself or a referring doctor is worried that the patient may have chest pain of cardiac origin. This is the reason a receiving doctor might write 'chest pain, rule out cardiac cause' as the overall 'impression'. However, there are other causes of acute chest pain, both common and rare. There is often a feeling that suggesting rare diagnoses opens avenues of investigations that are time consuming and expensive, but this is far from the truth. For instance, it may take only brief consideration that the patient may have a dissecting thoracic aortic aneurysm to return to the patient and clarify the character of the chest pain (dissecting aneurysms produce pain that is tearing in nature and clearly going through from front to back) and to check the blood pressure in both arms. Together with a simple chest X-ray, this may be sufficient evidence to exclude a dissecting thoracic aortic aneurysm without the need to resort to an emergency CT scan.

The most common cause of an acute headache is probably a tension headache. There is no useful test for this and the diagnosis will largely be made on history. Particularly in the emergency situation, there are some very serious causes of acute headache which must not be missed, such as a subarachnoid haemorrhage or a sagittal sinus thrombosis. Careful and accurate differentiation between these two is clearly imperative because anticoagulation for a suspected

Box 3.1 Samples of common emergency medical problems and the contrast between a simple 'Impression' and a full list of 'Differential Diagnoses'

Presenting problem	Impression	Differential diagnoses
Chest pain	Rule out cardiac cause	Acute coronary syndrome Pulmonary embolus Gastro-oesophageal reflux Musculoskeletal pain Dissecting thoracic aneurysm
Severe headache	Likely migraine	Tension headache Migraine Subarachnoid haemorrhage Temporal arteritis Sagittal sinus thrombosis
Apparent stroke	Cerebral infarction	Cerebral infarction (thrombus or embolus) Cerebral haemorrhage Carotid or vertebral dissection Hemiplegic migraine Brain tumour with haemorrhage Cerebral abscess Cerebral vasculitis

Box 3.2 Examples of key questions that help to confirm or refute specific diagnoses

Diagnosis	Key questions
Subarachnoid haemorrhage	■ Was it the worst headache you have ever had ■ Did it start extremely suddenly like a blow on the head
Diarrhoea due to irritable bowel	■ Does the need to open your bowels ever wake you from your sleep (rare in irritable bowel)
Cardiac chest pain	■ Does the pain feel like a weight pressing on your chest
Intermittent claudication or angina pectoris	■ Does the pain come on with a predictable amount of exercise

sagittal sinus thrombosis would be completely the wrong treatment for a subarachnoid haemorrhage.

The process of differential diagnosis does not mean that every single possible cause needs to be specifically excluded in every clinical situation. However, having the full list of differential diagnoses written down helps the doctor weigh the likelihood of each one and then clarify the situation as is appropriate to the particular clinical situation. This clarification will not necessarily mean arranging complex investigations. It might mean just a mental check that the right specific questions have been asked (such as the true nature of sudden headache) or making sure that particular physical signs have been checked (such as differential blood pressure suggesting dissecting aneurysm).

This reviewing, checking and clarification process which is mentally undertaken by the doctor clerking the patient is not something that needs to happen once the history and examination are completed. As the student and doctor become more experienced in the process of history and examination and the preparation of the differential diagnoses, they will begin to think through the patient's problems as soon as the consultation begins. The consultation will often be punctuated by key questions that are aimed at confirming or refuting a particular diagnosis that has occurred to the doctor during the course of the clerking process. Box 3.2 is a list of some key questions and the diagnoses to which they refer.

Management plan

Having obtained the history and examination and formulated a list of differential diagnoses, the student or doctor needs to decide on what should happen next. As with everything clinical, what the patient actually wants is of paramount importance. Box 1.16 in Chapter 1 gives a list of the general scenarios that may lie behind a consultation between patient and doctor. Of particular relevance to the process of differential diagnosis and planning management is the degree to which patients want answers to queries or want relief of symptoms. Quite a useful question can be 'Are you worried about your symptoms because of the trouble they give you and you want to be rid of them, because of what might be wrong, or both'. This can be quite a confusing question for the patient, but if explained carefully and answered specifically, it can avoid a lot of unnecessary investigation. In addition, starting out on the right track can make subsequent management much simpler, and it is often much easier to reassure a patient that there is nothing seriously wrong than to give him an exact diagnosis or full relief of symptoms. This process particularly applies to a patient who has a fear of cancer. In a relatively young patient with quite harmless symptoms, even if a serious diagnosis is not really suspected, it may be necessary to perform some sort of investigation (such as an endoscopy or a CT scan) to provide the necessary reassurance, even if it is not absolutely necessary for the process of resolving the differential diagnosis.

The priority of different investigations, the order in which they are done and the question of when treatment is given all have to be considered and planned carefully. There is often quite a strong temptation for the doctor making the initial plan to start off with quite a large series of investigations. This is often done because the doctor assumes the patient needs the reassurance of normal tests, and to some extent doctors need that reassurance themselves. There may even be a temptation to practice defensive medicine to avoid being accused in the future of under-investigating and missing diagnoses. However, this level of investigation is often not a productive way forward, can overuse resources, can sometimes prevent other patients having their tests in a timely manner, and according to circumstance, can be financially detrimental to the individual patient. However, there may also be drawbacks to a logical series investigation and planning out the next test only when the results of the first one are known. On occasions, this can seem a slow and tedious process for the patient, particularly if the health system allows only relatively infrequent patient review. Box 3.3 illustrates some clinical scenarios and the contrast in investigation style.

What to write in the case notes

Recording the possible differential diagnoses and the thinking behind them at the time of an initial consultation is a very important process and can be crucial in getting to the correct diagnosis and avoiding the very real risk of neglecting a diagnosis that seemed very possible at the outset but less so as clinical events change. This is particularly true if the relevant

Box 3.3 Example clinical scenarios and contrasting investigation styles

Clinical scenario	Logical investigation	Immediate investigation
Iron deficiency anaemia with dyspepsia in a man	Gastroscopy – if no ulcer then colonoscopy – if no colonic source of blood loss then do coeliac check and exclude or treat for parasites/worms	Gastroscopy and colonoscopy combined and a check for coeliac disease – exclude or treat for parasites/worms
Transient ischaemic attack	Carotid ultrasound – if no clear embolic source then cardiac ECHO for possible cardiac source of emboli – if normal then blood tests for hypercoagulability	Carotid ultrasound, cardiac ECHO and blood tests for hypercoagulability all arranged at the same time
Abnormal liver function tests without alcohol excess or medication side-effect	Blood tests for viral hepatitis and ultrasound – if no cause found then blood tests for rarer liver diseases	Do a full 'liver screen' in all patients including tests for viral hepatitis, fatty liver disease and rarer liver diseases

symptoms are likely to become less severe after the initial presentation. An example might be a patient who presents with chest pain and who is hypoxic. When reassessed later, the hypoxia may have resolved and if the original differential diagnosis is not reviewed, the diagnosis of pulmonary embolus might be overlooked. It is particularly good practice to write down the differential diagnostic list annotated either with confirmatory features for each possible diagnosis or any areas which lack confirmation. Such a list is given in Box 3.4.

Some items on a list of possible differential diagnoses may be more a result of a hunch on the part of the doctor rather than logical derivation from the available information. This might particularly apply to conditions that have relatively vague presentations rather than with a classical symptom complex. An example might be putting Addison's disease on the differential diagnostic list of a patient who presents with a specific condition but has also been non-specifically unwell, has a relatively low systolic blood pressure and a sodium concentration below the lower limit of normal. The initial focus would be on treating the specific presentation. However, having Addison's disease on the differential list will allow this to be reviewed later and investigation planned, such as a Synacthen test. Addison's disease would be a good example of

Box 3.4 A 'model' write-up of a differential diagnostic list in a patient presenting as an emergency with chest pain (see Box 3.1), with relevant positive and negative pointers written down for each possible diagnosis

Differential diagnostic list	Key features
Acute coronary syndrome	Many risk factors, mildly raised initial troponin
Pulmonary embolus	Sudden onset but pain not pleuritic, not hypoxic and no ECG change
Gastro-oesophageal reflux	Burning pain but no previous dyspeptic history
Musculoskeletal pain	Tender right lower anterior ribs
Dissecting thoracic aneurysm	Blood pressure same in both arms, no mediastinal widening on CXR

a good style of clinical practice which states 'once you have thought of it, you need to exclude it'. This is particularly true in many areas of medicine which now rely on teamwork and doctors changing their duties from day to day. If the first doctor had considered Addison's disease as a possible diagnosis, it would often be unwise for a second doctor to come along and discard that possible diagnosis without arranging the specific test or at least considering it very carefully. This clinical approach applies in many situations, although each consultation is a clinical episode in its own right, and the doctor must make the best judgement of the clinical circumstance relevant to that moment in time.

What to say to the patient

Every doctor has a duty to be truthful with patients. However, this does not mean there is duty to tell a patient 'the whole of the medical textbook'. This means that there is a duty to say what is likely and also what is serious, the two not always coinciding. For example, in a patient aged 46 attending a gastroenterology out-patient clinic with a change in bowel habit of 3 months' duration associated with some cramping abdominal pain and bloating and a few episodes of bright red rectal bleeding, the most likely diagnosis is of the irritable bowel syndrome accompanied by some haemorrhoidal bleeding. A full differential list would include as relatively likely diagnoses irritable bowel syndrome accompanied by some haemorrhoidal bleeding and also inflammatory bowel disease. A less likely but certainly a serious diagnosis would be the presence of colorectal cancer, which would be unusual at age 46 but certainly not unknown. Rare diagnoses might include gut vasculitis and ischaemic colitis. Good practice would be to say to the patient, 'I think you have the irritable bowel syndrome accompanied by some haemorrhoidal bleeding, but to exclude inflammatory bowel disease and the unlikely possibility of bowel cancer, I recommend that you have a colonoscopy' (the rarer diagnoses do not need to be mentioned at this stage).

What to do when the diagnosis is unclear

At the outset, the diagnosis relevant to any clinical situation is almost always unclear. Occasionally the doctor may make a 'spot diagnosis', such as when a patient walks into the consulting room with obvious and previously undiagnosed Parkinson's disease, although the patient may have come with problems and issues that have a different underlying cause. After history and examination, the student or doctor will prepare a list of Differential Diagnoses and a process of confirming or refuting those diagnoses will start, often with key investigations, or sometimes starting treatment and watching the effect of that treatment.

Doctors must be prepared for the not uncommon situation in which the diagnostic list appears to be exhausted and the patient's condition has not improved. It is at this point that the initial diagnostic list is particularly useful, to double check that it is complete and to rethink what level of testing is needed to confirm or refute any diagnoses. The list may well be reviewed in the light of how the clinical situation has evolved.

One particular issue will often arise which can be posed as the question, 'Which is more likely – a rare condition that has not yet been thought of or a common condition that has been missed on the first round of testing?' This way of looking at a problem will often lead to the repeat of an examination (e.g. an upper GI endoscopy) or an alternative look at the same problem (e.g. an abdominal CT scan following a normal ultrasound scan). It is certainly important to realise that every medical test has an error rate, even with the best quality control in laboratories and the highest standards in departments such as Radiology and Endoscopy.

Multiple causation

A common challenge facing the doctor is whether to accept the clinical findings on the basis of a single process or whether to invoke more than one bodily system or pathological process. This skill can be acquired only with time and experience but, in general, younger patients, shorter histories and examination findings confined to a single organ system tend to favour a single cause, whereas multiple causation is more likely among older patients with symptoms and signs in more than one bodily system.

Selecting appropriate investigations

As with history taking and physical examination, judicious selection of appropriate investigations to clarify a patient's diagnosis is a skill that is developed through teaching, practice and a willingness to learn from mistakes. This is increasingly true as access to high-definition radiological imaging becomes more widespread and the vast majority of haematological and biochemical investigations are automated and provided as a 'package' rather than individually selected. Although it might instinctively be thought by the student that the easy availability of such data could only be beneficial to a patient (i.e. lead to the fortuitous diagnosis of unsuspected disease), in many cases it can lead to unnecessary expense and patient anxiety. This is because asymptomatic benign lesions identified on imaging or minor disturbances of haematological/biochemical parameters necessitate further investigation and surveillance.

Ask yourself the following questions when considering which investigations to request:

- Will this test confirm/complement the information derived from the history and examination?
- Will this test provide new information (such as a chest X-ray in a patient with a productive cough and weight loss but no physical findings on examination)?
- Could this test provide useful information over a period of time as a marker of disease progression (e.g. the inflammatory markers erythrocyte sedimentation rate (ESR) and C-reactive protein (CRP) in a patient with infective endocarditis. Neither test is specific for the diagnosis but changes in both values may be useful markers of disease progression)?
- What are the possibilities of this test yielding clinically irrelevant/distracting information compared to a diagnostically informative result? A good example of this would be the indiscriminate use of cranial computed tomography (CT) scans in patients with ill-defined neurological symptoms (such as dizziness) before a detailed neurological examination has been performed. Meningiomas (benign tumours arising from the meninges) are not-infrequent findings in patients undergoing cranial imaging. In a patient with dizziness without other neurological symptoms or signs, such a finding is likely to be irrelevant and, because the meningioma will need routine surveillance, is likely to cause unnecessary anxiety. In contrast, the finding of a meningioma in a patient with a carefully taken history of focal seizures is likely to be highly relevant (and, in fact, a reassuring finding for many

patients as the differential diagnosis includes many other, more aggressive, brain tumours with a bleak outlook).

- What are the potential risks and discomfort to the patient of the proposed test (including the risk of unnecessary anxiety generated by an irrelevant finding demanding further evaluation)? In the case of routine haematological and biochemical tests requiring straightforward venipuncture, the immediate risk (aside from minor discomfort) is low. In the case of coronary angiography, the risk of death is around 0.1% and of serious complication (myocardial infarction, stroke, arrhythmia, cardiac perforation) approximately 1.7%. Following a kidney biopsy, the risk of a haemorrhage sufficiently severe to require an emergency nephrectomy is around 0.0003% (1 in 3000). In these and other situations, the clinician must balance benefit and risk. The benefit can be diagnostic information leading to targeted treatment of a serious illness, or excluding problems for which the treatment has significant risk. The risk is that of the investigation itself or of the anxiety or distress that it may provoke.
- What information does the laboratory and/or radiology department require to make this test maximally useful? A biopsy or surgical specimen sent to the pathology laboratory is likely to yield much more diagnostic information when accompanied by clinical details and a specific question than if delivered, speculatively, without either.

Ethical considerations 4

William M. Drake

Introduction

The cornerstone of a good relationship between doctor and patient is trust. In primary care, this relationship (often in the context of caring for the whole family) may be built up over several years, but in hospital practice or in an emergency, the patient and the doctor may be meeting for the first time. Patients expect a high standard of behaviour and care when they seek medical help. This includes the following expectations:

- They will be consulted about decisions bearing on their treatment.
- They will be informed about their illness.
- They will be informed about the likely outcome of any treatment offered.
- Their right to confidentiality will be respected.

Always assume that a patient is able fully to understand the nature of the medical problem and its implications, regardless of your impression of their educational level. Some patients like to discuss what they would like to know early in a consultation and many will say clearly what information they would like to be given to the family. Occasionally, family members may feel that the patient would not be able to comprehend medical information or ask that he be 'protected' from the full details of a serious illness. Patients may insist that they do not wish the family to know about their medical problems or, sometimes, that they themselves do not wish to know the diagnosis. In all such instances, the needs and rights of each individual patient should be considered paramount, over and above those of the family, in the event of conflict.

Autonomy

The fundamental principle underlying medical ethics is autonomy: the patient has the right to decide his own medical destiny. This gives rise to the concept of seeking the patient's consent for medical interventions, for research and for teaching. Only in the case of a minor or a mentally disturbed person may consent be sought from the patient's lawful parents or guardians. Assent, but not consent, may be sought from relatives, such as in the case of an unconscious patient in an intensive care unit. The doctor therefore has a duty not only to advise but also to explain. This principle crosses all religious and cultural boundaries.

Consent

The patient's consent should be sought for any treatment, however minor, even when that consent might appear implicit as, for example, by attendance at an emergency unit with injury. Sometimes assessment of a minor symptom discloses a separate, more serious issue. In such circumstances, consent to investigate the new problem is required.

In order to give consent, a patient must have sufficient, accurate information about the illness to make an informed judgement about whether its investigation and treatment are justified. There are four requirements of the doctor discussing an intervention with a patient:

1. The procedure itself must be described, including the technique and its implications and the intended benefit of doing it.
2. Information about the risks and complications must be given, which usually means all the risks, as well as some information about the consequences of the complication (e.g. perforation at colonoscopy is a rare occurrence but, if it happens, a laparotomy and colostomy may be needed).
3. Associated risks (e.g. from anaesthesia or from other drugs that may be necessary) should be described.
4. Alternative medical or surgical investigations or treatments should be discussed, so that the reasons for the specific advice given are clear. In addition, the implications of the 'do nothing' option should be discussed.

Obtaining consent

The amount of information divulged will vary according to the context of the discussion and according to the needs of the patient as they emerge in the consultation. The objective is not to place the patient in the situation of having to decide between conflicting medical data, but to explain why a particular investigation or treatment is being recommended. The patient must not feel under duress.

Setting the scene

Discussions regarding consent for investigation and treatment should be conducted in a suitable environment that is quiet, free of interruptions and away from unnecessary observers, such as other patients or unfamiliar nurses or students. Make time for the discussion and turn off pagers or mobile phones which, if they interrupt a discussion, can give the impression that you are rushed and fitting the patient into a busier, more important schedule. Use simple language that the patient can understand. Be patient. If necessary, and with the patient's permission, involve relatives. If there is likely to be a language problem, make sure that an interpreter (not a relative) is available. At the end of the discussion, check that the patient has actually understood. A written summary of the information supplied should be given to the patient for later consideration.

Implications of consent or refusal

Some patients, after detailed discussion, decline the recommended investigation or treatment. This should not result in the doctor being any less committed to their welfare. Discussions regarding alternative strategies should commence within the framework of what has been agreed and what is acceptable to the patient.

If explicit consent is given, the patient and doctor should both sign an appropriate consent form. This procedure should be followed for all serious interventions. In hospital, this will be a standardized form, and a similar form should be used in family or private practice to verify that the discussion took place. The act of both parties signing the form does not constitute proof that consent has been lawfully given but merely documents that a discussion took place. It is good practice to make a separate, contemporaneous note describing what was discussed.

Legal requirements for consent

There are three aspects of consent that are required in law:

1 The patient must be mentally and legally competent to give consent.
2 The patient must have been sufficiently well informed to be able to give consent.
3 Consent must have been given voluntarily, and not under duress.

Box 4.1 Criteria for having mental capacity

- The patient can understand what has been explained
- The patient can recall and repeat what has been explained
- The patient can discuss what has been explained and weigh information
- The patient can communicate the decision that he has made

Competence and capacity for consent

The definition of mental capacity is given in Box 4.1. If the patient does not have capacity to make a decision, the doctor must involve the relatives, although the doctor is still making the final decision. If the patient does not have capacity and has no relatives, in the UK the doctor must involve an independent mental capacity advocate (IMCA) to help with decision making, particularly if consenting for surgery or for decisions about change of living circumstances.

Special difficulties with consent arise when the patient is unconscious. If treatment is necessary in order to save life, it can and must be given without waiting for consent. If relatives are available, they should be consulted, but their wishes are not necessarily paramount in the decision to initiate life-saving therapy. The relatives may thus assent to treatment but cannot legally consent to it (in the UK). This limitation also means that relatives cannot legally refuse treatment that is medically in the best interests of the patient, although a conflict of this kind should be reason to consider, carefully and in detail with the relatives, the reasons for disagreement.

Consent for the treatment of children requires special consideration. In general, a minor (i.e. a person under the age of 16 years) can be treated without parental consent, provided that care has been taken to ensure the child understands the nature of the treatment proposed and its possible risks, adverse effects and consequences. However, this should be a most exceptional decision. In practice, the parents' agreement should almost always be sought. An obvious exception would be in an emergency, such as after a life-threatening head injury or when non-accidental injury is suspected. Difficult decisions sometimes arise, such as when the prescription of contraceptive drugs to a young girl is requested in circumstances she does not wish her parents to know or parents refusing to allow a bleeding child to have a blood transfusion for religious reasons.

Appropriately informed

The point at which a patient can be considered to be appropriately informed is a matter of judgement. Some patients make it clear that they do not wish for long and involved discussions whereas others are comfortable only when very full explanations have been given. It is often necessary to strike a balance. It is easy to frighten a patient by reciting unwelcome but rare possible complications of a procedure to such an extent that he refuses treatment. This should not be the objective of discussing treatment and is rarely in the patient's best interest. If a procedure is so risky that the doctor feels it is not justified and is therefore futile, the patient should be advised accordingly rather than being asked to decide for himself.

Confidentiality

The fact that all aspects of the encounter are confidential forms the foundation for the consultation, as it allows the patient freedom of expression in the knowledge that disclosures made within the confines of the consulting room will not be made available to others.

The principle of confidentiality applies also to the medical records. These are held by the doctor or the group practice or, in the case of hospital records, by the hospital itself. Medical records are not available to anyone other than the medical and nursing staff treating the patient, and are immune from police powers of search. They are made available, however, with the permission of the patient and, once disclosed, can be used as evidence in court in both civil and criminal cases. Patients have the right to inspect their own medical records after making a written application. In the UK, the principle of confidentiality is rigorously supported by the General Medical Council and its breach is regarded as a serious matter.

The main situations in which confidentiality can be relaxed include the following:

- When the patient or his legal adviser allows it.
- When it is in the patient's interests.
- If there is an overriding duty to society as a whole.
- In cases of statutory disclosure.
- Sometimes after death.

With permission

A common example of relaxation of confidentiality with the patient's permission occurs when a consultation is witnessed (e.g. by medical students or a nurse). The patient should be given the opportunity to ask that others leave.

In the patient's interests

When it is necessary that another family member be informed about the nature of a patient's illness, for example in order to obtain information essential for effective treatment, it may be judged in the patient's best interests to break confidentiality. Another example might arise if a patient was judged mentally incompetent and it became necessary to involve a legal adviser to handle their financial and legal affairs during a severe illness. This generally requires permission from a court.

An overriding duty to society

Occasionally confidentiality may be relaxed in the context of a known or possibly pending violent crime. In the case of an illness such as epilepsy or coronary heart disease that might impair the ability to control a vehicle, the responsibility to inform the authorities rests with the patient. Voluntary disclosure is encouraged, maintaining the principle of confidentiality between doctor and patient, but if the patient clearly does not make the disclosure, the clinician does have discretion to break this principle in circumstances that entail serious public risk (e.g. a patient having regular seizures who clearly has not informed the driving licensing authority).

Statutory disclosure

Confidentiality is breached in the case of certain infectious diseases, such as tuberculosis, that are statutorily notifiable to the public health authorities. There is also a statutory duty for a doctor to help in the identification of a driver involved in a road traffic accident who, for example, might have attended a surgery or accident and emergency department after the accident. The doctor in the witness box is in a state of privilege and is protected against any action for breach of confidentiality when instructed by a court to disclose potentially confidential information. Similarly, a court can ask that medical documents be released to it if they are regarded as necessary for the completion of a fair trial of an accused person.

Inspection of medical records

Patients have a lawful right to inspect their own medical records and can see any reports concerning their own medical condition that have been prepared before they are released to another party. Such reports can only be prepared with the permission of the patient or at the request of a statutory body, as in the context of an order under the Mental Health Act, or in the jurisdiction of a recognized court. Generally, persons other than the patient have no right to inspect the medical records of an individual in the absence of written permission or when the records are subject to a subpoena from a recognized court.

After death

Generally, the principle of confidentiality should extend to patients who have died. In the cases of a number of deceased public figures of recent years (e.g. Winston Churchill and John F. Kennedy), this principle was not adhered to on the grounds (not universally accepted) that there were matters of public interest involved.

Organ donation

When a tissue that can be replaced by the donor's own tissues, such as blood or bone marrow, is given to another patient, no special ethical problem arises. When a living donor gives an irreplaceable organ, such as a kidney, difficulties arise. The donor must be of sound mind, not under duress and must not be placed in a position to gain financially by the gift. The sale of organs for transplantation is forbidden in all developed countries and is rapidly becoming illegal in all countries. Similar considerations apply to the acquisition of donor organs from a minor, a practice about which it is particularly difficult to issue sound guidelines.

Resuscitation

Resuscitation is generally available in hospitals in the event that cardiopulmonary arrest occurs unexpectedly. However, this is not always successful, and many patients, recognizing the terminal nature of their illness, may request that resuscitation not be attempted. This is an entirely valid request which should be respected once it is certain that the options are clearly understood by the patient.

Not for resuscitation

Sometimes a patient is so seriously ill that resuscitation is deemed inappropriate by medical and nursing staff. Clearly, this implies a value judgement by those concerned that, in some way, the patient's life is not worth saving. The situation most frequently arises when a patient has terminal cancer; resuscitation followed by a few hours or days of further pain and discomfort might be regarded as an unnecessary prolongation of the illness.

The decision to withhold resuscitation is a matter for which it is proper always to seek the patient's full, informed consent. The patient's views are paramount and should be respected whatever the views of the clinicians and nurses or even the relatives. Relatives have no legal rights in a decision about the possible resuscitation of another individual. Although they may be consulted and their views noted, they should not be allowed to influence a decision once it has been made by the individual, unless it is decided that the patient is not competent by reason of dementia or some other impairment of judgement to reach a decision. Overt depression, for example, might be a reason for not accepting a patient's expressed wish not to be resuscitated.

Although it might be thought not helpful to a patient to discuss this issue openly, in fact the reverse is usually the case. Most patients near death are aware of their situation and welcome the opportunity for full discussion of the issues. The agreement of the patient and medical staff should be signed in the case record, and most hospitals now use a formal protocol to document this procedure. Patients should always be resuscitated when cardiopulmonary collapse is unexpected and their wishes are unknown.

Consent for autopsy

Explicit consent is required for autopsy, as tissue samples will be taken and examined and some may be retained for future use. If this is intended or is likely to occur, permission to retain the samples must be obtained as part of the consent for autopsy. This process of consent implies that the family will be given some idea of what studies might be undertaken on the retained samples in the future. It may be considered appropriate to consider whether any circumstances might develop in which the family might reasonably expect to be informed of the results of any such studies. For example, if information of a predictive or genetic nature were to be obtained in relation to the risk of vascular disease or of specific cancers, then the family might wish to know of this.

Other ethical problems

There are several other problems that arise in medical practice, many of which are likely to become more important in the coming years.

Medical negligence

Inadvertent adverse events are common in clinical practice, but few of these result in any legal action. Accusations of negligence often imply that a doctor-patient relationship has broken down. For the doctor, such an action is distressing and sometimes professionally damaging, even when shown to be unjustified.

In considering whether there has been negligence, it is necessary to establish breach of professional duty (whether the standard of care afforded the patient fell below what was expected). The standard expected is that of the ordinary skilled practitioner in the field in question, practising in the circumstances pertaining. It is not that of the greatest expert in the land. Thus, in assessing possible negligence, a court will need to establish:

- what the ordinary practice is
- that the doctor did not follow this practice
- that the doctor undertook a course of clinical management that no ordinarily skilled doctor in that specialty would have undertaken if acting with ordinary care.

A mistake in diagnosis is not necessarily negligent, and the test of the standard of care applicable to the ordinary practitioner in the specialty will be applied by the court in considering this.

Doctors are expected to keep up to date in their expertise by continuing medical education, and this is an aspect that is relevant to this judgement. Doctors in training are expected, by and large, to exercise an appropriate standard of care, and no patient should expect a lower standard of care simply because they are cared for by a junior doctor with less experience. This would clearly be wrong. It is imperative, therefore, that in treating a patient, advice and help should be sought from senior colleagues whenever relevant.

If negligence has occurred, the legal process will go on to attempt to establish what harm resulted from the negligence and that the harm would not have occurred if the negligent act had not been committed.

HIV

Testing for HIV requires the consent of the patient or individual. It is usual to counsel the individual about the consequences of a positive result before testing, as there are implications for lifestyle, future health and even employment hinging on the result of the test.

Genetics

The rapidly evolving availability of relatively accurate genetic testing for susceptibility to inherited diseases, based on the modern understanding of DNA and the genetic code, has raised a number of ethical problems for which most societies are not well prepared. For example:

- Who should have genetic tests done?
- What should be done with the results?
- Who, if anyone, should have access to the information, other than the patient?
- How should expensive treatments that may be possible for genetically determined disorders be made available?
- Is it socially and economically appropriate to prevent such disorders?

The application of genetic information to medical practice is a current major area of change. It can be expected to have profound implications for the management of most aspects of disease and for the ways in which all societies view the acquisition and availability of medical information.

Box 4.2 Declaration of Geneva propounded by the World Medical Association in Sydney (1968)

On admittance to the medical profession:

- I will solemnly pledge myself to consecrate my life to the service of humanity
- I will give my teachers the respect and gratitude which is their due
- I will practise my profession with conscience and dignity
- The health of my patients will be my first consideration
- I will respect secrets that have been confided in me, even after the patient has died
- I will maintain by all the means in my power the honour and noble traditions of the medical profession
- My colleagues will be my brothers
- I will not permit considerations of religion, nationality, race, party politics or social standing to intervene between my duty and my patient
- I will maintain the utmost respect for human life from the time of conception. Even under threat I will not use my medical knowledge contrary to the laws of humanity
- I make these promises solemnly, freely and upon my honour

Box 4.3 International Code of Medical Ethics

Duties of doctors in general

- To maintain the highest standards of professional conduct
- To practise uninfluenced by motives of profit
- To use caution in divulging discoveries or new techniques of treatment
- To certify or testify only those matters with which the doctor has personal experience
- To ensure that any act or advice that could weaken physical or mental resistance of an individual must be used only in the interest of that individual

The following are unethical practices

- Any self-advertisement except as expressly authorized in a national code of ethics
- Collaboration in any form of medical service in which the doctor does not have professional independence
- Receipt of any money in connection with services rendered to a patient other than a proper professional fee, even if the patient is aware of it

Duties of doctors to the sick

- There is an obligation to preserve life
- The patient is owed complete loyalty and all the resources of medical science. Whenever a treatment or examination is beyond the capacity of the doctor, the advice of another doctor should be sought
- A doctor must always preserve absolute secrecy concerning all he knows about a patient because of the confidence trusted in him
- Emergency care is a humanitarian duty that must be given, unless it is clear that there are others better able to give it

Duties of doctors to each other

- A doctor must behave to his colleagues as he would have them behave toward him
- A doctor must not entice patients from his colleagues
- A doctor must observe the principles of the Declaration of Geneva

Genetic counselling

Genetic counselling is relatively long established. The clinical geneticist will usually be asked to assess the risks of genetically determined disease in the context of statistical data or a known familial occurrence of a disease, for example Down's syndrome, Duchenne muscular dystrophy or cystic fibrosis. There is knowledge about the genetic causation of each of these conditions, and certain tests with various probabilities of accuracy are available to assess the risk for individuals in a family and for the risk that a planned pregnancy might result in an affected offspring. Major difficulties arise in deciding whether to inform someone who has been shown by genetic testing to be certain to develop a disease in later life, for example Huntington's disease. Such decisions should ideally be made before testing is undertaken at all. Even when offering counselling about the risks for planned pregnancies, similar difficulties arise. The social costs in terms of unresolved problems to individuals and their families of offering treatment or prevention for genetic disorders are largely undetermined at present. Practice in this context will change as knowledge and experience accumulate.

Principles of medical ethics

Several modern attempts have been made to encapsulate the principles of ethical medical behaviour in a series of simple statements. The Declaration of Geneva (Box 4.2) represents a modern attempt to restate the Hippocratic Oath in contemporary language. The International Code of Medical Ethics (Box 4.3) was derived from these principles and restates them in more direct terms. The Declaration of Helsinki (1975) sets out recommendations for the guidance of doctors wishing to undertake biomedical research involving human subjects. The recommendations of the Declaration of Helsinki are generally recognized as relevant to the design of research protocols. The UK General Medical Council's duties of doctors are listed at the end of Chapter 1.

SECTION 2

Assessment in particular groups

Women 5

Rehan Khan

Introduction

All medical history taking, examination, investigation and management plans are intensely personal matters for patients, although their consent to such involvement is implied by their presence in the clinic or ward. In obstetric and gynaecological practice, intimate details must be elicited; this requires tact, discretion, consideration and the maintenance of proper confidentiality. Women may have particular expectations of their doctors, and complying with these may not be easy. A gentle manner and a genuine interest in the patient help the development of a good professional relationship. Allow adequate time, but it is essential to keep a sense of direction and purpose so that the important is quickly separated from the trivial. You must be aware that there may be an expectation on the patient's part that she would be seeing a senior person throughout, so always be very clear about your status as a medical student or doctor in training. As with breast disease, gynaecological and obstetric cases are usually multidimensional in nature; the reported symptoms are experienced and reported against a backdrop of core aspects of the patient's lay beliefs. Developing the necessary skills to gather and interpret the relevant information requires considerable care, insight and reflection.

Gynaecological history

The usual preparations for history taking should be followed: courteous introduction; a statement as to your status as a student or trainee; and a careful check that you have the correct patient, that she understands the language and seemingly has competence. It may be that the patient is younger than the age of competence (16, or 18 if she is in care, in the UK), and awareness of this and its effect on management may be an issue. If a relative, such as a parent, insists on being present during the history, potentially sensitive questions may be reserved for a time when the other person has been asked to leave the room, such as during the examination. Sometimes, it is appropriate to revisit sensitive issues at a future appointment which the patient may feel more confident to attend alone.

In all consultations, you should describe the process that is about to take place and get an agreement or verbal consent. This will include history taking, an examination, an explanation of the findings and a discussion of a plan of action which will, of course, include an opportunity for the patient to ask any questions.

There are different systems for eliciting a history: the one outlined below is comprehensive and is the author's preferred one. It should, of course, be adapted to the individual patient. For example, in a postmenopausal patient with a urogynaecological problem, detailed menstrual and obstetric histories contribute little. In a younger patient, the history may be more related to menstruation, pregnancy and its complications and sexual activity in general. As a general rule, the introductory part of the history should be taken using open questions to allow a broader response.

Presenting complaint

This is a statement as to what the patient perceives to be the problem. As the consultation progresses and the relationship between doctor and patient develops, it may become apparent that the real presenting problem is something separate. Even so, it is important to start with the patient's chief concern as a way of building trust and rapport with someone who is likely to be anxious.

History of presenting complaint

Take a detailed description of the presenting complaint, with an emphasis on the timeline (when the problem started and how it developed over time) and the degree of symptomatology (how much the problem is affecting the patient).

In order to assess a woman's gynaecological wellbeing, certain areas of focused questioning are needed. Many students (particularly males) feel awkward taking a gynaecological history, but this is often unnecessary, as women with gynaecological problems will be expecting such questions. It may be helpful, at least initially, to use pre-prepared direct questions in order to overcome this initial self-consciousness.

Pain history

It can be very difficult to know from the history if lower abdominal pain has its origins in the gynaecological, alimentary or urinary system. The principles of eliciting a pain history outlined throughout this book apply in gynaecological practice. In addition, cyclical pain associated with periods is typically caused by endometriosis, whereas pain that was originally cyclical but later becomes continuous is often caused by adhesions. In all cases it is necessary to take an accurate history of bowel and bladder symptoms, as a substantial number of patients attending the gynaecology clinic with pain symptoms subsequently turn out to have bowel pathology (e.g. irritable bowel syndrome) or bladder pathology (e.g. interstitial cystitis). The two major gynaecological causes of chronic pain are endometriosis and pelvic inflammatory disease, and in both cases the symptoms may be caused by the formation of pelvic adhesions.

Menstrual history

For premenopausal women, a menstrual history is mandatory. This can be done quite quickly with practice but is usually dependent on direct questioning. Menstruation (the cyclical loss of sanguineous fluid from the uterus) is recorded as the days of menstrual loss and the duration of the interval from the first day of one period to the first day of the next, for example 5/28. Medical and 'lay' terminologies sometimes overlap confusingly in medicine although, in this context, the words 'period', 'menstrual period' and 'menstrual cycle' can be used interchangeably by doctor and patient alike. The aim of this section of the history is to establish if the patient's menstrual periods are problematic and, if so, in what way. Box 5.1 shows some examples of direct questions around the menstrual history, together with some points requiring clarification. In addition, Box 5.2 shows several other questions are required in order to check for bleeding problems not connected to periods.

If the patient is post- or perimenopausal, the history taking should reflect this. Some examples of direct, focused questions that could be asked are the following:

- Are you still having periods? or
- When did you have your last period?
- Has there been any bleeding since your last period? (This relates to a definition of postmenopausal bleeding – generally defined as bleeding 6 months after the last period, unless the patient is taking hormone replacement therapy, in which case it is important to establish which type. Exclusion of organic pathology is mandatory in this situation.)

Occasionally, gynaecological conditions may be associated with cyclical blood loss from the anus or urethra.

Vaginal discharge

Even if this is not the presenting symptom, it should be routinely enquired about. If there is a troublesome discharge, enquire about its colour, smell, amount, presence of blood, whether there is an associated vulval itch and, if so, if there are other sites of itching. In women with an abnormal vaginal discharge, questions relating to sexually transmitted disease naturally follow but can be difficult to pose. If the patient is in a sexual relationship, ask about symptoms in her partner(s) and whether either (any) of them are aware of the presence of warts.

Box 5.1 Some examples of direct questions around the menstrual history, together with some points requiring clarification

- How old were you when your periods first started? (Menarche.)
- What was the first day of your last normal menstrual period? (Patients may recall the last day of the period which is not contributory. Whether the period was normal or not is important, as sometimes vaginal blood loss may be that associated with an abnormal pregnancy.)
- How often do your periods come?
- How many days are there from the first day of one period to the first day of the next? (It could be that the cycle is irregular; many women keep a diary of their menstrual periods and it is often helpful to see this.)
- For how many days do you bleed?
- How many heavy days are there? (With these two questions you are trying to gauge the level of menstrual loss, so some estimate of the volume of flow is required.)
- Do you use tampons, pads or both? How often do you have to change them? (The use of both tampons and pads together is termed 'double protection' and is strongly indicative of menorrhagia.)
- Do you pass blood clots, and if so how large are they? (The second part of this question is difficult to answer without a frame of reference, and comparison to coins of different denominations can be helpful.)
- Do you ever bleed through your clothes? Is the bleeding like a running tap? (This is called 'flooding'.)
- Does the bleeding interfere with your usual daily activities, e.g. do you have to take time off work? (This is a very important question as it helps to judge the impact of the bleeding problem.)
- Are your periods painful? (Some assessment of the degree of pain is necessary here, e.g. is medication used and, if so, what and how much? Does the pain stop you from carrying out your normal activities?)
- Do you have any other symptoms with your periods? (This is an enquiry about premenstrual syndrome, in which a variety of symptoms can aggregate and then disappear as menstrual flow starts.)

Urinary tract and uterovaginal prolapse symptoms

Uterovaginal prolapse refers to a situation in which the uterus 'sinks' or 'slides' down from its normal position in the body. Frequently a woman will notice

Box 5.2 Several other questions are required in order to check for bleeding problems not connected to periods

- Do you have bleeding between your periods? (If so, how much and when does it occur?)
- Do you have any bleeding after sexual intercourse? (If so, ask for an estimate of how frequently this loss occurs and how heavy it is.)
- What form of contraception are you using? (In the last two questions, it is first necessary to establish whether the patient is in a sexual relationship; this requires additional tact. The pattern of menstruation may be influenced by use of various contraceptive methods including the combined oestrogen/progestogen pill (combined oral contraception, COC), the progesterone-only pill (POP), injectable progestogens, various intrauterine contraceptive devices and newer progestogen-containing rings placed in the vagina.)

a bulge ('a lump down below') at the introitus (entrance) of the vagina and may report urinary symptoms consequent upon changes in the pelvic floor muscles that alter the angulation and therefore reliability of the bladder neck. It is very unusual for symptomatic prolapse to occur in women who have not had vaginal deliveries. If this appears to be the presenting complaint, the history can be explored with carefully phrased direct questions (Box 5.3).

It should be clear to the history taker if the reason for any incontinence is in part due to mobility limitations, but a general enquiry should be made about the layout of the home and symptoms of cough or constipation that may lead to repeated increases in intra-abdominal pressure. Where the history is not clear or needs more objectivity, it is sometimes useful to recommend a simple frequency/volume chart on which the patient can record her symptoms and bring to a subsequent appointment.

Sexual symptoms

A full sexual history would not be appropriate at the first appointment unless the history taker has specific training in this area. If you know that the patient is in a sexual relationship, it is reasonable routinely to ask her whether she experiences or has experienced pain with sexual intercourse (dyspareunia). Sometimes the patient will present with painful sex on penetration; again, direct but sensitive questions are useful in this context (Box 5.4).

In addition, it is essential to ask whether the patient has had any previous sexually transmitted infections, particularly chlamydia and gonorrhoea, which are associated with pelvic inflammatory disease.

Cervical cytology history

A gynaecological history should always include details of any cervical smears, their dates and whether there have been any abnormalities or treatments. The opportunity also arises to ask if any other screening has taken place, such as mammography and chlamydia, and what the results were.

Box 5.3 Questions to ask if a prolapse is suspected

- Do you have a feeling of something coming down?
- Does the feeling go away overnight or when you lie down? (Symptomatic prolapse is gravity dependent except in the most severe cases.)
- Are there occasions when you don't make it to the toilet in time?
- Do you leak urine if you cough or sneeze?
- When you pass urine, do you feel you have completely emptied your bladder?
- When you are passing urine, can you squeeze hard enough to stop the flow? (Arresting flow mid stream is a good test of the strength of the pelvic floor.)
- How often do you get up at night to pass urine?
- Have you ever seen blood in your urine?

Box 5.4 Direct questions for patients presenting with pain on sexual penetration

- How severe is the pain – does sex have to stop?
- Does it happen every time you have sex or only on some occasions? (If intermittent, ask how often this happens.)
- Can you say if the pain is superficial (near the outside) or deep on the inside? (Typical causes of deep dyspareunia include endometriosis and chronic pelvic inflammatory disease.)
- Do you have any other pains in the pelvic region other than the one brought on by sexual activity?
- Is there any bleeding during or after penetrative sex?

Past obstetric history

It is inevitable that a gynaecological history will include a truncated obstetric history. This can be a sensitive issue, as medical and lay terminologies regarding lost pregnancies can cause potential confusion and inadvertent distress. Spontaneous abortion is no longer used as the medical term for a miscarriage, and what many women refer to as an 'abortion' is a termination of pregnancy in medical language. If the questions are incorrectly constructed, the boundaries of confidentiality can be breached if the history is taken in the presence of a third person. No pressure should be placed on a patient during this part of the history, especially in the presence of others, but it is important to know the number of pregnancies, their outcome (gestational ages and weights), mode of delivery, age of the children, whether there was any infertility at any time and, if so, the details of any investigations or treatments. Direct questions that may help assimilate this information are listed in Box 5.5.

Box 5.5 Direct questions that may help inform the obstetric history

- How many times have you been pregnant? (Be aware that some patients may not indicate that they have had terminations of pregnancy.)
- What was the weight of the heaviest and the lightest baby?
- How old were you when you had your first pregnancy?
- How old are the children now? or
- How old is the youngest and how old is the oldest?
- How old would he be if he had survived?
- Did you have any difficulty getting pregnant?

Past gynaecological history

With the passage of time, many patients forget certain aspects of their past medical history (e.g. tonsillectomy, cataract removal). Women with a gynaecological history do not often forget, so a simple question 'Have you had any gynaecological problems or procedures in the past?' is sufficient to establish any significant gynaecological background, which should then be explored.

Past medical/surgical/anaesthetic history

In order to get a broad view of the patient's medical background, you could ask a simple question such as 'Is there anything in your past medical or surgical history that I should know about?' This is a helpful introductory question which can be followed by more focused enquiry depending on the case. For example, complicated appendicitis may be related to infertility; or a previous blood transfusion, which has produced blood group antibodies, may be related to subsequent pregnancy loss. If an anaesthetic is anticipated as part of the patient's management, it is important to make an assessment as to whether this is likely to be problematic. Ask if she has had an anaesthetic in the recent past and whether there were any problems with it.

Medication or treatment history

These are standard enquiries and may be contributory. An awareness of medications taken in the past, with their success or failure, is a useful observation. Be aware that patients may take various kinds of supplements which they do not regard as medicines, but which may affect gynaecological health, for example Chinese herbal remedies, agnus castus, black cohosh. Allergic reactions should be recorded and clearly displayed.

Social history

Enquiry as to occupational history, present and past, is appropriate. Even during the course of the relatively short time to take a history, a picture of the patient may emerge indicating how well adjusted she is to her life, her relationships and external influences. These may affect her prospects for recovery from illness or when planning the support of a child. For instance, if the patient is the subject of domestic violence, a request for termination of pregnancy may be considered differently or this may be relevant to antenatal or postnatal care.

Family history

Few purely gynaecological conditions have a familial basis. In the context of infertility, it is important to check whether recurrent familial conditions are present, both on the patient's and her partner's side; recessive and autosomal dominant genetic conditions are often known to patients.

Gynaecological examination

Full awareness of the privacy of the examination is mandatory. A chaperone should be present during any intimate examination (breast or pelvic examination) whether the person performing the examination is male or female. General, abdominal and peripheral examination can be carried out without a chaperone, although it is preferable to have one present. Breast examination is not part of the gynaecological assessment in UK practice unless there is a specific complaint related to the breasts. It is important to ensure that the patient gets undressed in privacy without the doctor or student present, and that she has a suitable covering for the lower half of her body.

For a new consultation, a general examination is necessary and particularly relevant if an anaesthetic is anticipated. Details of the general physical examination are covered in other chapters. In the context of gynaecology, measurements of height and weight (giving the body mass index, BMI) and an assessment of body proportions (e.g. general or central obesity) are important. In 'gynaecological endocrinological' cases, the presence or absence of signs associated with hyperandrogenaemia (hirsutism, male pattern baldness, acne, increased muscle bulk) should be documented.

Abdominal examination

The system of examination described in Chapter 14 is recommended but should focus on inspection and palpation; percussion and auscultation are less important in gynaecological practice. The presence or absence of scars should be noted. Laparoscopic scars can be subtle, particularly if tucked within the umbilicus. Occasionally (usually to avoid the risk of perforation through adhesions in the lower abdomen) the entry point for laparoscopic surgery may be via Palmer's point in the mid-clavicular line, under the rib cage. Transverse suprapubic (Pfannenstiel's) incisions may also be difficult to see in the suprapubic crease unless specifically looked for.

Suprapubic examination is particularly important as a gynaecological mass arises out of the pelvis and

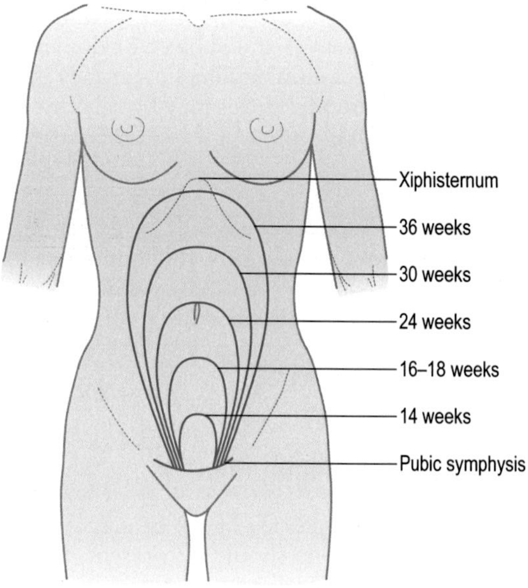

Figure 5.1 Approximate fundal height with changing gestation.

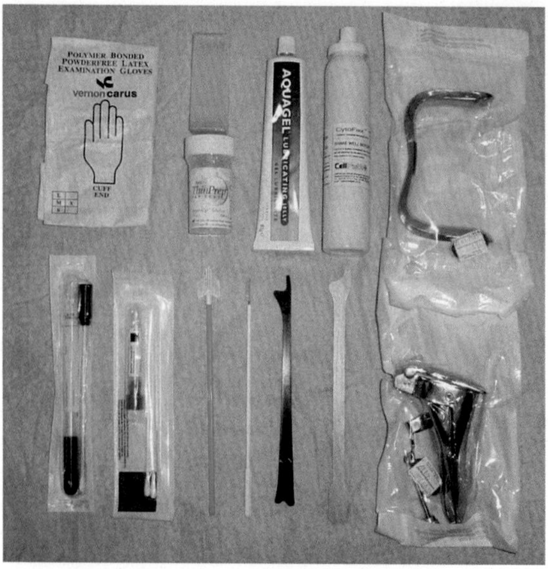

Figure 5.2 Equipment for the gynaecological examination.

the examining hand cannot get below it. Do this part of the abdominal palpation with the ulnar border of the left hand, starting at or around the umbilicus, and work your way down. When an abdomino-pelvic mass is present, its characteristics and size, either in centimetres measured from the symphysis pubis upwards or estimated as weeks' gestation of an equivalent-size pregnancy, are recorded (see Fig. 5.1). Note its consistency (hard if a fibroid, usually soft if a pregnancy), regularity (subserosal fibroids and ovarian masses are usually irregular) and the presence of any tenderness. It can sometimes be difficult to elicit such signs if there is a scar in the lower abdomen or if the patient is obese. If nothing is palpable arising out of the pelvis, it is reasonable to conclude that any pelvic swelling is less than the size of a 12-week pregnancy. If ascites is suspected, check the supraclavicular and inguinal lymph nodes and look for an associated hydrothorax.

Pelvic examination

In gynaecology, pelvic examination (PE) is usually undertaken vaginally but it may also be performed rectally. The instruments used are shown in Fig. 5.2. PE should always be preceded by abdominal examination. In order to reduce patient anxiety it is crucial to explain every step sensitively but clearly. Medical students should only undertake a PE in the presence of a supervisor; the same applies to trainees in gynaecology, except where specific permission has been granted by the trainer. In many centres, students begin to learn the technique of PE using artificial manikins and models.

PE commences with inspection of the perineum in the dorsal or left lateral position and is followed by internal digital examination, using the index and middle fingers (use one finger if the vagina does not accommodate two). Generally, but not always, a speculum examination precedes the digital examination (if it is important to visualize any discharge, take swabs or take a cervical smear, the speculum should always be passed first; Fig. 5.3). In the event of the patient experiencing undue discomfort (be it speculum or digital), the examination should cease immediately. Make note of any inflammation, swelling, soreness, ulceration or neoplasia of the vulva, perineum or anus (Fig. 5.4). Women from certain communities may have been circumcised in childhood: this is known as female genital mutilation (FGM) and can range from scarring of the labia to removal of the

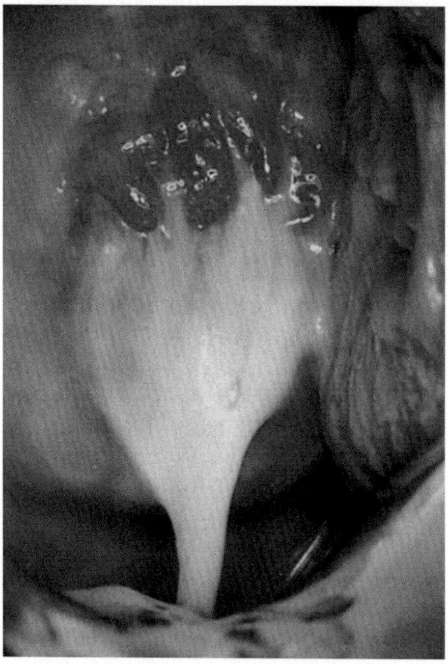

Figure 5.3 Discharge due to *Chlamydia trachomatis*.

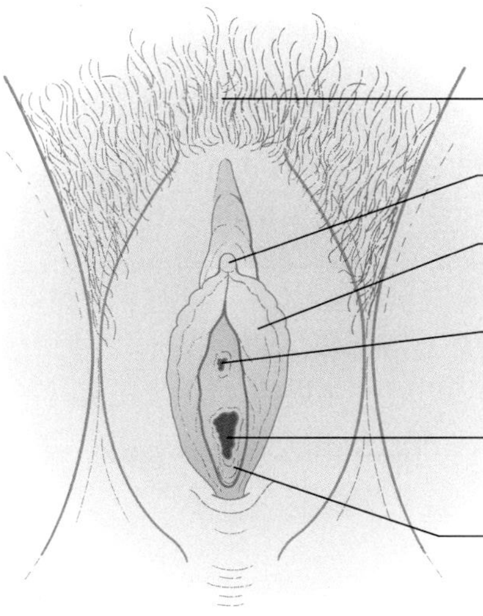

Figure 5.4 The vulva.

external genitalia. Small warts (condylomata acuminata) appearing as papillary growths may occur scattered over the vulva; these are due to infection with the human papilloma virus (HPV). Inspect the clitoris and urethra and ask the patient to strain and then cough to demonstrate any uterovaginal prolapse or stress incontinence. (Fig. 5.5 shows the various types of prolapse.) If the patient has given a history of involuntary incontinence, it is important that the bladder is reasonably full and that more than one substantial cough is taken, as the first cough frequently fails to demonstrate leakage of urine. It is kind to press on the anus with a tissue or swab to reduce the risk of involuntary flatus, indicating to the patient the reason for doing so.

For the digital examination, disposable gloves are used and the examining fingers should be lightly lubricated with a water-based jelly. With the patient in the supine position and with her knees drawn up and separated, the labia are gently parted with the index finger and thumb of the left hand while the index finger of the right hand is inserted into the vagina, avoiding the urethral meatus and exerting a sustained pressure on the perineal body until the perineal musculature relaxes. Watch for any sign of discomfort. The full length of the finger is then introduced, assessing the vaginal walls in transit until the cervix is located. At this stage, a second finger can be inserted to improve the quality of the digital examination or, alternatively, a speculum can be used if a cervical smear is required. The examination is continued with the left hand placed on the abdomen above the symphysis pubis and below the umbilicus – the bimanual examination (Fig. 5.6). The hand provides gentle directional pressure to bring the pelvic viscera towards the examiner's fingers in the vagina and serves to assess the size, mobility and regularity of masses. The cervix is then identified; it is approximately 3 cm in diameter, with a variably sized and shaped dimple in the middle, the cervical os. When the uterus is anteflexed and anteverted, the os is normally directed posteriorly. A retroverted uterus means the uterus is tipped backwards so that it aims towards the rectum instead of forward towards the belly. The consistency of the cervix is firm and its shape is irregular when scarred. Increased hardness of the cervix may be caused by fibrosis or carcinoma. As a 'soft' cervix indicates the possibility of pregnancy, even greater caution and gentleness is necessary. The mobility of the cervix is usually 1-2 cm in all directions, and testing this movement should produce only mild discomfort. If the cervix is moved when there is pelvic inflammation, particularly in association with ectopic pregnancy, extreme pain (cervical excitation) results.

It is possible to estimate the size, shape, position, consistency and regularity of the uterus and the relationship of the fundus of the uterus to the cervix (flexion). Uterine size is generally described as normal, bulky or in terms of weeks of gestation (e.g. 6 weeks, 8 weeks, 10 weeks size, etc.) even in the absence of pregnancy. Its mobility and shape (symmetrical or non-symmetrical) may be assessed and the ovaries and fallopian tubes (also known as the adnexae) palpated, although these can be difficult to feel in healthy women. Aside from the ovaries in some women, no other swellings should be palpable about the uterus in women of reproductive years. However, adnexal tenderness is an important finding. The pouch of Douglas is then explored through the posterior fornix via the arch formed by the uterosacral ligaments and the cervix.

Pelvic examination in special circumstances

Vaginal bleeding

In most cases, vaginal bleeding dictates that PE should be deferred to another occasion, but if a diagnosis of gynaecological malignancy is suspected, then a PE would be indicated in order to reduce the time taken to reach a diagnosis. As a general rule, consultations should not be cancelled because of vaginal bleeding; the patient can still have a history taken, a general and abdominal examination, preliminary investigations requested and arrangements made to complete the examination.

Cervical smear

Cervical smears can still be taken in the presence of bleeding and, if the result is inconclusive, it can be repeated. It is essential to involve the patient in the decision-making process. The inconvenience of a repeat visit can be avoided if the smear is taken even if there is bleeding. Patients who have had previous treatment for cervical neoplasia should not have

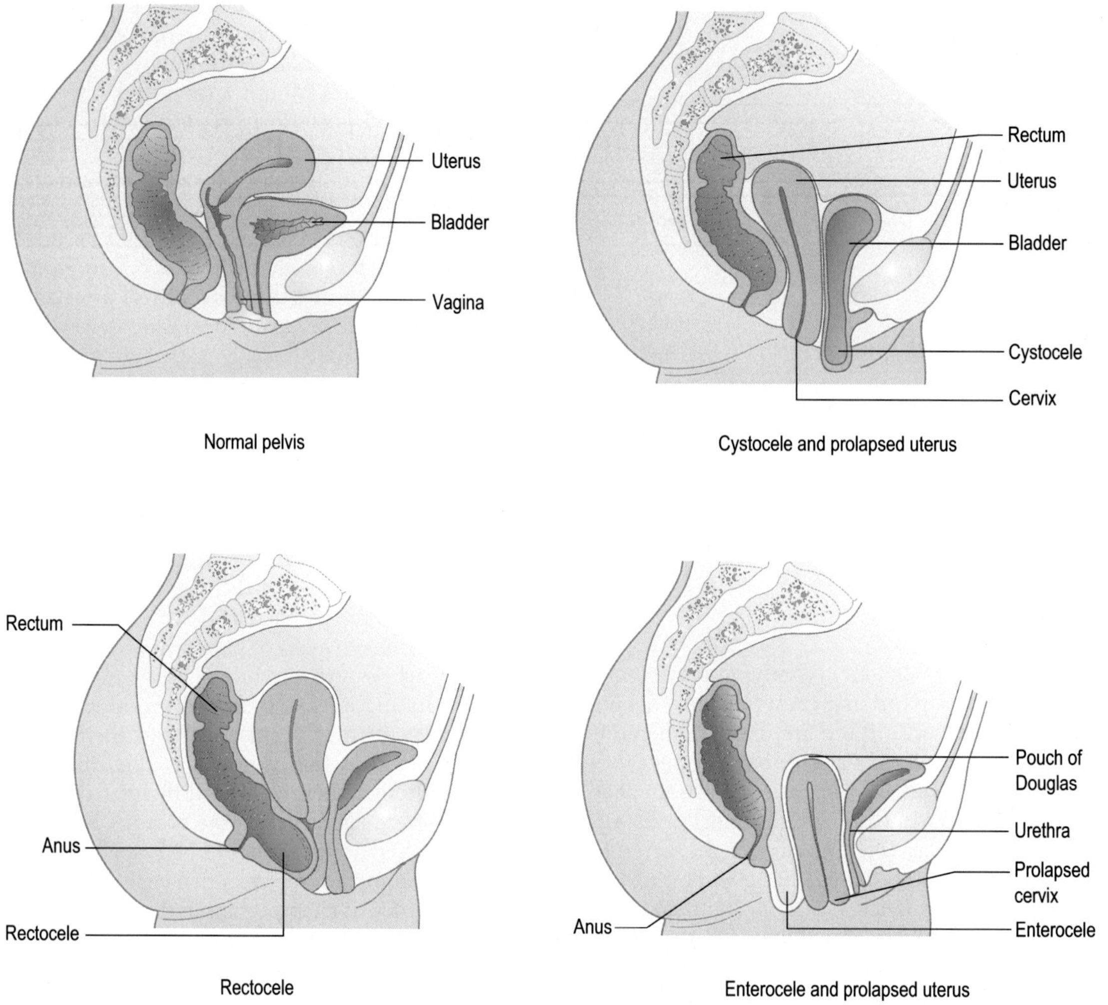

Figure 5.5 In cystocele, there is downward prolapse of the anterior part of the pelvic floor, straightening the angulation of the bladder neck and leading to urinary incontinence. In rectocele, the posterior part of the pelvic floor is mostly affected, sometimes with associated faecal incontinence. In some patients, the whole pelvic floor is weak, with double incontinence or prolapse of the uterus. In enterocele, there is a prolapse of viscera from the pouch of Douglas as part of a severe pelvic floor weakness.

follow-up smears cancelled because of vaginal bleeding.

Examination under general anaesthesia

In some situations, it may be necessary to perform PE under general anaesthesia. The technique for examination under anaesthesia (EUA) is the same as above, but additional care is needed to preserve the patient's dignity while she is unconscious and unable to take an active part in the proceedings.

Vaginismus

This term refers to the reflex adduction of the thigh muscles in response to an attempt at vaginal examination. In many cases, the examination has to be abandoned, but mild degrees of vaginismus can sometimes be overcome by asking the patient to clench her fists and place them under her buttocks. This tilts the pelvis in such a way that the examination becomes possible. It is worth attempting this manoeuvre if a cervical smear is required. In any event, a kindly and sympathetic approach by doctor and accompanying female nurse is always necessary.

Intact hymen

The possibility of rupturing or breaking the hymen during PE is an important consideration and is a particularly sensitive issue for women from some communities. In such situations, judicious use of ultrasound may often give the appropriate information.

Pregnancy

Vaginal examination in pregnancy is discussed later in this chapter.

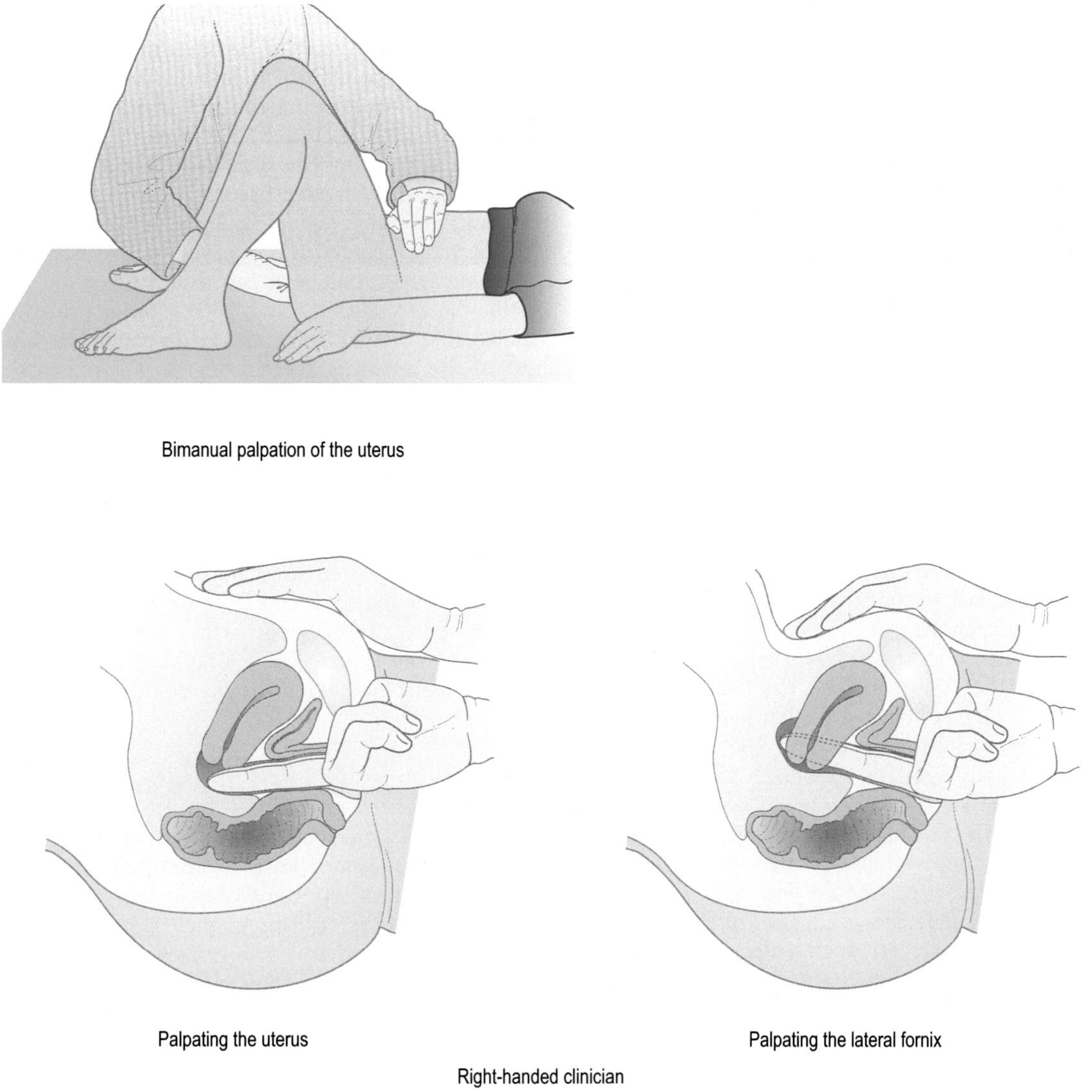

Figure 5.6 Bimanual examination of the pelvis.

Speculum examination

This is an essential part of a gynaecological examination. Several types of specula are available for use, including the bivalve type (e.g. Cusco's) used for displaying the cervix (Fig. 5.7) and the single-ended or double-ended Sims' (duckbill) speculum (Fig. 5.8) used to retract the vaginal walls. Occasionally, use is made of the Ferguson's speculum, which may be required to inspect the cervix when vaginal prolapse is so severe that a bivalve speculum fails to provide a sufficient view. If a cervical smear is to be taken, care should be taken not to get lubricant on the cervix, as this can compromise the quality of the sample, so the taking of the smear before digital examination is good practice without using excessive lubrication. The speculum should be warmed to body temperature and lubricated with water or a water-based jelly. All the necessary equipment, such as spatulas, slides, forceps,

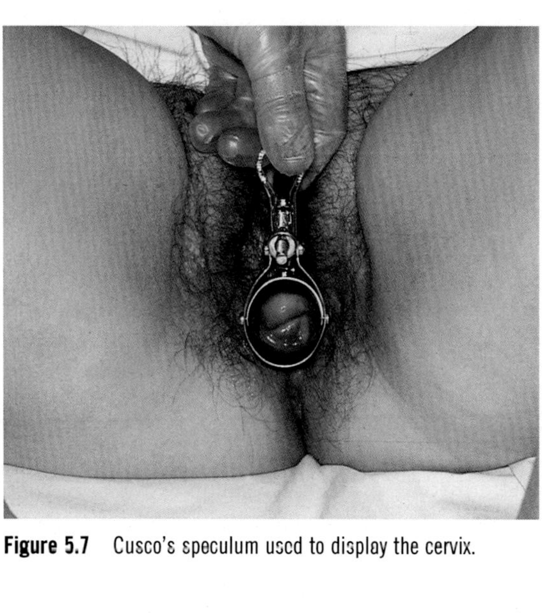

Figure 5.7 Cusco's speculum used to display the cervix.

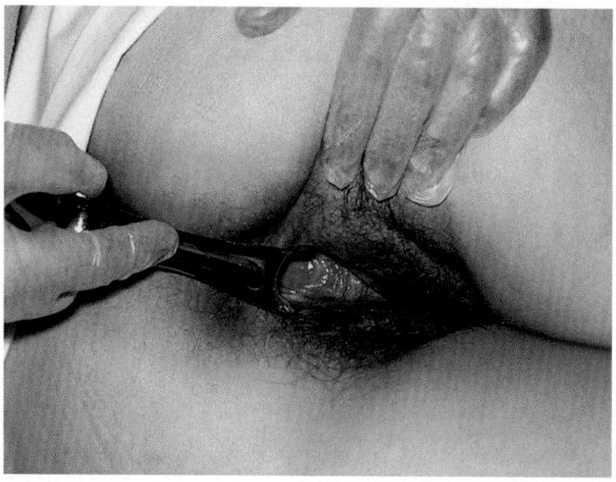

Figure 5.8 Sims' speculum used to display the anterior vaginal wall.

culture swabs, etc., should be prepared before the examination begins (see Fig. 5.2).

Carefully explain to the patient what will happen in the examination. Ask her to lie on her back with her feet together and knees drawn apart, as for the PE. Separate the labia and then the introitus with the thumb and index finger of the left hand and then insert the lightly lubricated bivalve speculum with the handle directly upwards, allowing it to be accommodated by the vagina. When it has been inserted to its full length, the blades of the speculum are opened and manoeuvred so that the cervix is fully visualized (the left hand should now be free to do this; see Fig. 5.7). The screw adjuster or ratchet on the handle is then locked so that the speculum is maintained in place. Any discharge (see Fig. 5.3) and the condition of the cervical epithelium, its colour, any ulceration or scars and retention cysts (nabothian follicles) should be noted.

Taking a cervical (Papanicolaou) smear

This involves the technique of liquid-based cytology, in which cells are obtained from the squamocolumnar junction (transformation zone). A spatula placed firmly in the cervical os and rotated through 360° or an endocervical brush may be used. If there is considerable discharge, with or without blood, the cervix can be cleansed using a cotton wool ball and a truer reflection of the cervix will result from the test. Taking a smear through a thick mucoid discharge may result in an unsatisfactory smear. Samples for *Candida, Trichomonas, Neisseria gonorrhoea, Chlamydia* and herpes may be obtained at the same time (see Ch. 17). The screw of the speculum is then released and the blades freed from the cervix so that the speculum can be gently removed.

Assessment for prolapse

Assessment of the vaginal walls for prolapse or fistula is performed using a Sims' speculum with the patient in the left lateral position. The best exposure is given by the Sims' position, in which the pelvis is rotated by flexing the right thigh more than the left, and by hanging the right arm over the distant edge of the couch. A Sims' speculum is inserted in much the same way as above, using the left hand to elevate the right buttock (see Fig. 5.8). The blade then deflects the rectum, exposing the urethral meatus, anterior vaginal wall and bladder base. Ask the patient to strain and note any vaginal wall prolapse. The level of the cervix is recorded as the speculum is withdrawn. The posterior vaginal wall can then be viewed by rotating the speculum through 180°. Uterine prolapse is called first degree if the cervix descends but lies short of the introitus, second degree if it passes to the level of the introitus and third degree (complete procidentia) if the whole of the uterus is prolapsed outside the vulva. Vaginal wall prolapse occurring with, or independent of, uterine prolapse consists of urethrocele, cystocele, rectocele or enterocele (prolapse of the pouch of Douglas). Several of these anatomical variations usually occur together (see Fig. 5.5).

After examination, it is courteous to help the patient to sit up, offer her appropriate wipes (avert your eyes as she uses them) and ensure that she receives any necessary assistance when she dresses.

History relating to current pregnancy

If a woman tells you she is pregnant, remember that some women may not wish to continue with the pregnancy so it is important to ascertain, as gently as possible, whether the pregnancy is welcome or not. Remember too that whatever the woman's initial reactions, by the time of their birth most babies are genuinely wanted. A review of the current pregnancy can be made. Record the date of the first day of the last menstrual period (LMP), with a note as to its likely accuracy. Ask about the menstrual pattern before conception and whether this was a natural cycle or due to the use of the contraceptive pill. The expected date of delivery (EDD) of the child can be calculated, assuming there has been a natural 28-day cycle for some months prior to the conception cycle. The EDD is then 9 months and 7 days from the onset of the last menstrual period (i.e. 280 days or 10 lunar months; alternatively, the EDD is 266 days from the date of conception). In some cases, the EDD should be altered at the time of the dating scan.

Later on in the pregnancy, ask about fetal movements. These are usually felt from about 28 weeks' gestation (there is no set number of movements, but it is important to ascertain if the woman suspects that the frequency of movements has reduced). Ask whether there have been any unusual pains or any bleeding. Data are usually assembled chronologically in 3-month episodes (the trimesters), as a healthy normal pregnancy has different characteristics and different problems occur at different stages.

If labour is suspected, ask if there has been a 'show' (a brownish or blood-tinged mucus discharge), breaking of the waters or contractions. If the waters have broken, ask about the colour of the water.

Relevant past obstetric history

Here, a reasonably in-depth history is needed. The course and outcome of previous pregnancies must be explored and recorded, as these are an essential guide to the progress of the current pregnancy. Where early loss of pregnancy has occurred, it must be established whether this was by miscarriage, ectopic pregnancy or therapeutic termination of pregnancy ('abortion') and on how many occasions it occurred. The gestation, symptoms leading to miscarriage, complications and any treatment must be noted. If a termination has taken place, ask about the method used (e.g. surgical evacuation or medical management with prostaglandin analogue), any complications and the time taken for the woman to return to a normal menstrual pattern afterwards.

The outcome of each previous pregnancy is recorded as a live birth, a neonatal death or a stillbirth. The birth of a child showing any signs of independent life is recorded as a live birth. This occurs beyond 24 weeks' gestation (or 500 g weight) but, with improved neonatal care, fetal viability may be obtained from an even earlier stage. If such a child dies, that event requires a death certificate in the UK. Also in the UK, a child born after the 24th week of pregnancy who does not, at any time after birth, breathe or show any signs of life is termed 'stillborn' and requires a stillbirth certificate. If the child is born dead at an earlier gestation, it is regarded as an abortion or miscarriage and certification is unnecessary. These are legal requirements.

Drug/smoking/alcohol history

As in the gynaecology history, these are all relevant. Prescribed and recreational drugs (including alcohol and tobacco) may harm both mother and fetus. There is evidence that some medicinal agents (e.g. methotrexate, both maternal and paternal) have a teratogenic effect when taken prior to the onset of pregnancy. The effect is greater when the relevant agent is taken early in pregnancy (an embryopathy as opposed to a fetopathy; as a general rule, the former has much wider ranging consequences) and when in doubt, a full history of exposure time, dosage and gestational age must be taken.

Family history

At some time in the history, taking a genetic history relevant to both partners is required and explored as indicated. Some couples may have had pre-pregnancy counselling if there is a strong family history of a particular disorder. Specific ethnic groups may have particular abnormal genetic predispositions and referral to a clinical geneticist may be indicated. It is especially important to determine whether there is a family history of hypertensive disorders or diabetes, as these can predispose to an increased risk of pre-eclampsia and gestational diabetes respectively.

Social history

This has been discussed under the gynaecology history-taking section and the principles are very similar.

Presentation of obstetric cases

It is common practice in obstetrics to present cases using particular language. Gravidity refers to the condition of pregnancy, regardless of outcome, including the one being presented. It therefore includes any ectopic pregnancies, spontaneous miscarriages and terminations of pregnancy. Para (to bring forth or bear) refers to the number of deliveries over 24 weeks' gestation or under 24 weeks showing any signs of life. Multiple pregnancies count as one delivery only. Thus, a pregnant woman with one previous healthy child and one previous termination of pregnancy would be described as gravida 3, para 1.

Obstetric examination

General examination

Again, this should follow the approach outlined in Chapter 2. In obstetric practice, height and weight (and calculated BMI) are important. As a general rule, labour is more efficient if the woman is above 152 cm in height, and hypertension, hyperglycaemia and anaesthetic difficulties are more common if the BMI is above 30 kg/m^2. Record the blood pressure (it should be 140/90 or lower in a normal pregnancy) and examine carefully for oedema, not only in the ankles but also in the fingers (can she remove her rings easily?) and face. Breast examination is not indicated unless there is a complaint related to the breasts themselves, although it is common for women to ask questions related to breastfeeding.

Abdominal examination in pregnancy

Ask the patient to empty her bladder before the abdominal examination. Make sure the light is good, the room comfortably warm and that there is maximum exposure of the area to be examined (Box 5.6). Look for striae gravidarum ('stretch marks'), linea nigra (a dark coloured midline abdominal stripe), previous caesarean section or other scars and any visible fetal or other movements (unlikely before 30 weeks' gestation but usually indicative of good health). Ideally the patient is examined semirecumbent. It is not usually an uncomfortable examination except in certain pathological situations. If part of the examination is likely to be painful, this should be left to the very end.

Box 5.6 Abdominal examination in pregnancy

Inspection

- Striae gravidarum
- Linea nigra
- Scars
- Fetal movements

Palpation

- Fundal height
- Fetal poles and fetal lie
- Presentation: breech, head, etc.
- Attitude
- Level of presenting part
- Fetal movements
- Liquor volume

Auscultation

- Fetal heart rate

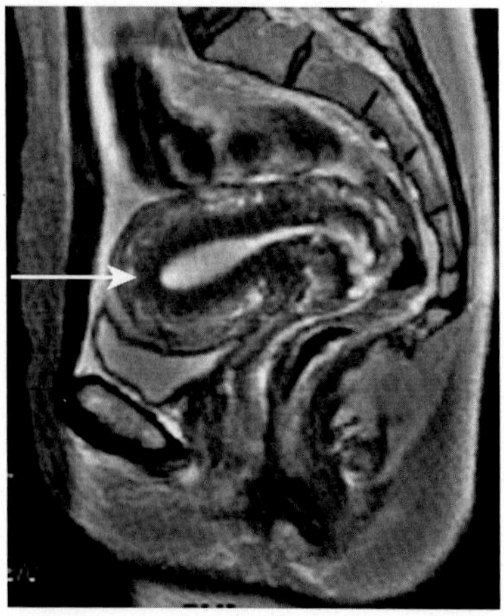

Figure 5.9 Magnetic resonance image of the female pelvis. The uterus is arrowed.

Ask about any tender areas before palpating the abdomen. Using the flat of the hand as well as the examining fingers can enhance comfort and gentleness; this allows the outline of the pregnant uterus to be delineated more readily. In late pregnancy, palpation may produce uterine contractions, which can obscure details of the uterine contents. Remember that, for women in their first pregnancy, the abdominal musculature (particularly rectus abdominis) has not been previously stretched, such that it is sometimes difficult to be sure about findings on palpation.

The size of the uterus (Fig. 5.9 is an MR scan of a normal uterus) is traditionally estimated by the fundal height (see Fig. 5.1), the distance from the symphysis pubis to the fundus (top portion) of the uterus. This is a useful measure, even though it is only one dimension of a globular mass. In a normal pregnancy, the fundal height is just above the symphysis pubis at 12 weeks' gestation, at the umbilicus at 22 weeks and at the xiphisternum at 36 weeks. When the fundus is equidistant from the symphysis pubis and the umbilicus, the gestation is 16 weeks,

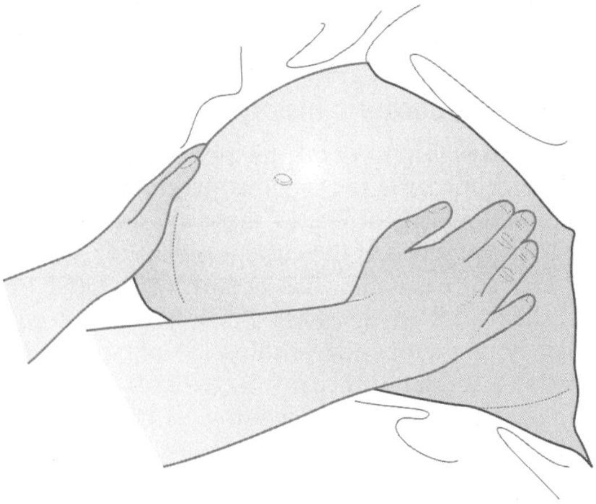

Figure 5.10 Method of abdominal palpation to determine fetal lie and location of back.

and when equidistant from the xiphisternum and umbilicus, it is about 30 weeks. From 36 weeks, the fundal height is also dependent on the level of the presenting part, and therefore decreases as the presenting part descends into the pelvis. This is the phenomenon of a 'lightening' sensation experienced by the mother. The height of the fundus above the symphysis is usually recorded in centimetres and, from 20 weeks onwards, the number of centimetres above the symphysis is approximately in accord with the number of weeks of pregnancy, plus or minus 3 cm, up to 38 weeks. This measurement is generally accepted to be objective and, importantly, is reproducible when different healthcare professionals participate in the same woman's care. Common causes of deviation from these measurements include multiple pregnancies, multiple fibroids, maternal obesity, fetal growth restriction and excess or reduced amniotic fluid volume (poly-hydramnios and oligohydramnios respectively).

Next, determine the lie of the fetus (this is the relationship of the long axis of the fetus to the maternal spine – longitudinal usually, but sometimes oblique or transverse). To confirm the lie, the location of the fetal limbs and back should be identified (Fig. 5.10).

The presentation (the part of the fetus that occupies the lower pole of the uterus) can usually be determined by abdominal palpation if it is cephalic (head), breech (buttocks or feet) or shoulder (Fig. 5.11). Other types of presentation, such as cord and compound, cannot be determined by palpation. At term, over 95% of babies present by the head, but at 30 weeks, because of the greater mobility of the fetus and the relatively larger volume of amniotic fluid, only 70% do so. The breech can usually be distinguished by its size, texture and ability to change shape. However, an ultrasound examination may be needed to confirm this.

The presenting part refers to the part of the fetus that is felt on vaginal examination through the cervix

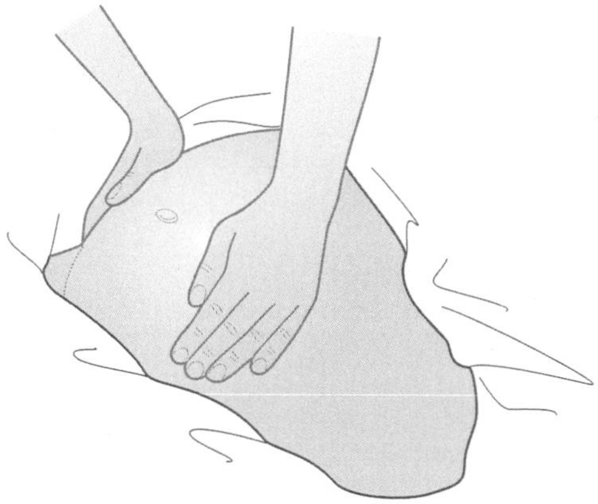

Figure 5.11 Method of abdominal palpation to determine presenting part.

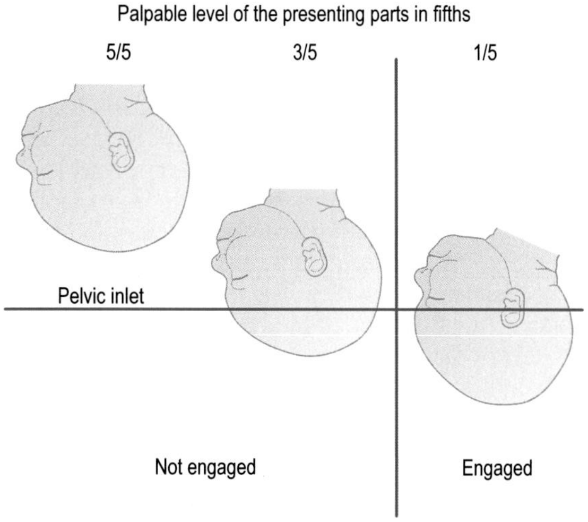

Figure 5.12 The vertical relationship of the presenting part to the pelvic inlet (the level).

(see vaginal examination in labour, below). The head may be presenting but the flexion of the head, or the extension of it, will govern what the presenting part is. In cephalic presentations, the smallest diameters presented to the pelvis occur when the head is well flexed. Thus, in a flexed head, it will be a vertex presentation, and in a deflexed head, it will be the brow or even the face. Flexion of the head is termed the attitude. These observations are not usually possible to ascertain on abdominal examination. For a breech presentation, an equivalent assessment is made to determine whether the breech is extended (frank), flexed (complete) or footling (incomplete). Once the presenting part has a relationship to the pelvis, that relationship can be vertical (the level) or rotational (the position). When the flexed head presents, the fetal occiput is termed the denominator. When the face presents, the denominator is the mentum (chin) and when the breech presents, it is the sacrum.

The presenting part is said to be engaged when the largest diameter has passed through the pelvic brim. It is conventional to estimate the number of fifths of the head that can be palpated through the abdominal wall and this indicates its level (Fig. 5.12). Thus, if there are three or more fifths palpable, the baby's head will be unengaged. If less than three-fifths are palpable, then the baby's head is probably engaged in the pelvis, but this does depend on the overall size of the fetal head and of the pelvis. Remember that the pelvic brim has an angle of approximately 45° to the horizontal when the mother is lying flat. If the abdominal wall is reasonably thin, the unengaged head can be palpated by the examiner's fingers passing round its maximum diameter (a manoeuvre known as a 'Pawlik grip'). This means it is above the pelvic brim. When this does not occur, the widest diameter must be below the examining fingers, and fixity of the baby's head in the pelvis is also a guide. This means it is engaged. Engagement will usually occur as the leading edge of the baby's head, on vaginal examination, reaches the level of the ischial spines (zero station).

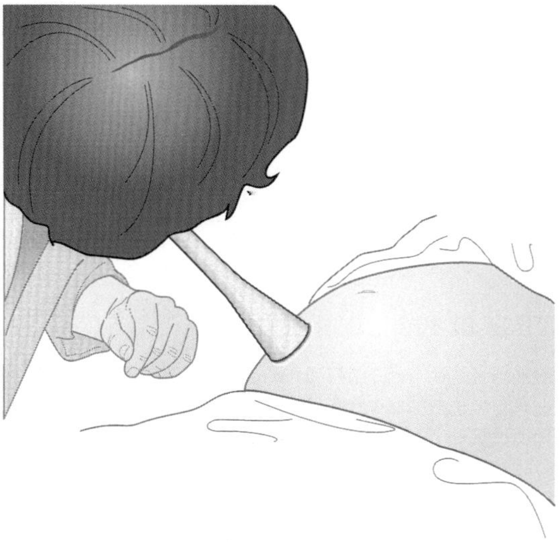

Figure 5.13 Listening over the fetal back to the fetal heart with a Pinard stethoscope (now largely historical).

Fetal movements, both as reported by the mother and observed by the examiner during the examination, are noted. An estimate is made of the fetal size and volume of liquor by a combination of palpation and ballottement. This requires considerable practice. Last, the fetal heart rate (FHR) (normally between 115 and 160 beats/min) is recorded either using a Pinard stethoscope (Fig. 5.13) or now more often with a handheld Doppler device.

Vaginal examination in pregnancy

Vaginal examination (VE) is not usually recommended in early pregnancy. If there is bleeding or retention of urine, it may provide useful information, but the widespread availability of ultrasound scanning has made diagnosis in this situation far less intrusive. In the situation of a threatened miscarriage, it is more appropriate to perform a detailed ultrasound examination, even on the next working day if necessary, than to undertake a VE that may not be particularly helpful and may lead to anxiety (and, possibly later, accusations that the examination contributed to fetal loss). Exceptions to this approach include a suspected ectopic pregnancy with haemodynamic instability or the situation of considerable vaginal blood loss in early pregnancy, in which it is important to quickly diagnose the presence of (and remove) the products of conception at the cervical os. Cervical smears are rarely indicated in pregnancy, unless there is suspicion of a cervical malignancy or one is required for follow-up of known cervical neoplasia.

A case for VE can be made in the situation of possible cervical incompetence. This is a situation in which previous surgery or loop diathermy has led to thinning and dilatation of the cervix such that the weight of the pregnancy sac is too great for the cervix to withstand. The patient, usually somewhere between 16 and 24 weeks into pregnancy, may complain of a small vaginal loss and irregular contractions. If the natural history is allowed to progress, there will be rupture of the membranes followed by a short and painful labour, with subsequent delivery of a fetus (almost always non-viable). Scanning of the cervix in cases at risk has replaced these examinations to some extent but it remains a difficult problem to diagnose.

Vaginal examination in labour

Assessment of whether a woman is in labour is not always straightforward. A VE may help, but is contraindicated if there is painless loss of blood and/or it is known that the patient has a low-lying placenta; potentially dangerous blood loss can occur if a VE disturbs a low-lying placenta.

Vaginal examination in labour should always be preceded by an abdominal examination as described above, together with observation of any contractions, their intensity, frequency, length of time and whether and how much pain they provoke. The VE aims to answer the questions listed in Box 5.7.

The Bishop score is an amalgam of the these findings (excepting the presenting part) at VE and is used to determine whether a woman is in labour. A low score is indicative of an 'unfavourable cervix' (firm, posterior, long, closed cervix with a high presenting part). In contrast, a 'favourable cervix' is one which is associated with an efficient labour – anterior (easy to reach), soft, open, thinned, with a low presenting part.

By repeating abdominal and vaginal examinations at intervals, the diagnosis and progression of labour can be ascertained. Vaginal examination is a potential introduction of infection and can be unpleasant and uncomfortable, so it is usual to not perform this more frequently than every 4 hours. Once labour is established (i.e. the cervix is fully effaced and dilated at least 4 cm), the cervix should progressively dilate at a rate of at least 0.5 cm per hour.

Box 5.7 Reasons for vaginal examination in suspected or actual labour

- Is the cervix anterior, mid position or posterior?
- What is the consistency of the cervix – hard, firm or soft?
- Is the cervix dilated?
- Is the cervix effaced (thinned)?
- What is the presenting part? Assuming a head/cephalic presentation, is the presenting part a vertex (posterior fontanelle palpable through the cervical os), a deflexed head (anterior fontanelle palpable) or, unusually, a brow (supraorbital ridges palpable) or face (mentum or chin)?
- What is the station? The station is the relationship in centimetres between the dominator as above and the ischial spine of the pelvis and is measured in centimetres above or below the spines – thus the depth of the presenting part is low when the tip of the presenting part is 2 or 3 cm below the spines.

Investigations in obstetrics and gynaecology

A variety of investigations is available in gynaecological and obstetric practice. The principles of some commonly requested ones are described here.

Pregnancy testing

Most pregnancy tests depend on the detection of human chorionic gonadotrophin (hCG) or its β subunit in urine or blood respectively. As the chorion produces increasing amounts of hCG from about 10 days postfertilization, pregnancy diagnosis is possible even before the first missed period. Urine pregnancy test kits may be used at the bedside.

Bacteriological and virus tests

Bacteriological and virus tests used in gynaecology and obstetrics include the following:

- Swabs from the throat, endocervix, vagina, urethra and rectum may be needed to diagnose sexually transmitted diseases (see Ch. 17 for more detail).
- Cervical scrape brush or liquid cytology samples for human papilloma virus.
- Mid-stream urinalysis (MSU).
- Serum tests for toxoplasma, rubella, cytomegalovirus and herpes simplex (TORCH) detect antibodies from previous infections and may indicate risk of congenital infection in a future pregnancy.

Imaging

Ultrasound

Transabdominal ultrasound enables a wide field of view, greater depth of penetration and transducer movement. Transvaginal ultrasound, with higher frequency transducers, gives increased resolution and diagnostic power but over a more limited area. More recently, 3-D scanners have been introduced, and these give improved image quality.

In obstetrics, the integrity, location and the number of gestation sacs can be viewed in early pregnancy. By 11 to13 weeks, mono- or dichorionicity, nuchal translucency, nasal bone development and gross fetal abnormality can be detected (Figs 5.14 and 5.15).

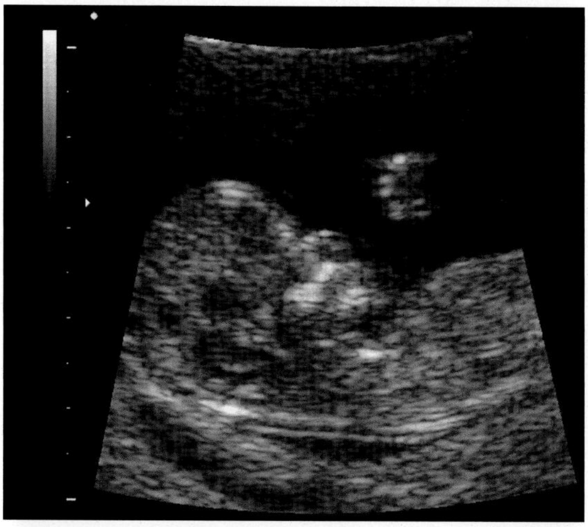

Figure 5.14 Ultrasound scan for early dating.

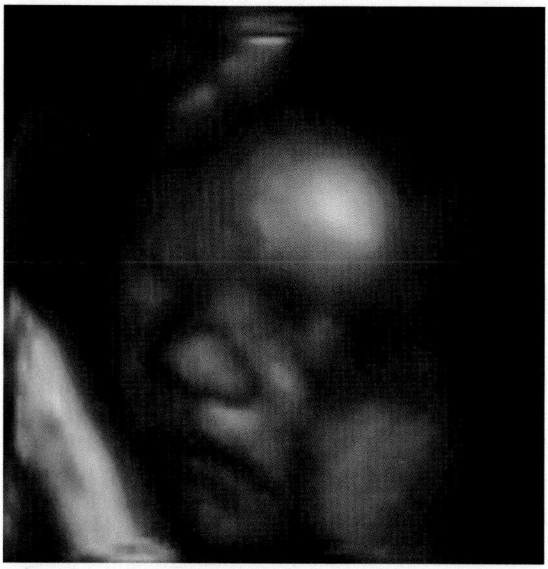

Figure 5.15 An ultrasound image with shading which gives an impression of three dimensions. Its use scientifically is not yet determined, but patients love it for the view it gives of their babies.

Cervical length can be measured, giving an indication of risk of possible late miscarriage or early premature labour. Fetal anatomy surveillance can be carried out using ultrasound from 18 weeks, and if indicated this can include fetal echocardiography. By 20 weeks, uterine and placental blood flow can be assessed in the form of a uterine artery Doppler test, which can help predict risk of fetal growth restriction and pre-eclampsia. Ultrasound scans in the second and third trimester can be used to measure fetal growth velocity, amniotic fluid volumes, and Doppler examination of blood flow through fetal arteries can be used to ascertain fetal wellbeing.

In gynaecology, ultrasound is useful in the diagnosis of uterine and ovarian pathology and in the assessment of bladder function, by measuring residual urine volume and bladder neck activity. It is also helpful in the preoperative preparation for repair of anal sphincter damage.

Computed tomography and magnetic resonance imaging

Computed tomography (CT) scanning has proved less useful in gynaecology than was originally anticipated and is now used mainly for staging and follow-up of malignancies. Magnetic resonance imaging, where available, is a better option (see Fig. 5.9). It does not use ionizing radiation and is particularly good at staging gynaecological malignancies.

Hysterosalpingography

Imaging the uterine cavity and Fallopian tubes with X-ray hysterosalpingography (Fig. 5.16) has largely been replaced by the contemporary technique of hysterosonography (hysterosalpingo contrast sonography, HyCoSy), in which the flow of saline or galactose microparticles through the tubes and uterus is visualized with a vaginal ultrasound probe, thereby avoiding exposure to radiation.

Endometrial sampling (biopsy)

Sampling of the endometrium is often diagnostically useful (Fig. 5.17). An adequate representative sample

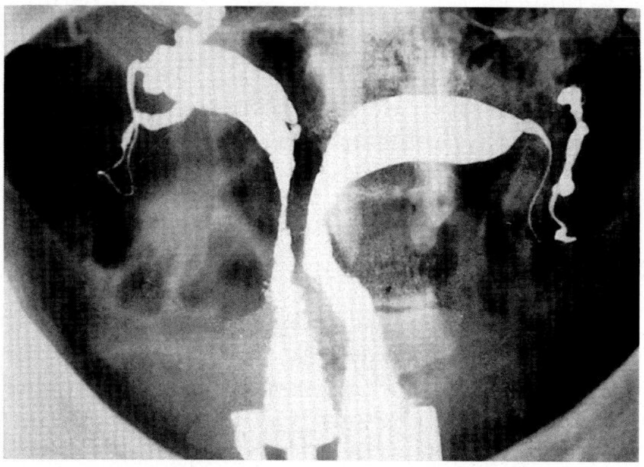

Figure 5.16 An abnormal X-ray hysterosalpingogram; uteri didelphys (double uterus).

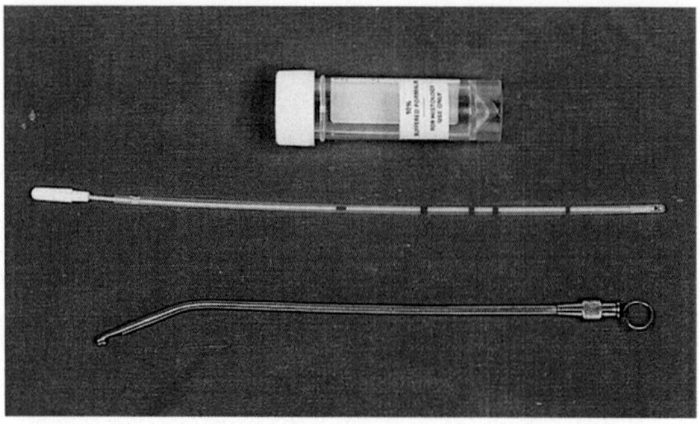

Figure 5.17 An endometrial biopsy curette, a pipette cell sampler and fixing medium.

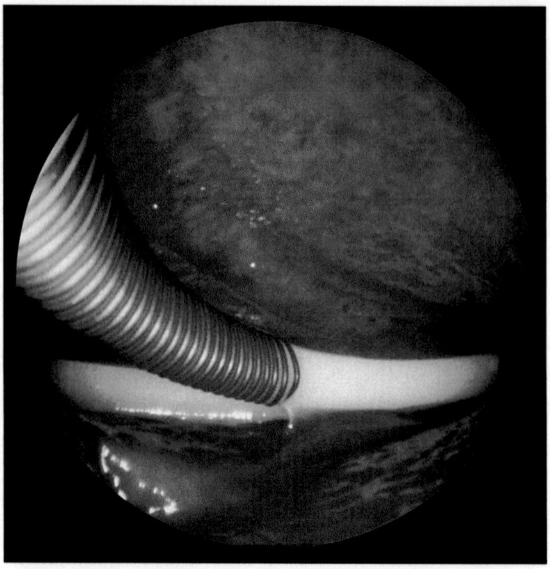

Figure 5.18 Hysteroscopic view of an intrauterine device in situ.

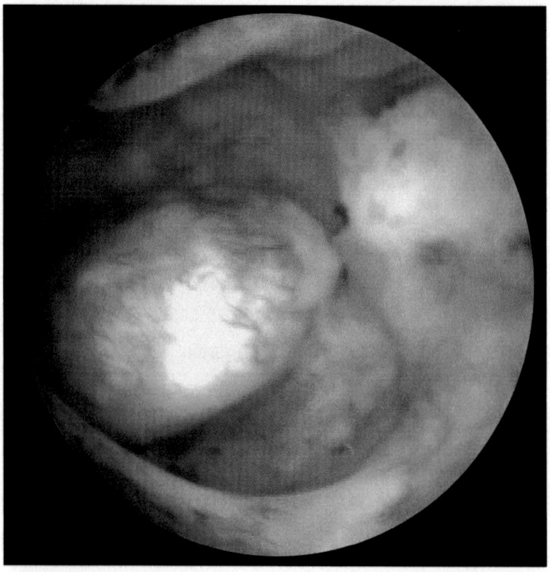

Figure 5.19 Hysteroscopic view of submucosal fibroids.

of endometrium can be obtained using a Vibra or Pipelle sampling system in the outpatient setting. The definitive assessment of the endometrium is usually by hysteroscopy and directed biopsy. With current miniature fibreoptic systems, this can be done under local analgesia in an outpatient setting.

Colposcopy

Colposcopy permits visualization of the cervix, the vaginal vault (vaginoscopy) or vulva (vulvoscopy) with an illuminated binocular microscope to detect precancerous abnormalities of the epithelium. It can be undertaken on an outpatient basis, by accessing the cervix with a speculum, treating it first with acetic acid then with Lugol's iodine. This aqueous solution of iodine and potassium iodide causes the cervix and the normal mucous membrane, which contain glycogen, to stain dark brown. Those areas of abnormality that fail to take up the stain can then be identified (Schiller's test). The whole cervix is viewed through a colposcope, which gives binocular magnification, to identify the degree, site and extent of the cervical pathology.

Hysteroscopy

In this technique, the cavity of the uterus is viewed using small-diameter fibreoptic instruments (Fig. 5.18). Diagnostic hysteroscopy using a 4-mm hysteroscope can be performed as both an inpatient and an outpatient procedure for disorders such as abnormal bleeding and subfertility. This technique can also be adapted with larger hysteroscopes to be used operatively for the resection of uterine adhesions, polyps, septae, submucous fibroids (Fig. 5.19) and endometrium.

Cystoscopy and cystometry

The pressure/volume relationships of bladder filling, detrusor and sphincter activity and urethral flow rate can be assessed with a cystometrogram. The bladder is catheterized and slowly filled with sterile saline. The volume and pressure at which bladder filling is perceived, and at which a desire to micturate is felt, are noted. The urinary flow rate and postmicturition bladder volume are recorded. Electromyographic (EMG) activity in the external urethral sphincter and/or real-time ultrasound assessment of bladder neck activity and descent may provide further information. In stress incontinence, urinary flow commences at low bladder pressures because of sphincter incompetence; in urge incontinence, urinary flow develops at low bladder volumes because of uninhibited detrusor activity. Reflux and overflow also show as urethral leakage. Incontinence can also result from a defect in the anatomical integrity of the urinary tract, such as a congenital abnormality or fistula. Viewing the interior of the bladder by cystoscopy gives information about its condition and allows biopsy of the mucosa or the removal of foreign bodies.

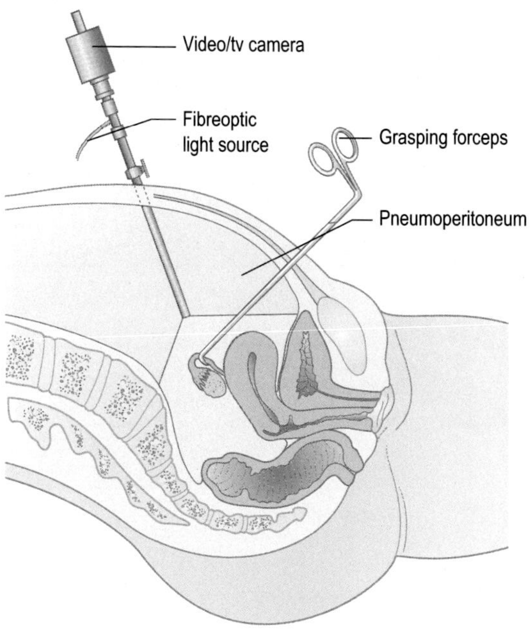

Figure 5.20 Diagram of a diagnostic laparoscopy.

Laparoscopy

Visualization of the pelvic and abdominal viscera is particularly valuable if it can be done without a major injury to the abdominal wall (Fig. 5.20). The abdomen is inflated with carbon dioxide under general or local anaesthesia, so that the anterior abdominal wall is lifted away from the viscera, allowing inspection of the abdominal and pelvic contents using a fibreoptic telescope illuminated by a light source remote from the patient. Laparoscopy may be useful diagnostically (e.g. in the investigation of pelvic pain or infertility) and therapeutically (e.g. sterilization procedures, ectopic pregnancy, division of adhesions, treatment of endometriosis and hysterectomy).

Tests of fetal wellbeing

Besides 'standard' tests of maternal health (haemoglobin, blood glucose, etc.), various investigations may be used to assess fetal wellbeing. In the UK Hepatitis B and HIV testing is offered to all pregnant women, and particularly to those in known risk groups, and may also be checked anonymously in order to obtain an estimate of the community prevalence of these infections.

Biochemical tests

Early pregnancy markers

α-Fetoprotein (AFP), unconjugated oestriol, βhCG, inhibin A, PAPP A

These are normal fetal proteins or hormones that pass into the amniotic fluid and maternal serum. The maternal concentration of these substances varies in a predictable way with gestation. For example, at 16 weeks' gestation, increased levels of AFP suggest fetal spina bifida or anencephaly. However, similar levels can be caused by several other conditions, including threatened miscarriage, multiple pregnancy and exomphalos. Decreased levels are associated with Down's syndrome. A computed risk of Down's syndrome can be produced from maternal weight, gestation, parity and race, measured against βhCG and unconjugated oestriol, and the results matched against ultrasound findings. The 'integrated test' for Down's syndrome predicts a risk ratio that depends on such a comparison. Alternatively the 'combined test' uses the same information plus fetal nuchal translucency at 11 to 13 weeks' gestation.

Late pregnancy

Fetal health in labour can be estimated by checking for the presence of meconium, the responsiveness of the fetal heart rate and by counting fetal movements. In addition to these simple clinical tests, fetal pH measured on a scalp blood sample can be used to detect acidosis and is particularly useful if labour is prolonged, complicated or known to be high risk. Once the membranes are ruptured, the fetal scalp is displayed using an amnioscope and a small sample of capillary blood obtained from a puncture site. If the pH of the sample is below 7.2 then delivery is an urgent priority.

Biological tests

Although biochemical tests provide useful information as the likelihood of a problem with a fetus, biological tests are generally more specific and accurate. It is important before commencing these tests that the woman's attitude to the possible outcomes is explored. Detailed counselling by a trained professional may be required.

Chorion biopsy (chorionic villus sampling, CVS)

This is a method of obtaining chorionic material at 9-13 weeks of pregnancy (usually through the abdomen) so that the genetic constitution or biochemical function of fetal cellular material can be determined. It is useful for the diagnosis of Down's syndrome, thalassaemia and a number of other hereditary conditions. Early and rapid diagnosis allows the possibility of therapeutic termination of an abnormal pregnancy, thereby increasing the safety and acceptability of that procedure. There is a small but definite increased risk of spontaneous miscarriage after CVS.

Amniocentesis

Samples of amniotic fluid may be used for the following:

- Chromosome analysis: amniotic fluid is sampled at 13 to 18 weeks' gestation and is currently safer than chorion biopsy. The amount of

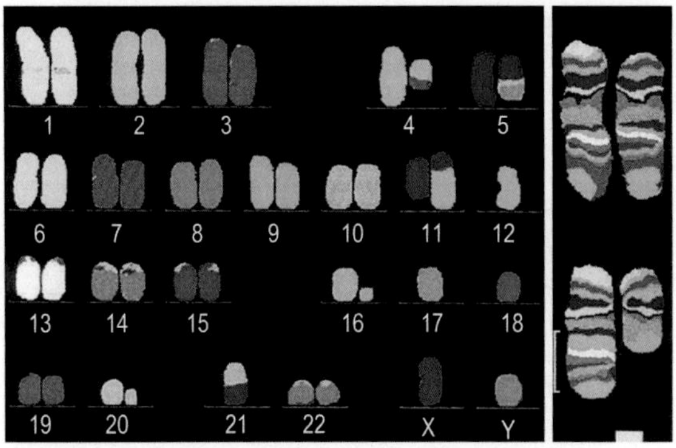

Figure 5.21 Multicoloured FISH. The FISH technique is 'fluorescent in situ hybridization'. The picture is not meant for detail but to show the overall multicoloured appearance of the specific nucleic acid sequences on metaphase chromosomes, which allows the antenatal diagnosis of Down's syndrome, X-linked disorders, Turner's syndrome, Klinefelter's syndrome and trisomies 13 and 18.

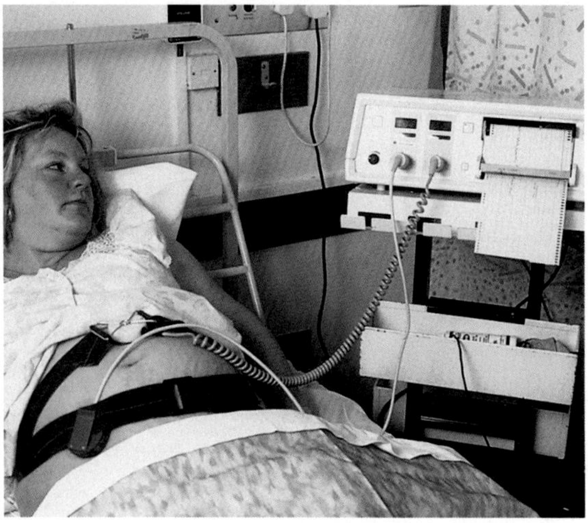

Figure 5.22 Cardiotocography equipment.

desquamated fetal cells obtained is much smaller than from chorion biopsy, and cell culture is necessary, so chromosomal analysis is not immediately possible. However, rapid preliminary results can be obtained using the fluorescent in situ hybridization (FISH) technique (Fig. 5.21). This test is mostly used for prenatal diagnosis of Down's syndrome and other chromosomal abnormalities.

- DNA analysis: fetal cells obtained by amniocentesis, CVS or cordocentesis (see below) can be used for DNA analysis of nuclear chromatin in order to test directly for a number of genetically determined diseases in families known to be at risk. DNA testing and chromosomal studies should only be carried out with fully informed parental consent, and with the help of a genetic counselling service.
- Cordocentesis: in this procedure, a needle is inserted through the abdominal wall and into the amniotic sac to obtain fetal blood from the placental insertion of the cord. It is used in special centres when chromosomal abnormality, haemophilia, haemoglobinopathies, inborn errors of metabolism, fetal viral infections or fetal anaemia are suspected. Although the procedure carries more risk than amniocentesis, it is less traumatic than fetoscopy (which views the amniotic sac contents directly) while still permitting rapid diagnosis.

Non-invasive prenatal testing

Technological advances have meant that it is now possible to detect fetal nucleic acid in maternal plasma, and as this technique removes the risk of miscarriage associated with invasive testing, it is likely to enter general obstetric practice once cost-effectiveness is established.

Biophysical tests

Fetal movements

In some cases of placental insufficiency, fetal movements decrease or stop 12 to 48 hours before the fetal heart ceases to beat. In a healthy pregnancy, fetal movements generally increase from the 32nd week of pregnancy to term. Subjective reports of reduced movements are likely to be more significant than attempting to use a counting system. A report of reduced fetal movements may indicate that sophisticated and detailed surveillance is required.

Cardiotocography (CTG)

Assessment of the fetal heart rate and its variation with fetal and uterine activity can be recorded antenatally or in labour with ultrasound using the Doppler principle (Figs 5.22 and 5.23). A pressure transducer is attached to the abdominal wall so that variations in uterine activity can be matched with the ultrasound recordings. In labour, once the membranes rupture, a more accurate recording of the fetal heart rate can be achieved by an electrode attached to the fetal scalp (Fig. 5.24). The recording is triggered by the fetal electrocardiogram. The information received may be further refined by computerised analysis of the ST segment of the foetal ECG.

Ultrasound visualization

Sequential real-time ultrasonic scanning to detect the presence of symmetrical or asymmetrical growth retardation or changes in fetal activity, breathing, movements, etc., can be used to assess placental function. If it becomes clear that fetal growth has halted or the child's survival in utero is in doubt, then urgent assessment of blood flow by Doppler and delivery with neonatal medicine support should be planned.

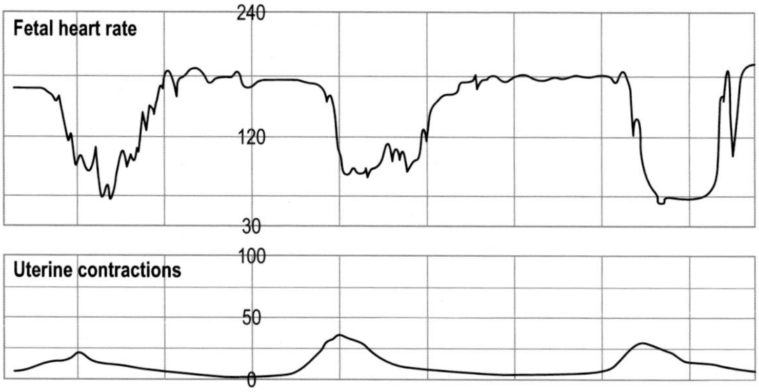

Figure 5.23 An abnormal cardiotocograph showing late variable decelerations during uterine contractions with fetal tachycardia.

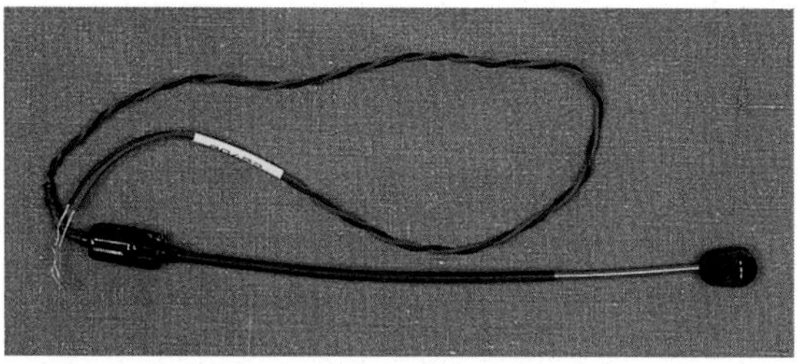

Figure 5.24 Fetal scalp electrode.

Doppler blood flow

Studies of changes in the uterine circulation (uterine artery Doppler) may predict the later onset of pregnancy-associated hypertension. Changes in uteroplacental blood flow (absence or reversal of end-diastolic flow in the umbilical arteries) and those in the cerebral fetal circulation (especially the middle cerebral artery) and fetal ductus venosus give further clues to the state of the fetus, or even imminent fetal death, especially in already compromised circumstances.

Children and adolescents 6

Anna Riddell

Introduction

The skill of clinical examination is the true art of medicine and nowhere more seen than in the examination of children. Children are not small adults and as such the approach to their examination is different. The examiner needs to be flexible, opportunistic and able to tailor the examination to the individual infant, child or young person. In order to maximize the success of the examination, time must be spent trying to gain their confidence. During most of the examination the child should be contented and any discomfort minimized. Do not give false reassurances as this will result in a loss of trust which will hinder the examination. It helps if the consulting room has a range of toys suitable for all ages. Younger children may be happier sitting on their parent's lap. If old enough, the child should be allowed to explore the room freely.

As the family enters the room they should be greeted in a friendly manner and introductions made. Adapt the approach according to the age of the child. An adolescent may want to be the focus of the consultation from the start. Younger children usually will want to have time to observe and assess their surroundings before being observed themselves. They will often take a cue from their carer's response. If everyone relaxes and laughs in the first few minutes, the child will relax and the subsequent history and examination will be easier. Ascertain who is with the child. It may not be the mother or father but another family member. Establish at the onset if you will need the help of an advocate to communicate effectively with the family.

For the experienced clinician, much of the information needed to reach a diagnosis for a child is gleaned from careful observation. While talking to the parent, watch and listen to the child. Assess their behaviour and use this information to adapt the approach. Does the child look unwell? Is the child interested in the surroundings and exploring them, or apathetic? Watch the child running around: are there any obvious abnormalities in the gait? Is the face normal, or are there features of abnormal development? Are there any obvious physical abnormalities? Is the breathing unusually noisy? Does the child seem well nourished, or wasted? What is the child's interaction with their carer like?

History

The history (Box 6.1) will normally be taken from the accompanying carer, but an older child can be invited to give their version of events first. It is appropriate to give an adolescent the opportunity for a few minutes of confidential time during the consultation. Use this to ask questions about alcohol, drugs and sexual activity which young people may be uncomfortable discussing in front of their parents. Even younger children should be asked simple things in words they can understand. Involve them by asking relevant questions such as the site of the pain, etc. Remember that the carers are giving their versions of the problem, not the child's. Parents may also welcome an opportunity to talk in private away from the child, and it is often during such discussion that the real reason for the consultation emerges. Always take notice of what the carers are saying, and listen to their concerns. Any interruptions should be to clarify rather than try and direct the history. Make sure they are given full attention and that they feel their concerns are being taken seriously. All the time

Box 6.1 Structure to history taking in children

- Presenting problem(s)
- History of the presenting complaint
- Previous medical history:
  - birth and the newborn period
  - immunizations
  - specific illnesses, accidents, etc.
  - development and behaviour (including milestones)
  - school
  - contacts and travel
- Family history:
  - consanguinity and genetic risk
- Social history
- Drug history (including allergies)

Box 6.2 Pregnancy and infancy

- Did the mother have any particular illnesses or infections, or was she taking any drugs during the pregnancy (including alcohol)?
- Was the baby born at term?
- What were the birth weight and type of delivery?
- Were there any problems in the newborn period: jaundice, breathing problems, fits, feeding difficulties?
- Has the baby had any illnesses?
- How was the baby fed? When were solid foods introduced?
- Were there any intolerances to food?
- Was the weight gain satisfactory?
- What immunizations has the child had?

they are talking, keep watching everything that the child is doing and his reactions.

The structure and focus of the history is slightly different from that of an adult. The core elements of the presenting complaint, a history of the present illness and a history of any previous illness are the same; however, greater emphasis will be placed on aspects such as the developmental history and less on the systems enquiry. Much of the key information will be collected in the history of the presenting complaint. Most children have a single system involved, and enough time needs to be spent evaluating this carefully. Consider the timing of the symptoms: do they tend only to occur at school? Are there any associating or triggering factors? Are the symptoms interrupting daily activities such as sleep, school attendance, participation in sport or play? Is the child's perception of the symptoms different to that of the parent? Ask about symptoms from other systems in relation to the presenting history rather than as abstract questions. For example, a child presenting with cough may be asked about symptoms of gastro-oesophageal reflux which may be an underlying cause for the cough.

In children, the previous medical history starts from birth and specific attention should be paid to the pregnancy and newborn period (Box 6.2). Is the child fully immunized? This can be checked in the child health record, held by the parent, which should have documentation of child health clinic attendances, weights, immunizations, etc. Enquire into the nature and severity of previous illnesses and the age at which they occurred, for example common childhood infections such as chickenpox, admissions to hospital (in particular to intensive care), significant injuries and accidents. Is the child taking any regular medication or allergic to anything? It is important to ask about the child's developmental progress: when did the child first sit up, smile, crawl, walk and talk? Fuller details regarding the 'milestones of development' are given in Table 6.1. Some useful general questions are outlined in Box 6.3.

Box 6.3 General questions

- What are the child's present habits with regard to eating, sleeping, bowels and micturition?
- What sort of personality does he have – e.g. extrovert, moody?
- Behaviour: anything unusual which the parent is worried about?
- How does he get on with other children?
- How does the child compare with siblings or friends of the same age?
- School: which school, does he like it, academic achievement, does he miss much school?

Family history

Ask about parental age and consanguinity. Find out who are the other children in the family, with age and sex, and who else lives in the family home. Find out if there have been any stillbirths, miscarriages or childhood deaths in the family. Ask if there are any illnesses in the siblings, parents or any near relatives, and if there is any background of inherited disease.

Social history

Approach the social history with diplomacy; sometimes it is more prudent to leave deeper probing to a later occasion in order to develop an initial rapport. The depth of enquiry in a paediatric social history must always be judged on an individual basis. It is useful to know about living conditions and whether either or both parents are employed. Who is the main carer for the child? Is the child in any form of day care? If the child has been separated from the main carer in the past or there is difficulty in the parent's relationship, this may be the basis of a variety of behavioural difficulties. Is there a supportive family structure involving other relatives, for example grandparents? Has the family moved between or within the country frequently and how many languages are spoken in the family?

Examination

After forming an impression of the child, the family and their relationship, the examination can now proceed. By now, younger children should have found the occasion so fascinating that they will be prepared to cooperate in most parts of the physical examination, or they may even have fallen asleep. If the child is now crying loudly, things will be difficult and strategies to calm him down to allow examination will be needed.

A key principle in the examination of children is that most of the information needed to make a diagnosis will be gleaned from careful observation, including listening to the child and playing with the child. Findings can then be consolidated with the

Table 6.1 Normal developmental milestones

Age	Movement and posture	Vision and manipulation	Hearing and speech	Social behaviour
6 weeks	When pulled from supine to sitting, head lag is not quite complete When held prone, head is held in line with body When prone on couch, lifts chin off couch Primitive responses persist	Looks at toy, held in midline Follows a moving person	Vocalizes with gurgles	Smiles briefly when talked to by mother
4 months	Holds head up in sitting position, and is steady Pulls to sitting with only minimal head lag When prone, with head and chest off couch, makes swimming movements Rolls from prone to supine	Watches his hands Pulls at his clothes Tries to grasp objects	Turns head to sound Vocalizes appropriately Laughs	Recognizes mother Becomes excited by toys
7 months	Sits unsupported Rolls from supine to prone Can support weight when held, and bounces with pleasure When prone, bears weight on hands	Transfers objects from hand to hand Bangs toys on table Watches small moving objects	Says 'Da', 'Ba', 'Ka' (babbling)	Tries to feed self Puts objects in mouth Plays with paper
10 months	Crawls Gets to sitting position without help Can pull up to standing Lifts one foot when standing	Reaches for objects with index finger Has developed a finger–thumb grasp Object permanence (knows an object exists even when it is removed from view)	Says one word with meaning	Plays 'peep-bo' and 'pat-a-cake' Waves 'bye-bye' Deliberately drops objects so that they can be picked up Puts objects in and out of boxes
13 months	Walks unsupported May shuffle on buttocks and hands	Can hold two cubes in one hand Makes marks with pen	Says two or three words with meaning	Understands simple questions such as 'Show me your shoe?' Tends to be shy
15 months	Can get into standing position without support Climbs upstairs Walks with broad-based gait	Builds a tower of two cubes Takes off shoes	Will say around 12 words but often understood only by parents	Asks for things by pointing Can use a cup
18 months	Climbs stairs unaided holding rail Runs and jumps Can climb onto a chair and sit down	Builds tower of three cubes Turns pages of a book two or three at a time Scribbles Takes off gloves and socks Can undo a zip	Is beginning to join two words together	Recognizes animals and cars in a book Points to nose, ear, etc. on request Aware of when needs the toilet but not clean and dry Carries out simple orders

remaining techniques requiring laying on of hands. Try to get down to the level of the child in order to appear less threatening. Ideally the child should be fully undressed, but young children often do not like being fully exposed and children of all ages can be modest. Older children will usually cooperate sufficiently to be examined lying down, and routine physical examination is similar to an adult examination. A younger child should be examined sitting on their carer's lap, as any attempt to get the child to lie down may result in distress. Always talk to children, however young; do not be afraid of looking silly if the result is a cooperative child. Those parts of the examination that are unpleasant should be left until last; if an attempt is made to examine a child's throat at the outset, the rest of the examination could be jeopardized. Offer the child something to play with – even a stethoscope will be a source of amusement

Box 6.4 Scheme for examination of children

- Face
- Head
- Neck
- Feet
- Hands and pulse
- Abdomen
- Chest
- Neurological
- Eyes and fundoscopy
- Genitalia, groins, anus
- Ear, nose and throat
- Routine measurements and simple clinical tests

to a young infant. Children often find it amusing if their toy is examined first. The scheme set out in Box 6.4 can be adapted opportunistically, provided all areas are covered.

Always wash your hands before and after the examination in front of the parent. This will inspire confidence and show that you take infection control seriously. The examination techniques include the usual methods of inspection, palpation, percussion and auscultation; however, no set routine can be followed, and the examination is by regions rather than by systems. The older the child, the more the examination will be akin to that for an adult. Bear in mind the child's age and level of understanding and ability to cooperate when planning the examination. Infants and younger children will need alternative strategies and adapted techniques to elicit clinical signs. The examination may have to be opportunistic, as each child will dictate the order of the examination by his reactions to various procedures.

General examination

Note the state of nutrition. Are there any obvious rashes to be seen? Are there any naevi or other skin anomalies? Look at the colour of the child's lips: is there cyanosis or pallor? Listen to the child. Are there any audible noises such as stridor, wheeze or stertor? Is the speech appropriate for the age of the child? Has the child come with any pieces of equipment such as a feeding pump or portable oxygen? Are there any obvious devices to be seen such as a central venous line, gastrostomy tube or ventriculoperitoneal shunt? Is the child interacting with the parent and with you as expected for his age? If not, why not? There could be a sensory deficit or a behavioural problem as a reason for this.

The head, face and neck

Look at the child's face and ask the following questions:

- Does it look normal? If not, try to identify which features seem unusual and describe them. There are many syndromes diagnosable by particular facial features.
- If the baby looks dysmorphic, then do not forget to look at the parents to correlate with any family traits. If the appearance is still not clear, ask who the baby looks like.
- Does the child have a large or protruding tongue?
- Are the ears in the normal position, or are they low set and abnormal in any way?
- Are the eyes small (microphthalmus)? Are they set close together or wide apart (hypo- or hypertelorism)?

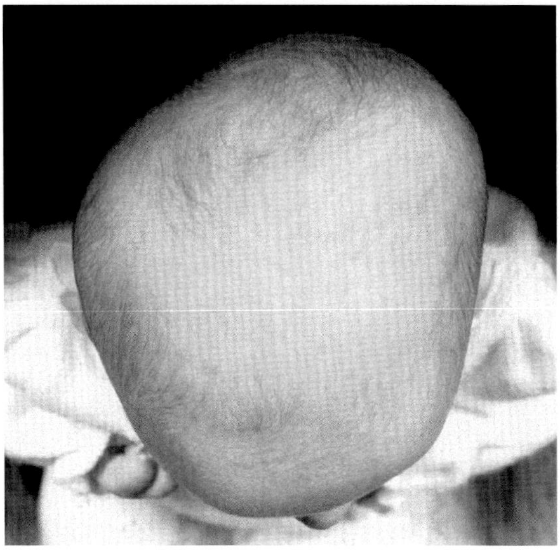

Figure 6.1 Plagiocephalic skull.

Next note the shape of the head. This needs to be done by viewing the child's head from the front, sides and from above. It may be small if the baby is microcephalic, globular if the baby is hydrocephalic, sometimes with dilated veins over the skin surface, or brachycephalic (flattened over the occiput), for example in trisomy 21. It is often asymmetrical (plagiocephalic) in normal infants who tend to lie with their heads persistently on one side (Fig. 6.1). This is now much more common because babies are placed on their backs to sleep in order to reduce the risk of sudden death in infancy. It becomes much less noticeable as the child grows older.

Having gained the child's confidence you can now feel his head for fontanelles and sutures. The anterior fontanelle is normally small at birth, enlarges during the first 2 months, and then gradually reduces until final closure at around 18 months. It can close much earlier and has been reported as staying open in a few normal girls until 4 years of age. Delayed closure may be seen, however, in rickets, hypothyroidism and hydrocephalus. An assessment of the tension of the anterior fontanelle is important. In health, it pulsates and is in the same plane as the rest of the surrounding skull. A tense, bulging fontanelle indicates raised intracranial pressure, but it does also become tense with crying. A sunken fontanelle is a feature of severe dehydration. The posterior fontanelle is located by passing the finger along the sagittal suture to its junction with the lambdoid sutures. It should normally be closed after 2 months of age. Sometimes, when passing the finger along the sagittal suture, a small notch is felt over the vault of the cranium. This is the third fontanelle and, although it can be normal, it is seen in some chromosome abnormalities and in congenital infections such as rubella. While feeling the head, any ridging of the sutures should be noticed, suggesting premature fusion (craniostenosis). In the neonatal period, the sutures tend to be separated, and there is sometimes a continuous gap from the forehead to the posterior part of the posterior fontanelle. Sutures close rapidly and are normally ossified by 6 months of age. Leave the measurement of the head circumference until near the end of the examination, as some babies find this a little threatening and may start crying.

Having assessed the skull, the neck can be checked, paying particular attention to the presence of lymph nodes. It is common in childhood to feel small lymph nodes in the anterior and posterior triangles of the neck. They can persist for some years and change in size in response to local infections such as tonsillitis (reactive lymphadenopathy). Lymph nodes of greater than 1 cm diameter or rapidly increasing size may indicate significant pathology and should be investigated. Examination of other lymphatic areas can be carried out at a later stage of the examination – the inguinal nodes when the napkin area is checked, and the axillary nodes when the chest is examined. In young babies, the sternomastoid muscles should be checked for the thickened area known as a sternomastoid tumour. This is a benign lesion occurring usually as a result of birth trauma but can lead to difficulties with neck movement and an abnormal head and neck posture. Torticollis is a potentially more sinister sign and can be associated with posterior fossa tumours, vertebral osteomyelitis and urinary tract infections.

The limbs

The feet need to be checked for a variety of problems, such as minor varus deformities, overriding toes or flat feet. It is helpful to feel the surface of the legs with your hands to detect muscle wasting or tenderness. Note any bony abnormalities and examine the movements of the knee and ankle. Feel for any swelling or warmth of the joints which may be suggestive of an arthropathy. At the same time, an assessment of the muscle tone can be made. This part of the examination may be made easier as part of a game. It is easy to notice at the same time whether the skin is dry or lichenified (as in eczema) and to note any skin lesions. All the time the child's reactions should be watched. Is the child still friendly? Be prepared to stop the examination if the child seems to be getting upset, and spend a few minutes trying to re-establish the previous rapport.

The examination can now proceed to the rest of the body. The arms can be examined in the same way as the legs. Do the hands have a single palmar crease, as seen in children with trisomy 21 (Down's syndrome)? Is there any clubbing leading to suspicion of underlying cyanotic congenital heart disease or chronic lung disease such as cystic fibrosis? Are there any limb abnormalities such as syndactyly (fusion of the digits) or polydactyly (extra digits)? Feel the wrists for widening of the epiphyses of the radius and ulna – a sign of rickets. Try to feel the pulse and count it. This is best done at the brachial pulse in a plump, young infant.

The abdomen

The abdomen can be a little difficult to examine if the child is crying, which is why it is important to have gained the child's cooperation by this point in the examination. Most infants and toddlers will need to be examined while sitting on their carer's lap (Fig. 6.2). It is sometimes possible to quieten a crying infant by placing him over his mother's shoulder and examining from behind. Small infants can be given a feed to quieten them. Older children can be asked if they would be happy to lie on an examination couch.

The examination needs to be structured along the three essential components of looking (observation), feeling (palpation) and listening (auscultation). During the first 3 years of life, the abdomen often gives an impression of being protuberant due to the laxity of the rectus muscles. Causes of true abdominal distension are shown in Box 6.5. Look for any obvious distension or for peristaltic waves (intestinal obstruction or pyloric stenosis). Note the umbilicus and whether or not there is a hernia. Palpation should be gentle initially. Always ask the child if his tummy hurts anywhere and watch his facial expression during palpation. The liver edge can be felt in normal children up to the age of 4 years; it can be anything up to 2 cm below the costal margin. When enlarged, the

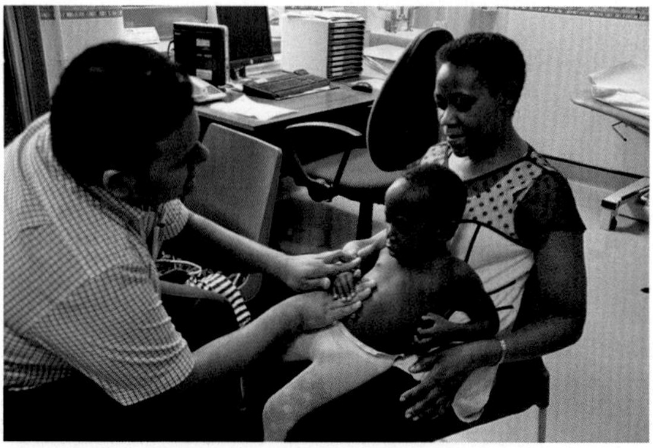

Figure 6.2 Baby sitting on mother's lap while the abdomen is examined.

Box 6.5 Causes of abdominal distension

- Obesity
- Faeces (constipation, Hirschsprung's disease)
- Ascites (nephrotic syndrome, cirrhosis)
- Gas (intestinal obstruction, swallowed air)
- Pregnancy in adolescent girls
- Distended bladder (lower abdomen)
- Pyloric stenosis (upper abdomen)

Box 6.6 Reasons for a thoracotomy

- Lung surgery
- Persistent ductus arteriosus repair
- Pulmonary artery banding
- Coarctation of the aorta repair
- Blalock–Taussig shunt (also results in unequal radial pulses)

Table 6.2 Causes of hepatomegaly and splenomegaly in children

Hepatomegaly	Splenomegaly	Hepatosplenomegaly
Glycogen storage disorders Congenital infections Heart failure Haemolytic disease of the newborn	Sickle cell disease Spherocytosis Malaria	Leukaemia Lymphoma Mucopolysaccharidoses Thalassaemia Alpha-1-antitrypsin deficiency

Table 6.3 Normal observation values at different ages

Age	Respiratory rate (breaths per minute)	Pulse rate (beats per minute)	Blood pressure (systolic/diastolic mmHg)
Newborn	40-60	140-160	65/45
1 year	30-50	110	75/50
3 years	20-30	100	85/60
8 years	15-25	90	95/65
11 years	15-20	80	100/70

spleen may be felt below the left costal margin, and in infancy it is more anterior and superficial than in the older child or adult. Slight enlargement of the spleen can occur in many childhood infections (EBV, CMV). Causes of hepatosplenomegaly are listed in Table 6.2. Faecal masses can be felt in the left iliac fossa in constipated children. They often feel like a sausage which can be rolled underneath the fingertips. A full or distended bladder presents as a mass arising from the pelvis. Deep palpation of the kidneys can be carried out last. Although it would be logical to examine the groin area at this time, it is often better to do this at a later stage. If the child has cried persistently, it is still possible to examine the abdomen. When the baby breathes in and the abdominal muscles relax, the abdominal viscera and other masses, if present, can be palpated.

The chest

Examining the chest in a child takes in both the respiratory and cardiovascular systems. The basic structure remains the same, at first looking then feeling then listening with the stethoscope. It helps to have let the child play with the stethoscope at an earlier stage of the examination to alleviate any worries about this strange instrument. Observation will give much of the information required for the diagnosis, particularly in younger children and infants. On observation, check for abnormalities which are fixed and those which become obvious on movement. Static deformities in children include pectus excavatum and carinatum which are a source of great anxiety to many parents but are not usually of any clinical importance. Fixed indentation of the lower ribs at the line of insertion of the diaphragm (Harrison's sulcus) may be seen in obstructive airway disease, due either to asthma or to a nasopharynx blocked by adenoidal hypertrophy or in conditions leading to increased pulmonary blood flow. Look from the side for an increased anteroposterior diameter of the chest, which could be a sign of a chronic lung disease such as cystic fibrosis. Thickening of the costochondral junction is felt in rickets (rachitic rosary). Note any scars as a result of cardiac surgery. It is important to look for the thoracotomy scar under the arms or even round the back; otherwise you will miss it (Box 6.6). Sternotomy scars usually indicate the child has had major heart surgery involving valves or closure of septal defects. Asymmetry of the chest becomes more obvious on movement (dynamic deformity) and may indicate an underlying pneumothorax or empyema. Look for any increased work of breathing. This may be indicated by seeing recession (intercostal or subcostal), tracheal tug or flaring of the nares when breathing. The infant may be using accessory muscles such as the sternomastoids which results in head bobbing. Count the respiratory rate (Table 6.3) which, in infants, must be done over a minute to be accurate, due to periodic breathing. Listen for grunting respiration which is audible in infants who are attempting to prevent alveolar collapse by creating their own positive airway pressure. The grunting expiration is followed by inspiration and then a pause.

Palpate the anterior chest wall for the cardiac impulse and for thrills. In children under the age of 5 years, the apex is normally in the fourth intercostal space just to the left of the mid-clavicular line. Midline shift can be assessed in this way as palpation for the trachea in the suprasternal notch can be difficult and unpleasant for the child. Vocal fremitus is of less

Table 6.4 Chest signs of some common respiratory disorders of children

Disorder	Chest movement	Percussion (if carried out)	Auscultation
Bronchiolitis	Restricted, with hyperinflation Often tracheal tug and subcostal recession	Hyper-resonant	Widespread crackles, or wheezing
Pneumonia	Rapid, shallow respirations with audible grunt May be reduced on affected side	Dull or normal	Localized bronchial breathing or crackles May have no abnormal signs
Asthma	Restricted with hyperinflation Use of accessory muscles, and subcostal retraction	Hyper-resonant	Expiratory wheeze
Croup	Inspiratory stridor, with subcostal recession	Normal	Inspiratory coarse crackles

clinical value the smaller the child. This is because of difficulty with cooperation and the small size of the precordium. Expansion is also better assessed by observation for the same reasons. The axillary nodes may now be felt in the same way as in adults.

Percussion of the chest is useful in older children, but in young children and infants it is rarely of value. Tell the child 'I am going to make you sound like a drum'. Percuss very lightly in babies, directly tapping the chest wall with the percussing finger rather than using another intervening finger. The chest is more resonant in children than in adults.

A stethoscope with a small bell chest piece is suitable for auscultation of the child's chest. Do not use adult-sized chest pieces, as it is impossible to localize added sounds accurately with a chest piece covering such a wide area in a small child. Often it is less threatening to examine the back of the chest first, and much more information about the lungs can be acquired in this way. Listen for the breath sounds and adventitious sounds. Because of the thin chest wall, breath sounds are louder in children than in adults, and their character is more like the bronchial breathing of adults (puerile breathing). Upper respiratory tract infections in children often give rise to loud, coarse rhonchi, which are conducted down the trachea and main bronchi (transmitted upper airway sounds) (Table 6.4). All is not lost if the child is crying, as this is accompanied by deep inspiration giving an opportunity to listen for the character of the breath sounds.

When you are auscultating the front of the chest, the child's immediate instinct is to push the stethoscope away. You can ask the parent to hold the child's hands or try to distract the child with toys held in the hand (Fig. 6.3). It is a good idea to examine a doll or teddy bear first if the child is playing with one. The normal splitting of the first and second sounds is easier to hear in children than in adults. Venous hums and functional systolic flow murmurs are often heard in normal children (Box 6.7). If the murmur does not fit into this classification, remember that most cardiac problems in children are as a result of congenital heart disease and not acquired as in adults (Table 6.5). Count the heart rate in young children (see Table 6.3). Arrythmias are uncommon in children unless they have had cardiac surgery.

Box 6.7 The five S's of an innocent murmur

- Short
- Soft
- Systolic
- Sitting/standing (varies with posture)
- Symptom free

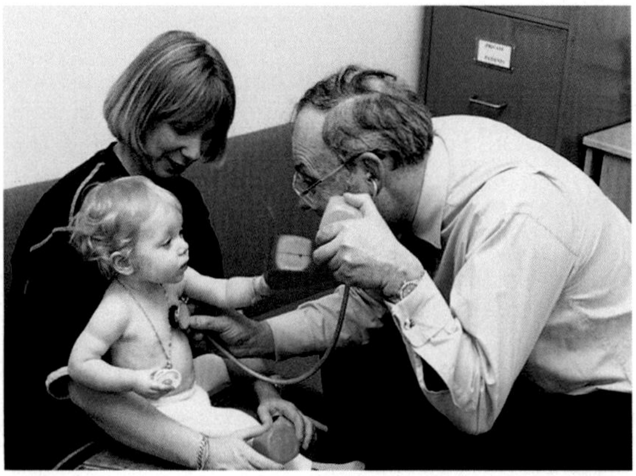

Figure 6.3 Attracting the attention of a 10-month-old baby while examining her heart.

Neurological examination

The neurological examination can usually be carried out in the normal way in older children, but in younger children the extent of the neurological examination will depend on the child's age and willingness to cooperate. Although a great deal should have been learned already from initial observations, still look at the child's static and dynamic posture. Asymmetry may indicate a hemiparesis. A hypotonic child may sit on his back rather than his bottom and an infant may display a 'frog leg' posture when lying down. Children with cerebral palsy may have a characteristic 'windswept' posture (quadriplegic) or have uncoordinated continuous movements (ataxic or dyskinesic). If the child is walking, the gait should have been

Table 6.5 Categories of key congenital heart disease lesions

Acyanotic (presents with hyperdynamic circulation in heart failure)	Cyanotic (presents with respiratory distress and cyanosis)	Outflow tract obstruction (presents grey and shocked)
Ventricular septal defect (VSD) (pansystolic murmur at left sternal edge) Atrial septal defect (pulmonary flow murmur with fixed splitting of 2nd heart sound) Persistent ductus arteriosus (continuous 'machinery' murmur)	Pulmonary stenosis (PS) (ejection systolic murmur at the left 2nd intercostal space) Tetralogy of Fallot (murmur of PS ± VSD and right ventricular heave) Transposition of the great arteries (no murmur)	Coarctation of the aorta (pansystolic murmur at left sternal edge)

observed already. Look for toe walking (spasticity), wide-based gait (seen in cerebellar ataxia but normal in toddlers) and limping (antalgic gait or hemiplegia). Hemiplegia may become more obvious on running as the affected upper limb is brought up closer to the body.

Note any abnormal movements. Tics or habit spasms are repetitive but not purposeful movements, such as shrugging of the shoulders or facial grimacing. Choreiform movements are involuntary, purposeless jerks that follow no particular pattern. Athetoid movements are writhing and more pronounced distally. Fits may be seen as lip smacking or flickering eye movements.

Take the opportunity to check for spinal abnormalities such as scoliosis or kyphosis or any evidence of spina bifida such as a tuft of hair. Be careful to pick up on any signs of a neurocutaneous disorder such as café-au-lait spots or telangiectasia.

Coordination can best be checked by watching a child at play. It is useful to have toys available that require a degree of coordination, such as a toy farm or garage. Otherwise, a modification of the finger–nose test using a toy held in the hand can be used. If the child is old enough, watching them dressing or doing up shoelaces is a good way to assess coordination.

Check muscle tone if this has not already been done. Pick the child up if there is still a friendly relationship. This gives a good idea of the feel of a child and of the muscle tone. A hypotonic infant will feel as though they are slipping through your hands. Muscle power is difficult to check in young children except by watching playing habits and assessing power by ability at a variety of lifting games. Always remember to check for neck stiffness by testing resistance to passive neck flexion rather than by testing for Kernig's sign.

Testing of sensation is difficult in young children and less likely to yield useful information. Unless there is a strong suspicion of neurological disease, it is usually omitted. Touch can be tested by observing the reaction when the skin is touched with a cotton wool ball.

Testing the cranial nerves takes a little ingenuity. Eye movements are relatively easy using a toy moved in different directions in front of the baby's face. Young infants will often copy poking out the tongue at them, which will check the 12th cranial nerve. If the child can be made to smile, and even if he is crying, any asymmetry of facial movements can be seen. If a child is able to bite on a wooden spatula, the trigeminal nerve is probably intact.

Getting a child's limbs into the correct position to test tendon reflexes may take some time. Often they can be elicited by using a finger rather than a patellar hammer. Tendon reflexes in young infants tend to be brisk, and up to 18 months of age the plantar responses are extensor. The persistence of an extensor response beyond the age of 2 years indicates an upper motor neurone lesion. Note whether primitive reflexes have persisted (Box 6.8) indicating significant neurodevelopmental dysfunction.

Box 6.8 Primitive reflexes

Rooting reflexes

On touching a baby's cheek, he will turn his head towards the stimulus. Sucking itself is a reflex, and failure of the sucking response beyond the 36th week of gestation suggests significant neurological impairment.

Palmar and plantar grasp

A finger placed across the child's palm or plantar surface of the foot will cause flexion and grasping of the finger. Lost by 2 months of age.

Stepping reflex

When lowered vertically onto a hard surface, the foot presses down and the other leg flexes at the hip and knee in a stepping movement. As this response is alternated from one leg to the other, the baby makes a walking movement. Lost by 2 months of age.

The Moro reflex (see Fig. 6.11)

On dropping the head a few centimetres, the upper limbs abduct and extend symmetrically and then flex. Lost by 6 months of age.

The eyes

The eyes should now be checked. There are signs critical to other systems to look for such as pallor and jaundice. Inspect the eyes for ptosis, conjunctivitis, cataracts or congenital defects such as colobomata. Watch for spontaneous nystagmus or roaming eye movements which may indicate a visual impairment. It is very important to check for squints, as ophthalmological referral is necessary, particularly in an infant over 3 months of age. Squints are checked for by shining a light in the eyes from in front of the face and observing the position of the light reflex; it should be at the same position in each cornea. A cover test should then be used (see Ch. 20), using a doll or some other appropriate toy on which the child can focus his gaze. Pupillary accommodation and light reactions can be noted at the same time. Examination of the fundus is particularly difficult in infants and will require dilatation of the pupils. It should be possible to see the red reflex which, if absent, is suggestive of a corneal, lens or vitreous opacity, such as cataract or retinoblastoma. Usually, enough of the disc can be seen to detect papilloedema. The testing of vision in young children is included in the section on developmental screening examination (see page 78).

With the possible exception of the eye examination, nothing so far should have upset a baby unduly. The following examinations should be carried out at the end of the consultation, as they are more likely to upset the child.

The genitalia, groins and anus

The nappy or underpants can now be removed if it is necessary to examine the groin or anus. In boys, notice the penis. The lack of retraction of the foreskin can be a source of worry to parents but it is normal for it not to retract under the age of 5 years. Forcibly attempting retraction is not only painful but can also result in balanitis. Check the hernial orifices and see whether the testes have descended. To feel the testes, make sure that the examining hand is warm and place a finger in the line of the inguinal canal; advance the finger towards the scrotum. This will stop the cremasteric reflex causing the testes to disappear into the inguinal canal, which tends to happen if the scrotum is approached from below. In young babies, it is not unusual to find a testis in the inguinal canal, but it can usually be pushed into the scrotum without too much difficulty. The testis can be expected to descend into its normal position with increasing maturity.

In girls, check the vulva for redness, soreness or discharge which are commonly seen in vulvovaginitis. Fusion of the labia is not uncommon, so check that they separate normally. Enlargement of the clitoris may suggest an endocrine disorder. It is important to note that examination for possible sexual abuse should be left to an expert. Check for inguinal lymph nodes and palpate the femoral arteries (simultaneously with the radials) to exclude coarctation of the aorta.

Examination of the anal margin can best be carried out by gently separating the buttocks with one hand on either side; the anal orifice can then easily be seen and inspected for fissures which are commonly associated with constipation. Rectal examination is rarely necessary in children and, if carried out, should be done with a well-lubricated, gloved little finger, which should be advanced very slowly.

In older children and adolescents puberty is assessed using the Tanner stage (Table 6.6). This will involve examination of the genitalia and looking for breast development and body hair.

The nose, ears, mouth and throat

The worst parts of the examination as far as the child is concerned are the nose, ears, mouth and throat.

The nose need only be examined superficially, looking for nasal patency, any deviation of the septum or the presence of polyps or inflamed nasal turbinates. Older children are quite good at sniffing, and this will give some idea of nasal patency.

A cooperative child will allow a look into his ears but, if not, the child should be held by the mother, as shown in Fig. 6.4. Held in such a way, the child can be kept still long enough for the eardrums to be inspected. Look carefully for the light reflex, which can be lost if the child has chronic secretory otitis media ('glue ear'). In acute suppurative otitis media, the drum may be bright red and bulging.

The mouth and throat can be examined by encouraging a cooperative child to 'show me your teeth'; an open mouth will then allow a clear view of the mouth and fauces. If uncooperative, the child will

Table 6.6 Tanner staging

	Boys (external genitalia)	Girls (breast)	Boys and girls (pubic hair)
Stage 1	Prepubertal	Prepubertal	Prepubertal
Stage 2	Enlargement of scrotum and testes	Breast bud stage	Sparse growth of long, slightly pigmented hair
Stage 3	Enlargement of penis length	Enlargement of breast and areola	Darker, coarser and more curled hair, spreading sparsely over junction of pubes
Stage 4	Increased size of penis with growth in breadth, scrotum skin darker	Areola and papilla form a secondary mound above level of breast	Hair adult in type, but covering smaller area than in adult
Stage 5	Adult genitalia	Mature stage	Adult in type and quantity

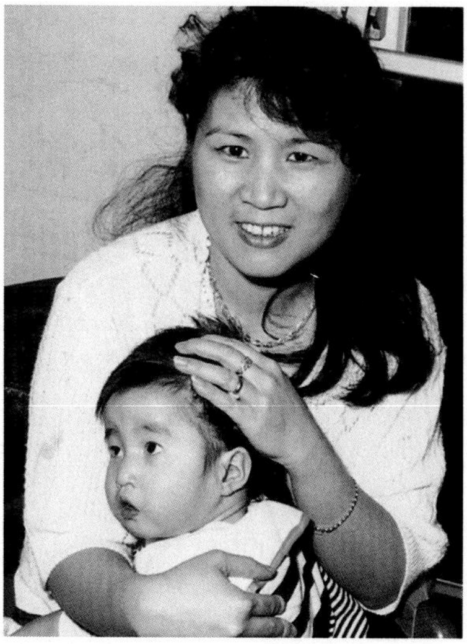

Figure 6.4 How to hold a baby to allow the ears to be examined. The mother faces the baby to one side and holds him firmly, with one arm around the head and the other around the upper arm and shoulder.

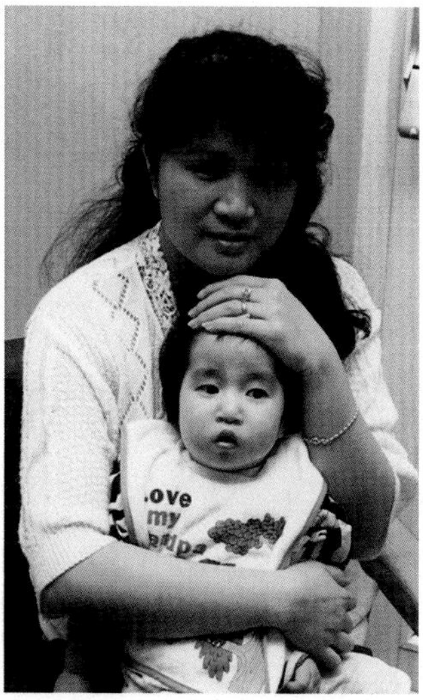

Figure 6.5 How to hold a baby to allow the mouth and throat to be examined. The baby faces the examiner, with the mother holding him firmly with one hand on the forehead and the other holding both arms.

need to be held as shown in Fig. 6.5. Sometimes it is not too disastrous if the child cries at this point, as this will give a very clear view of the teeth, the tonsils and sometimes even the epiglottis. A spatula is a terrifying instrument to the average child, causing most to clamp their teeth shut. If this happens, the spatula should be advanced to the back of the tongue to induce a gag reflex. Look for the presence of the white patches of candida infection, ulcers seen in inflammatory bowel disease and the Koplik's spots seen in measles.

The general physical examination has now been completed. Hopefully the child is still friendly. Once the child is dressed, the examiner should sit with the parents and explain what has been found. It is always best for the child to have finished dressing before talking to the parents: they are more likely to listen and take in what you have to say if they are not worrying about buttons or shoelaces. Always involve older children in the discussion, as they have every right to know what you have found. Even young children can be given information in terms they will understand. Never under any circumstances deceive a child. The eventual truth will result in his losing confidence in you and with later medical attendants.

Signs associated with abuse/child neglect

During the examination of the child you may pick up signs which lead you to be concerned about the possibility of non-accidental injury or other forms of child abuse. These should be noted and considered as part of the differential diagnosis. Detailed definitions of the four categories of abuse (physical, emotional, sexual and neglect) can be found in Working Together to Safeguard Children: March 2015 (HM Government; http://www.workingtogetheronline.co.uk/). Box 6.9 lists some alerting features of abuse which will help you recognize if abuse is occurring. It is now recognized that safeguarding children is everyone's responsibility, however challenging that may feel. If you do have concerns, make sure you are aware of your organization's policies and procedures and that you have someone you can discuss them with.

Routine measurements

Height and weight

Childhood is a period of growth, the pattern of which may be adversely affected by many disturbances of health as well as social deprivation. Serial measurements of height and weight are therefore essential in the examination of children. In children able to stand, height can be measured against a wall-mounted gauge. Younger children can be measured lying down on special measuring boards. Measurements should be made under standard conditions, and children should be weighed unclothed. If the child keeps any clothes on, this should be noted against the weight so that subsequent weights can be taken with the child wearing the same quantity of clothing. Heights and weights should be compared with those of healthy children of similar sex, age and build on percentile charts. Figs 6.6 and 6.7 show standard height, weight and head circumference charts for UK boys and girls from birth to 18 years developed by the RCPCH/WHO/Department of Health. Other charts for body mass index (BMI), puberty monitoring and Down's syndrome can be obtained from the RCPCH website.

Comparison should also be made against the parents' height by calculating the mid-parental height. This is done by adding together the height of the

Box 6.9 Symptoms and signs to help with recognition of abuse/neglect (from NICE guidance 'When to suspect child maltreatment' 2009)

	Consider maltreatment	Suspect maltreatment
Physical abuse	Any serious/unusual injury with absent/unsuitable explanation; oral injuries; burns or scalds; lacerations	Bruising in specific shapes; human bites; lacerations on protected areas of the body; retinal haemorrhage without another medical explanation; bruises on non-bony parts of the body or face including the eyes, ears and buttocks
Emotional abuse	Fearful/withdrawn; excessive clinginess; overfriendliness; enuresis/encopresis; signs of deliberate self harm; behavioural or emotional change that has no medical explanation	A combination of several concerning symptoms or signs
Neglect	Severe infestations; dirty clothing/unwashed child; faltering growth/obesity; animal bites; poor school attendance; unimmunized; failure to attend for developmental checks; dental decay	Cold injuries; hypothermia; medical advice not sought; repeated reports of poor living environment, lack of adequate food
Sexual abuse	Gaping anus; anogenital warts; anogenital injury; anal fissure with constipation; vaginal discharge; persistent dysuria	Persistence of anogenital symptoms or signs with no explanation; pregnancy in a child; hymenal injuries; significant anogenital trauma; unusual sexualized behaviours

father and mother (cm) and dividing by 2. Add 7 cm for a boy and take away 7 cm for a girl. Plot the final value in centimetres at the final adult height line (either at 18 years or 20 years depending on the chart used) to find the child's expected final centile. A child who fails to grow at an appropriate velocity (growth rate) needs to be investigated further. The term 'failure to thrive' is used to denote children whose weight gain is below that expected (fallen across 2 centiles on the chart). The child will need a very careful history and examination to be carried out. It is important to pick up any markers of potential chronic disease. There are as yet no satisfactory growth charts for children of Asian origin born in the UK. They tend to be smaller than Caucasian children at least in the first few years of life; as a rough guide, the mean percentile for an Asian child is the 25th percentile on the standard UK charts. Children of African origin tend to be larger than Caucasian children. There are special growth charts for children with Down's syndrome and Turner's syndrome.

The meaning of the term '10th percentile' is that 10% of all children in the measured population are respectively lighter or shorter at the age concerned. Slightly different standards are applicable in different races and in different countries. Preterm infants should be plotted according to their corrected age (chronological age minus the number of weeks born early) up until the age of 2 years.

Head circumference

In infants under the age of 2 years, the head circumference is a good proxy for linear growth and a much more reliable measurement than height or length. The standard measurement is the largest occipito-frontal circumference out of three using a paper tape.

Box 6.10 Causes of microcephaly and macrocephaly

Microcephaly

- Perinatal insult
- Fetal alcohol syndrome
- Craniostenosis syndromes

Macrocephaly

- Hydrocephalus
- Mucopolysaccharidosis
- Excessive brain growth (Canavans and Sotos syndromes)

As applies to height and weight, it is the rate of growth rather than a one-off abnormal value which usually gives cause for concern. Some causes of microcephaly and macrocephaly are listed in Box 6.10. Rather than using a chart showing the head circumference alone, it is more useful to use one that combines head circumference and length and weight percentiles, so that the proportions of each individual child can be compared.

Blood pressure

Abnormalities of blood pressure are uncommon in childhood and, because the measurement of blood pressure can be frightening and technically difficult, it is often only measured when cardiovascular or renal disease is suspected. An electronic monitor will be used in most paediatric settings as manual methods can be inaccurate in small children. There should be a variety of cuff sizes available and the largest cuff which will fit around the upper arm but not extend to the elbow joint should be used. The use of cuffs which are too small will give erroneously high readings. Doppler techniques more accurately measure blood

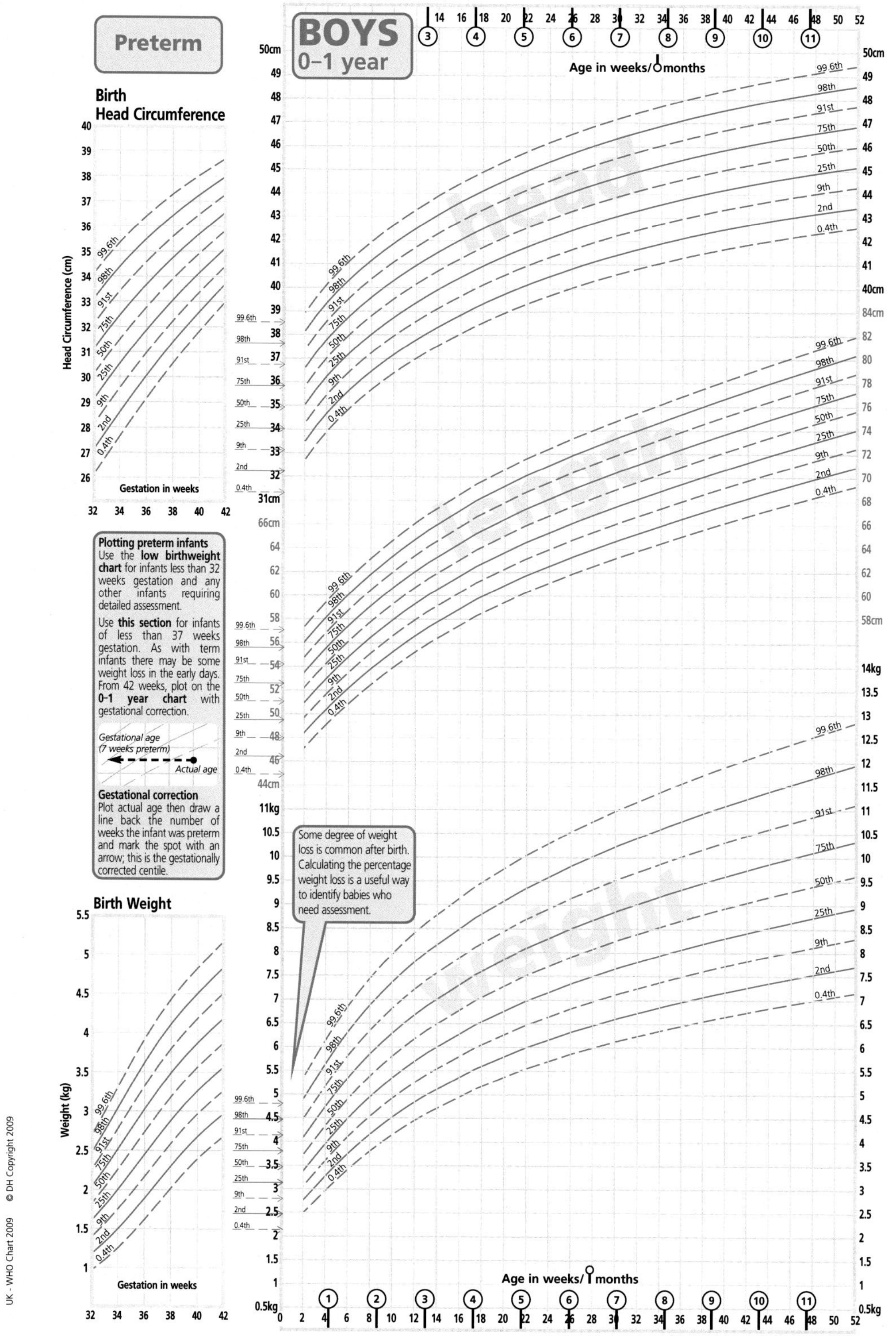

Figure 6.6 Height, weight and head circumference: boys aged 0-4 years. (© 2009 Department of Health Charts developed by RCPCH/WHO/Department of Health. Reproduced with permission.)

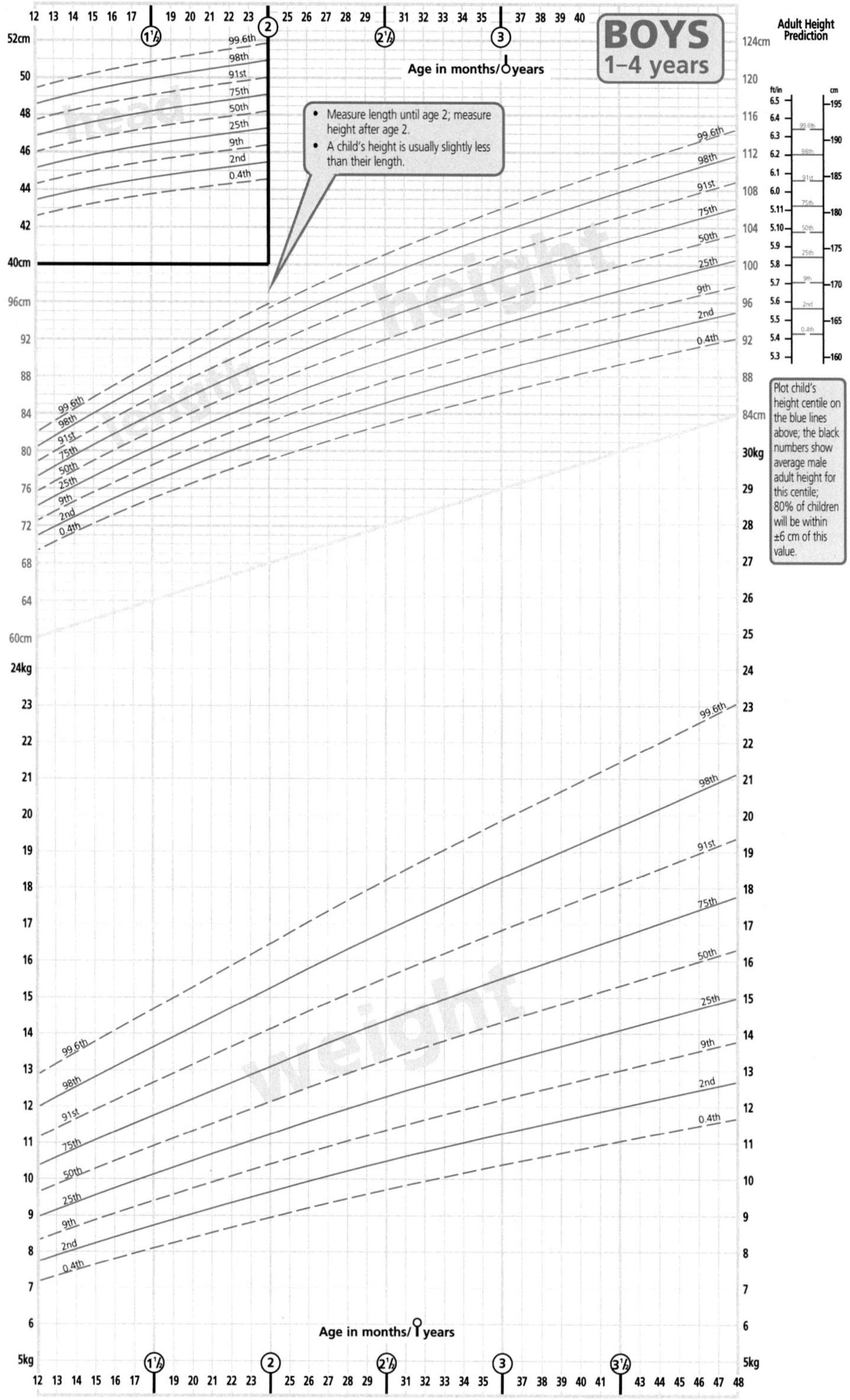

Data Recording

Birth Measurement
- Recording Date
- Weight
- Head Circumference
- Length/Height
- Location
- Health worker name

Measurement 2
- Recording Date
- Weight
- Head Circumference
- Length/Height
- Location
- Health worker name

Measurement 3
- Recording Date
- Weight
- Head Circumference
- Length/Height
- Location
- Health worker name

Measurement 4
- Recording Date
- Weight
- Head Circumference
- Length/Height
- Location
- Health worker name

Measurement 5
- Recording Date
- Weight
- Head Circumference
- Length/Height
- Location
- Health worker name

Measurement 6
- Recording Date
- Weight
- Head Circumference
- Length/Height
- Location
- Health worker name

Measurement 7
- Recording Date
- Weight
- Head Circumference
- Length/Height
- Location
- Health worker name

Measurement 8
- Recording Date
- Weight
- Head Circumference
- Length/Height
- Location
- Health worker name

Measurement 9
- Recording Date
- Weight
- Head Circumference
- Length/Height
- Location
- Health worker name

Measurement 10
- Recording Date
- Weight
- Head Circumference
- Length/Height
- Location
- Health worker name

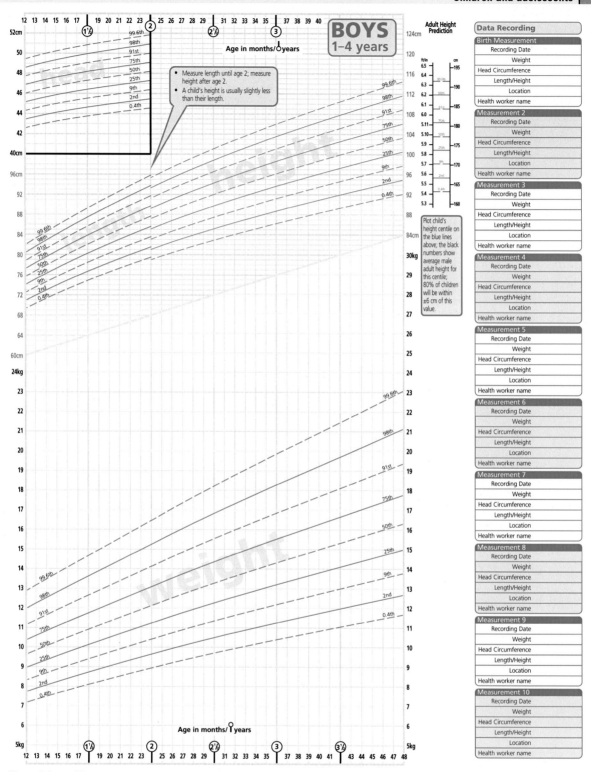

Figure 6.6, cont'd

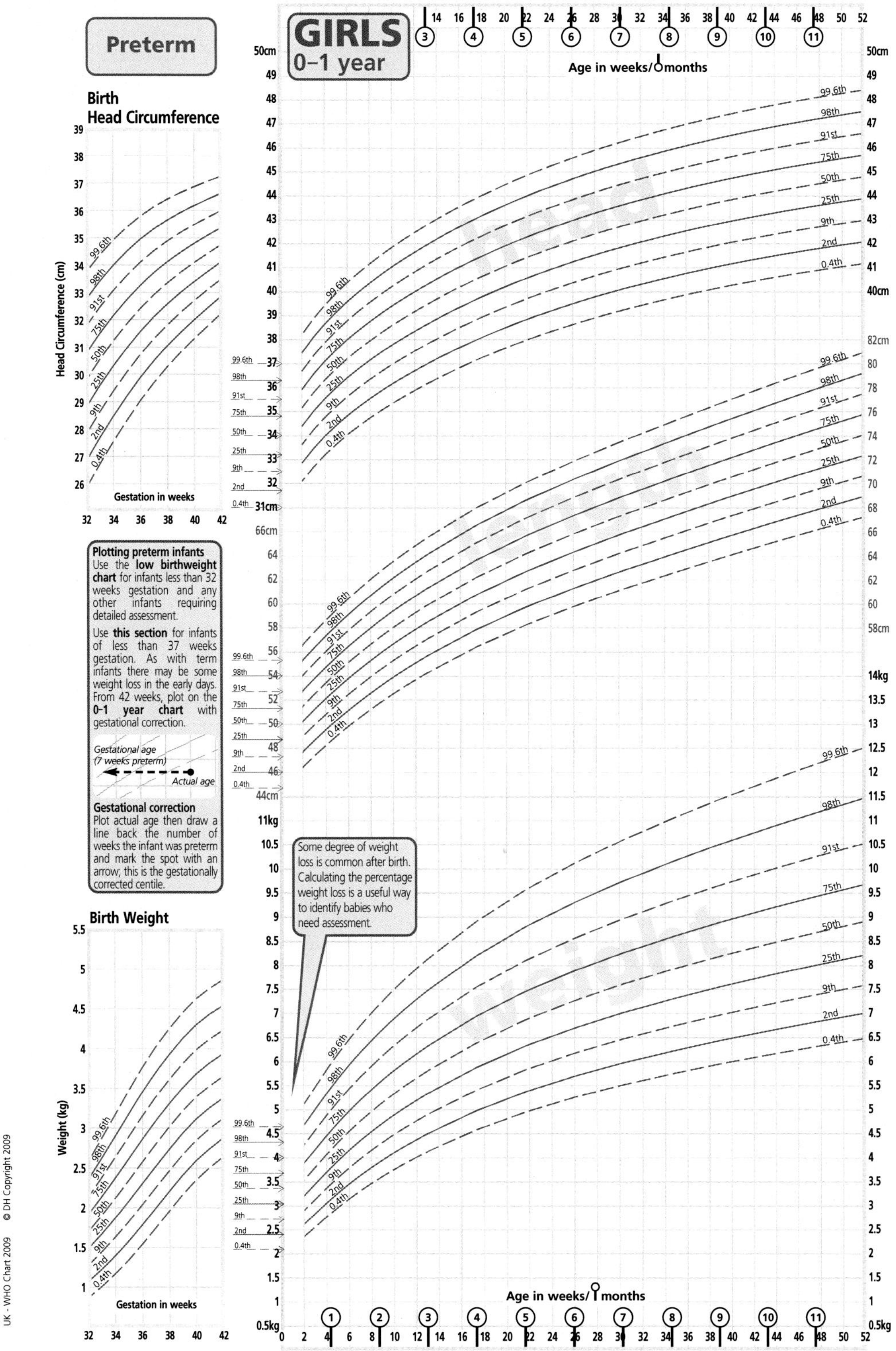

Figure 6.7 Height, weight and head circumference: girls aged 0-4 years. (© 2009 Department of Health. Charts developed by RCPCH/WHO/Department of Health. Reproduced with permission.)

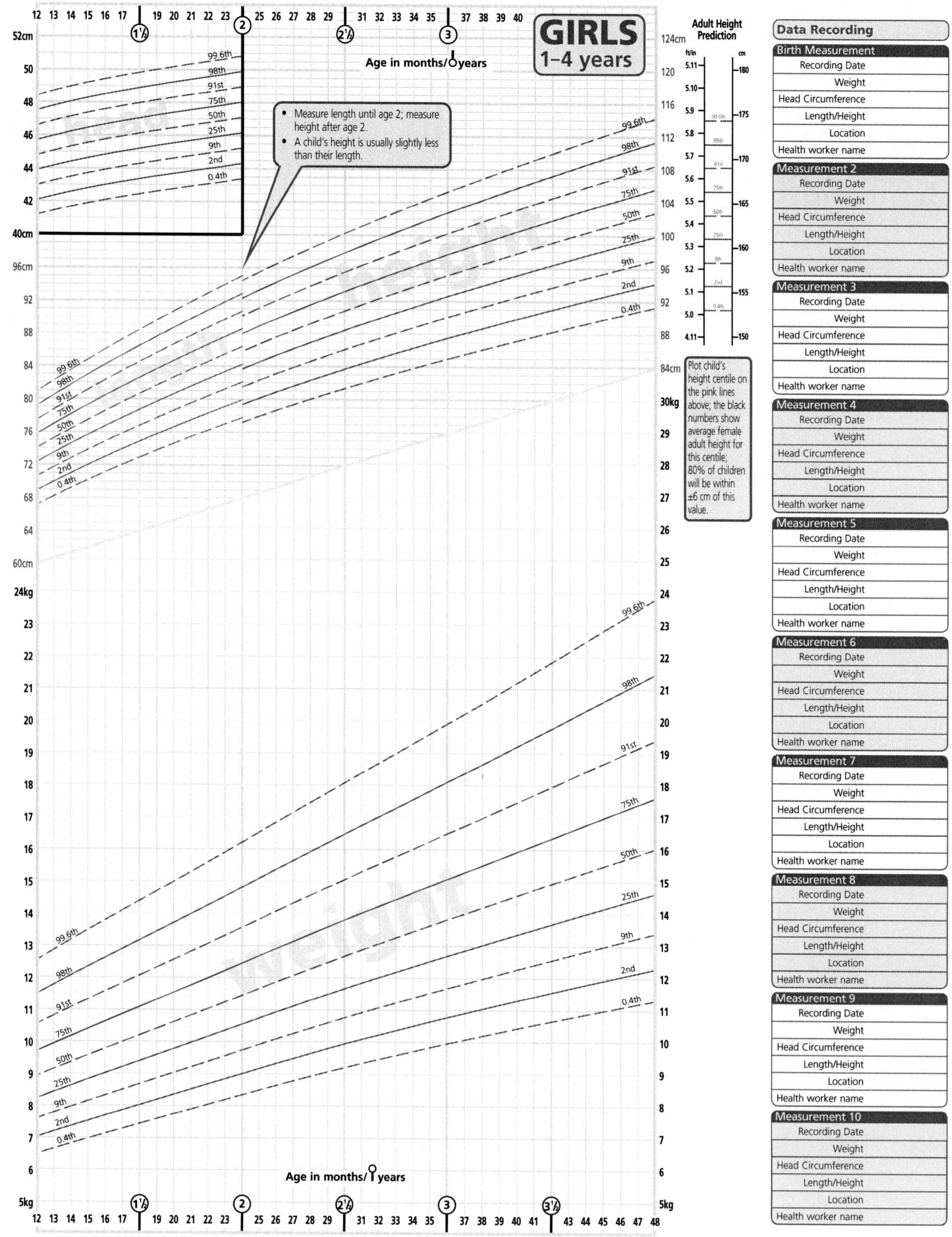

Figure 6.7, cont'd

pressure in children, but these are not always available. The blood pressure should be checked in all four limbs to exclude coarctation of the aorta when congenital heart disease is suspected. Normal values of blood pressure at different ages are listed in Table 6.3.

Temperature

The temperature should be taken if there is a suspicion of an underlying infection or if there is a report from the parent of the child having been hot. Fever is a very common finding in children and may be due to exercise and minor infections, as well as severe infections and other serious illnesses. Small infants often respond to infection with low temperatures.

The most common methods used in current practice are axillary measurements using chemical dot strips, or electronic devices giving tympanic membrane readings. These methods are the easiest to use but readings should be interpreted according to the method used. For example, axillary temperatures are 0.5-1.0°C below core body temperature. Rectal temperature is the best approximation to core temperature but is seldom, if ever, taken. Febrile convulsions may occur in children between 6 months and 6 years of age when the temperature rises rapidly to 39.5°C or above.

Stools

Never be afraid to see a dirty nappy or stool. This is part of the examination of a baby, and it is important to know the normal appearance of stools in childhood. The stools of a breastfed infant are usually loose and have yellow seeds in them with a characteristic odour. Infants fed on cows' milk formulas pass stools that are a paler yellow colour and more pasty. The character of the stool in older children is more variable than in adults. Some healthy children pass frequent, loose stools containing undigested vegetable matter – 'toddler's diarrhoea'. The stools of children with coeliac disease or cystic fibrosis are bulky, particularly smelly and quite characteristic.

Urine

Urine can be tested easily and reliably using modern reagent dipstick methods, but collection of the specimen can be difficult in the younger child. Specially designed collection bags can be attached to the perineum but these are prone to faecal contamination and should never be used to test for a urinary tract infection. This should be done using a 'clean catch' sample specimen into a sterile bowl or other container. Urine samples from children under the age of 2 years should always be double checked for infection in the laboratory. Modern techniques use flow cytometry and results will be available within a few hours. In a septic infant when a specimen is required urgently and an accurate diagnosis needed, the urine may be obtained by suprapubic aspiration of bladder urine, a procedure which is not too difficult in infants as the bladder sits relatively high in the pelvis.

Developmental screening examination

The developmental examination assesses the acquisition of learned skills. Development progresses from head to toe (a child needs to be able to hold his head up before being able to sit unsupported). Progress also requires the loss of primitive reflexes (see Box 6.8) at the appropriate age (a child cannot transfer objects between his hands if he still has a grasp reflex). Developmental progress can be affected by emotional difficulties, environment (e.g. lack of stimulation due to neglect) and illnesses.

All infants should have a simple developmental screening examination at regular intervals. Table 6.1 lists the important milestones. Detailed developmental assessment is a specialist subject, but it is important for all those who examine children to be able to carry out a simple developmental screening examination, and to be aware of all the basic milestones.

It is usual to consider development under four main headings:

1 Movement and posture.
2 Vision and manipulation.
3 Hearing and speech.
4 Social behaviour.

Screening for developmental delay involves testing the child's performance of a few skills in each of the four fields of development, and comparing the results with the average for children of the same age. The range of normal developmental progress is wide, and the milestones shown in Table 6.1 are those of an average normal child. Delay in all fields of development is more significant than delay in a single modality, and severe delay is more meaningful than slight delay. Allowance must always be made for those infants who were born prematurely, at least until the age of 2 years, by which time they should have caught up.

By 18 months of age, obvious deviations from normal development should become apparent. Beyond this age, developmental testing is more specialized, and is beyond the scope of this chapter. A baby who appears to have delayed development on screening will need further specialized assessment to establish the cause and subsequent management.

Techniques used

The same rules apply to the techniques used in developmental screening as to those of general physical examination. As with all parts of the examination, much more is learned by simply watching a child play and watching his reactions to the surroundings. Time has to be spent gaining the friendship of the child. For example, when offering a 10-month-old baby a small toy, watch to see how he grasps it and reacts to it. Let the baby play with the toys and bricks while sitting on the mother's lap, and if the child remains suspicious, get the mother to offer the various objects.

In the UK, routine developmental screening is usually carried out by a health visitor who is trained in developmental skills and who will refer to a doctor babies about whom there is any suspicion. There is always an assessment at 2 weeks (the newborn review), 6-8 weeks, 9-12 months and 2 and a half years of age. If at any point concerns are raised, then the child will be referred to a specialist community team for further assessment. Once at school age, the school nursing team supports their health and development.

Head control

By 4 months, babies can normally keep their head in line with the trunk when pulled from supine to sitting and, when held in the sitting position, will keep their head upright. Before this age, the head lags behind the trunk (Figs 6.8 and 6.9).

Testing vision

Much will be learned about a child's vision by observation. Note whether the child is looking around the room and at particular toys, or staring at nothing in particular, especially if there are random or nystagmoid eye movements, the latter suggesting that the child is unable to see. When he picks toys up, is accommodation normal? The routine examination of the eye has been dealt with in the first part of this chapter.

Checks of visual acuity are not easy in young babies. By 6 weeks of age, babies should be following their mother with their eyes, and by 6 months they should be able to follow a rolling ball at 3 metres. This is the basis of one method of visual testing at this age. The ability of the child to follow rolling balls of differing diameters gives an accurate assessment of visual acuity. At the 8-month check, the baby should be able to see and pick up an object the size of a raisin at arm's length. From the age of approximately 2 years, the Sheridan-Gardiner test is used. This is a simple comparison test, with the examiner indicating letters or familiar toys on a board and asking the child to indicate a similar object on a board held by the mother. The acuity is the ability of the child to pick out the smallest objects (see Ch. 20).

Testing hearing

In the past, it was usual to check the hearing for the first time between 6 and 8 months of age using the distraction test (Fig. 6.10). This can still be used as a screening method but has a large observer error and has largely been replaced by a national screening programme for all newborn babies, based on oto-acoustic emissions. This measures vibration reflected from the normally functioning cochlea. Additionally, brainstem auditory evoked potentials are used to assess the more vulnerable babies with the risk factors detailed in Box 6.11. This measures electrical activity in the baby's brain in response to sound. Audiometry and tympanometry are methods used in older children

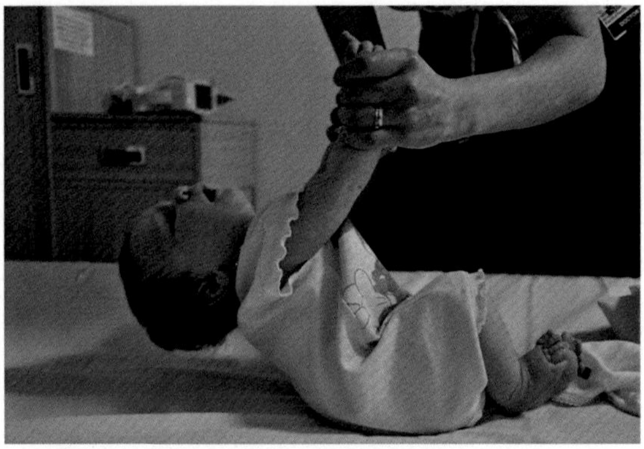

Figure 6.8 Head control at 6 weeks of age.

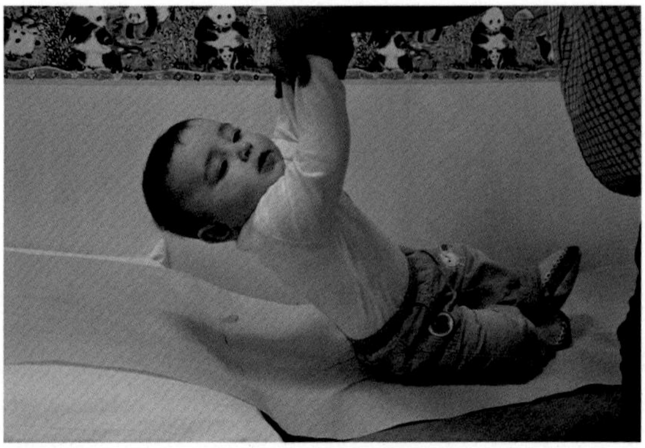

Figure 6.9 Head control at 4 months of age.

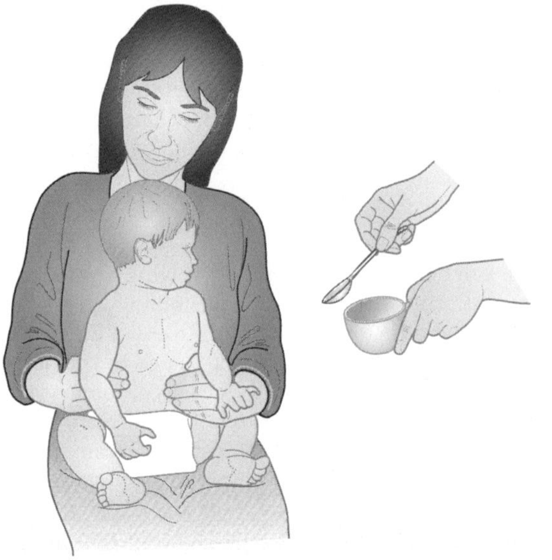

Figure 6.10 Testing hearing at 8 months: the child is held upright and forward on his parent's lap and distracted by an examiner in front of him. An examiner then presents sounds at 35 dB at different frequencies behind him and observes if the child turns towards the direction of the sound.

Box 6.11 Risk factors for hearing impairment

- Family history of deafness
- Congenital malformations (particularly ear, facial and spinal)
- Congenital infections (rubella, cytomegalovirus)
- Perinatal illness (gestation below 32 weeks at birth, low birth weight, jaundice)
- Postnatal illness (meningitis)

Box 6.12 The Apgar score

In each of the five categories, a score of 0, 1 or 2 is awarded, to give a maximum of 10. A score of 7-10 is good, 3-6 is moderate CNS depression and 0-2 is severe CNS depression:

- Heart rate
- Respiratory effort
- Muscle tone
- Reflex irritability
- Colour

Box 6.13 Checklist for examination of the newborn

- Weight, length, head circumference
- Alertness and wakefulness
- Skin colour: cyanosis, jaundice, birth marks
- Face: ears, dysmorphic features
- Head: skull and fontanelles
- Eyes: red reflex
- Mouth and tongue
- Neck: branchial cysts
- Limbs: digits and palmar creases, talipes
- Chest: murmurs
- Abdomen and umbilicus
- Perineum and genitalia
- Spine: sacral development
- Neurological assessment: posture, movements and tone, reflexes, the cry
- Hips

who can cooperate with the tests. They are useful for detecting middle-ear disease or glue ear which is more common in this group of children (see Ch. 21).

Examination of the newborn

The Apgar score (Box 6.12) is a combined cardiorespiratory and neurological score used immediately after birth and will be the first assessment a baby will have in his life. An Apgar score of 6 or less at 5 minutes after birth is associated with neurological deficit in about 10% of cases. Assessment of gestational age can be carried out clinically using the Dubowitz score (not detailed here). With more reliable dating scans, this method of assessment is rarely used now.

Every newborn baby is examined within the first 24 hours of life and again before the end of the first week. This is a very important examination designed to assess the general state of health and to detect congenital abnormalities (Box 6.13). It must always be interpreted in the context of the history of the pregnancy and birth and in the knowledge of any known history of inherited disorders in the family.

Weight is measured routinely at birth; the head circumference (occipitofrontal) may not be measured before 48 hours, to allow for moulding to subside. Note whether meconium, the dark green, sticky stool of the newborn baby, has been passed within the first 24 hours. If not, consider the possibility of Hirschsprung's disease (agangliosis of the rectum).

It provides reassurance to the baby's mother to conduct the examination in front of her. Ask the parent to undress the baby in a warm place and treat the baby gently, leaving the most unpleasant parts of the examination until last. Initially watch the baby, noting the state of awareness. If the baby is awake, seemingly looking around and not crying, take the opportunity to examine the nervous system at this point.

The skin

Note the colour of the skin. Peripheral cyanosis is a common finding in the normal newborn, but central cyanosis may indicate the presence of cardiac or respiratory disease. The head and neck may appear plethoric due to confluent petechial haemorrhages as a result of prolonged or obstructed labour. Jaundice is common after 48 hours in most preterm and some term babies and is considered physiological. Any baby jaundiced before 48 hours or after 7 days of age needs to be investigated. The commonest cause is haemolytic disease of the newborn due to ABO blood group incompatibility.

Look for birthmarks, which are either pigmented lesions or haemangiomata. Many babies have a collection of dilated capillaries on the upper eyelids and nape of the neck (sometimes called 'stork bites'), which fade after a few weeks. Some babies develop a crop of small erythematous papules with a surrounding red flare on the trunk during the first week (erythema toxicum or urticaria neonatorum) which look alarming to the first-time parent but do not have any pathological significance and usually fade after a few days. Superficial peeling of the skin, especially over the periphery, is common and is most apparent in post-term and some small-for-gestational-age babies. Milia are whitish pinhead spots concentrated mainly around the nose. They are sebaceous retention cysts and can be felt with the finger. They usually disappear within a month. Lanugo hair may cover the body, especially in preterm babies and some dark-haired babies. It usually disappears over the first 2 or 3 weeks. Mongolian blue spot is the name given to the normal dark blue areas of pigmentation commonly seen over the sacrum and buttocks or back of the legs in black and Asian babies, as well as some from the Mediterranean region.

The face

Look at the face for obvious dysmorphic features. Accessory auricles are small, pedunculated skin tags, usually just in front of the ears. Note any lip defect which may indicate an underlying cleft palate.

Once the superficial examination has been completed, more formal examination takes place. As for older babies, this should be regional rather than by systems, starting with the head and working down.

The head

Inspect and palpate the head. The caput succedaneum is an area of oedema of the scalp over the part of the head that presented during labour. It pits on pressure and is not fluctuant. A cephalhaematoma is a subperiosteal haematoma which appears a few days after birth as a large, cystic swelling limited to the area of one of the skull bones. It tends to resolve relatively slowly over a few months and may leave a calcified edge. It should be distinguished from a meningocoele which is usually midline and occipital and associated with an underlying bony defect. The anterior fontanelle varies in size considerably at birth.

The eyes

The eyes are best examined when they are open spontaneously. A bluish tinge to the sclera is usual. Even though newborn infants can see, eye movements tend to be random, often giving the impression of a transient squint. Subconjunctival haemorrhages show as dark red patches covering the sclera, sometimes ringing the cornea, and can occur following normal deliveries. Look for evidence of conjunctivitis which could be secondary to maternally transmitted infections, and check for other abnormalities as described earlier in this chapter. In particular, check for the red reflex, as its absence could indicate a major ophthalmic problem, such as a retinoblastoma or cataract.

The mouth and tongue

Make sure that there is no cleft of the palate, and note particularly whether the uvula is normal. A bifid uvula indicates a submucous cleft of the palate, which requires surgery. Epithelial pearls are small white areas, best seen on the hard palate. Occasionally teeth are present at birth. They are usually incisors, and can be green in colour. If loose, they are best removed. True macroglossia is seen in babies with congenital hypothyroidism, Beckwith's syndrome and in mucopolysaccharidosis. Children with trisomy 21 appear to have large tongues because their mouths are small, resulting in protrusion.

The neck

The neck of a newborn baby seems rather short and can be difficult to visualize. Rarely, cystic swellings are seen: dermoid cysts and thyroglossal cysts in the midline or branchial cysts just in front of the upper third of the sternomastoid muscle.

The limbs

Examine the limbs for abnormalities. Extra digits on the hand are not uncommon and may be familial but are rarer on the feet. Look for a single transverse palmar crease, which is classically seen in babies with trisomy 21, syndactyly (partial fusion of two or more digits) and clinodactyly (in-turning of the tip of the digit). Talipes equinovarus is a serious abnormality of the arrangement of the tarsal bones and requires an orthopaedic referral.

The chest

The general appearance and shape of the chest should be noticed. Breast enlargement with exudation of a milky fluid from the nipples is sometimes seen in newborn infants of either sex. This is due to transferred maternal hormones and disappears in a few days without causing problems. Listen for stridor which may be secondary to laryngomalacia or an anatomical obstructive defect. Listen also for grunting. Note the symmetry of the chest wall, the pattern of respiration and whether there is any in-drawing on inspiration. Neonatal breathing is predominantly abdominal and quiet. Palpation, percussion and auscultation are of almost no value in the neonate. Transient systolic murmurs are extremely common in the first few days and may reflect the closing ductus arteriosus or non-specific flow murmurs, as discussed earlier.

The abdomen

The abdomen of a newborn baby usually seems a little distended and moves with respiration. Slight divarication of the rectus muscles may occur, and this exaggerates this abdominal bulging. True abdominal wall defects may be present, such as exomphalos. The liver edge is palpable up to 2 cm below the costal margin, and the lower poles of both kidneys can be felt. A very enlarged bladder could suggest a neurological problem such as spina bifida. Check the umbilical stump: it should contain two arteries and one vein. A single umbilical artery is associated with an increased incidence of congenital abnormalities of the renal tract. Sometimes excess granulation tissue accumulates over the stump to form a small granuloma; this can be treated by local application of a silver nitrate stick.

The perineum and genitalia

Examine the perineum for hypospadias, hydroceles, inguinal hernias or undescended testicles. Look for patency of the anus: an imperforate anus is easily overlooked unless it is specifically checked for. While looking at the buttocks and anus, inspect for a sacral dimple. This is a blind-ending pit which is usually of no significance. Make sure that the back is straight and that there are no gross spinal lesions, especially spina bifida. Check female external genitalia for clitoral enlargement, which would suggest a virilizing condition such as congenital adrenal hyperplasia, and for labial fusion. It is not unusual for girls to have a mucus vaginal discharge and sometimes bleeding. This is the result of transferred maternal hormones and is usually transient. Make sure that the femoral pulses are palpable.

Neurological assessment

Combine a formal neurological examination with observation of the baby's behaviour. Spontaneous movement normally consists of alternating flexion and extension. Any marked difference between the two sides is abnormal.

The normal position of a newborn baby is one of flexion. If the baby is crying, look for any weakness or paralysis in the face, suggesting injury to the facial nerve, or any deficiency of arm movements suggesting injury to the brachial plexus which may have occurred during delivery (Erb's palsy). Note the limb and truncal tone. Assess power from resistance during undressing. Tendon jerks are difficult to elicit at this age but can be checked, using a finger rather than a tendon hammer.

Primitive reflexes

Primitive responses are present in the normal newborn infant and disappear at variable times in accordance with developmental progress (see Box 6.8). The absence of one or more of these reflexes in the newborn infant may indicate some abnormality of the brain, a local abnormality in the affected limb or a neuromuscular abnormality. The most well-known startle reflex is the Moro reflex (Box 6.8 and Fig. 6.11). As it is a startle reflex and may make the baby cry, it should be left until the end of the examination. A clearly unilateral response suggests some local abnormality, such as a fracture or brachial plexus injury in the arm on the side that does not respond. Persistence of primitive reflexes beyond the fourth month of life should alert you to the possibility of developmental delay.

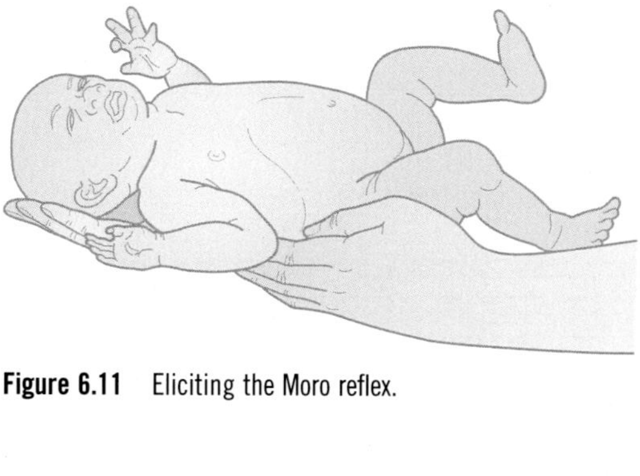

Figure 6.11 Eliciting the Moro reflex.

Examination of the hips

Examination of the hips is essential but should be left to the end because it can be uncomfortable for the baby. It is performed by carrying out two provocation manoeuvres to demonstrate that the femoral head can be dislocated and then lifted back into the acetabulum, as illustrated in Figs 6.12 and 6.13. It is usual to differentiate between a tendinous 'click' and the typical 'clunk' of a hip moving in and out of its socket. The latter is more a feeling than an actual noise. Asymmetry of skin creases on the upper posterior thigh and limitation of abduction are signs which do not develop until 6 weeks of age. If there is any doubt about possible congenital dislocation of the hip, ultrasound examination should be carried out. This is routine for all at-risk newborn babies (breech delivery, a family history of congenital dislocation of the hip (especially if female) and any baby in an unusual intrauterine position).

Having now completed the examination, the baby should be dressed and, as in every examination of

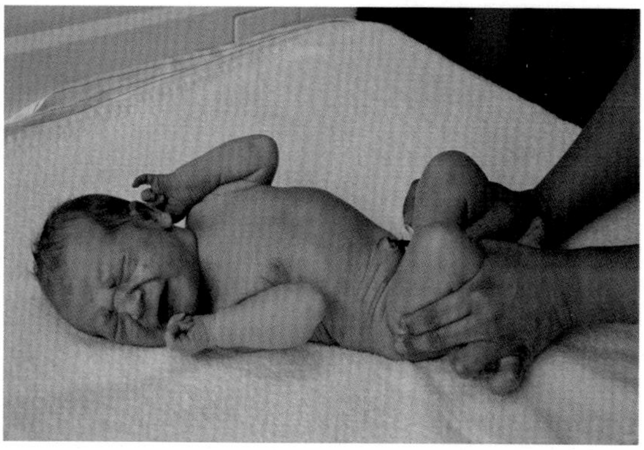

Figure 6.12 Stage 1 of the examination of the hips: the hips are flexed, rotated medially and pushed posteriorly. This will dislocate dislocatable hips.

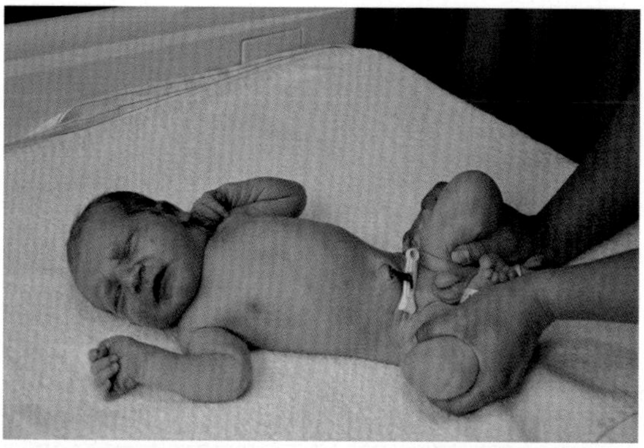

Figure 6.13 Stage 2 of the examination of the hips: the hips are abducted and a 'click' or a 'clunk' is felt for (see text). Note the position of the examiner's hands, with the thumbs on the medial aspect of the thigh and the fingers over the lateral trochanters.

children, your findings must be conveyed to the parents.

Summary

Throughout this chapter, emphasis has been placed on getting to know the child and treating him as gently as possible. Time has to be spent gaining the child's confidence. Students and doctors new to working with children have a natural anxiety when approaching young children, and it is only by playing and being with them that confidence in examining them will develop. Developing and practising the skills of the examination of children is a challenge that is immensely rewarding when completed satisfactorily.

Older people 7

Adam Feather

Introduction

'In the end, it's not the years in your life that count. It's the life in your years.'

Abraham Lincoln

At the turn of the twentieth century, there were 65 000 people in the UK aged 85 or older. By 2050, it is projected there will be more than 3 million. Old age is still associated with frailty, disability and loss of independence. The positive aspects of ageing, such as sagacity, maturity and experience, are too often neglected. One hopes that these commonly held negative beliefs about growing old will gradually disappear as the period between the average age of onset of disability in the old and the average age of death narrows and the elderly enjoy healthier lives.

Age is traditionally defined in terms of chronological age. Older people are considered in three distinct chronological groups: the young old (65-74), the old (75-84) and the very old (85+). However, older people are a very heterogeneous group and each old person should be respected as an individual, not merely classed according to chronological age. Frailty, disability and dependency are not synonymous with getting old. The accumulation of disability resulting from chronic disease and environmental insults must be separated from the process of merely getting older, i.e. senescence. People age at different rates, and it is the interplay of environmental, genetic and acquired pathological processes that determines an individual's biological age. Functional age takes into account the combination of a person's biological and chronological ages and, although difficult to define, this concept circumvents the negative implications of grouping individuals together because of arbitrary socioeconomic or statutory definitions, such as 'pensioner'. With an increasingly healthy and longer-lived population, these concepts will require redefinition according to functional ability.

Presentation of disease in older people

Two major factors influence the recognition of disease processes in older people:

1 Acceptance of ill health, with delay in seeking help.
2 Atypical presentation of disease processes.

The acceptance of ill health and disease as 'ageing', with its resultant disabilities, means that many older people expect to be frail, rarely complain and often seek help late. Coming to terms with some disability or change is necessary at all ages, and acceptance is part of survival. However, the tacit acceptance of inevitable deterioration – for example in vision, hearing, teeth and feet – may lead to treatable conditions being ignored and result in loss of independence. Table 7.1 illustrates what may be regarded as normal ageing and what is pathological.

The range of presentation of disease in old age is an essential element for the student and practitioner to comprehend. The term 'geriatric giants' (Box 7.1) refers to a set of symptoms and signs that occur in old age which may have as their cause many different disease processes. In normal day-to-day circumstances, ageing organs are able to maintain normal metabolic function. However, when major stressors are experienced, as in acute illness, functional capacity is exceeded and rapid clinical deterioration may occur. In the elderly patient, multiorgan failure may develop rapidly in the context of illness, especially infections. Another important concept is that of multiple comorbidities, which may be causally linked, although more typically they are not. Iatrogenic illness, most commonly due to polypharmacy, often exacerbates disability in the older person.

Recognition of the social presentation of disease is of major importance in older patients. The 'social admission' to hospital and the subsequent failure to cope with this upheaval, often termed 'acopia' (a made-up word), usually indicates a poor level of information gathering in the process of history taking, examination and investigation. The likelihood of the disease process leading to social decompensation, for example relatives leaving a person in the emergency department or the breakdown of the older person's level of physical and mental function during hospitalization or illness at home, can usually be predicted and hence often prevented, thereby avoiding secondary disability.

Proper diagnosis and management in older people requires the identification and treatment of amenable

Table 7.1 Normal ageing and changes in body systems

System	Normal ageing	Pathophysiological changes common in older age
Cardiovascular	Slight increase in heart size Normal stroke volume and left ventricular ejection fraction Exertional oxygen consumption declines 7.5-10% per decade; thus exercise tolerance is reduced	Ischaemic heart disease Heart failure Valvular heart disease Peripheral vascular disease Aneurysms
Respiratory	Vital capacity: 40% reduction by age 70 FEV_1 and FVC: 30% reduction by age 80 Progressive reduction in PEFR after age 30	Haemoptysis Chronic obstructive pulmonary disease (COPD) Lung fibrosis Lung cancers
Alimentary	Reduced and abnormal peristalsis: 'presby-oesophagus' Slower colonic transit Reduced absorption of some nutrients; reduced energy requirements	Weight loss Dysphagia Change in bowel habits Bleeding from the upper or lower GI tract
Hepatobiliary	Reduced hepatic mass and metabolic reserve but maintenance of normal function	Jaundice Deranged liver function tests, including abnormal clotting
Renal	Reduced GFR and numbers of functional tubules and glomeruli Reduced serum creatinine due to loss of muscle mass	Renal impairment with raised serum creatinine Haematuria
Genitourinary	Men: Reduced testosterone Normal FSH/LH 50% of men over 70 have 'abundant spermatogenesis' Women: Postmenopausal low oestradiol; raised FSH and LH Loss of female reproductive capability Atrophic vaginitis due to low oestrogen levels Loss of sexual interest may also occur, but this is complex and multifactorial	Erectile dysfunction Prostatic enlargement Bladder outflow tract symptoms Postmenopausal bleeding (PMB) Urinary incontinence Painful intercourse
Nervous system, including higher senses	High-frequency hearing loss Vision: close focusing declines from age 40 Distinguishing fine detail (reduced acuity) declines after 70 years Loss of muscle mass leads to decline in strength Reduced mental agility and minor loss of mental ability	Deafness, tinnitus and vertigo Glaucoma, macular degeneration Cataracts Dementia and delirium Hemiparesis, paraparesis Many other factors, including reduced distal sensation, vascular disease, poor balance
Endocrine	Pituitary dysfunction Abnormal thyroid function Abnormal pancreatic function Reduced adrenal response to stress	Hyponatraemia Hypothyroidism Impaired glucose tolerance and frank diabetes mellitus
Musculoskeletal	Increased body fat and loss of muscle mass (although this may be retarded with exercise)	Osteoarthritis and vertebral spondylosis Osteoporosis
Dermatological	Loss of collagen in the skin leads to thin, paparaceous skin Ecchymoses and senile purpura	Basal and squamous cell carcinoma Solar keratoses Malignant melanoma
Haematological and immune system	Loss of T-cell function with age may be associated with late-onset autoimmune disease Possible link between changes in immune system and: (a) age-related cancers (b) response to disease	Anaemia Myelodysplasia Haematological malignancies Chronic lymphatic lymphoma and myeloma

FEV_1, forced expiratory volume in 1 second; FSH, follicle stimulating hormone; FVC, forced vital capacity; GI, gastrointestinal; GFR, glomerular filtration rate; LH, luteinizing hormone; PEFR, peak expiratory flow rate.

Box 7.1 The 'geriatric giants': major clinical syndromes that may result from any disease process

- Immobility, instability/falls
- Incontinence
- Intellectual impairment/confusion
- Pressure ulcers
- Impaired senses: vision, hearing, speech and language

clinical problems and recognition of the special needs and the specific clinical presentations of older people. Thus, social aspects of care may be as important as the disease process itself. Understanding this encourages a patient-centred multidisciplinary team approach. Caring for older people requires clinical acumen and much skill. Geriatricians not only recognize diseases and their presentations in older people but perhaps equally importantly act as their patients' advocate in all areas of healthcare.

Box 7.2 History taking: points to note

- The introduction – observation as they enter; greeting
- Cadence and interest
- Position and comfort of patient
- Vision, hearing, cognition
- Environment
- Autonomy and respect
- Use of multiple sources of information
- Interview versus interrogation

Box 7.3 Observations during the introduction

- Can the patient see and hear you?
- Is behaviour normal?
- Is language normal?
- Does the patient understand your role as a doctor?
- Is the patient at ease, or in pain?
- Is there evidence of support from family or friends?

History

Taking a good history is always essential but requires particular sensitivity in the elderly. Respect for autonomy should always be afforded, just as for the young. 'Don't talk about patients, talk with them', especially when dealing with carers. Negotiate how much information the patient would like to share with carers when giving investigation results or trying to obtain corroborative information. Avoid being judgemental and paternalistic. The grey-haired are not necessarily disabled or confused! Even severely physically disabled people, no matter what their age, may have the brightest minds.

There are several universal practical points in the way the history is approached which are particularly important when taking a history from an older patient (Box 7.2). The first contact is extremely important (Box 7.3). Eye contact, a greeting, an outstretched hand (expecting a returned handshake), your name and the purpose of the meeting are all that are required to begin with. These relatively simple gestures can provide a wealth of information in the first few minutes. Depressed and very anxious patients may avoid eye contact. The handshake is often revealing. Some patients with dementia may not respond, not recognizing the meaning of the social gesture. Frightened older patients may continue to clutch one's hand. Giving your name and purpose puts people at ease and can also be used later to assess short-term memory. Ask the person 'What is your name?' Be alert for hearing impairment. The reply will indicate how a person wishes to be addressed; alternatively, the patient may be specifically asked this.

The environment should be changed to suit the individual patient, particularly if he is in a wheelchair, has multiple carers or is deaf. Ensure the patient puts on any spectacles or hearing aid. If he is hearing impaired, try to sit in a well-lit area to aid lip reading. Hearing impairment is such a common problem that any setting where older people are seen regularly should have a communication aid available. Talking at the bedside in a busy environment is accepted practice, but be sure the patient is really at ease, especially if any delicate or personal issues need to be discussed. Drawing the bed curtains offers some privacy and dignity to the patient but does not ensure privacy.

The cadence of the history may be slower than with younger people. Try to avoid interrupting the patient. There may be multiple medical and social issues, and it is important to let patients tell the story in their own way, as they will often prioritize issues. Learning to interrupt politely and redirect the conversation is a necessary but difficult skill to learn. Only when the patient has given consent should you attempt to corroborate information with relatives or carers.

The social history and social networks

The social history has extra significance in older people. Routine questions regarding occupation, smoking and alcohol are often forgotten but should provide a familiar stepping-stone to discussing the patient's home, how he is managing and what support he has. Find out the kind of home he lives in, the number of internal and external stairs, where the toilet and bathroom are situated, and who does the cooking, shopping and cleaning. Remember that most older people, including many of those with severe functional impairment, live in private households. Many are dependent to a greater or lesser extent upon friends and relations who contribute to their social networks, whether informally or formally.

Box 7.4 Social networks

Informal

- Family, friends and neighbours: available, concerned and committed, familiar, flexible

Formal

- Financial entitlements: pension and other income
- Statutory services: healthcare and social services
- Voluntary services: church and charity

No assessment of an older person with even a slight disability is complete without a description of the people who are available to help. The informal network of support consists of both direct and extended family and friends and neighbours (Box 7.4). This network is usually limited in size but often has a long history of contact. Although perhaps less skilled than a formal network, it has the great advantage of being flexible, familiar and continuous. The formal network consists of any basic financial entitlements, such as pensions, statutory agencies and in the UK, the NHS, which includes a community multidisciplinary team, and the local social services, e.g. home care, meals-on-wheels and day care facilities. Local availability of these organizations will vary. Finally, voluntary organizations, religious authorities and other organizations can provide valuable help.

Activities of daily living

An enquiry about activities of daily living (ADL) provides useful information in patients with multiple disabilities and health problems (see Table 7.2) and informs the planning of treatment and future care. In general, patients who can dress, get about outdoors, are continent, can do their own housework and cooking and manage their own pension do not require much immediate enquiry other than about their presenting problem. Among the old and the very old, such patients are the exception. If a daily living task cannot be carried out, a detailed enquiry focusing on the reason for this must be made.

It is useful to obtain a 'premorbid' picture of the patient's ADLs. This provides a rough goal for the outcome of treatment. A patient who previously had limited functional abilities and needed a lot of help to remain independent is unlikely to return to an independent lifestyle after a serious illness. One cannot assume that an older person was free from disability before the onset of an acute illness, and a corroborative history of premorbid ability is essential in planning future needs.

Drug history

Older people are prescribed more medication than any other age group. A treatment history checklist is useful when enquiring about current and past medications (Box 7.5). This is applicable to any patient with

Table 7.2 The Barthel ADL Index (total score 20)

Item	Categories
Bowels	0 = incontinent (or needs to be given an enema) 1 = occasional accident (once per week) 2 = continent
Bladder	0 = incontinent/catheterized, unable to manage 1 = occasional accident (max once every 24 h) 2 = continent (for over 7 days)
Grooming	0 = needs help with personal care 1 = independent face/hair/teeth/shaving (implements provided)
Toilet use	0 = dependent 1 = needs some help but can do something alone 2 = independent (on and off, dressing, wiping)
Feeding	0 = unable 1 = needs help cutting, spreading butter, etc. 2 = independent (food provided in reach)
Transfer	0 = unable – no sitting balance 1 = major help (one or two people, physical), can sit 2 = minor help (verbal or physical) 3 = independent
Mobility	0 = immobile 1 = wheelchair independent (includes corners) 2 = walks with help of one (verbal/physical) 3 = independent (may use any aid, e.g. stick)
Dressing	0 = dependent 1 = needs help, does about half unaided 2 = independent, includes buttons, zips, shoes
Stairs	0 = unable 1 = needs help (verbal, physical), carrying aid 2 = independent
Bathing	0 = dependent 1 = independent (may use shower)

The Barthel Index should be used as a record of what a patient does, not as a record of what he was able to do previously. The main aim is to establish the degree of independence from any help, physical or verbal, however minor and for whatever reason. The need for supervision means the patient is not independent. Performance over the preceding 24-48 hours is important, but longer periods are relevant. A patient's performance should be established using the best available evidence. Ask the patient or carer, but also observe what the patient can do. Direct testing is not needed. Unconscious patients score 0 throughout. Middle categories imply that the patient supplies over 50% effort. Use of aids to be independent is allowed.

Box 7.5 Areas to cover in a treatment history

- Current medications
- Previous hospital and family doctor medications
- Treatment from 'alternative' practitioners
- Self-medication
- Past bad experiences with medicines
- Other non-drug treatments
- Medicines kept in the home
- Compliance and help: dosette box; nurses; carers

chronic illness or multiple comorbidities. Many patients do not take all (or even any) of their prescribed medications. Checking dates on bottles, and a tablet count, is a rough guide to compliance. Medicine cabinets often contain old medications kept for use in the event of future problems – patients will sometimes change a new medication for an older, trusted remedy without telling the doctor. Compliance may be improved by the use of dosette boxes or by carers giving the patient his medications. The local pharmacist and GP will also be useful contacts when checking adherence to a treatment regimen.

Review of systems

The systems enquiry used for younger patients may produce spurious symptoms, many of which are not immediately relevant. However, do not be too hasty to dismiss them. If they are a concern to the patient, they may be important to your diagnostic search. The traditional review of systems may also be used as a 'medical sieve' when there are multiple, seemingly unconnected symptoms. In patients with cognitive impairment or in the acutely unwell, it may be necessary to check key points in the history from collateral sources. Always obtain all the old case notes. After obtaining permission from the patient, if this is possible, talk to a close relative or friend. The telephone can be a vital piece of equipment for history taking with disabled older patients. Ensure that any information you obtain is based on recent contact with the patient and is not anecdotal and several years out of date. Always try to check with the patient that the information is reliable.

Examination

General

Examination starts at the first contact and continues throughout the consultation. Useful information may be gathered at any point in your assessment, particularly with regard to functional abilities and cognition. The examination of an older person should be thorough, appropriate and respectful but may be limited by the patient's disability or cognitive impairment or by lack of appropriate privacy. Be guided by the principle of 'appropriateness and need'. For example, a frail, severely disabled or cognitively impaired patient will find it very difficult to cooperate with a formal neurological assessment and will tire rapidly. The examination thus becomes impossible, invalid and inappropriate. Likewise, a digital rectal examination may normally be considered part of a comprehensive examination but may simply be inappropriate or impossible in such patients. The answer to the question 'How will this part of the examination contribute to the management of this patient?' should then direct further assessment. However, disability and cognitive impairment should not be used as an excuse for not performing a complete assessment. Older people may present many years after they last visited a doctor. The examination should therefore include screening tests such as body weight, urinalysis, breast examination and digital rectal examination, including assessment of the prostate. Remember, the patient has the right to refuse these seemingly irrelevant examinations, and full explanations are needed.

Where appropriate, ask the patient to undress himself. Consider whether he can reach his feet and manage buttons. Can he get on to the examination couch unaided? If the patient does have obvious weakness or disability, help him to undress, making sure there are grab rails around the couch or bed, the height of which should be adjustable, or there is a step provided for the patient to get on and off. Once the patient is undressed, make sure comfort and dignity are preserved. If the patient is agitated or if you are intending an invasive examination, a nurse must be present to assist.

Special considerations

Skin

Wrinkles are mainly due to past exposure to ultraviolet light and hence are not usually seen in covered areas. The skin of the elderly bruises easily (senile purpura); some people have skin like transparent tissue paper, described as paparaceous, especially on the backs of the hands and the forearms (Figs 7.1 and 7.2). The skin around the eyes may show yellow plaques – Dubreuilh's elastoma. Some solar-induced changes to be aware of include keratoacanthoma, basal cell carcinoma, squamous cell carcinoma and malignant melanoma. The most common skin lesion noted is the small red Campbell de Morgan spot, a benign lesion seen most often on the trunk and abdomen.

Leg ulcers resistant to healing are common in old age: 50% are due to venous stasis (Fig. 7.3), 10% to arterial disease and 30-40% are of mixed origin.

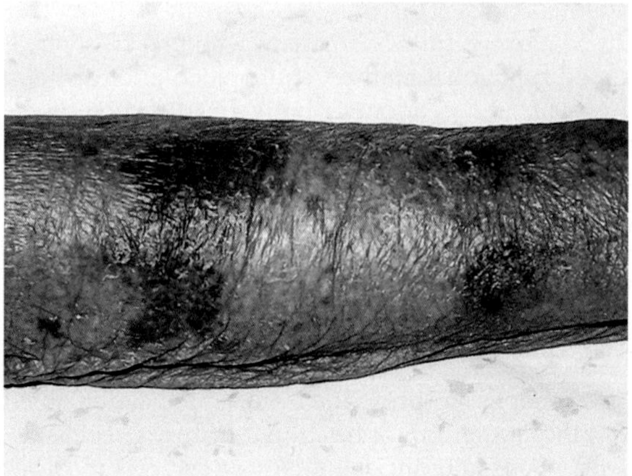

Figure 7.1 Transparent 'paparaceous' skin and senile purpura.

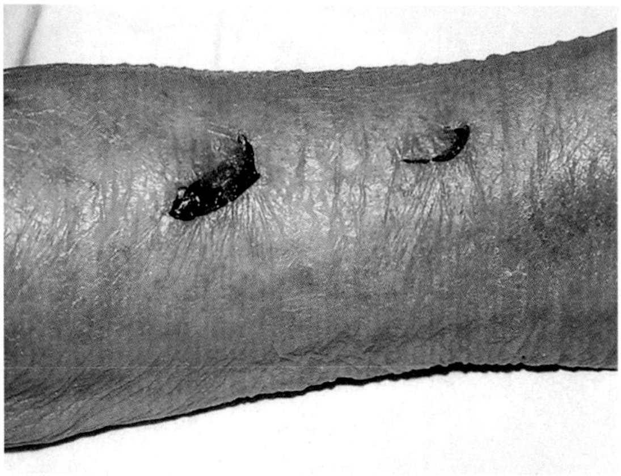

Figure 7.2 Transparent 'paparaceous' skin. The surface has been broken by trivial trauma.

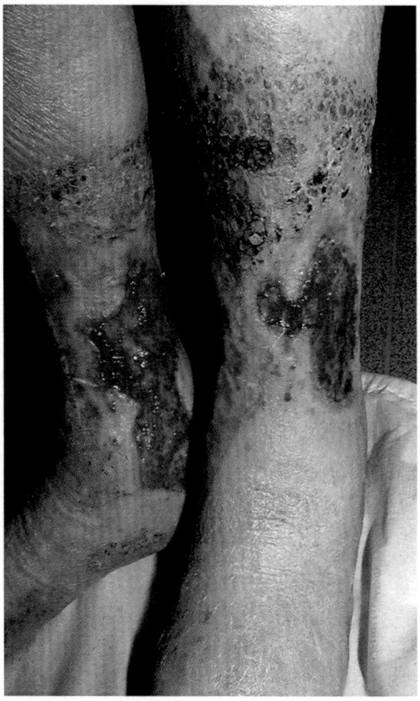

Figure 7.3 Leg ulcers.

Examination should include sensory (neuropathic ulcers) and vascular (ischaemia and varicose veins) examinations of the lower limbs. Measure the ankle and brachial blood pressures using a Doppler meter and sphygmomanometer cuff, the Doppler meter being used instead of a stethoscope at the feet. The ankle–brachial pressure index (ABPI) is calculated using the formula:

$$\text{ABPI} = \frac{\text{Ankle systolic pressure}}{\text{Brachial systolic pressure}}$$

An ABPI of 1.0 is normal; an ABPI below 1.0 may indicate arterial disease. An ABPI <0.8 indicates compromised distal circulation, and so pressure bandaging for leg ulceration should be avoided.

Check cutaneous pressure areas, especially the heels, hips and sacrum, for signs of skin breakdown (pressure or decubitus ulcers).

Cardiovascular system

Cardiovascular examination in older patients is no different from that in younger adults, but there are a number of important factors to take into account. Bradyarrhythmias and tachyarrhythmias are common in sick, older patients and may lead to cardiovascular collapse despite similar rates being well tolerated in the young. The increase in heart rate in response to stress (e.g. exercise, illness or pyrexia) is reduced in advanced old age, and this may be exacerbated by medications such as β-blockers and other antiarrhythmics.

A lying and standing (or sitting) blood pressure is extremely useful, but may not be obtainable in the more disabled patient. Postural hypotension, defined as a drop in systolic blood pressure of more than 20 mmHg on standing, is a considerable cause of morbidity in old age, often caused or exacerbated by medications. The sitting or standing blood pressure should be measured immediately prior to and then 1, 3 and 5 minutes after changing position. Age-related structural and functional changes in the cardiovascular system account for a slight increase in mean blood pressure with increasing age, although adult hypertensive guidelines should still be applied.

Heart valves, especially the aortic valve, can become less mobile, exacerbated by calcification. This is known as aortic sclerosis and is characterized by a non-radiating ejection systolic murmur, heard loudest in the aortic area. Degeneration and calcification of the mitral valve can result in either apical ejection murmurs or the more common pansystolic mitral regurgitant murmur (see Ch. 11).

Arterial abnormalities such as an aortic aneurysm, arterial bruits and evidence of peripheral vascular disease should be sought. Palpation of the pulses can be difficult because of atheroma or oedema and, in the lower limbs, Doppler measurement (see above) may be necessary to assess the peripheral circulation. Assessment of retinal vessels for signs of disease, as in hypertension and diabetes, can prove difficult in old people owing to the frequent presence of cataracts.

Respiratory system

Kyphosis, resulting from intervertebral disc degeneration and osteoporosis, and calcification of the costal cartilages make the chest wall more rigid and less expansible. A reduction in pulmonary elasticity with age may be responsible for some hyperinflation on a chest radiograph, but this is principally due to pathological hyperexpansion associated with chronic obstructive pulmonary disease (COPD). Generally, the physical signs of respiratory system disease are the same in the old as in the younger patient.

Measurements of peak expiratory flow rate (PEFR) and vital capacity (VC) are reduced (see Table 7.1) but, despite these changes, normal oxygenation is maintained and the normal adult ranges for oxygen saturation should be used.

'All that crackles is not necessarily heart failure or pneumonia.' Coarse basal crackles caused by air trapping owing to loss of pulmonary elasticity can make the interpretation of breath sounds difficult. It is important to note their presence when the patient is well so that inappropriate therapy is not initiated if and when he becomes ill. In this situation, a chest radiograph is essential, regardless of the presence or absence of other signs and symptoms of cardiopulmonary disease. Common changes on the chest radiograph include calcification from old tuberculosis, calcification in chondral cartilages and major blood vessels, pleural calcification from past pneumonia and old rib fractures. Pleural effusions, cardiomegaly, areas of collapse and consolidation, interstitial changes and pleural thickening should not be accepted as normal at any age.

Gastrointestinal system

The older patient should be weighed at every visit. As in younger patients, nutritional assessment includes estimation of the body mass index (BMI): weight (kg)/height (m^2). Because of osteoporotic vertebral collapse and other age-related changes, height may reduce in the old and so trends in weight are a more useful benchmark. If a true nutritional assessment is required, skin folds at the biceps, triceps, waist and thigh should also be measured.

The majority of older people are edentulous. If dentures are used, they should be worn during the examination so that problems with fit, for example poor speech or eating difficulties, can be corrected early. Oral candidiasis is common in the unwell older patient and is easily treatable. Leukoplakia appears as small white patches on the oral mucosa. It is associated with repeated mucosal trauma and may become malignant. Varicosities on the underside of the tongue are seen in about 40% of older people; their significance is unknown, but vitamin C deficiency has been implicated.

Abdominal examination may be limited by patients' orthopnoea, kyphoscoliosis or other disabilities. However, always try to perform an appropriate assessment. If abdominal examination is limited by such disabilities, the patient will also find it difficult to lie supine for investigations such as computed tomography (CT) scanning or colonoscopy. The indications for digital rectal examination are the same as for younger patients, but this may not be feasible or appropriate, particularly in the very disabled or frail older patient. Constipation severe enough to cause faecal impaction is not uncommon and can have serious consequences (Box 7.6). This is often iatrogenic but if of recent onset should be investigated appropriately.

Box 7.6 Faecal impaction may cause

- Faecal incontinence (ball-valve effect, with spurious diarrhoea)
- Intestinal obstruction
- Restlessness and agitation in the confused (but never itself causes confusion)
- Retention of urine
- Rectal bleeding

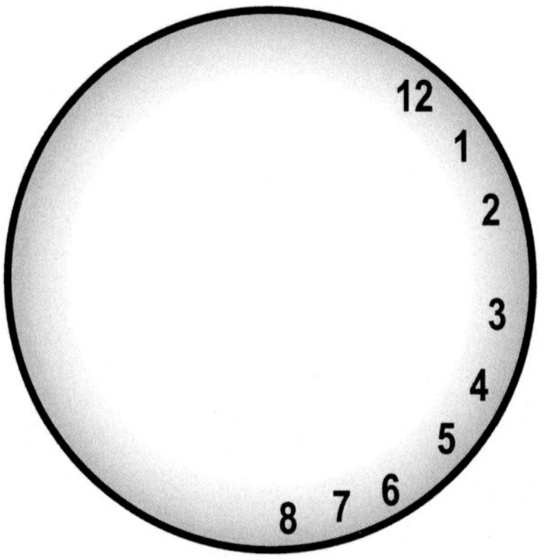

Figure 7.4 Clock-face drawing.

Nervous system

Central nervous system examination should routinely include an assessment of higher cortical function (language, perception and memory). If cognitive impairment is suspected, assess the mental state early in the interview before the patient tires and record the result in the clinical notes (see below). As well as the Abbreviated Mental Test Score (AMTS) and Mini-Mental State Examination (MMSE) (see below), use the 'clock test'. The patient is presented with a drawn circle, about 10-15 cm in diameter, and asked to fill in the numbers of a clock face (Fig. 7.4). Abnormalities may be due to visual impairment, agnosia (owing to right parietal lobe lesions) or cognitive impairment. This test is easily reproducible and less influenced by cultural and language problems than the AMTS or MMSE. A newer test, the Test Your Memory (TYM), has recently been introduced for patients attending diagnostic memory clinics or outpatient clinics to fill in prior to being seen by medical staff.

It is important to recognize difficulties with communication. Communication is a two-way process that involves understanding and comprehension as well as the production of appropriate speech. Communication problems can be considered in terms of:

- disorders of language (dysphasia)
- disorders of articulation (dyspraxia, dysarthria)
- disorders of voice (dysphonia) or of fluency (dysfluency).

Dysphasia, that is difficulty in encoding and decoding language, is usually associated with a left hemisphere lesion (see Ch. 16). Dyspraxia is difficulty initiating and carrying out voluntary movements, for example of the tongue, and hence can affect speech. Dysarthria has many causes, including local factors in the mouth and dentition, stroke, Parkinson's disease and other neurological disorders. Dysphonia, an abnormality of the quality of the voice (e.g. hoarseness), can be due to anxiety, vocal abuse, local disease of the larynx and pharynx or hypothyroidism. It is common after throat surgery and intubation. Dysfluency (stammer) is found in people of all ages.

The formal assessment of the peripheral nervous system by examining muscle bulk, tone, power, sensation and tendon reflexes is something the inexperienced clinician often finds difficult. In older, disabled patients, where judgements about normality and abnormality may be more subjective, this can be especially difficult. As with all clinical skills, such judgement is acquired only with practice. As part of this assessment, it is useful to ask the patient to hold his upper limbs fully extended and supinated, at shoulder height, with his eyes closed. Observe for pronator drift, which is a sign of pyramidal weakness. The reflexes should be examined in the normal manner. It is not uncommon for the ankle jerks to be diminished or hard to elicit in very old people but, as with all clinical signs, this should be viewed in the context of other findings and not in isolation.

It is essential to observe the walking or gait pattern wherever possible. This may reveal subtle evidence of hemiparesis, poor balance (Box 7.7) or the furniture-clutching gait of the patient with long-standing mobility problems. When observing the gait, always have someone walk alongside the patient to offer a helping hand in case he stumbles or falls. Occasionally patients claim that they are capable of carrying out activities when in reality they cannot. Always check the feet for chiropody problems (e.g. onychogryphosis), which cause a 'painful' or antalgic gait.

Vision and the eyes

Age-related loss of periorbital fat may give the eyes a sunken appearance; this may be severe enough to cause drooping of the upper lid (ptosis) and redundant skin at the lateral borders. The loss of fat can also cause the lower eyelid to curl in (entropion) and irritate the cornea, causing redness and watering (epiphora) or to fall outwards slightly (ectropion). A whitish rim around the iris (arcus senilis) is a zone of lipid deposition around the periphery of the cornea.

Visual acuity should be assessed and any loss of vision noted, together with the history of development of the visual disorder. Acute and chronic causes of loss of vision should be considered during the examination (Box 7.8). If the patient wears glasses, ask to see them. A state of disrepair may be an indication

Box 7.7 The causes of falls in elderly people

Premonitory

- Forerunner of acute, usually infectious, illness

Medication

- Multiple drug therapy
- Psychotropic drugs
- L-dopa
- Antihypertensives

Postural hypotension

- Drugs
- Alcohol
- Cardiac disease
- Autonomic failure/dysfunction

Neurological disease

- Neurocardiogenic syncope
- Multiple strokes
- Transient ischaemic attack
- Parkinson's disease
- Cerebellar disease
- Epilepsy
- Age-related loss of postural reflexes
- Spastic paraparesis (usually due to cervical spondylosis)
- Peripheral sensory or motor neuropathy
- Situational and postprandial syncope

Cardiovascular disease

- Carotid sinus syndrome
- Brady- and tachyarrhythmia: second-degree and complete heart block, sick sinus syndrome, atrial and ventricular tachyarrhythmias
- Structural abnormalities: valvular stenosis and regurgitation, hypertrophic obstructive cardiomyopathy
- Myocardial infarction and ischaemia

Musculoskeletal disease

- General muscle weakness (e.g. due to systemic malignancy)
- Muscular wasting due to arthritis
- Unstable knee joints
- Myopathy (e.g. osteomalacia)

Miscellaneous

- Drop attacks
- Hypoglycaemia
- Cervical spondylosis
- Alcohol
- Elder abuse (e.g. physical mistreatment)
- Poor vision
- Multisensory deprivation:
  - deafness
  - poor vision
  - labyrinthine disorder
  - peripheral neuropathy

Box 7.8 Common causes of acute and chronic loss of vision

Acute

- Retinal detachment
- Vascular (central retinal artery/vein thrombosis)
- Angle-closure glaucoma

Chronic

- Cataract
- Macular degeneration
- Open-angle glaucoma
- Diabetic retinopathy

of cognitive impairment and/or their underuse, thereby explaining falls and misinterpretation of the environment. The visual fields should always be assessed. It is common to see irregular, asymmetrical pupils due to previous iridotomy. Pupillary responses are normal in the well, older patient, but stroke and medication may cause abnormal size and responses. Abnormalities such as Horner's syndrome and palsies of the third, fourth and sixth cranial nerves are relatively common in the elderly, related to stroke and neoplastic disease. Funduscopy should be attempted wherever necessary but may be difficult when there are cataracts.

Hearing

Communication is often compromised in the older patient by hearing impairment. Patients are described as confused when in fact they are simply hearing impaired. If deafness is detected, the external ear should be inspected for wax. This should be softened with bicarbonate drops and then removed by gently syringing the external auditory canal. Hearing loss is often due to presbycusis an age-related degeneration of the cochlear hair cells. If a hearing aid is being worn, make sure it is switched on. This is easily tested by placing one's hand over the aid. If it is on, it will let out a shrill whistle. Communication is aided by raising your voice (but *not* by shouting), obtaining attention, sitting face to face, reducing background noise and speaking slowly and clearly. When the patient has severe hearing impairment, you may need to use written communication, provided his vision is good enough.

The 'geriatric giants'

Professor Bernard Isaacs drew attention to the four 'geriatric giants' (see Box 7.1) – immobility, instability (falls), incontinence and intellectual impairment – in the mid 1970s. Impaired senses (vision, hearing, speech and language), iatrogenesis and pressure ulcers are now commonly included. These are important causes of disability and illness but are not diagnoses in themselves so much as presentations of disease. In any older person presenting with one of the geriatric giants, the underlying causes must be considered.

Box 7.9 Abnormalities of gait

- The broad-based, unsteady gait of cerebellar ataxia
- The high-stepping, foot-slapping unsteady gait of sensory ataxia
- The apraxic gait, with rapid small steps like a slipping clutch, or with feet apparently glued to the floor
- The parkinsonian gait, with loss of postural reflexes, festination, a fixed posture, tremor, rigidity, hypokinesia of face and limbs, excess salivation and seborrhoea
- The gait of stroke with dragging of one leg
- The myopathic waddling gait due to weak proximal muscles, e.g. from osteomalacia
- The tentative antalgic or painful gait of patients with acute pain from e.g. arthritis, injury or ulceration

Immobility

Impaired mobility is one of the most common clinical presentations in the elderly. It is almost invariably multifactorial, and frequently the patient has several other medical problems. A careful history is necessary to elucidate the likely underlying issues and in separating cause from effect. The essential information is the onset of symptoms. Sudden immobility should be straightforward to diagnose, yet stroke and impacted subcapital femoral fractures are easily missed. A steady deterioration in mobility over several years implies a chronic process, for example Parkinson's disease or osteoarthrosis. A stepwise decline indicates a disease that has periods of exacerbation and remission, for example recurrent strokes or rheumatoid arthritis. Rapid deterioration from full mobility to total immobility over a few days indicates a serious acute medical problem. The most difficult patients are those in whom the disease process caused immobility a long time ago and the clinical picture has become clouded by the complications of immobility.

Within the bounds of common sense, the patient should be asked or helped to stand up and attempt a few steps, during which the gait can also be assessed (see above). Always have someone in close attendance in case of falls. The patient may be able to mobilize but unable to get out of a chair or bed unaided. Look for signs of distress on standing that may not have been mentioned by the patient. Tentative steps or clutching helpers may indicate loss of confidence or apraxia. Sometimes a diagnostic gait pattern is found (Box 7.9).

Instability/falls

It is said that 'young people trip, but old people fall'. With age, muscle strength is lost and postural reflexes become impaired. Falls are therefore common in old age, especially in the very old. Several causes may coexist (see Box 7.7). Even a single fall should lead to a detailed history and examination, and a corroborative history sought from spouse or friends. In a patient who was previously well, a search should be made for new acute illness. If none is present, the fall may be deemed 'accidental' due to environmental or mechanical factors, although this is a diagnosis of exclusion. Information about the pattern of any previous falls can be helpful: frequency, relationship to posture, activity or time of day, prewarning and residual symptoms following the fall, and any avoiding steps taken by the patient should be ascertained. The absence of any warning implies a sudden event, usually neurological or cardiovascular in nature. Sinister symptoms associated with falling include loss of consciousness (although, notoriously, this is poorly reported), focal neurological deficit, features of seizure, chest pain, palpitations or other cardiorespiratory symptoms. The most useful clinical investigation in older fallers is to watch them walking. Patients may also require 24-hour ambulatory electrocardiograph monitoring, a CT head scan and sometimes tilt-table testing.

Incontinence

Incontinence is an involuntary and inappropriate voiding or leakage of urine or faeces. Continence depends on intact sphincter mechanisms and the functional ability to toilet oneself or at least to acknowledge the need for toileting. Age-associated changes in the lower urinary tract predispose older people to incontinence but, despite these changes, most well older people are continent. Incontinence should not be regarded as a normal part of ageing and is more specifically associated with sphincteric damage, loss of neurological control mechanisms, especially in dementia or stroke, and with severe disability, chronic illness and frailty. Among the institutionalized older population, as many as 50% may suffer urinary and/or faecal incontinence.

When taking a history of urinary of faecal incontinence, try to differentiate between loss of ability to control voiding and failure to identify or reach an acceptable place. Find out how socially disabling the incontinence has become: many patients become isolated or afraid to go out because of the associated anxiety and potential embarrassment. Clinical examination should include rectal and vaginal examinations, assessment of the prostate gland, evaluation of the pelvic floor muscles and culture of a mid-stream specimen of urine. An incontinence chart kept for a few days may suggest a recognizable pattern of urinary and/or faecal incontinence. The specialist help of a continence adviser is often useful. Causes of urinary incontinence are shown in Box 7.10.

Faecal incontinence is relatively rare in well older men but is principally associated with severe chronic disability or cognitive impairment. In women, it is relatively more frequent but still rare. It may result from pelvic floor weakness. In both sexes, it may occur with carcinoma of the rectum, diverticular disease, laxative abuse and excess, faecal overloading with impaction and neurogenic bowel.

Box 7.10 Common causes of urinary incontinence in the older person

- Pelvic floor weakness
- Sphincter defects from injury in childbirth
- Pelvic floor neuropathy
- Urinary tract infections
- Bedridden state with immobility
- Dementia and delirium
- Neurological disease, e.g. stroke, myelopathy
- Autonomic neuropathy

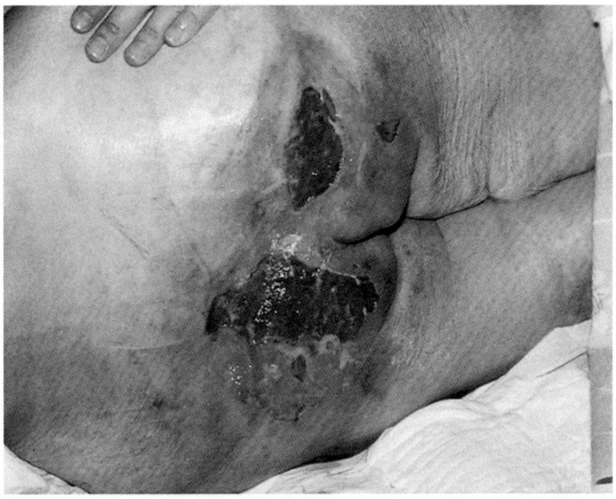

Figure 7.5 Superficial pressure ulcers.

Pressure ulcers

The mean capillary pressure in the skin of healthy young adults is approximately 25 mmHg. A bedridden patient or a person lying on the floor generates pressures in the skin in excess of 100 mmHg, especially over the sacrum, heels and greater trochanters (96% of 'decubitus' pressure ulcers occur below the level of the waist). Such pressures lead to occlusion of cutaneous blood vessels, causing the surrounding tissues, including the skin, to become hypoxic. In such circumstances, necrosis of the skin, adipose tissue and muscle may develop in as little as 4 hours. About 80% of pressure ulcers are superficial (Fig. 7.5). They occur mainly in dehydrated, immobile and incontinent patients exposed to sustained pressure. People with impaired sensation or with diabetes are especially vulnerable. Decubitus ulcers are always potentially preventable but will occur in any setting if skin care is disregarded. Any superficial ulcer will deepen if the pressure is not relieved. Deep ulcers (Fig. 7.6) are formed when localized high pressure applied to the skin cuts off a wedge-shaped area of tissue, usually adjacent to a bony prominence.

All at-risk patients should have active skin care management, including good nursing care and adequate hydration, started immediately when a new illness or injury occurs, whether at home or in hospital. All pressure area sites must be inspected at the first

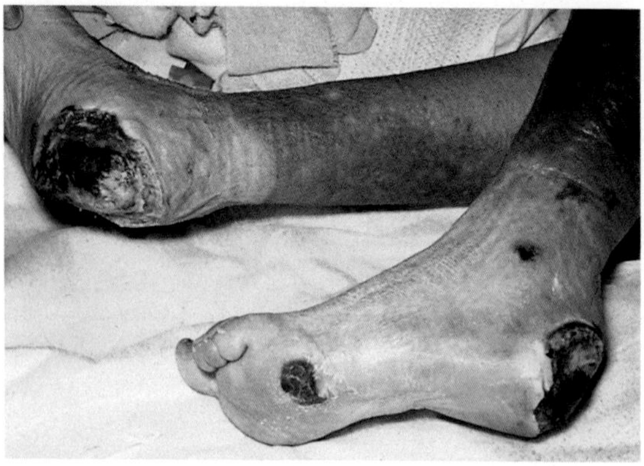

Figure 7.6 Deep pressure ulcers.

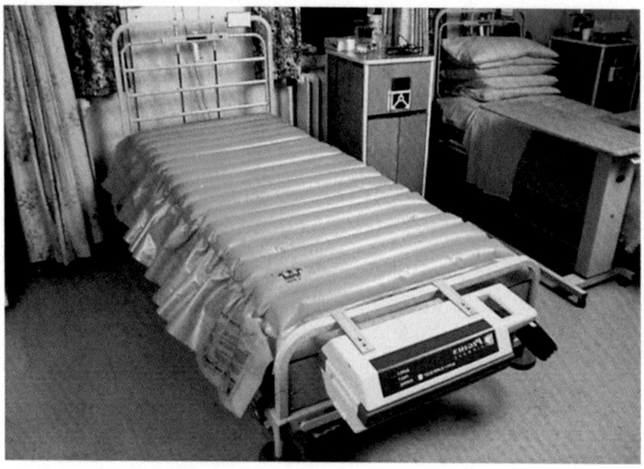

Figure 7.7 An alternating-pressure air mattress (APAM).

clinical assessment and again at regular intervals during the illness. An alternating-pressure air mattress (APAM) in which horizontal air cells (Fig. 7.7) inflate and deflate over a short cycle, constantly supporting the patient, provides periods of low pressure at all pressure sites, and good protection.

Confusion

Delirium is an acute confusional state that occurs in the context of a depressed level of consciousness. Delirium may occur in patients with underlying brain disease, such as dementia, often termed 'acute on chronic confusion' but more often occurs acutely in the previously unimpaired. Often there are several underlying causes, including pneumonia, toxic states and metabolic abnormalities, for example uncontrolled diabetes or hyponatraemia. Failure to recognize delirium and therefore to diagnose and treat the underlying condition can have fatal consequences. During any hospitalization, a person's level of cognitive functioning should be monitored periodically.

Dementia is a chronic confusional state associated with loss of higher mental function, for example judgemental capacity, memory and language, but unlike delirium it is not associated with altered consciousness. There are, however, reversible causes even of long-lasting confusion – for example drugs, depression and endocrine abnormalities – and appropriate diagnosis and treatment may produce improvement. Dementia is increasingly common in old age (10% above age 65 years, 20% above age 80 years) but is not a component of normal ageing. Regardless of age, a search for the cause is warranted. The differential diagnoses include benign senescent forgetfulness, amnestic syndromes and depression (pseudodementia).

Box 7.11 Abbreviated Mental Test (AMT): total score 10 (1 point for each item)

A score of 7 or less implies significant cognitive impairment and should be followed up, if persistent, with an MMSE* and further investigation

- Age
- Time (to nearest hour)
- Address for recall
- Year
- Where do you live (town or road)?
- Recognition of two people
- Date of birth (day and month)
- Year of start of First or Second World War
- Name of present monarch/prime minister
- Count backwards from 20 to 1

*MMSE was copyrighted by its author's university and has hence fallen out of day to day use. Commonly used in its place is the Montreal Cognitive Assessment (MOCA) and other cognitive assessment scores.

The confused older patient

'Patient confused, no history available' is a phrase that should never be used. It is crucial to establish whether the patient is oriented in place, time and person, and whether he is alert. A corroborative history from a friend or relative and thorough clinical examination will help decide whether the confusional state is acute or chronic. It is important to use a standard test of mental function (Box 7.11). Explain to the patient that you wish to test his memory. With experience, it is possible to check most of the items in the mental test score by working them into your introductory conversation. Hearing and speech impairments (such as nominal dysphasia) can make people appear very cognitively impaired but should be easy to recognize. Depressed patients tend to perform poorly on mental test scores. If a problem is detected with a simple test, proceed to a more in-depth assessment using the MMSE. Assessment of mental state is most valuable when applied serially over a period of time.

Management of suspected dementia should aim to confirm the diagnosis, to identify potentially reversible causes and to determine a management plan with the patient and carers. This is best achieved in a diagnostic memory clinic, where a multidisciplinary approach involving a geriatrician, psychiatrist, psychologist and nurse specialist may be taken. As with any other group of patients, examination and investigation should be appropriate and directed towards helping with the management plan.

Assessment of capacity

This is an important part of medical practice in general but particularly important in the field of elderly care medicine. Although similar principles apply in most countries, the following text refers specifically to the UK. Legally, competent adults (relatives or carers) are not able to make any decisions about the medical management or social care of another adult unless they have been made their legal representative through a lasting power of attorney (LPA) or are a court-of-protection appointed deputy. Similarly, cognitively impaired patients may be unable to make a valid and consistent decision. Such patients require assessment of their mental capacity when making important decisions about their health or social care. A person lacks capacity if he is deemed to have a temporary or permanent impairment of, or a disturbance in the functioning of, his mind or brain. The Mental Capacity Act (MCA; 2005) (see the Department of Health Web site for more information: http://www.dh.gov.uk/en/Publicationsandstatistics/Bulletins/theweek/Chiefexecutivebulletin/DH_4108436) defines a person as lacking capacity (i.e. someone who is unable to make a valid decision) if he is unable to:

- understand the information relevant to the decision
- retain that information
- use or weigh that information as part of the process of making the decision, or
- communicate their decision (whether by talking, sign language or any other means).

If one or more of the four criteria are not present, then the patient is deemed to lack capacity. Such patients require an advocate from family or friends (or an Independent Mental Capacity Advocate (IMCA) may be appointed). An IMCA advocates for the patient and supports the decision-making process, trying to ensure the patient's 'likely' wishes, feelings, beliefs and values are taken into account. However, IMCAs cannot consent for or deny access to treatment unless they have previous LPA (they must have evidence of this; verbal confirmation is not good enough) or the patient has a court-of-protection order in place.

When considering whether a patient retains mental capacity, one should also bear in mind the following:

- Is the patient consistent in his decision? – Often demented patients make different decisions each time they are asked a given question. Consistency is NOT part of the MCA definition but pragmatically becomes important if they keep changing their mind.
- Does the patient personalize the information to himself? This is not part of the MCA definition but important.
- Capacity is decision-specific; a patient may retain capacity around one decision and not around another; for example, they may retain capacity around the dangers of going home but not around receiving a therapeutic intervention such as major surgery.
- Do not assume that patients with a reduced score on the AMTS (especially around scores of 6-8/10) do not retain capacity.

When discussing 'acting in a person's best interest' (as a health or social care professional), the Act also encourages a dialogue with any parties who may be involved with the person's care or wellbeing. This is extremely important when negotiating with relatives and carers about medical and social care. In the Emergency Department you should ensure that several senior, experienced medical, nursing or therapy staff are involved in any decisions around a patient's mental capacity; such decisions should not be made in isolation.

Other issues

Ethnic elders

Ethnic minority elders form a small but significant proportion of the older population in many contemporary societies. Older ethnic populations may have a racial predisposition to certain conditions but often develop diseases similar to those of the indigenous population within one to two generations. Indeed, environmental excesses, such as the Western diet, alcohol and cigarettes, may contribute to an increased incidence of premature death compared to their own indigenous population. The availability of health services for this group is often inadequate and insensitive to their specific needs. Any healthcare professional must always try to understand and respect the cultural background of the patient and his family. Find out about the beliefs and cultural background of your patients – you will find it interesting as well as helpful in your work.

Inadequate care and elder abuse

There are many types of abuse and any older person can be a victim. About 5% of older people suffer abuse. The most vulnerable are female partners, those living with adult children, perhaps because of financial difficulties or unemployment, and older people in poorly run institutional care homes. In the domestic setting, abusers are often dependent on their victims for finance. They may themselves have health and financial problems, especially alcohol and psychological difficulties, and frequently their relationship has been dysfunctional for a long time. In institutions, inadequate staffing levels, poor staff training, repeated complaints, and poor client and environmental hygiene are all indicators of potential abuse.

Potential elder abuse should be considered if carers make frequent visits to doctors, are preoccupied with their own problems and often seem to indicate their inability to cope, perhaps using non-verbal cues. Marked changes in a carer's lifestyle (bereavement, unemployment, illness) may also precipitate abuse. Recognition of elder abuse is made more difficult by the physiological and the pathological changes that occur with ageing (e.g. senile purpura). However, abrasions, pressure ulcers and poor nutrition should raise the possibility of abuse. Assessment requires a history that includes open questions about the possibility of violent behaviour. Enquiry regarding the full social background is important, including a sympathetic description of the carer's role. A thorough physical examination should be made and the patient's mental state assessed and recorded. If abuse is suspected, expert help from senior colleagues, social services, psychiatrists or clinical psychologists may be necessary for recognition, disclosure and management. It may be necessary to involve the police. Elder abuse is a complex phenomenon which is only beginning to be recognized. We fail the most vulnerable people in our society, however, if we are not sufficiently aware of the problem.

Psychiatric assessment 8

Trevor Turner

Introduction

Psychiatry is the medical specialty that concerns itself with the diagnosis and management of mental illness. Many people, even fellow doctors, often feel confused about the distinction between psychiatry and other disciplines in which the prefix 'psych' appears, for example psychology and psychotherapy. The distinction is quite clear though, since psychiatry is practised by medically qualified practitioners who deal with diseases of the mind (i.e. psychiatrists are doctors), just as gastroenterology is concerned with diseases of the gut and cardiology with diseases of the heart. The proper practice of psychiatry involves an understanding of the normal workings of the mind and brain and a thorough knowledge of psychopathological manifestations of the mind and the behaviours that accrue when mental illness is present. It embraces therefore not only full medical training (and postgraduate clinical practice) but also a knowledge of psychology and personality structure and a wider understanding of sociology, culture and belief systems.

As in any medical specialty, the cornerstone of becoming a successful practitioner is clinical experience and the mastery of taking a detailed history and performing an examination of the mind, referred to as a mental state examination (MSE). It is also often essential to perform a general physical examination. History taking follows a similar structure to that adopted in any branch of medicine, with some additions and adaptations. The MSE is unique to psychiatry and involves learning a systematic way of observing and recording all aspects of how the patient behaves and appears in the consultation, what he says and how he says it.

Thus the clinical symptoms, signs and presentations of abnormal experience (often referred to as phenomena) are recorded in a systematic way, and this is the basis of the diagnosis. It is, therefore, crucial to understand how to perform the MSE properly and how to be rigorous and systematic in recording both normal ('no abnormality detected' – NAD) and abnormal phenomena, which point to a particular diagnosis. Gaining experience in this technique is vital to psychiatric expertise.

The process of history taking and examination should be seen as an exploration akin to detective work (literally, solving problems) during which items of evidence for the diagnosis are unearthed. Sometimes the evidence will be in the form of the patient's narrative (i.e. a particular constellation of symptoms) or particular themes in their thinking. Sometimes it is the way the patient talks – for example, a patient's speech can reveal thought disorder of the mind (a symptom of schizophrenia) – whereas at other times it may be the patient's own experience – for example third-person auditory hallucinations (see below). These are a hallmark of schizophrenia, whereas visual hallucinations are strongly suggestive of an organic brain disorder.

Psychiatric diagnoses are syndromal diagnoses (i.e. they are based on clusters of symptoms and overlap to a degree). There are very few clinical signs in psychiatry (for example, abnormal postures or overt thought block when the patient suddenly stops talking). There are also no confirmatory investigations such as blood tests or X-rays, but such investigations may be crucial to excluding organic conditions (e.g. hypothyroidism, brain tumour). If, after taking a history and performing an MSE the clinician suspects the patient has schizophrenia, it cannot be confirmed with a definitive blood test or piece of imaging. The diagnosis rests solely on eliciting the typical cluster of symptoms of schizophrenia, and observing the abnormalities of behaviour (not necessarily present), speech, thought and experience which are typically seen in the schizophrenia syndromes.

It is therefore clear that in psychiatry, the importance of meticulous history taking (and in particular obtaining a collateral history, since patients may not be able to give a clear account of themselves) as well as a detailed MSE is paramount. There is nothing else upon which to base a diagnosis, and diagnosis is the basis of appropriate treatment. It is also vital that the history and symptoms are accurately recorded, because the illness may have evolved in a patient who has been ill for some while. It can be vital to the diagnosis to know how the illness has evolved, the effects of treatment, and, for example, changes in insight (see below). Despite the lack of so-called 'objective' testing, trained psychiatrists are extremely reliable in their diagnoses (greater reliability for example than diagnoses of an acute abdomen), but it is a speciality that requires accumulated clinical experience as well as background knowledge.

The main purpose of this chapter is to teach the skill of taking a psychiatric history and performing an MSE in the context of the typical diagnostic presentations (e.g. depression, anxiety, schizophrenia) that are encountered.

History taking

As in all of medicine, the history if properly elicited should provide the basis for a diagnosis, which the clinical examination (including the MSE) is used to confirm and/or clarify. Furthermore, in psychiatry the history taking and MSE should begin the development of a therapeutic rapport with the patient upon which effective management rests. Possibly more than in any other specialty, there are steps to be taken even before starting to talk to a patient. The first step is to consider the context of the interview (emergency, routine, legal) and where it will take place. The second is to think about what background information is accessible and necessary, since a good referral letter from a GP can so outline the history that going onto the specialist part of psychiatric examination (the MSE, for example) can be expedited.

Context of the interview

There are important factors which will tend to be different in different settings, for example, outpatients, the emergency department, the medical or psychiatric ward, the home or even the street.

Patient factors

Is the patient aware of the referral? Is he expecting to see a psychiatrist? What does he think of seeing a psychiatrist? The assessment may be of a patient following an overdose or who has been brought in by the police under the Mental Health Act section, who may have no wish to engage in any kind of psychiatric assessment. A patient may have presented with what has been assumed to be a medical problem, and all too often a psychiatric referral may not even have been discussed with the patient beforehand. Clearly the approach to the interview in these situations will be very different compared to that of a patient voluntarily attending a psychiatric outpatient clinic, having sought specific help. It will require a careful and skilful engagement of the patient in the assessment. How successful this will be will determine the extent of the history taking that is possible.

Factors in the physical environment

Psychiatric assessment requires a suitable interview room, in terms of safety, privacy, and confidentiality. Quiet surroundings, in which a patient can be listened to and engaged with, are essential although not always possible.

Safety

The doctor should sit nearest the door and neither the patient nor any obstacles should block the doctor's ability to exit. There should be an alarm buzzer and someone available to respond to the alarm. In the emergency department where patients have been brought to hospital in a disturbed state, other safety measures may also be needed, for example checking for weapons and having a security presence or a chaperone.

Privacy

The patient should be interviewed in a quiet private space where he is not likely to be overheard by other patients and staff. Clearly there is a balance to be struck, and the need for police or security presence nearby may sometimes outweigh the privacy and confidentiality requirement. However, such situations are exceptional since most psychiatric consultations can be conducted privately and confidentially, although many people like to have a family member or friend with them as support, and this should be encouraged.

Collateral history

Psychiatry is unique in requiring more than the patient's account of problems. Previous medical or GP notes or information on the mental health record system provide valuable information. For example, in a patient with unexplained physical symptoms, a history of previous presentations with unexplained symptoms can point to a particular diagnosis (e.g. a somatoform disorder, in which patients experience a range of physical symptoms which have no physical basis but which cause them distress and anxiety).

It is also important to check for a history of previous violent behaviour, as the best predictor of future violence is previous violence. It is vital that any violent behaviour (to self, others or the environment) is recorded accurately in the notes and electronic recording systems.

As noted above, the other valuable source of information is talking to informants who know the patient well, for example partners or friends. This requires the patient's permission, and if the partner or friend is not accompanying him, then it may need to take place after the interview. In the inpatient setting it is appropriate to talk to other health professionals (e.g. nurses, social workers) who have been working with the patient.

The psychiatric history

Introduction

Introduce yourself, shake hands (if appropriate) and tell the patient clearly who you are, who has referred the patient to you, the purpose of the interview and how long it is likely to take. Obviously physical contact should be avoided with a patient who seems very fearful or likely to strike out. Sensitivity to a patient's body language helps to judge the most appropriate way in which to greet him. It is worth asking if he was even expecting to be seen and how he feels about this, reassuring him that you are a doctor, for example just like his GP.

Confidentiality and note keeping

Always inform patients that the conversation is confidential, but that information will be shared with other healthcare professionals as appropriate, for example a letter to the referring GP or to the physician or surgeon who has made a referral.

Where patients object to information sharing, be clear that some note keeping and communication is essential, but details of very sensitive issues can be avoided in letters. However, patients have to know that information cannot be withheld from others if it is likely to place them or others at risk.

Notes taken (whether written or typed) can be brief but should be an outline of the key features, while not intrusive to the flow of the interview. It is important to write some of the patient's statements verbatim to illustrate his state of mind, and this can provide evidence of the presence of certain symptoms with respect to the MSE and what aspects to focus on.

Interviewing a patient who does not speak English

Patients should always be offered an interpreter as they may feel more able and willing to discuss feelings in their own language. Try not to use family members as interpreters (except in emergencies where no alternative is available) as it raises confidentiality issues. Conducting an interview via an interpreter requires more time, and there are pitfalls. Sometimes patients may feel suspicious of someone from their own community and may fear that the information will not remain confidential. Some interpreters impose their own views and advice, and the interviewer should be alert for this. It is important to make clear that you, the clinician, need to hear just what the patient has been saying, not any elaboration or inappropriate summary.

Interviewing technique

As with any patient, aim for an open, empathic and non-judgemental approach and try to maintain non-threatening eye contact (for example, looking at the lower half of the face) as much as possible. Start with open questions, avoid loaded questions, encourage patients to tell their story in their own words and follow the approaches for general history taking detailed in Chapter 1. Another way of questioning is to use a normalising statement. This is employed when you are asking about symptoms or behaviours that the patient may find embarrassing or difficult to acknowledge. For example, you might say something like 'Sometimes when people have been feeling very depressed or have been under great stress, they may have odd experiences which they cannot explain. For example, they may hear or see things which are unusual – has anything like this happened to you?' Further examples of these are provided in the appropriate sections. Finish with a summary of what you have understood and check with the patient if you have missed anything that he feels is important.

Structure of the psychiatric history

This section details all the areas of history taking which need to be covered in a full psychiatric history. There may be situations where, in the initial assessment, they cannot all be covered, usually because the patient is too disturbed to engage with the interview process or too disorganised in his thoughts to produce comprehensible information. In these situations, the omitted information can be gathered when the patient is somewhat better. Sometimes patients do not (understandably) feel comfortable sharing all aspects of their personal background at a first meeting with a stranger. The interviewer needs to be sensitive to this and to check with the patient as to how he feels and whether he is comfortable discussing a particular topic.

Order of sections

The order in which the sections of the history are covered is suggested in Box 8.1 and followed in the text. However, if it is impossible to complete the interview on a single occasion, it is more useful to have found out about previous psychiatric illness, current contact with mental health services, medication and important medical conditions than it is to know the patient's father's occupation or career details.

It can be useful to present the information obtained as a life chart which illustrates, in adjacent columns, years, patient's age, social history, family history, relationship/psychosexual history, medical history and psychiatric history as a way of illustrating possible predisposing factors, precipitating factors and maintaining factors in a patient's illness.

Presenting complaint

Start by establishing the main problem for which the patient is seeking help. In psychiatry, there will be situations in which the patient does not have any complaints and denies any problems ('you tell me Doc!'). In this situation, the details of the presentation and behaviour, as reported by others, as well as the concerns of others (especially the family) should be

Box 8.1 Suggested order for psychiatric history

- Presenting complaint (C/O)
- History of presenting complaint (HPC)
- Previous medical history – psychiatric and physical (PMH)
- Current medication/treatment
- Family history
- Personal history
  - Childhood
  - Schooling
  - Occupation
  - Psychosexual history including relationships and marriage
  - Reproductive history (in women)
  - Children
  - Present social circumstances
  - Social support
  - Forensic history (if relevant)
- Premorbid personality

Box 8.2 Features supporting a diagnosis of depression

- Persistent/pervasive low mood, often tearfulness
- Diurnal variation of mood, typically worse in the morning
- Loss of motivation/interest
- Anhedonia, i.e. inability to experience pleasure in things
- Irritability and/or poor concentration
- Lethargy, fatigue and lack of energy
- Sleep disturbance, usually early-morning waking
- Appetite and weight loss (increased in atypical depression)
- Constipation and/or loss of libido
- Ideas of hopelessness, worthlessness, guilt, persecution, nihilism
- Loss of confidence and social withdrawal
- More severe depression
- Self-deprecation and/or self-neglect
- Motor retardation, leading to depressive stupor
- Retardation of speech, or muteness
- Paradoxical agitation
- Psychotic symptoms with mood
- Congruent delusions and auditory hallucinations

recorded as the basis for your interview. If the patient is being formally held on any section of the Mental Health Act, this must be recorded. If the patient cannot define a problem, then telling him what others have reported and why they are concerned can open up the conversation and allow him a chance to give his version of events.

History of presenting complaint (HPC)

Obtain a detailed description of how symptoms began (e.g., 'when did you last feel well?'), inquiring about the relationship to any life events that might have kicked things off. Establishing if the symptoms are new, that there has been a change in their condition or they are longer lasting helps to clarify if the current presentation is part of, for example, long-standing personality traits or due to the acute onset of a psychiatric disorder. The nature and persistence of symptoms and their impact on day-to-day functioning should be clarified. In order to fulfill diagnostic criteria for a psychiatric disorder, symptoms should persist across different circumstances and be severe enough to have an impact on a patient's functioning in daily life.

For example, with low mood it is important to establish whether the low mood is a brief fluctuation or whether it has persisted for a period of time. (The *International Statistical Classification of Diseases and Related Health Problems, Tenth Revision – ICD-10* specifies 2 weeks of low mood for a formal diagnosis of depression.) How reactive is it to circumstances? Moods unreactive to day-to-day events are generally indicative of a greater severity of depression. The evolution of symptoms over time, any help sought or given and any treatment received should all be clearly noted.

Patients may volunteer symptoms associated with the presentation, for example, finding it hard to get up in the morning or to focus on problems, but if none are volunteered a systematic inquiry is essential. Thus, in a patient presenting with depression, inquire about other symptoms in the depressive syndrome (Box 8.2) such as concentration, memory, things not enjoyed (anhedonia) and social withdrawal. Taking patients through a typical 24-hour day in terms of sleep, waking, what they do and how they feel can be very helpful. Anxiety and depression frequently coexist and so either presentation should lead to a systematic inquiry about symptoms of the other. Somatic and psychic symptoms of anxiety are outlined in Boxes 8.3 and 8.4. An acute onset of these will generate what is known as a panic attack.

Biological symptoms are important in all mental disorders, so inquiry should always be made about sleep, appetite, weight and energy levels. Particular note should be taken of any abrupt change to sleep pattern, as this is more significant in diagnosis than a chronic sleep problem. Inquire about sleep onset. Delay in getting to sleep is described as initial insomnia, and initial insomnia of 1 or 2 hours or more is pathological. It is often due to intrusive anxiety, perceptual experiences such as voices (see below) or pain. Inquire about waking in the night, since this is a pattern sometimes seen in anxiety. Waking regularly in the early hours (e.g. 3 or 4 in the morning) and being unable to get back to sleep is a pattern described as 'early morning wakening' and is indicative of a depressive disorder. Sometimes patients have a shifted sleep phase (sleep lag syndrome, just like jet lag) so, although they do not get off to sleep until late into the night and will complain about this, they will sleep on until later in the morning, say midday.

Box 8.3 Somatic symptoms of anxiety

- Headaches and other muscular aches and pains
- Palpitations
- Breathlessness (typically feel unable to get breath in)
- Tachypnoea
- Chest pain
- Urinary frequency
- Faintness and light-headedness, dizziness
- Blurred vision, dry mouth
- Fatigue
- Pins and needles, tremor
- Diarrhoea
- Abdominal discomfort, 'butterflies in stomach'
- Nausea and vomiting
- Flushes or pallor, sweating
- Insomnia, classically difficulty getting off to sleep

Box 8.4 Psychic symptoms of anxiety

- Feelings of anxiety
- Irritability
- Inability to relax
- Inability to concentrate
- Worry/anxious rumination
- Feeling of impending doom
- Depersonalisation
- Panic episodes (sudden onset of panic, sense of doom, fears of dying/collapsing/having a heart attack, with pounding heart and/or shortness of breath and hyperventilation, with an urge to flee one's situation)

If there is a distinct sleep problem, you should ask about sleep-related behaviours (e.g. bedtime routines, if children share the bed) or phenomena such as sleepwalking or hypnagogic hallucinations (see below). Establish if sleep is refreshing. Chronic fatigue patients describe unrefreshing sleep and waking still tired, but this is also seen in patients with anxiety. Even so, most patients underestimate how much sleep they actually get.

Ask if the patient's appetite has changed. In typical depression appetite is poor, but in atypical depression there may be an increase in appetite and a craving for carbohydrate-rich foods. Some patients without depression will describe eating to cope with brief episodes of low mood or to cope with upsetting events. Ask if the patient's weight has changed. Significant weight loss (more than 5%) in a depressed patient indicates moderate to severe depression. Weight increases can indicate a major problem of mood-related eating or bulimia (impulsive eating and self-induced vomiting), while very low weight may indicate anorexia nervosa (morbid fear of weight gain and severe weight loss).

Cycling of weight gain and loss can occur in eating disorders, such as bulimia and anorexia. It is also very important to inquire into changes in weight in relation to starting psychotropic medication. Many psychotropic medications (e.g. some antidepressants, antipsychotics and anticonvulsants) tend to cause weight gain. This should not be ignored and consideration should be given to stopping the relevant drugs as well as to clear dietary advice.

History of psychiatric disorder

Inquiry should be made about the lifelong history of mental health problems. The questions need to be asked in terms the patient will understand. For example, you could ask 'Have you ever had any problems with your nerves or mental health in the past?' or 'Have you ever suffered with a very low mood or with worrying too much or had any kind of nervous breakdown?' Ask about previous contact with mental health, counselling or psychology services. In women who have had children, inquire as to whether they experienced any mental health problems during or after pregnancy. Ask about previous use of psychotropic medication: 'Have you ever been prescribed any medication for your nerves or mental health, for example, taken an antidepressant, sedative or sleeping tablet?' Establish what previous medication has been effective in similar episodes or any medication to which they have reacted adversely. Establish whether the patient is currently in contact with any mental health professionals.

Past medical history

Inquire about any current or previous physical health problems, including operations. Note childhood operations or chronic childhood illness, which can be pointers to a tendency to somatise (i.e. to experience physical symptoms when anxious or distressed). Any chronic debilitating conditions or acute life-threatening events, such as a myocardial infarction, are important risk factors for depressive and anxiety disorders. A number of neurological illnesses have important psychiatric manifestations. Ask about all contacts with health services. Frequent consultations with many different specialists for a variety of symptoms in the absence of a definite medical diagnosis indicate a distinct somatoform disorder.

Current medication

Record all the medication a patient is currently taking (including over-the-counter medications, any recently 'borrowed medications' and herbal products). Overuse of some over-the-counter medications can exacerbate a problem (e.g. analgesic overuse headache). Record any allergies clearly.

Family history

Ask about parents: their ages, whether they are alive and, if so, whether they have any physical or mental health problems, where they live and the nature of the patient's current relationship with them. Inquire about the parents' occupations and personalities and the patient's relationship with them during childhood. Establish if the parents are separated or divorced and, if so, how old the patient was at the time. If the parents have died, inquire into when they died, their age at death, the circumstances of their death, how old the patient was at the time and how the patient has coped with the grieving process.

Establish how many siblings there are, whether full or half siblings, and the patient's order in the family. As for the parents, inquire into any siblings' mental and physical health, place of living, marital status, occupation, personality and the patient's relationship with them.

Some family structures can be very complicated, with parental separations, remarriages or re-partnerships and half- or stepsiblings from different parental relationships. In this situation, it can be helpful to draw a family tree and annotate it with the above information. Circles are used for women, squares for men; a line through the symbol denotes death. Marriage or permanent liaisons are indicated by a line connecting the symbols and divorce or permanent separation by two oblique lines through the connecting line.

Considerable information can emerge about relationships with parents, siblings, etc. while taking the family history, which can be explored further in the personal history. Specifically inquire whether there is any family history of mental health or psychological problems. When considering the heritable component of a condition, obviously you are only interested in first-degree relatives and not in relatives by marriage.

Personal history

Birth and early developmental milestones (in most patients only a brief outline is required)

This begins with inquiry about the patient's birth. Was it a normal delivery or were there any medical interventions or birth complications requiring specialist care? This is relevant to assess the possibility of any early brain injury. It can also be relevant if there were problems in early maternal bonding. Were developmental milestones reached within the normal range (see Ch. 6). Patients may not have any knowledge about their birth and milestones. If a patient tells you about some problem surrounding their birth and early milestones, this may be significant and is worth recording. If no problems are identified, it is possible that the patient just does not know. Clearly an informant, such as the patient's mother, may have more accurate information.

Family milieu, childhood health and early relationships with caregivers

Start with an open question such as 'How do you remember your childhood?' 'Was it a happy or unhappy time of life?' Cover the family atmosphere during early upbringing, relationships between parents and relationships with parents or alternative caregivers such as grandparents or foster carers. It is important to note any periods of separation from parents and the quality of alternative caregivers. Inquire about and record any loss of parents or other caring figures through death, separation or divorce. These factors are important in understanding whether there has been any early disruption of attachment bonds for the individual. Childhood health is important. Ask about operations, hospitalisation or chronic illness in childhood and about family attitudes to any illness. Asking how much time was missed off school due to illness is a good indicator of childhood health, whether organic or non-organic. A happy childhood can be covered quickly, with more time spent exploring causes of an unhappy childhood experience.

Specifically ask about physical or sexual abuse. This may seem difficult at first as these feel like taboo topics. Make sure the questions are in an appropriate context (i.e. when inquiring about the patient's experience of childhood). Then you can ask, in a matter of fact though sensitive way, questions such as the following:

- Did you ever have any experience of being badly treated as a child?
- Were you ever neglected and not provided with adequate physical care?
- Was anyone persistently mean or cruel to you in what they said?
- Were you ever hit?
- Were you ever physically abused in any way?
- Were you ever sexually abused by anyone as a child?

If the rapport with a patient is poor for any reason, or if you are seeing a very psychotic disorganised patient, just asking a general question and deferring exploration may be better. Sometimes patients will indicate that they did experience abuse, in which case it is important to test out sensitively how much to explore this in an initial interview. It is usually best not to do so, but useful to ascertain if this is the first time abuse has been disclosed.

A patient who has undergone a period of therapy, for example, and has discussed abusive experiences at length beforehand may be comfortable recounting such experiences at a first interview. A patient however who has never disclosed such abuse before may find it difficult to discuss it at all, and an agreement to talk more about this subsequently may be more appropriate. Patients should never feel coerced, either overtly or covertly, by the whole context of the interview to talk about issues which cause pain or distress. If they do, the interview itself can feel like an abusive experience.

Schooling

A person's experience of school can be very important in terms of understanding the development of their peer relationships and indicating whether there were any behaviour problems as well as finding out what educational level has been attained. Inquire about both primary and secondary school, what sort of schools were attended, whether school was enjoyable and any experience of bullying. Likewise, things enjoyed, peer relationships, ease of friendships and whether friends from school are still part of the friendship group should be inquired about. Truancy, school refusal, exclusions from school and referral to any children's service are all important to clarify.

Truancy refers to a child missing school deliberately, usually without parental knowledge, and doing something else such as working or playing with other truants. School refusal describes a situation in which a child stays at home refusing to go to school despite persuasion from parents, usually due to an anxiety disorder. Sometimes parents keep children at home due to the parent's health or practical needs (the parent may need practical help due to physical illness or with looking after other children).

Establish the patient's level of academic achievement (qualifications attained). Ask about further education or training on leaving school and their experience of this (college or university). Further education is an important point in a person's developmental trajectory as it is often the point at which an individual starts to live independently. How successfully this major milestone is negotiated is an important indicator of psychological health and can reveal information about emotional attachments and functioning. Inquire specifically about the transition from home to living independently, even if not for further education, or whether the patient still lives in the parental home.

Time may not allow all aspects of schooling to be covered but always record age at start and end of full-time education, any problems encountered and the highest level of qualifications attained. This information can be important in evaluation of cognitive state.

Occupational history

Take a history of the first job patients have had after their education, what other jobs they have had, how long they have stayed in those and the reasons for leaving. It is not necessary to go into exhaustive detail, but it is important to establish if the individual is able to sustain long-term periods of employment. Use a shortened approach by asking about total number of jobs, longest period of employment and highest level of employment, longest period of unemployment, difficulties at work and relationships at work. If a pattern emerges of frequent job switches after brief periods of employment, it is important to establish the reason for this pattern: is there a pattern of repeated behaviour (e.g. getting bored) or a particular problem (e.g. difficulty with authority figures or other problems in interpersonal relationships). This can give important information about ability and personality. Ask about his current job (if the patient is employed) such as the hours worked, what it involves and if it is enjoyable as well as any particular current work stressors. If a patient is unemployed, establish when he last worked and the reasons for not working (e.g. illness, redundancy).

Psychosexual history, including marital/relationship history and children

The psychosexual history can be a source of embarrassment for students and patients, but this is unnecessary if handled in a straightforward way. If there is a problem, patients may even be relieved to be asked about this, since they may have been afraid to mention such a topic. Many psychotropic drugs have psychosexual side effects (e.g. erectile dysfunction or loss of libido with some antidepressants), but patients often do not mention such side effects unless asked. How much detail is needed will vary depending on the presenting complaint. Obviously, if the patient is complaining of marital or psychosexual difficulties, a full history of this area is relevant. The level of detail outlined in Box 8.5 is usually not necessary, but you should routinely gather basic details of the psychosexual history. In the relationship history, do not make an assumption about sexual orientation. Ask about sexual orientation in an open non-judgemental way. Look for patterns that may be indicative of relationship problems (lots of brief

Box 8.5 The psychosexual history

- Women: age at menarche, menstrual history, sex education at home/school
- Men: puberty, sex education at home/school
- For both sexes, a full sexual history would also cover sexual fantasies, masturbation and deviant sexual behaviour (this level of detail is inappropriate unless the problem is specifically a psychosexual one)
- Boyfriends/girlfriends in adolescence, age at first sexual relationship
- Marital history: age at marriage, how they met, parental attitude to marriage and quality of marital relationship – confiding, conflict, separations. Establish age, occupation and health of spouse. How and why relationships ended
- Current relationship: any conflict? What is the partner's attitude to the patient's illness? Are they supportive?
- Children: how many, names, ages, who the biological parents are, who cares for them. Any worries about the children's health, behaviour, schooling or relationships with the patient
- Reproductive history in women: did they get pregnant easily? Fertility treatment? Were the pregnancies planned? History of miscarriages, terminations of pregnancy or stillbirths. Mental health problems during pregnancy or after childbirth or related to menstruation

relationships, a repeated pattern in intimate relationships, repeatedly entering into abusive relationships). Be aware of domestic violence and the need to ask about this if there is a very difficult or aggressive relationship. Basic details about children (also in Box 8.5) can be important later if child-protection issues are raised.

Current social situation (Box 8.6)

Forensic history

Details of a full forensic history are beyond the scope of this chapter. It is useful to inquire routinely if the patient has ever been in any trouble with the police. You should then record the nature of any charges, court appearances, convictions and prison sentences. It is particularly important to record in detail, highlight and pass information to other health professionals about violent offences. As noted above, the best predictor of future violent behaviour is past violence, and there is a real risk that this information gets buried in notes and forgotten.

Use of alcohol and non-prescribed recreational drugs

Alcohol

Ascertain quantity and frequency of alcohol intake. If the level of alcohol use is above safe drinking limits (Box 8.7), or if there are other indicators of a problem with alcohol (Box 8.8), a full drinking history should be taken and symptoms of alcohol dependence should be sought (Box 8.9). A very brief and commonly used screen for alcohol dependence is a questionnaire called the CAGE (Box 8.10). Alcohol misuse is drinking which causes physical, social or psychological harm to the drinker. Alcohol dependence is said to exist when the criteria for a dependence syndrome are met (Box 8.9).

Box 8.6 Current social situation

- Type of accommodation: council, private rented or homeowner, any problems
- Who else lives in the home, quality of relationship with them, whether the partner is very possessive
- Friends and social support: with whom does he confide and share problems?
- Financial situation: earnings, debts, benefits, worries
- Locality: are they settled in the community? Is it familiar to them? Happy to live there, or wanting to move?

Box 8.7 Units of alcohol and safe drinking limits

1 unit contains 10 g of pure alcohol and is equal to half a pint of beer, one small glass of table wine or one bar measure of spirits (for more detail, see Box 1.12):

- Safe limits (debated still):
  - men <21 units/week
  - women <14 units/week
- High risk of social/health problems:
  - men >50 units/week
  - women >35 units/week

Box 8.8 Features suggesting alcohol misuse

- Excessive consumption (if acknowledged)
- Secret drinking and drinking alone
- Morning drinking
- Amnesia for events (i.e. blackouts) during episode of drinking
- Drunk driving convictions or other alcohol-related crime
- Violent behaviour related to consumption
- Marital problems related to consumption
- Employment problems related to consumption
- Alcohol-related physical illness (e.g. abnormal liver disease, neuropathy) or abnormal investigations such as raised gamma GT or MCV
- Patient is evasive or vague when questioned about intake
- Patient in a high-risk occupation, e.g. bar worker, publican, armed forces, entertainers, journalists, company directors
- Family history of alcohol problems
- Any of the features of dependence listed in Box 8.9

Box 8.9 Features of alcohol dependence

- A strong desire or sense of compulsion to drink alcohol (craving)
- Difficulty controlling intake of alcohol in terms of not being able to control starting, stopping or amount taken
- Withdrawal symptoms when alcohol intake is reduced or stopped and drinking to relieve withdrawal symptoms
- Tolerance, i.e. increased amount of alcohol is required to achieve same effects as previously obtained with a lower amount
- Neglect of alternative activities when drinking or recovering, e.g. leisure activities, work, time spent with family
- Continued drinking despite harm caused (either physical, mental or social)

Box 8.10 The CAGE questionnaire

- C – Have you ever felt you needed to *C*ut down on your drinking?
- A – Have people *A*nnoyed you by criticising your drinking?
- G – Have you ever felt bad or *G*uilty about your drinking?
- E – Have you ever had a drink first thing in the morning to steady your nerves or get rid of a hangover (*E*ye-opener)?

Two or more positive replies are indicative of alcohol misuse and should lead the interviewer to take a full drinking history.

Taking a full drinking history

You need to obtain as accurately as possible an estimate of the quantity, type and pattern of alcohol consumption as well as the effects of alcohol on day-to-day life. Patients are frequently in denial and will underestimate their intake. The most efficient way to take the history is to ask about a typical drinking day or week. Go through the day ascertaining type, quantity and context of alcohol intake. Cover the features listed in Boxes 8.8 and 8.9 to establish if there is alcohol misuse or dependence. Never forget that most patients underestimate their alcohol intake by at least 50%.

After establishing current drinking level and problems, ask about the lifetime history of drinking such as when the patient started drinking, pattern over the years, episodes of dependent drinking, previous attempts to abstain and previous treatment for alcohol problems. Remember, alcohol use is often an attempt by the patient to self-medicate other psychiatric disorders such as depression, anxiety or post-traumatic stress disorder (PTSD).

Recreational drugs

Routine inquiry should be made into previous or current use of recreational drugs (and do not forget excessive coffee intake). The question can follow on from inquiry about medication using a question such as 'Have you ever used any other non-prescribed drugs, such as cannabis ('pot', 'ganja'), cocaine, amphetamines ('speed'), LSD ('acid') or anything like that?' The phrase 'designer drugs' or 'recreational drugs' can be used, judging the appropriate terminology for the patient. The criteria for drug dependence and problem drug use are the same as those for alcohol. The same structure can be used for taking a history of drug misuse as was outlined for alcohol, with the addition of inquiring about method of administration of the drug. This can lead on to asking about needle sharing, source of needles, HIV and hepatitis C status. Taking a full substance misuse history can be complex and time consuming if patients are polysubstance abusers, since often they will be vague about how much they have been using of each drug, but each drug must be dealt with in turn.

Personality assessment

Do not rely too heavily on a patient's self-assessment of personality, although it is important to hear how he views himself. Depressed patients may paint a picture of themselves as incompetent, blameworthy and lacking in confidence, which may be far from their premorbid personality. To avoid such misrepresentations, try to rely on objective information in the history, and where possible talk to an informant who knows the patient well and what he is usually like. The important areas to cover in assessing personality are shown in Box 8.11. In this area of assessment a collateral history is mandatory.

Box 8.11 Personality assessment

- Usual mood
- Pessimistic and worrying or optimistic. Stable mood or mood swings.
- Relationships with others
- Deep and enduring or superficial short-term relationships, quality of marriage, work relationships, conflict with authority figures.
- Character
- How they describe themselves, e.g. shy, sensitive, introvert, extrovert, quarrelsome, laid back, dependent, controlling. Any obsessional traits, e.g. tidy, rigid.
- Leisure activities and habits (including drug and alcohol use)
- Risk-taking activities, collecting, passive spectator or active participant, solitary pursuits or very sociable, party going, time spent on leisure versus workaholic
- Personal standards and attitudes
- Religious beliefs and participation, moral views, attitudes to health and body, level of acculturation (if from an ethnic minority), e.g. traditional or Western attitudes, dress

The mental state examination

The MSE is the cornerstone of the psychiatric assessment. It enables a systematic observation of clinical symptoms and signs on which a differential diagnosis is based. Students often feel that they do not know where to start and it seems a very unfamiliar genre. However, in essence it is simple: look at and listen to the patient carefully and observe in a systematic way. The examination is a word portrait of how the patient appears, using clinical observation, informed questioning, empathic listening and accurate recording. It is helpful sometimes to take verbatim notes of what the patient says and record these in quotation marks.

Observations and interpretations should be recorded separately. An MSE consisting solely of the doctor's interpretations is of little use. For example, a patient may say that the police are in a conspiracy against him and are monitoring his flat with listening devices in the walls. It is inadequate just to record that the patient has paranoid delusions. It may not be a delusion. It could be true, or he could be intentionally creating fantasy stories. The record should include what the patient actually says and then state 'This belief seems to be a delusion'. A basic comprehensive structure is outlined in Box 8.12 with a detailed outline of what should be recorded under each heading.

Appearance and behaviour

Appearance

Describe how patients appear and whether their dress and general presentation seems appropriate for

Box 8.12 The mental state examination

- Appearance and behaviour
- Speech
- Mood: subjective and objective
- Thought: form and content
- Perception
- Cognitive assessment: including orientation, attention and concentration, registration and short-term memory, recent memory, remote memory, intelligence, abstraction
- Insight

their age, culture, occupation and social class. Severe weight loss (e.g. ill-fitting clothes) may indicate the loss of appetite as a result of depression or even dementia or failure to eat because of delusional ideas or anorexia. It may represent simple social disorganisation in those with schizophrenia, or it may be due to a distinct physical illness. Excess weight by contrast can also occur in schizophrenic illness (secondary to medication, typically) or can indicate an eating disorder such as bulimia or excessive alcohol intake (in some people). Poor self-care indicated by body odour, lack of shaving and dirty clothes can be due to depression, or patients with schizophrenia or dementia may become too disorganised and lose the capacity to care for themselves.

A lowered level of consciousness indicates an organic brain disorder. Suspected altered consciousness should be checked out early on with tests of orientation, as the interpretation of the MSE will be different if the patient is confused or severely cognitively impaired. This situation calls for a simplified interview, with careful observation of behaviour and an attempt to interview an informant.

Behaviour

Essentially this is a description of how the patient behaves, in relation to the environment and the interviewer. Is the behaviour socially appropriate or is it unusual in some way? Included in this section would be the following:

General demeanour

Is the patient relaxed or anxious? Is he agitated (fiddling or wringing hands), angry or behaving as though suspicious? Patients with severe depression may be slow to respond or (paradoxically) may need to pace about, unable to stay still because of agitation. Excitability due to mania or schizophrenia looks like agitation although will usually be more disorganised. Angry or suspicious behaviour may be due to persecutory delusions, without any natural fear of being examined. A distracted or preoccupied patient may just be very anxious (due to inner fearfulness or fearful thoughts) or may be experiencing auditory hallucinations or may be seen actively responding to auditory hallucinations (e.g. muttering inexplicably), visual hallucinations (looking away suddenly) or tactile hallucinations (reacting as if hit or bitten).

Rapport

Does the patient engage comfortably or seem nervous, awkward and troubled with the interview? He may be warm or indifferent, suspicious, ingratiating, dismissive, supercilious or hostile. The patient's way of relating to you could be defined by personality or mental illness. Patients with severe depression may be apathetic and indifferent. Those with schizophrenia may be suspicious and hostile. Patients with mania may be dismissive, impatient and supercilious, being readily irritated by the interruption of whatever important task they may be engaged in.

Eye contact

Does the patient establish good eye contact, exhibit an avoidant gaze or look suspiciously around? There may even be an abnormal staring eye contact or a hostile frown or grimace when looking at people. Wearing dark glasses indoors may just be fashionable but could imply a sense of fearfulness, a visual problem or, not uncommonly, drug withdrawal.

Gait

Note any abnormalities of gait when a patient walks in. There may be a manneristic gait (see mannerisms below) where the patient walks in an exaggerated posing way. There may be functional gait problems, so look for inconsistencies in what can be done when a patient is asked to walk and what may be elicited on examination. Asking someone to walk as if on a tightrope, heel to toe, can clarify whether or not they are ataxic.

Reduced motor activity

In bradykinesia (patients seeming to act in slow motion), voluntary movements are reduced and abnormally slow. The face and arms tend to be particularly affected. Bradykinesia is most commonly caused by parkinsonism due to Parkinson's disease or medication, particularly antipsychotics. Slowness and paucity of movement may also occur in psychomotor retardation, which is a feature of depression and indicates quite severe depression. In stupor, there is severe paucity of movement and mutism. This occurs in severe depression, catatonia and organic brain disease. Catatonia is characterised by a stuporous state with additional features (see Boxes 8.13 and 8.14).

Increased motor activity

Note any excessive activity and whether it is purposeful or not. Manic patients may just be overactive and distractible. Agitation has a different quality, being driven by an unpleasant inner sense of tension. It is a general restlessness in which there may be apparently purposeful activity but it is not carried through properly. There may be repetitive

Box 8.13 Movement changes in the mental state examination

- Dystonia: due to older major antipsychotic drugs
- Choreiform: Huntington's chorea – common with L-dopa therapy (for Parkinson's disease)
- Tics: quite frequent in childhood and during periods of emotional stress
- Mannerisms:
  - habitual repetitive voluntary movements or behaviour patterns
  - can be part of normal behaviour, e.g. frequent raising of eyebrows
  - bizarre occurrences in schizophrenia, e.g. saluting frequently or raising one leg every few strides. They can be voluntarily controlled
- Stereotypies: repeated uniform movements or utterances, purposeless (unlike mannerisms), regularly occurring (unlike unpredictable tics), e.g. rocking to and fro on a chair. Stereotypies are found most commonly in patients with learning difficulties
- Tardive dyskinesia: syndrome of abnormal movements, e.g. facial grimaces, writhing movements, abnormal rolling of tongue. It can be a delayed side effect of older antipsychotic medication. Onset may be months or years after starting the medication and, paradoxically, it can worsen initially after stopping it
- Catatonia: (see also Box 8.14) striking condition characterised by stupor, sometimes alternating with excited motor and behavioural features. Motor excitation can be extreme and lead to injury or exhaustion, which can be lethal

Box 8.14 Variable features of catatonia

- Waxy flexibility: the patient maintains a posture in which he has been placed by the examiner
- Negativism: the patient seems to behave in the opposite way to that requested by the examiner
- Aversion: the patient turns away when addressed
- Mannerisms: see Box 8.13
- Grimacing: common in schizophrenia. Schnauzkrampf is a facial grimace in which the nose is wrinkled down and the lips drawn up towards it in a pout
- Stereotypies: see Box 8.13
- Posturing: the patient adopts an unusual posture for a prolonged period, e.g. symbolic like a cross
- Automatic obedience: the patient shows excessive compliance (opposite of negativism)
- Echopraxia: the patient exactly imitates the interviewer
- Advertence: the patient frequently turns to the interviewer in an exaggerated way
- Mitgehen: the interviewer can move the patient's limbs with fingertip pressure
- Ambitendence: the patient will start and then reverse a movement, e.g. putting out a hand and withdrawing it

purposeless behaviour such as hand-wringing, scratching, rubbing hands on knees and pacing up and down. See Box 8.13.

Speech

This is divided into two components: rate and structure of speech.

Rate

Slowed speech with a long latency between question and answer may be a component of psychomotor retardation in depression; it can occur in dementia or in psychosis due to distraction by hearing voices or in the very anxious patient. Lack of spontaneous speech occurs in depression, as a negative symptom of schizophrenia and in some dementias. It may be due to expressive aphasia caused by a cerebral lesion. There may be excessive spontaneous speech, as in a manic patient or also in some dementias, where there is a loss of appropriate social understanding of reciprocal speech. 'Pressure of speech' refers to an increase in both the rate and amount of speech, characterised in particular by patients being very difficult to interrupt, and is typical of manic states. Sometimes speech is so pressured and driven that it becomes incomprehensible. By contrast, mute patients will not speak at all, as in states of stupor due to severe depression, schizophrenia or organic brain disease but occasionally as a hysterical symptom. Elective mutism (the patient will speak in some situations but not in others) occurs mostly in children.

Structure

This can be disrupted in a variety of ways and due to a range of disorders (Box 8.15).

Other abnormalities of speech that should be noted are any evidence of dysphasia or dysarthria, which would indicate neurological disease, or that may be due to drug or alcohol side effects.

Mood

This is usually divided into subjective and objective mood. Some clinicians separate mood ('My description of how I feel') from affect (how the patient's mood affects the interviewer). For subjective mood, record how the patient actually feels, for example 'I'm really fed up', or 'I'm feeling sad' etc. It is most useful to record this verbatim. Interpreting mood is particularly difficult in people whose first language is not English, given the limited range of mood-related terms in other languages.

Ask an open question first, for example 'How have you been feeling in yourself?' or 'How have your spirits been lately?' If there is no clear response, ask a more closed question: 'Have you been feeling low, sad or miserable recently?' or 'Have you been feeling depressed?'

If the patient acknowledges low mood, you should explore severity and persistence. Persistently low

Box 8.15 Disorders of structure of speech

- Circumstantial: frequent digressions, taking a long time to get to the point ('over-inclusive thinking'), as in OCD or forms of epilepsy and organic brain disorders
- Tangentiality: answers seem unrelated or only slightly related to questions, e.g. in schizophrenia, severe anxiety
- Disorders of the form of thought: abnormality of the structure of thought manifest in speech. There are three main types of formal thought disorder – flight of ideas, loosening of associations or perseveration:
  - Flight of ideas: speech jumps from one idea to an associated one but with loss of the end goal. The associations can be based on meaning or on similarities of sound ('clang associations'), for example 'head – red – dead in bed'.
  - Loosening of associations: jumps from one idea into another apparently unrelated one, making understanding very difficult, e.g. 'Knight's Move' speech in schizophrenia and, in extreme forms, a mixture of unrelated words ('word salad')
  - Perseveration: repetition of a theme or answer when no longer appropriate (in 'echolalia', the patient repeats what the interviewer says), e.g. in organic brain disease and some forms of schizophrenia

mood indicates more severe depression than mood which is reactive to events. Is it worse at any time of day? Feeling very depressed on waking with mood lifting later is called diurnal mood variation and is a good marker for significant depression. Thoughts related to depression are considered below.

To assess elated mood after the initial open question about mood, ask 'Have you been feeling in very good spirits, unusually happy or very elated for no reason recently?' If the patient says yes, you can ask 'What is that like? Can you describe it to me?' Do not take what patients say at face value; always try to get a good description of what they are actually experiencing. Thoughts related to an elated mood are considered below.

Inquire about irritability, as this often accompanies a lowered mood and can occur both in depression and mania. Its effects may be noted only by taking a collateral history, for example, from a partner. If present, explore its severity and in particular note any related physical violence, for example domestic violence, and there may also be child protection issues. Inquire also about anxiety: 'Have you been feeling very nervous, frightened or shaky recently?' A particular type of anxious foreboding accompanies both anxiety and depression, and in this the patient constantly feels a sense of dread, as though something awful is going to happen, while also being perplexed since it is not clear what this might be.

Sometimes patients describe a sense of feeling flat and numb. They may describe no longer feeling love for a spouse or child, and this in itself they find distressing. Such psychological numbness is seen in depression, depersonalisation and (as a key symptom) in post-traumatic stress disorder (PTSD).

An objective assessment of mood should be recorded, for example whether a patient is distinctly depressed, anxious or angry. An overall level of wellbeing may be helpful on a rough self-rating scale of $^{1}/_{10}$ to $^{10}/_{10}$ to enable patients to sum up their overall outlook. Observe and record objective indicators of mood during the interview, for example body language, and facial expressions (e.g. weeping, frowning or laughter). Opinion varies as to whether biological symptoms of depression or somatic symptoms of anxiety should be recorded in the mental state or as part of the history.

Important features of mood to observe are variation and whether it is appropriate to the circumstance. Mood may be appropriately reactive to what is being described, or a persistently low mood may indicate severe depression. Mood may be excessively reactive and labile, switching from laughing and joking to floods of tears, which is strongly associated with organic brain disease and sometimes manic-depressive illness. Incongruous affect (e.g. a patient laughing while talking about his baby's death) is a feature of schizophrenia. It can be worth asking a patient why he smiled or laughed while discussing something upsetting. Blunting of affect, also seen in schizophrenia, describes the loss of the normal variation of mood.

Thought

Attention should be paid to both the way people think as well as thought content. Thought form (when impaired this is known as 'formal thought disorder') refers to whether a patient's thoughts are ordered in a logical way or whether his thinking jumps about, with discontinuities and moving from topic to topic, making it hard for the listener to follow or understand. (Such a reaction in the interviewer in itself is often diagnostic, just like feeling a lump when examining the abdomen.) In particular it is the flow of a patient's speech that will indicate the presence of thought disorder, and these abnormalities of form of thought have therefore been described above in the section on speech. However, the presence of formal thought disorder should be recorded in this section.

Attention should be paid to the content and theme of what patients discuss, as it gives a window into what is on their minds. Consider the overall theme of what is being discussed as this will indicate mood (e.g. depressive, manic, persecutory). Often the content of thought will have already emerged from the history taking. However, there are some questions worth asking to explore specific issues in more detail or to raise them if they have not already come up.

The exploration of depressive thoughts is described in Box 8.16. It is important always to establish whether or not a patient experiences suicidal thoughts, and this is part of risk assessment. It is negligent to perform

Box 8.16 Exploration of depressive thoughts

Guilt

- Do you ever feel guilty about anything, or blame yourself for things or feel ashamed?

Self-esteem/self-worth

- What is your opinion of yourself compared to other people?
- Are you as good as other people?
- Do you run yourself down?

Hopelessness

- How do you see the future?
- Do you ever feel hopeless about your situation?

Suicidal thoughts

A good time to ask these questions is after exploring depressive cognitions with the questions suggested above. It is best to ask about suicidal feelings with a graded series of questions:

- Do things ever get so bad that you feel you don't want to carry on?
- Do you ever wish you did not wake up in the morning (passive suicidal feelings)?
- Do you ever have thoughts about doing something to harm yourself?
- Do you ever have thoughts about ending your own life?

a psychiatric assessment without a basic risk assessment. Medical students and doctors may feel uncomfortable asking about suicidal ideas or may fear that asking about suicidal thoughts increases the likelihood that the patient will act upon them. Research has shown that the opposite is the case. Patients are often relieved to share these feelings and welcome this opportunity.

Some patients self-harm for reasons other than wanting to end their life. For example, patients may deliberately self-harm by cutting themselves as a way of getting a sense of release from unpleasant emotions, or they may overdose to draw attention to their distress. A suitable question covering both suicidal ideas and self-harm might be 'Have you ever had thoughts of harming yourself in any way, for example by taking too many tablets or by cutting yourself?'

It is important to pursue a risk assessment to determine the likelihood of a patient acting on thoughts of suicide or self-harm. Ask what he has thought of doing and whether he has done anything specific to prepare (e.g. saving up tablets). Look for protective factors by asking what it is that stops him from acting on his suicidal thoughts and how he copes with such thoughts. Box 8.17 summarises important risk factors for completed suicide; the student should know about and explore these in assessing risk.

Exploring thoughts in elevated mood

Patients with elevated mood states (mania or hypomania) will often mention all kinds of grandiose ideas

Box 8.17 Features suggesting increased risk of suicidal behaviour

- Previous self-harm, especially:
  - poison
  - stabbing
  - hanging
  - jumping from heights
  - falling under vehicles
- Continuing suicidal thoughts
- Current depressive or schizophrenic psychosis
- Male, aged over 40 years
- Social isolation, especially in adolescence or the recently bereaved or divorced
- Chronic painful illness
- Alcoholism and drug abuse
- Family history of suicide

Box 8.18 Exploring thoughts in elevated mood

- You may find some of these questions a bit unusual and they don't apply to everyone, but I need to ask them just to check whether you have had any of these experiences:
  - Do you ever feel as though you can do some things much better than other people?
  - Have you seemed especially efficient at work or in other activities?
  - Do you ever feel you have special abilities, talents or powers which other people do not have?
  - Have you got any new projects in mind or new plans for the future?
  - Have you ever had the thought that you may be a special person and, if so, who?
  - Have you had thoughts of doing rather reckless things which are out of character and you would not normally do, for example planning to spend a lot of money on a shopping spree, or thinking of starting affairs or relationships which may not be wise?

while you are taking a history and may have disinhibited behaviour. Specific questions to ask if they have not already come up are listed in Box 8.18.

Obsessional thoughts

Obsessional thoughts are repeated, stereotyped thoughts that intrude into a person's mind – they are usually experienced as unpleasant, silly and even irrational. Patients ask themselves 'why do I keep thinking this?' for example. Such thoughts are not delusional, but the patient is unable to stop them from occurring, despite attempts at resistance which often produce anxiety. Patients are clear that these are their own thoughts, as distinct from the experience of thought insertion when there is a sense of something 'not you' being imposed on your mind. Common obsessional thoughts are those of contamination (e.g. patients feel their hands are dirty and feel compelled

Box 8.19 Definition of delusion and overvalued ideas

A delusion is a fixed false belief, held with complete conviction, which dominates a patient's outlook, which is not amenable to alteration by any argument and which is not shared by others of the same social and cultural background.

Overvalued ideas are beliefs which are intrusively prominent in the patient's mind and with which he is unreasonably preoccupied (e.g. his hair does not feel right and needs constant attention), but the patient is able to acknowledge that the belief may not be true and may be open to an alternative explanation.

constantly to wash them) or even infection (they may reek of antiseptics), and many patients constantly worry that they have not, for example, shut the front door or locked all the windows before going out. The compulsive motor act that accompanies the thought (e.g. hand washing or door checking) is called an obsessional ritual.

Obsessional thoughts and other obsessional phenomena are part of the normal range of experience, and careful checking makes, for example, a good clinician. However, when severe and disabling, they form the central psychopathology in obsessional compulsive disorder (OCD), and it is important to ask screening questions for obsessional symptoms (which may not be volunteered, because of individual embarrassment about such habits). If a patient acknowledges any of these problems, explore their frequency, severity, and the attempts to resist and the extent of functional disability as a result. For example, washing and checking rituals take time, people are late for work and some people find it hard even to leave the house.

Abnormal beliefs

The main types of abnormal belief are primary and secondary delusions, overvalued ideas and sensitive ideas of reference (Box 8.19).

Primary delusions (also called true delusions) are delusions that are not secondary to other abnormal mental processes such as abnormal mood or hallucinations. A particular example of a primary delusion is a delusional perception in which a patient has a normal perception to which is attached a delusional significance. For example, a patient may see a waiter pick up a glass (a normal perception) and the patient realises immediately that the waiter is an envoy of the devil (delusional significance). Primary delusions are generally associated with schizophrenia provided they occur in clear consciousness (i.e. they are not occurring in an organic confusional state). Indeed they are one of the Schneiderian first-rank symptoms of schizophrenia (see Boxes 8.20 and 8.21).

Secondary delusions (also called delusion-like ideas) are secondary to an abnormal mood state or hallucinatory experience. Unlike primary delusions, they are

Box 8.20 Diagnosis of schizophrenia

Schneider described what he called first-rank symptoms of schizophrenia. The presence of any one symptom in the absence of organic brain disease is regarded as diagnostic of schizophrenia, but first-rank symptoms are not always present. This is not a comprehensive list of the clinical features of schizophrenia, but they are symptoms which are quite specific to it (as long as there is no organic disease). The first-rank symptoms are:

1 Audible thoughts: auditory hallucination of hearing thoughts while thinking them (Gedankenlautwerden) or as an echo immediately after thinking them (echo de la pensée)
2 Argumentative voices: two or more voices referring to the patient in the third person in an argumentative manner, e.g. 'He's an odd sort of fellow', 'No, he is evil'
3 Auditory hallucinations of running commentary on behaviour referring to the patient in the third person, e.g. 'Now he is opening the door'
4 Thought insertion or thought withdrawal
5 Thought broadcasting
6 Passivity 'made' experiences, including impulses, feelings, and actions occurring without the patient initiating or controlling them
7 Delusional perception

Box 8.21 Distinction between positive and negative symptoms of schizophrenia

Positive symptoms (i.e. experiences additional to the norm)

- Tend to occur in the acute phase and generally respond to antipsychotic medication
- Hallucinations including thought echo
- Delusions, primary and secondary, including delusions of thought control and passivity experiences
- Disturbance of emotional control – there may be outbursts of emotion, e.g. laughter or anger, without appropriate cause
- Disturbed thinking with thought disorder or neologisms

Negative symptoms (i.e. loss of normal experiences)

- Tend to be chronic and accumulate as the illness progresses
- Poverty of speech – the patient has little to say and very little spontaneous speech
- Poverty of thought and movement – speech indicates loss of richness and complexity of thought. Movement is lacking and slowed
- Blunting of affect – absence of normal modulation of mood and lack of emotional response
- Lack of volition – loss of motivation; can be extreme when patient neglects basic self-care
- Social withdrawal

understandable in the light of the patient's mood and life history. For example, a severely depressed mother may become convinced that she is evil and that she is not worthy to bring up her child. Secondary delusions lack diagnostic specificity but their content may relate to the diagnosis.

Sensitive ideas of reference can be described when patients falsely believe that things actually occurring in their environment are specifically referring to themselves. These experiences typically occur in depression, body dysmorphic disorder (BDD), paranoid states and paranoid personality types. For example, patients may feel that others are looking or laughing at them. In delusions of reference, patients are completely convinced that people are talking about and laughing at them (and may react). Sometimes patients will be convinced that a TV presenter is speaking directly to them or talking about them. Questions to elicit these sorts of ideas might be 'Have you felt that other people are too interested in you?', 'Do you feel that people comment on you or say things behind your back?' or 'Do people seem to drop hints for you or say things with double meaning?'

When eliciting delusional beliefs, and because psychotic symptoms are often very bizarre, it is wise to put patients at ease by making some kind of normalising statement and asking a very open general question first. For example, you might say 'Some people find that when they are feeling very stressed or having difficulties with how they are feeling, they have some rather odd experiences. Has anything very odd or unusual happened to you recently?' Follow up on any positive responses with open questions, asking the patient to describe experiences in detail. If there are no positives, you can screen for certain sorts of delusions. Some of these, and suggested screening questions, are given in Box 8.22.

Box 8.22 Types of delusional ideas

Persecutory delusions

'Do you ever have the feeling that people are against you or out to get you in some way?' They may occur in organic psychoses such as confusional states, dementia, alcohol and drug-induced psychoses, in stress-induced psychogenic psychoses and sometimes in people with paranoid personalities, particularly with advancing age and in whom sensory deficits such as visual and hearing impairment occur. They may also occur in schizophrenia.

Delusional misinterpretation

This is a type of delusion of reference. Patients will ascribe particular significance to normal objects in their environment. For example, they will see a coded message intended for them in a car number plate.

Delusions of grandeur

Patients are delusionally convinced that they are special in some way, for example they have been given a special purpose by God or that they are famous. It is characteristic of syphilitic general paralysis of the insane (now rarely seen). They can also occur in mania and schizophrenia but are uncommon.

Hypochondriacal delusions

Patients believe that some part of their body is abnormal or diseased. This is common in depressive psychosis, as are delusions of guilt, self-blame and poverty.

Nihilistic delusions

Seen in severe psychotic depression, they involve a delusional belief that parts of one's body (internal organs usually) are rotting away or even no longer exist ('no stomach').

Delusions of jealousy

This is a delusional conviction that one's spouse or partner is being unfaithful. It occurs in substance misuse (especially alcohol misuse), in schizophrenia and in people with a suspicious/possessive personality style. It is important to take these delusional beliefs seriously and do a full risk assessment.

Erotomanic delusions

Patients hold delusional beliefs that someone (usually famous) is in love with them. They occur mainly in schizophrenia and in organic psychoses. They may lead to stalking behaviour, so take these delusions seriously and do a full risk assessment.

Fantastic delusions

These are bizarre delusions – for example, that aliens have landed and are causing things to change in some way or they are involved in some other attempts to interfere with the patient's life. These occur in schizophrenia.

Delusional memory

The patient describes remembering things which are clearly delusional. For example, the patient remembers and can give graphic descriptions of being abducted by aliens and experimented upon.

Delusions of passivity

These are a group of bizarre phenomena in which the core experience is of loss of the normal sense of boundary between the self and the outside world (ego boundaries). They include thought insertion (the experience that one's thoughts are not one's own) and the accompanying belief that thoughts have been inserted into one's mind; thought broadcasting (where the patient experiences his mind as open to others so that thoughts can leave it and be picked up by others); and thought withdrawal (where patients feel that thoughts are actually extracted from their heads). These experiences are very specific and, in the absence of organic brain disease, are diagnostic of schizophrenia.

Perception

There is a wide range of abnormal perceptual experiences, some of which can be part of normal experience and others which are indicative of mental illness or organic disease of the brain. It may be obvious from their behaviour that patients are seeing things or attending to auditory hallucinations ('voices'). Gentle inquiry about what the patient sees or hears will often elicit a description of the experience. Record as much detail as possible. Patients may be embarrassed to mention having had abnormal experiences, so specific inquiry is needed. For patients who have not had these experiences, being asked about them can be quite threatening as they may feel the doctor is suggesting they are 'mad'. To deal with this, it may be appropriate to make a normalising statement first, and then ask a screening question for abnormal perceptual experiences: 'It is quite common for people to have unusual experiences which may puzzle them. For example, some people may hear noises, music or voices when there is no one there, or people may see things which others are not able to see. Have you ever had any experiences like these?' If the patient has had such experiences, they can then be explored in more detail (Box 8.23).

Abnormal perception

Abnormal perception can occur in any of the sensory modalities: hearing, vision, smell, taste and somatosensory modalities (touch etc.). When perception is distorted, the perceived object is correctly recognised but altered in some way, such as alteration of intensity of sound, quality, colour or distortions of form. These occur in psychiatric disorders but also in many organic conditions such as epileptic seizures or toxic/metabolic states or alcohol withdrawal. A well-known phenomenon, namely hypnagogic or hypnopompic hallucinations (when you are falling asleep or waking up) does not usually indicate any kind of psychopathology, but rather your brain being variably aware when half-asleep/half-awake.

Illusions occur when the object is real but is misperceived, usually due to particular conditions in the perceptual environment, for example, an anxious person in a dimly lit street seeing a tree as a figure in pursuit. They are often caused by sensory deficit (partial blindness or deafness) or a lowered level of consciousness (common in acute confusional states).

Hallucinations are perceptions that are not based on any real external stimulus. They can occur in any sensory modality but the commonest are auditory, for example, a voice being heard by the patient but no one else hears it. Auditory hallucinations occur in many disorders including schizophrenia, organic brain disease and bipolar disorder. Voices can be heard speaking in the second or third person. In severe depression, voices are often second person and the content may be mood congruent, for example 'Look at you, you're useless, why not do away with yourself?'. By contrast, manic patients may hear God's voice telling them they have special powers or that they have been chosen to do something special. Third-person hallucinations (e.g. the patient being addressed as 'He' or 'She') in the absence of organic disease suggest schizophrenia (see Box 8.20 for first-rank symptoms).

Visual hallucinations are uncommon in psychiatric illness and are more suggestive of organic conditions, particularly an acute brain syndrome (e.g. delirium), illicit drug use (e.g. LSD) or drug withdrawal (e.g. delirium tremens). However, they do occasionally occur in schizophrenia or bipolar disorder.

Visual hallucinations vary from the elementary, for example flashes of light (from visual pathways and the occipital lobe) to complex visions of objects or scenes (from visual processing areas and the temporal lobes). In confusional states, small animals are often seen, typically at the periphery of vision. In temporal lobe epilepsy, complex visual hallucinations (scenic) may occur as may polymodal ones (involving multiple sensory modalities).

Hallucinations may also occur in other sensory modalities, for example olfactory, gustatory and tactile. Some patients with epilepsy commonly have olfactory and gustatory hallucinations (smelling odd smells or tasting unusual tastes). These experiences often precede an epileptic seizure. Patients with severe depression may have olfactory hallucinations, perceiving themselves as smelling unpleasant (cacosmia).

Tactile hallucinations are difficult to distinguish from illusions. In cocaine psychosis, patients may complain that insects are crawling over them (formication). Patients with schizophrenia may describe tactile hallucinations which may be incorporated into their delusional beliefs, for example, a patient may feel sensations on the skin and believe this is due to, for example, an animal or insect biting them. A specific subcategory of illness, delusional parasitosis, leads to constant dermatological referrals and the conviction of some persisting infestation. In the absence of organic brain disease, tactile hallucinosis is otherwise a first-rank symptom of schizophrenia (see Box 8.20).

Hallucinations can occur in the absence of mental illness, for example in extreme fatigue or in between

Box 8.23 Details of hallucinations

- When they started
- In what context
- Frequency
- Stereotypical or not
- Disturbing/frightening or pleasant/amusing
- Internal or external (auditory)
- Recognisable voice
- What voices say (record verbatim)
- Commands to do harm (part of risk assessment)

Box 8.24 Abnormal experiences of self and environment

Déjà vu

Patients feel that they have been in their current situation before – it can be normal or occur in temporal lobe epilepsy.

Capgras' syndrome

The patient asserts that people are not who they claim to be but are their double – occurs most commonly in schizophrenia but also in dementia.

Sense of a presence

This reflects a sixth sense of someone being around but not actually seen or heard. It is seen in schizophrenia, drug-induced states and simple fatigue.

Depersonalisation

An unpleasant sense that one is altered in some way and as if one is no longer completely real – patients will struggle to describe it. Often a manifestation of heightened anxiety and occurs in depression and severe fatigue.

Derealisation

Patients say that their surroundings feel unreal or grey or colourless. Some patients say it is 'as if' they are on a stage set and the world no longer feels real. This often accompanies depersonalisation, in a similar context of heightened anxiety, or depression or severe fatigue.

sleep and waking, and can occur in bereaved individuals, usually being experiences of either seeing or hearing the lost loved one and are generally experienced as comforting. They are a normal part of grief in some people and do not indicate psychopathology. Some people complain that, when alone, they feel the presence of someone else beside them. This may occur in grief reactions, when the patient is frightened, as a manifestation of hysteria or in organic brain disease and schizophrenia.

Abnormal experiences of self and environment are listed in Box 8.24.

Cognition

An assessment of cognitive function is a routine part of any MSE. It is impossible to interpret the significance of a variety of other symptoms, such as hallucinatory experiences or paranoid ideas, unless a basic assessment has been done of the state of consciousness and the presence of grossly normal brain function. In elderly people, or when organic brain disease is suspected (e.g. in acute confusional states), the assessment of the cognitive state is the most important part of the examination.

It can be difficult to perform a full assessment of cognitive function at a first interview, and in general only an outline of concentration, orientation and memory should be attempted. Many patients will be too disturbed, or there may be poor rapport, and some will resent an implication that there is something wrong with their brain. Even where formal cognitive testing is impossible or undesirable, a minimum assessment should be attempted, as follows:

- What is the patient's level of consciousness?
- Does it fluctuate?
- Is he fully alert and behaving appropriately for the context?
- Does he seem to be oriented to time, place and person?

In the majority of patients, it is possible to conduct a basic assessment of cognitive function. This should be preceded by an explanation that it is important for you to do a check of their memory and concentration, with a normalising statement that this is routine with all patients.

Basic assessment of cognitive function

A useful and commonly used semi-quantitative measure is the Mini-Mental State Examination (MMSE) (Box 8.25). Scores are to some extent dependent on educational level. The test has subcategories related to orientation, registration, attention, recall and language. The maximum score is 30, and scores lower than 21 are associated with cognitive impairment. The MMSE cannot differentiate multifocal from diffuse organic brain disease, but it provides a useful baseline assessment of a patient's cognitive performance.

Level of consciousness

The patient's level of alertness or, if unconscious, the level of unconsciousness, may be assessed. Some patients have fluctuating levels of consciousness; the mental state may then fluctuate between lucidity and gross abnormality. This is a manifestation of an acute organic confusional state. For a fuller account of the examination of the unconscious patient, see Chapters 9 and 16.

Orientation

The patient's orientation in time, place and person should be formally assessed by direct questioning and the answers written down verbatim. Disorientation is an important sign of organic brain disease, whether chronic or acute, but may also occur in chronic institutionalised schizophrenics and in hysterical dissociative states.

Time

Ask about the day, date, month, year and time of day. If the patient does not know the month, ask about the season. All patients should know the year and either the month or season and the approximate time of day (e.g. morning, afternoon, evening or night). However, not knowing the exact date is not

Box 8.25 Mini-mental state examination

Orientation

1 point for each correct answer.

What is the:
- time
- date
- day
- month
- year?

(Maximum 5 points)

What is the name of this:
- ward
- hospital
- district
- town
- country?

(Maximum 5 points)

Registration

Name three objects.

Award 1, 2 or 3 points according to how many the patient can repeat.

Resubmit list until patient is word perfect in order to use this for a later test of recall.

Score only first attempt.

(Maximum 3 points)

Attention and calculation

Have the patient subtract 7 from 100 and then subtract 7 from the result a total of five times; 1 point for each correct subtraction.

(Maximum 5 points)

Recall

Ask for the three objects used in the registration test, 1 point being awarded for each correct answer.

(Maximum 3 points)

Language

1 point each for two objects correctly named (e.g. pencil and watch) (2 points).

1 point for correct repetition of 'No ifs, ands and buts' (1 point).

3 points if three-stage commands correctly obeyed: 'Take this piece of paper in your right hand, fold it in half and place it on the floor' (3 points).

1 point for correct response to a written command, such as 'close your eyes' (1 point).

Have the patient write a sentence. Award 1 point if the sentence is meaningful, has a verb and a subject (1 point).

Test the patient's ability to copy a complex diagram of two intersecting pentagons (1 point).

(Total score 30)

uncommon these days, especially in those with unstructured timetables. Long stays in hospital, where one day is much like the next, however, are not conducive to an awareness of which particular day it is or the exact date of the month.

Place

Patients should know where they are (e.g. home or hospital) and approximately where it is situated (e.g. what town or part of the town). They should know the way to places such as the bathroom or toilet. Some patients with acute confusional states may say they are in hospital but that the hospital is part of their own home.

Person

If disorientation is suspected, patients should be asked their name and address. Ignorance of such basic details would indicate a relatively severe dementia or dissimulation, for whatever reason.

Attention and concentration

The patient's behaviour during the interview will have shown whether he is easily distracted (by internal or external stimuli) or have been paying attention to and concentrating on the questions you have asked. Attention and concentration can be tested more formally by tasks which involve keeping track of familiar sequences of information and so do not involve new learning. A basic test of attention and concentration is to ask the patient to repeat the days of the week or months of the year backwards and unobtrusively note how long it takes him. Another useful test is to ask the patient to spell 'world' backwards: the impaired patient often transposes the central letters of the word. Remember that literacy is implied in this test. Another test is to ask the patient to do serial sevens, for example 'Starting at 100, take 7 away and keep taking 7 away for as long as you can'. If the patient finds this too difficult, you can do the same thing with serial threes starting at 20. Performance in these mathematical tasks is more dependent on formal schooling than the first tasks, so this must be borne in mind. Repeating a sequence of digits (digit span) is also useful (see memory testing below).

Memory

In order to remember anything it must be registered, and this depends on attention and concentration. Where attention and concentration are very impaired, the patient will not be able to attend to memory tests so it is probably pointless to proceed with them. A basic subdivision of memory in clinical practice is into registration and immediate recall, short-term memory (about 5 minutes) and long-term memory (which encompasses recent memory going back a few days and remote memory of the more distant past and childhood).

In chronic organic brain disease, memory for recent events is diminished, whereas early in the illness the patient often remains able to remember events that have happened in the past and can give a coherent account of the family and early personal history. In Korsakov's psychosis due to thiamine deficiency, often associated with heavy drinking, the patient may confabulate, apparently recounting in great detail things which never happened. Confabulation is not deliberate invention but consists of the inappropriate recall of recent or distant past experiences, illustrating a defect in the process of recall of memories. In the case of head injuries or in epileptic attacks, a detailed attempt should be made to assess the presence of retrograde (time from insult to return of memory) and anterograde (period prior to the insult in which memory was absent) amnesia.

Memory impairment may be simulated for gain by some manipulative patients (so-called 'Ganser syndrome'), some of whom give approximate answers such as, to the question 'what colour is grass?' they answer 'green', and to the question 'how many legs has a cow?' they answer 'five'. Hysterical amnesia may occur in dissociative states in which there is a sudden total loss of memory. In contrast, in organic amnesia, even in dementing illnesses, long-term memory and personal identity are usually spared until the later stages of the disorder. Patients who are depressed may appear to have memory impairment, depressive pseudodementia, which may only become recognised when the depression lifts and the memory improves.

Testing registration and immediate recall

This can be tested using digit span. The interviewer asks the patient to repeat a series of digits immediately after the interviewer has said them. They should be said evenly about one per second with no particular grouping or emphasis. The patient then repeats the whole series. Start with three digits and build up the number of digits until the patient makes a mistake. Note the maximum that can be repeated without a mistake. This can be done repeating the digits backwards. An unimpaired person of average intelligence can repeat seven forward and five backward. Being able to repeat five or less forward suggests definite impairment.

Another test of registration and immediate recall is to read out a sentence and ask the patient to repeat it immediately. Standardised sentences exist (e.g. the 'Stanford Binet sentences').

Testing short-term memory

A useful test of this is to give patients fictitious details to remember. Tell them that as a test of their memory, they will be given a person's name, address and the name of a flower the person likes. Immediately after finishing, the patient is asked to repeat back the information and their response is recorded. If the patient makes a mistake, repeat the same information. Keep going until it is repeated correctly, and record how many tries this takes. When the patient repeats it correctly, ask that it be remembered, since it will be asked for again later. Continue with another part of the interview and, after 2 minutes, ask the patient to repeat the information, record the response and ask again after a further 3 minutes. Three or more mistakes at 5 minutes indicate a short-term memory problem.

Testing longer term memory – recent

A useful approach is to ask the patient about recent television programmes, such as the events in a popular soap opera or the fortunes of a favourite football team. Other recent events will include details about the hospital itself and how the patient got there (the interviewer needs to be able to corroborate the answers). Current affairs should also be asked about, such as the names of top politicians and details of any recent happenings of major importance. A less direct approach is to ask the patient what has been going on in the world or in this country recently, or (if there is a partner or friend present to corroborate) what they had for supper.

Testing longer term memory – remote

Autobiographical memory (ask about past experiences) is useful, but the interviewer needs to be able to corroborate the information (e.g. name of primary and secondary schools, teachers' names, date and place of marriage). Another approach is to ask about general events (e.g. the dates of the First and Second World Wars, the names of UK cities or capital cities). This kind of information is general knowledge and so will depend on education and intelligence as well as memory.

The patient's answers to all specific questions about memory should be recorded. Where there is evidence of potentially significant memory impairment, the patient often needs a formal assessment using detailed tests, often performed by a neuropsychologist.

Intelligence

An assessment of the patient's intelligence is one objective of the interview. Not only will this help to determine suitable treatment, it will also affect the interpretation of the MSE itself. In a patient with intelligence below the normal range, bizarre behaviour and abnormal ideas may occur as part of a normal fantasy life or as a result of stress or conflict and may not represent psychiatric illness. An approximate assessment of intelligence can be obtained from the educational and occupational history and from an assessment of general knowledge. Alternatively, intelligence can be tested more formally, especially by using the National Adult Reading Test (NART), as reading ability correlates closely with intelligence in the absence of other disabilities (see below). If in doubt, inquire whether patients can read and write and see whether they can solve simple mathematical problems, especially where these are related to daily activities such as shopping. Thus 'what change would you get from a pound coin, if you bought something that cost 35p?'.

Abstraction

Tests of abstraction are rarely used in routine practice but can be helpful in indicating patients who have very concrete thinking as seen in organic impairment (particularly frontal lobe disorders). Responses can also elicit florid thought disorder indicating schizophrenia. A useful test is to give patients proverbs of increasing difficulty and ask what the meaning is, for example 'Too many cooks spoil the broth'. An appropriate answer would be something like 'if too many people get involved in something it doesn't go very well' as compared to a concrete answer, for example 'too much cooking gets you angry'. Record the answers. Again, intelligence level is important in such tests.

Insight

This is an important section of the MSE since it informs the decision of how to manage a patient. Insight refers primarily to a patient's capacity to understand his problems and that they arise from a mental illness. It also relates to his understanding of specific symptoms (e.g. realising that his 'voices' are not real) and to being willing to comply with treatment such as medication.

There is a tendency for doctors to consider insight as either present (the patient is aware of having a mental illness) or absent (the patient has no awareness of illness). However, patients' views are generally more nuanced, and their own understanding of an illness can give a much richer and more useful assessment of insight. This will often involve an understanding of the patient's background culture and, for example, religious beliefs. Asking what patients think can be done to help the problem will always assist in forming a management plan, and working with a partner or family (and their insight) will also be of benefit.

Ending the interview

Ending the interview properly is nearly as important as how it begins. Some minutes before the end, inform patients that you are nearly finished and ask what else would they like to ask or talk about. Asking patients what they think is wrong, for example, should help with clarifying insight. Let the patient know that a report will be sent to the referring doctor and/or the GP.

Any psychiatric consultation should end with a clear outline to the patient about what you, the doctor, think is the problem and what should be done in terms of treatment. This stage may need negotiation, and it is important to leave a patient feeling that the history taking was part of a helpful process, showing that you do understand his problems and out of which useful interventions can arise.

Be clear about the management plan and give a specific follow-up appointment or advise that no follow up is required, given your view of his state of health. It is important to avoid a situation where patients feel they have shared a lot of very private information but cannot see the reason for this and will not get anything out of it. A good interview will act in the way of a detective explaining 'who did it?' to the assembled crowd in a standard detective story.

Final reflection

It can be very useful to spend a few moments thinking about how the patient made you feel. This can tell you something about the patient as well as about yourself. This is part of a process called countertransference. Countertransference is used in some forms of psychotherapy. Consider whether any difficulties the patient described to you may be due to the fact that they engender certain reactions in others. Likewise, your own feelings may be diagnostic, for example considerable sadness (and even at times tears in your eyes) when assessing a depressed patient, or intrusive anxiety when a very anxious patient outlines a stream of troubling symptoms which make you think of lots of physical diagnoses. By and large, however, the more symptoms a patient presents, the more certain you can be that it is not a specific organic illness.

Further investigations

Extended information gathering during further interviews, continuing assessment of the mental state, some laboratory investigations, psychological testing, brain imaging, social inquiry and occupational therapy assessment are all important.

Mental state evaluation

The evaluation of the mental state is a continuous process and should be carried out at each interview. The behaviour on admission wards of patients in hospital should always be regularly observed and documented. Two or three days' appropriate nursing observation, medical assessment and review can be diagnostically as clarifying as a laparotomy for an unknown surgical condition. Observation includes the way patients relate to other patients as well as to staff and visitors, and whether there are any signs of sleep or appetite disturbance or other abnormal behaviour (e.g. talking to themselves at night). Questionnaires and structured interview schedules may also aid quantitative assessment of the mental state and evaluation of progress and response to treatment.

Neuropsychological testing

Psychological tests can be used quantitatively to assess the patient's cognitive state, behaviour, personality and thinking process. Tests can be given to assess the level of intelligence, either briefly with the Mill Hill test or Raven's Progressive Matrices or in more detail with the Wechsler Adult Intelligence Scale (WAIS). In behavioural disorders, it is useful to carry out a thorough behavioural analysis that must be designed to be relevant to the individual problem. These investigations require the specialised skills of a clinical psychologist. If there is a question of localised organic brain dysfunction, neuropsychology tests that aim to explore specific cognitive processes or the functions of individual brain regions will be employed by the clinical neuropsychologist. A detailed neuropsychological assessment may be indicated to establish the presence of current cognitive functioning when cognitive decline is suspected. By comparing performance against expected premorbid levels and against comparable population norms, the abnormality may be defined. Repeat testing after an interval of several months may help to clarify an unclear diagnosis or support a more detailed prognosis when a diagnosis of dementia has been reached. Repeat testing may also help to distinguish the relatively static cognitive deficits arising from chronic depression in the elderly from the deteriorating scores in dementing illness. Patients with schizophrenia, at least in the acute stage, do not normally have cognitive decline, so if there is some clinical evidence of disturbed cognition then formal cognitive assessment may help to establish whether a condition other than schizophrenia is present.

Brain imaging

Electroencephalography (EEG), computed tomography (CT) and magnetic resonance imaging (MRI) are sometimes appropriate when exploring the possibility of a demonstrable organic cause for behavioural signs and symptoms, such as epilepsy or a space-occupying lesion. Indications for these techniques include periodicity in the behavioural changes, the presence of an altered level of consciousness or the finding of abnormalities on neurological examination. In the absence of any of these and in the presence of a typical psychiatric presentation, the chances of finding any contributory structural brain anomalies are small. However, if a clinical presentation is atypical, if the course of the illness does not proceed as expected or if a diagnosis of dementia is questioned, then structural brain imaging may be helpful. In the future, however, functional brain imaging may increasingly be of diagnostic value.

Patients presenting as emergencies

9

Geraint Morris

Introduction

A medical emergency requires swift recognition and prompt action. Recognition of urgency does not necessarily require a precise diagnosis; the fact that the patient is dangerously unwell is usually obvious due to an abnormality revealed by the internationally recognized assessment system for critically ill people of Airway, Breathing, Circulation, Disability and Exposure of the patient (ABCD and E). When an abnormality is found it should be acted upon and followed by a reassessment to establish if the intervention was useful. The clinician simultaneously needs to make a decision during this time as when to summon help if available.

The importance of clinical assessment

High-quality history taking and clinical examination will usually identify a diagnosis in a timely fashion and enable the initiation of appropriate investigation and management plans. In modern medicine, much has been made of the awareness of 'vital observations' or 'vital signs', which are often recorded by nursing staff and are usually available prior to a doctor's clinical assessment. It should be remembered that observations support clinical diagnosis and management and do not replace them.

The relationship between good history taking, sound examination skills and the ordering of appropriate investigations is as important in an emergency situation as in any other clinical setting. Many could try to argue that with the advancement of science, history taking and clinical examination should be superseded by simple awareness of available investigations. A poorly taken and rushed history, followed by numerous irrelevant investigations, is poor-quality medicine. Such an approach often leads to a wrong or missed diagnosis and some abnormal results of uncertain significance. Investigations are not always risk free, and patients should not be exposed unnecessarily to interventions such as ionizing radiation without serious thought.

This chapter deals with conditions requiring assessment and management within the first hour and focuses on the presenting complaint. Recognising the nature of an emergency presentation begins with how the patient comes to medical attention. This may be from information provided by the patient himself or witnesses such as paramedical (e.g. ambulance) staff, friends, family or concerned members of the public. The clinician will make an initial assessment by simply observing the patient; no apparent signs of life should initiate a life support response. If the patient is alive, then the general impression of how sick a patient appears is a reasonably accurate judgement of urgency. The experienced clinician will make these decisions in seconds. A particular clue will be in the respiratory rate and effort. An increased respiratory rate and work of breathing are the first physiological parameters to be altered in the shocked state and are often the subtle clues that alert a clinician to an unwell patient even from the end of the bed. Observing and recording this parameter for all patients is a fundamental part of developing a sound clinical method in emergency situations.

Urgency of response is dependant upon responses to assessment of the ABCD and E system of assessment. A talking patient has a patent airway, can maintain sufficient respiratory effort to make the vocal cords vibrate and move enough air to allow gas exchange. Similarly, if the patient is talking he must be perfusing his brain with sufficient oxygen to undertake the processes of speech as well as being responsive enough to do so. The clinician therefore has a degree of time with which to make further assessments and management decisions in this situation.

It should be stressed that the aim of this chapter is to help the reader develop a logical method for the clinical assessment of the acutely presenting patient. Although the topics covered here relate to common acute presentations, greater detail relevant to these presentations has not been provided, as much of this will be dealt with elsewhere in this book. It is also hoped that the reader will not look on this chapter as an amalgamation of lists but rather as an approach to logical thinking.

Diagnosis versus resuscitation

Sometimes, the severity of illness dictates that life-saving resuscitative treatment should begin before any diagnosis is reached, especially in acutely ill patients with problems such as shock or breathlessness. However, it should be possible to make an underlying diagnosis (or a differential diagnosis) in the majority of cases, and an acutely ill patient may not clinically improve until the treatment based on the correct diagnosis is provided. Acute resuscitation and the formulation of diagnoses will often be performed successfully in tandem.

The pyrexial and septic patient

Patients frequently present to emergency departments with signs and symptoms of infection, as do existing inpatients, irrespective of the cause for initial hospital admission. Severe infections have the potential for significant morbidity and mortality, and it is vital that they are identified and diagnosed promptly. Although the majority of patients presenting with fever will have an infective cause that can be easily elicited from the history and examination, it is also well recognized that there are many non-infective inflammatory causes (Table 9.1).

The concept of 'systemic inflammatory response syndrome' (SIRS) is widely recognized, in which an acute-phase response (such as pyrexia or hypothermia, tachypnoea, tachycardia, leucopenia or leucocytosis) indicates underlying inflammation. If these features are present in the face of infection, the term 'sepsis' is often used. The term 'severe sepsis' is used if there is evidence of sepsis with additional physiological upset, such as new or increased requirement for oxygen, hypotension, acute oliguria, delayed capillary refill or mottling or deranged laboratory values (e.g. raised serum creatinine, coagulation abnormalities, raised serum lactate, thrombocytopenia, raised bilirubin). Severe sepsis leading to shock ('septic shock') is discussed below.

The history will often suggest the source of sepsis (cough, abdominal pain, dysuria, headache). Other important features include details of any recent travel (country and duration of residence), a drug and lifestyle history (including any recreational drug use), weight loss, chronic illness and any risk factors for immunosuppression such as recent chemotherapy, steroid therapy and the possibility of HIV infection.

The examination should initially focus on critical issues that need immediate action. If the patient has a raised pulse or heart rate, respiratory rate, prolonged capillary refill, hypoxia or hypotension, oxygen, fluids and appropriate antibiotics should be administered urgently before embarking on a detailed examination. In searching for a source, look for exudate or pus at the back of the throat. Lung auscultation may reveal features of acute bronchitis (wheeze) or consolidation. Heart murmurs in the presence of fever may indicate infective endocarditis. The abdominal examination should identify any tenderness (e.g. right upper quadrant in cholecystitis, loin in pyelonephritis). If a patient has obvious cellulitis, look carefully for skin bites, lacerations or tinea pedis as a possible route of entry. If the patient complains of headache, look for features of meningism. Lymphadenopathy and superficial or skin abscesses should be noted.

Immediate investigations may include those which lend support to an inflammatory process (white cell count, C-reactive protein), severity of infection (blood cultures), consequences such as dehydration (urea and electrolytes), underlying predisposition (blood sugar) and source (urinalysis, urine culture, blood culture, chest X-ray). In response to the history and examination, one may proceed to throat swab, blood films for malaria, faeces analysis (toxin or culture), lumbar puncture, transthoracic echocardiogram or abdominal imaging (ultrasound or CT scan).

Table 9.1 Logical thinking for patients presenting with fever

Mechanism	Common or important examples
Infection	Viral (upper respiratory, lower respiratory, infectious mononucleosis, hepatitis A); bacterial (less common causes include infective endocarditis, meningitis, tuberculosis, spontaneous bacterial peritonitis, pleural empyema, cholangitis); parasitic (malaria, schistosomiasis); fungal
Systemic inflammation	Rheumatoid arthritis; systemic lupus erythematosus (SLE); polymyalgia rheumatica; Wegener's granulomatosis; inflammatory bowel disease; malignant neuroleptic syndrome; blood transfusion reaction
Malignancy and granulomatous disease	Solid tumours; lymphoma; leukaemia; amyloidosis; sarcoidosis
Drugs	Prescription; recreational (e.g. ecstasy)

The patient with chest pain

Although the majority of patients who present to the emergency unit with chest pain will not have clinically significant coronary artery disease, it is this potential diagnosis that often dominates the initial thoughts of the assessing doctor. This is why patients with chest pain who appear unwell or in need of immediate resuscitation should have an ECG recorded before the initial history and examination are complete. The outcome from attempts to open an occluded coronary artery depends on the speed with which

Table 9.2 Logical thinking for patients presenting with chest pain

Potentially life-threatening conditions – all usually causing central chest pain	Other causes of central chest pain	Causes of pleuritic chest pain
Coronary artery disease (myocardial infarction or acute coronary syndrome) Massive pulmonary embolus (PE) Thoracic aortic dissection: severe, tearing in nature, radiating to interscapular area Pneumothorax (particularly tension) Oesophageal rupture	Pericarditis Gastro-oesophageal reflux disease (GORD) Muscular or skeletal Anxiety	Pericarditis PE (more likely to be smaller and more peripheral) Pneumothorax Pneumonia (reactive pleuritis) Empyema Viral pleuritis Malignant involvement of chest wall (including mesothelioma) Rib trauma, fracture or metastases Inflammatory pleuritis (e.g. rheumatoid arthritis, systemic lupus erythematosus)

arrangements can be made for either thrombolysis or angioplasty, so there is little to be gained (and much to be lost) from a prolonged assessment. In many countries, paramedical staff are trained to recognize acute myocardial infarction on an ECG and take patients direct to the nearest centre that provides round-the-clock acute angioplasty services. However, such facilities are not universally available and in some patients with critical coronary artery disease the initial ECG recording may be normal, so it is essential that a careful history and examination are performed on all patients with chest pain not obviously in immediate need of resuscitation or intervention. Patients with chest pain are, understandably, often anxious about the possibility of underlying serious heart disease and an important part of the doctor's role is to project calm reassurance.

Chest pain that has a life-threatening cause (Table 9.2) is usually central and of sudden/rapid onset. Certain features may be diagnostically helpful; these include radiation of the pain to the left arm and/or jaw (myocardial ischaemia) or the interscapular area (aortic dissection); accompanying breathlessness (massive pulmonary embolus or pneumothorax); or a clear temporal association with prolonged vomiting (oesophageal rupture). In pericarditis, the pain may be 'classic' (central pain relieved by sitting forward) or pleuritic. The features of chest infections and viral infections should be obvious. Pneumonias are not infrequently associated with headache. Important examination features to note during the initial, rapid assessment of an ill patient with chest pain include the fine crepitations of pulmonary oedema, the hyperresonant percussion and tracheal deviation of pneumothorax and the asymmetric blood pressure readings consistent with thoracic aortic dissection.

If 'ABC' interventions are not required for resuscitation, if the patient is stable and there are no other features requiring immediate action (e.g. peripheral cyanosis), a more considered assessment is appropriate. In addition to the history, the risk factors for coronary artery disease and pulmonary embolism (PE) may be factored into the diagnostic process (Box 9.1 and Table 9.3). The blood pressure should be taken in both arms, particularly if the arm pulses are unequal. Unequal blood pressure measurements in the arms raises the possibility of aortic dissection and serious consideration should be given to appropriate urgent imaging (usually thoracic CT scanning). A raised jugular venous pressure may suggest early heart failure. Precordial auscultation may reveal a pericardial rub. There may be classical signs of pneumonia. It can be difficult to differentiate between pleuritic and

Table 9.3 Modified Wells criteria for assessing the risk of pulmonary embolism (PE) in a patient with symptoms consistent with pulmonary embolism

Clinical parameter	Score
Clinical evidence of deep vein thrombosis (DVT)	3
No alternative diagnosis likely other than PE	3
Heart rate greater than 100 per minute	1.5
Surgery or immobility in preceding 4 weeks	1.5
Previous confirmed DVT or PE	1.5
Haemoptysis	1
Active malignancy	1
Total score	**Risk**
>6	High
2-6	Moderate
<2	Low

Box 9.1 Risk factors for coronary heart disease

- Age
- Blood pressure
- Smoking
- Cholesterol
- Diabetes
- Racial grouping
- Family history of coronary artery disease or stroke before the age of 60
- Girth (obesity)

musculoskeletal chest pain from the history, but pain exacerbated by palpation and posture changes more than by inspiration is more likely to be musculoskeletal. Signs of deep venous thrombosis automatically raise the clinical suspicion of pulmonary embolism.

The serious nature of many of the diagnoses that present with chest pain dictates that the threshold for certain investigations is often low. In addition to being a crucial test at the moment of initial assessment, the ECG has additional value when it is repeated over a period of time, looking for any evolution in its appearance (often called 'dynamic changes'). Detailed description and explanations of the possible ECG features of myocardial infarction and pulmonary embolism are given elsewhere. The chest X-ray may show features of pneumothorax, pneumomediastinum (from oesophageal rupture), heart failure, widened mediastinum (often seen in thoracic aortic dissection), pneumonia, rib fractures/destruction and pleural effusions. In the emergency unit, measurement of troponin in blood (a protein released when cardiac myocytes undergo ischaemic necrosis) is performed on many patients with chest pain. It is not a diagnostic test of cardiac chest pain, but 'negative' results (below a certain threshold) indicate that the risk of a serious acute cardiac event in the ensuing 30 days is extremely low. A negative troponin test does not obviate the need to make a detailed clinical assessment; a patient with a typical history of 'crescendo angina' (worsening in severity and/or frequency, occurring at rest or on minimal exertion over days to weeks) should still be treated as an emergency even if the troponin result is reassuring.

The breathless patient

When life-threatening conditions present with breathlessness, it should be rapidly established whether immediate and resuscitative interventions are required whilst simultaneously making a clinical assessment to establish the cause (Table 9.4). The patient should be placed in a safe, monitored (ECG and pulse oximetry) environment and clinicians should act quickly if there is evidence of visible distress, the usage of accessory muscles of respiration, high respiratory rate, high pulse rate, cyanosis or observable low oxygen saturations. The immediate response should be to administer high-flow oxygen to the patient with any of the above findings, unless there is good evidence that this has on this occasion, or previous occasions, caused breathing difficulties (most commonly patients with chronic obstructive pulmonary disease, COPD). In the majority of cases, arrangements for urgent ECG and chest X-ray (CXR) will be made immediately, before the initial clinical assessment is complete. There may even be certain clinical scenarios (e.g. upper airway obstruction, tension pneumothorax) in which immediate clinical intervention is necessary.

Table 9.4 Potentially life-threatening conditions presenting as breathlessness

Clinical assessment	Potentially life-threatening conditions
Stridor (may be mistaken for wheeze)	Partial obstruction of trachea or major airway
Audible wheeze (one should listen very carefully, as it may be very quiet)	Severe asthma Anaphylaxis Acute bronchitis Pulmonary oedema
Diffuse features	Pneumonitis Widespread pneumonia Pulmonary oedema
Significant asymmetry of findings in a whole lung on percussion and/or auscultation	Pneumothorax Massive pleural effusion Total lung collapse
Focal features of consolidation	Lobar collapse from tumour, foreign body or mucus plug Pneumonia
No obvious abnormality	Pulmonary embolism (hypoxia often present) Metabolic acidosis (hypoxia often absent)

General principles

A rapid clinical assessment will establish if detailed history taking is going to be realistic. A conscious, alert patient who is able to speak in full sentences is reassuring. Features suggestive of an obstructed airway include complete absence of airway sounds (complete obstruction) or added sounds of laboured breathing where air entry is diminished (partial obstruction). Tachycardia and tachypnoea may reflect respiratory distress. Use of accessory muscles of respiration is typical in the partially obstructed airway, and signs include a tracheal tug (a slight downward movement of the trachea with each inspiratory effort), paradoxical chest and abdominal movement ('see-sawing' – the chest wall moves inwards during inspiration and outwards in expiration and there is dyssynchrony between rib cage and abdomen), with supraclavicular and intercostal 'in-drawing'. Irritability, agitation and reduced consciousness level may reflect hypoxaemia and carbon dioxide retention. Do not rely on cyanosis as a feature in identifying an obstructed airway as this is a very late preterminal sign. Observe or ask about 'best breathing position'. Be aware that the patient may have positioned himself for optimal airflow in the setting of airway obstruction; moving the patient into a supine position may precipitate loss of the airway altogether. Low pulse oximetry readings (SpO_2) reflect inadequacy of oxygenation, although it is important to remember that pulse oximetry provides a measure of oxygenation and is

Table 9.5 Logical thinking for conditions causing breathlessness, including the emergency conditions

Clinical assessment	Classification	Condition
Stridor	Large airway disease	Partial obstruction of trachea or major airway
Bilateral or diffuse wheeze	Small airway disease	Asthma Acute bronchitis (including bronchitic component to chronic obstructive pulmonary disease) Anaphylaxis Pulmonary oedema (presenting as bronchial oedema) Obesity hypoventilation syndrome (though often the wheeze from obesity-related airflow limitation is not heard)
Asymmetric features in whole lung field (tracheal deviation, hyper-resonance to percussion and diminished breath sounds)	Pleural disease	Pneumothorax
Asymmetric features in whole lung field (tracheal deviation, stony dullness to percussion and diminished breath sounds)	Pleural disease	Massive pleural effusion
Asymmetric features in whole lung field (tracheal deviation, dullness to percussion and diminished breath sounds)	Large airway disease	Total lung collapse (tumour, foreign body, mucus plug)
Diffuse bilateral abnormalities (crepitations)	Diffuse parenchymal disease	Pneumonitis Pulmonary oedema Pulmonary fibrosis
Diffuse bilateral abnormalities (bronchial breathing)	Diffuse parenchymal disease	Multilobar or bronchopneumonia
Focal abnormality (bronchial breathing)	Focal parenchymal disease	Pneumonia Lobar collapse Bronchiectasis
Focal abnormality (dullness to percussion and diminished breath sounds)	Pleural disease	Pleural effusion
Bilateral, focal abnormalities (basal stony dullness and diminished breath sounds)	Pleural disease	Bilateral pleural effusions
Bilateral, focal abnormalities (bronchial breath sounds)	Parenchymal disease	Bilateral pneumonia (e.g. bibasal pneumonia)
Thoracic deformity	Chest wall skeletal disease	Scoliosis Thoracic surgery
No obvious abnormality	Pulmonary vascular disease	Pulmonary embolism Pulmonary hypertension
	Respiratory muscle weakness	Diaphragm paralysis Neuromuscular disease
	Compensatory effort	Metabolic acidosis Anaemia
	Psychogenic	Psychogenic hyperventilation

This table is not intended to be an exhaustive list. It is aimed at assisting logical thought, particularly with regard to clinical features.

not the same as ventilation. Arterial blood gas sampling may be helpful but should not delay management. Respiratory acidosis, with a high carbon dioxide tension ($PaCO_2$) and reduced pH, reflects alveolar hypoventilation. When assessing patients, look carefully for these signs and symptoms and always call for help early from an anaesthetist if airway compromise is suspected. The young can compensate well initially, masking impending desaturation and hypoxaemia. Be mindful of injuries that will compromise the airway, such as facial burns, bleeding and foreign bodies obstructing the airway. Always provide high flow oxygen with a reservoir bag at 15 litres/minute, and reassess frequently, looking for signs of deterioration.

In the emergency situation of the acutely breathless patient it is helpful to consider the potential problem in one of two 'groupings': upper airway obstruction and cardiopulmonary pathologies that affect ventilation and/or gas exchange (Table 9.5).

Airway obstruction

Most commonly, airway obstruction occurs in a patient with a decreased level of consciousness with resultant loss of the cough reflex used to clear normal bronchial secretions. Such patients are also at risk of aspiration of gastric contents because of depression of other reflexes that control the competence of the tracheo-oesophageal junction. Pragmatically, this can be easily inferred by the patient's response to insertion of an adjunct such as an oropharyngeal (Guedel) airway. Fully conscious patients, in whom laryngeal reflexes are present, will not tolerate this airway and inserting one may precipitate gagging, vomiting and laryngospasm. In a patient with reduced consciousness and a threatened airway, the adjunct is tolerated, with consequent relief of backward tongue displacement and soft palate obstruction. Insertion of a Guedel airway should usually be combined with manoeuvring the patient into the recovery (lateral) position (the effect of which is to push the tongue and jaw forward under gravity, thereby improving the airway) (Fig. 9.1).

The second, less common scenario of airway obstruction is the patient presenting with stridor – the term used to describe the harsh high-pitched musical breathing noise caused by narrowing of the upper airways with impending complete obstruction. It may be inspiratory, expiratory or biphasic, although it is most commonly heard just during inspiration. Inspiratory stridor indicates laryngeal obstruction, since the negative intrathoracic pressures exacerbate extrathoracic obstruction during inspiration. Intrathoracic obstruction may cause expiratory stridor, as the airways are compressed during expiration. Common causes of stridor include tumours (usually laryngeal/tracheal but also mediastinal and oesophageal), peritonsillar and retropharyngeal abscesses, inhalation of a foreign body and laryngotracheobronchitis ('croup'). Children are more susceptible to the latter two causes due to the narrower diameter of their airway and the fact that normal inquisitive behaviour often leads to objects being inserted into their mouths. In developed countries, vaccination programmes that include *Haemophilus influenzae* type B vaccine have led to a sharp reduction in the incidence of acute epiglottitis – an important cause of stridor in children in which infection by this organism of the valve at the tracheo-oesophageal junction causes fever, dysphagia, sore throat and (classically) drooling of saliva as the pain of swallowing dictates that the child will try to avoid doing this. If stridor as opposed to wheeze is considered, the cause may be evident from the history (airway cancer, foreign body exposure or anaphylaxis). The examiner's ear should be placed carefully close to the mouth of the patient to try to establish the source of airflow limitation. Stridor of any cause in any age group is frightening to patients; the attending doctor's demeanor needs to be calm and gentle whilst simultaneously arranging emergency assistance from colleagues (e.g. ENT and/or anaesthesia) to establish a secure airway. Acute stridor is an airway emergency, and the teams of intensive care and ear, nose and throat specialists should be mobilized as quickly as possible.

Specific mention should be made of burn victims in whom inhalation of superheated gases and toxins of combustion causes swelling of the lining of the tracheobronchial tree with consequent obstruction. The history will usually be obvious, but important clinical signs that suggest airway injury include a hoarse voice, singed hairs of the nasal passages and soot and erythema in the upper airway. Recognising this promptly should initiate measures to secure the airway early with an endotracheal tube. The stridor associated with the severe upper airway oedema of anaphylaxis will be dealt with later in this chapter.

The importance of recognizing airway obstruction as the cause of acute breathlessness is self-evident; although provision of supplemental oxygen is a crucial therapeutic intervention, it will not resolve the underlying problem of hypercapnia associated with hypoventilation.

Acute breathlessness due to ventilatory and/or oxygenation defects

The sensation of breathlessness is poorly understood. In normal respiration active inspiration is followed by passive expiration, but in breathlessness of any

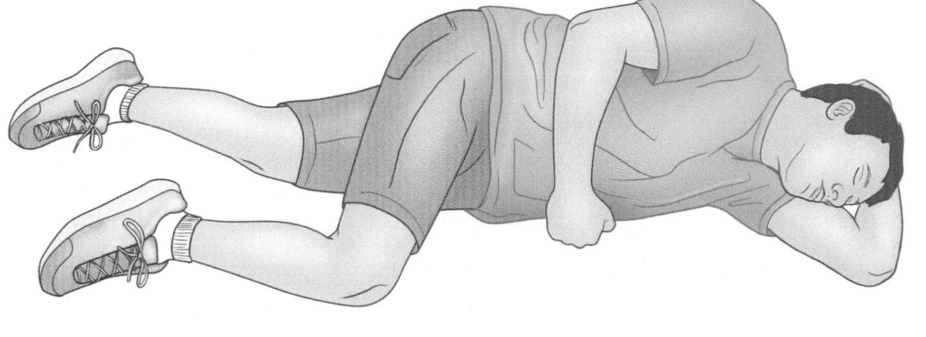

Figure 9.1 The recovery position.

cause there is active expiration and a change in the normal inspiration:expiration time ratio. The diaphragm works at a mechanical disadvantage when this ratio changes and hypoxia added to this situation may contribute further to the discomfort of breathlessness. The usual cause is of loss of lung compliance/elastic recoil which requires active expiration to compensate. This is seen either with chronic damage to lung parenchyma or acutely when the alveolar spaces are filled with material which is less compressible than aerated lung such as interstitial fluid, pus or blood. In some conditions (classically acute asthma) severe overinflation of the lungs reduces their ability to expire effectively. Finally the sensation of breathlessness may occur with conditions completely unrelated to the heart or lungs, such as diabetic ketoacidosis. Here, a change in blood pH is sensed by chemoreceptors in the brainstem leading to Kussmaul's breathing ('air hunger') as an attempt is made to hyperventilate and blow off carbon dioxide, thereby improving the acidosis.

History taking is often limited in breathless patients. Accompanying friends, relatives or carers may be able to provide collateral information and it may be possible to elicit certain key features by asking simple 'yes/no' questions ('Do you have asthma? Have you eaten something you are allergic to?). It may be impossible to differentiate between the wheeze of acute asthma, anaphylaxis, bronchitis or, rarely, pulmonary oedema, but a history of previous asthma and atopy, fever or chest pain may help direct the clinician to a working diagnosis. If asthma is suspected, then early administration of a beta-2-adrenergic agonist can be lifesaving and will rarely cause harm. The ability to administer this medication either via nebulizer or metered dose inhaler and spacer device is a fundamental skill that should be familiar to all clinicians. If it is ineffective due to severe bronchoconstriction, then intravenous administration can be considered by experienced clinicians.

Clinical examination of the breathless patient may reveal significant asymmetry in chest expansion, percussion and/or auscultation. In general, the side that moves less has the pathology within it. The deviated trachea will be ipsilateral to the side of lung collapse or focal fibrosis and contralateral to a tension pneumothorax or very large pleural effusion. These are differentiated by the percussion note which will be hyper-resonant in tension pneumothorax and dull (some say 'stony dull') in the presence a massive effusion. Breath sounds may be absent or poorly heard in the affected lung in all of these conditions. Relief may be immediate with minimal aspiration of either air (tension pneumothorax) or fluid (pleural effusion) prior to formal drainage.

Diffuse polyphonic wheeze or indistinct widespread coarse crackles with acute on chronic shortness of breath is typical of an exacerbation of COPD. Widespread bilateral unchanging fine crepitations are most often heard with acute pulmonary oedema. Focal features such as tactile fremitus, dullness to percussion, increased vocal resonance and bronchial breathing provide evidence of consolidation and/or collapse and can usually be confirmed by an urgent chest X-ray.

It may be impossible to differentiate between the wheeze of severe asthma, anaphylaxis and acute bronchitis. One should try to establish a history of asthma or exposure to potential allergens. There may be historical features of infection. Examination may identify other features of anaphylaxis, such as swollen facial tissue (orbital areas, lips, tongue). The wheeze of pulmonary oedema occurs when there is compression of the major bronchi by oedematous parenchyma (when diffuse features are heard in addition to wheeze) or when there is predominant bronchial oedema (when the diffuse auscultatory features may not be heard). The patient with pulmonary oedema manifesting as wheeze may share other clinical features seen in 'classical' pulmonary oedema.

If there are no obvious examination abnormalities in the acutely breathless patient, then the history will need further clarification. Chest pain and/or breathlessness in the presence of relevant risk factors raise the possibility of pulmonary embolism (PE) (Table 9.3). Investigation with an arterial blood gas is useful in determining oxygen and carbon dioxide exchange alongside any disturbances in pH. Most conditions causing breathlessness are exacerbated by lying flat and relieved by sitting up, though this 'orthopnoea' is most obvious with pulmonary oedema and respiratory muscle weakness. Breathlessness relieved by lying flat (platypnoea) is relatively rare and is most often associated with PE; in this case, the supine posture improves pulmonary perfusion and provides relief. A cough acutely productive of purulent sputum may support a working diagnosis of pneumonia. Longer-standing cough may be associated with non-purulent sputum production (asthma, chronic obstructive pulmonary disease and bronchiectasis) or non-production (interstitial lung disease and lung cancer). An absent or weak cough may suggest respiratory muscle disease. Acute, frothy sputum (occasionally tinged with blood) may be seen in pulmonary oedema. Frank haemoptysis may occur in PE, lung cancer, pulmonary vasculitis, pneumonia, tuberculosis and acute bronchitis.

The patient with hypotension or shock

There are numerous definitions for 'shock' but a useful one may be considered to be 'a failure of blood flow to provide sufficient perfusion of the major organs'. It is often associated with hypotension. Hypotension and shock are clinical emergencies and require appropriate and immediate intervention. Hypotension may be defined as 'abnormally low blood pressure for that given patient', which means interpreting the documented blood pressure in context. For one patient, a 'normal' recorded blood pressure may be significantly lower compared to previous readings. In another, a 'low' blood pressure may be entirely normal for that specific patient. If in doubt, a low blood pressure should always be acted upon. For the purposes of this chapter, it will be accepted that hypotension and shock encompass similar pathologies and belong on the same spectrum. Severe hypotension may lead to shock. It is essential, therefore, that, irrespective of aetiology, this is seen as a medical emergency, and a joint effort is made simultaneously to initiate resuscitative treatment and make a diagnosis. This involves administering intravenous fluids while other clinical features and vital observations are elicited. The fluids may be subsequently stopped if pulmonary oedema becomes evident. The organ that is most sensitive under perfusion is the brain; confusion and decreased levels of consciousness in the context of shock indicate poor oxygenation, so patients should usually be nursed lying flat to promote cerebral perfusion.

Teamwork is paramount. If more than one clinician is available, one may focus on taking a history while another may take responsibility for examination and institution of treatment. Examination findings, irrespective of the cause, may include a rapid pulse and heart rate and a third heart sound. It should be noted that in otherwise fit individuals, in the face of severe hypovolaemia, there may be a prolonged period of 'compensation', in which the healthy heart maintains cardiac output and a normal blood pressure by increasing the heart rate and the force of contraction. Therefore, the patient with unexplained tachycardia should be examined and investigated thoroughly, and impending shock should not be missed.

During resuscitation, a quick starting point is needed when assessing the causes of shock, as a correct diagnosis will dictate the most appropriate intervention. One way to categorize shock is to differentiate causes into those with a wide or a narrow pulse pressure ('pulse pressure' is the difference between systolic and diastolic blood pressure) (Table 9.6). As a general rule, patients with widened pulse pressure will present with warmer peripheries, and the palpable peripheral pulse may be more 'bounding' in nature. Patients with narrowed pulse pressure often have cooler peripheries, with weak, 'thready' peripheral pulses. Although 'normal' pulse pressure is often quoted as 40 mmHg, it should be noted that during hypotension this figure should be interpreted with caution. For example, a blood pressure of 75/40 mmHg could be interpreted as having a widened pulse pressure of 35 mmHg, as this is in the context of a low systolic blood pressure.

There are varying types of shock, which need general discrimination to apply definitive treatment (Box 9.2). One type of shock may evolve into another, leading to a mixed clinical picture requiring more than one treatment strategy. For example, it is not uncommon for septic shock (ordinarily presenting with a widened pulse pressure) to lead rapidly to cardiogenic shock (usually characterized by a narrow pulse pressure) in patients with coexisting heart disease. Septic shock is also often associated with hypovolaemic shock. It is not uncommon for cardiogenic shock to improve with treatment but then be superseded by infection and septic shock. If it is not possible to categorize a pulse pressure into narrow or wide, other features described below may help identify the cause of shock.

Narrow pulse pressure associated with shock is almost always a consequence of cardiac failure ('cardiogenic shock') or hypovolaemia ('hypovolaemic shock'). Examination findings, in addition to specific features described below, may include cold and pale limb peripheries. Although there are many general causes of widened pulse pressure (including aortic regurgitation, thyrotoxicosis, fever, anaemia, pregnancy, patent ductus arteriosus, aortic dissection, raised intracranial pressure, vasodilating drugs, Beriberi heart disease and old age), wide pulse pressure *with shock* is almost always a consequence of profound vasodilatation, usually with warm limb peripheries. The most common cause is infection ('septic shock'); less common causes include anaphylaxis ('anaphylactic shock') and loss of neurogenic vasomotor tone ('neurogenic shock').

Hypovolaemic shock

Conceptually, this is the easiest to understand as simply insufficient circulating volume to provide for the oxygen demands of the organs. Typically, this is due to haemorrhage and may be divided into four classes (Table 9.7). External haemorrhage is usually clinically obvious, either from the history or from visual evidence of blood loss. The source of internal bleeding may be more difficult to diagnose, although

Table 9.6 Logical thinking in shock

Mechanism	Common or important examples
Narrow pulse pressure	Hypovolaemic shock (haemorrhage, fluid losses from enteral tract, fluid losses from renal tract, fluid losses from skin (burns)); cardiogenic shock from myocardial failure (coronary ischaemia, acute myocarditis)
Widened pulse pressure	Septic shock; anaphylactic shock; neurogenic shock

Box 9.2 Types of shock

Hypovolaemic
Cardiogenic
Distributive
Obstructive

Table 9.7 Classes of haemorrhage

	Class I	Class II	Class III	Class IV
Blood loss (ml)	Up to 750	750-1500	1500-2000	>2000
Blood loss (% Blood volume)	Up to 15%	15%-30%	30%-40%	>40%
Pulse rate	<100	>100	>120	>140
Blood pressure	Normal	Normal	Decreased	Decreased
Pulse pressure (mmHg)	Normal or increased	Decreased	Decreased	Decreased
Respiratory rate	14-20	20-30	30-40	>35
Urine output (ml/hr)	>30	20-30	5-15	Negligible
CNS/Mental status	Slightly anxious	Mildly anxious	Anxious, confused	Confused, lethargic

Table 9.8 Internal bleeding sites

Pelvis	Pelvic fracture Ectopic pregnancy
Abdomen	Liver Spleen Kidney
Thorax	Massive haemothorax
Gastrointestinal	Oesophageal and/or gastric varices Duodenal ulcer
Retroperitoneal	Ruptured abdominal aortic aneurysm
Peripheries	Long bone fractures

the prevailing clinical picture is common to both (Table 9.8). Cool peripheries and corresponding changes in heart rate, blood pressure and respiratory rate are key indicators. Simple assessment through testing the capillary refill time and provocative testing such as a postural blood pressure is useful in unmasking compensated shock. In the initial period following a haemorrhage, it should be remembered that the blood haemoglobin concentration may be preserved. Once bleeding is suspected as the cause of hypovolaemic shock, the clinical approach is straightforward and intuitive; replace the blood that has been lost (as it is the best resuscitative fluid) and stop the bleeding. External bleeding can be controlled in most situations by locally applied pressure. Internal bleeding often necessitates surgical intervention, although interventional radiology techniques are increasingly being applied in a number of situations and specialist institutions.

Although external and internal bleeding are the most common causes of hypovolaemic shock, non-haemorrhagic causes also exist. In developing countries gastrointestinal fluid loss (e.g. due to cholera) is a leading cause of death, especially in children. Other volume-losing conditions include salt-wasting renal conditions, burns, sequestration of fluid into the bowel and adrenal failure (Addison's disease). As a rule, hypovolaemic shock in the context of these conditions takes longer to develop than, for example, acute intra-abdominal blood loss, so a carefully taken history is likely to be diagnostically informative. Replacement of fluid with crystalloid in the first instance is the most important intervention.

Cardiogenic shock

Cardiogenic shock refers to a failure of the heart to pump blood effectively to meet peripheral oxygen demands. It is most frequently due to a large myocardial infarction but may also be due to cardiac dysrhythmias, other causes of cardiac muscle pump failure (e.g. myocarditis, cardiomyopathy) or acute cardiac valve problems. In this situation, as with hypovolaemic shock, there will usually be a narrow pulse pressure. Cardiogenic shock may be associated with a preceding history of chest pain, palpitations or breathlessness (in particular orthopnoea). There are frequently auscultatory features of pulmonary oedema. Patients with brittle cardiac function may present with cardiogenic shock irrespective of the initial trigger. An ECG is often informative and may show changes of recent infarction, dysrhythmia and nonspecific changes of pericarditis, myocarditis and cardiomyopathy. Treatment will largely depend on the cause; inotropic support and invasive measures are frequently required.

Distributive shock

Distributive shock is due to inappropriate distribution of a normal or elevated cardiac output. Invariably there is profound vasodilatation with associated capillary leakage. The most common cause is severe sepsis, in which an overwhelming cascade of inflammatory mediators causes distribution of blood to inappropriate areas. The clinical history may suggest an obvious source of infection and examination findings may include a fever, observed rigors, auscultatory features of lung consolidation or abdominal features of peritonitis.

Anaphylactic shock is usually clinically easily apparent (respiratory distress, agitation, urticarial rash, face, mouth, tongue and orbital swelling and wheeze), but there may not be a history of allergy or hypersensitivity. Accompanying hypotension is frequent, due to marked vasodilatation, pooling of blood and a consequent reduction in venous return to the heart. Knowing the common causes of the allergy and the ability to recognize urticaria are important. Once recognized, detailed clinical assessment is inappropriate; immediate resuscitation is required with intramuscular adrenaline (epinephrine) and intravenous fluids.

Neurogenic shock is another form of distributive shock and is very rare. It is due to disruption of the vasomotor tone of blood vessels causing inappropriate dilatation and pooling of blood with a marked reduction in venous return and consequently cardiac output. A history of either spinal trauma or medical intervention (e.g. epidural anaesthesia or autonomic blocking agents) will usually prompt its consideration as a diagnosis.

Obstructive shock

Most commonly, obstructive shock occurs with massive pulmonary embolism in which obstruction to blood flow through the pulmonary circulation reduces venous return to the left atrium and ventricle so markedly that cardiac output into the systemic circulation falls and hypotension develops. Patients will be breathless and usually have chest pain. The combination of clinical signs of right heart strain with hypotension and hypoxia should prompt consideration of massive pulmonary embolism. Obstruction to the outflow of the left ventricle occurs with severe aortic stenosis, although usually this condition develops over a prolonged period of time.

The patient with diminished consciousness

The definition of 'consciousness' may be the (waking) state of awareness of oneself and environment. The absence of awareness, therefore, even when one is stimulated, may implicate diffuse or multifocal brain dysfunction and may be defined as 'coma' or 'diminished consciousness'. Although the last two terms may be seen as synonymous, the term 'coma' may have widespread and conflicting implications. In these situations, ambiguity should be avoided, and the patient should be described as having 'diminished consciousness'.

Consciousness is controlled by the brainstem through a system of nerve cells and fibres known as the 'reticular activating system' or the 'ascending arousal system'. The cerebrum helps maintain consciousness and alertness and at least one hemisphere, as well as the reticular activating system, must be functioning normally to maintain consciousness. The brain's ability to adjust its activity and consciousness levels can therefore be impaired in several ways, particularly when both cerebral hemispheres are suddenly and severely damaged, when the reticular activating system malfunctions, when blood flow or the amount of nutrients (such as oxygen or sugar) supplying the brain decreases or when toxic substances impair brain function.

There are several ways to objectively describe the conscious state, though perhaps the two best known 'scores' are the Glasgow Coma Scale (GCS) and the 'AVPU' score (Tables 9.9 and 9.10). The GCS

Table 9.9 The Glasgow Coma Scale

	1	2	3	4	5	6
Eyes	Does not open eyes	Opens eyes in response to painful stimuli	Opens eyes in response to voice	Opens eyes spontaneously	N/A	N/A
Verbal	Makes no sounds	Incomprehensible sounds	Inappropriate words	Confused, disoriented	Orientated, converses normally	N/A
Motor	Makes no movements	Extension to painful stimuli (decerebrate response)	Abnormal flexion to painful stimuli (decorticate response)	Flexion or withdrawal to painful stimuli	Localizes painful stimuli	Obeys commands

Table 9.10 The 'AVPU' score (a simplification of the Glasgow Coma Scale)

Alert	Voice	Pain	Unresponsive
A fully awake (although not necessarily oriented) patient This patient will spontaneously open eyes, will respond to voice (although may be confused) and will possess motor function	The patient makes some kind of response (eyes or voice or motor) when prompted by questions, e.g. 'Are you ok?' The patient's eyes may open, or the response may simply be a moan or slight movement of a limb	The patient makes some kind of response (eyes or voice or motor) when pain stimulus is used on them	No response to voice or pain

attributes a score, ranging from 3 to 15. It was originally devised to assess the level of consciousness after head injury, although now is used for almost all acutely presenting patients. When faced with a poorly conscious patient, the usual pairing of resuscitation and diagnostics should be followed. Severe neurological conditions may affect upper airway tone, respiratory drive (e.g. Cheyne–Stokes respiration), vasomotor tone and cardiac rhythm. Also, if the cause of the brain dysfunction is systemic (Table 9.11), this will need to be dealt with. Therefore, it is paramount that the 'airway, breathing, circulation' (ABC) algorithm is given due respect. The airway should be supported appropriately (if necessary with endotracheal intubation), the 'recovery' lateral position may be required in the unintubated patient to prevent aspiration, hypotension may require vigorous intravenous fluids and monitoring will be required for hypertension and cardiac dysrhythmias.

After resuscitation, one should focus on rapidly identifying the cause of brain dysfunction (Table 9.11). If there is an obvious systemic cause, this should already have been dealt with. A brief history from witnesses may reveal preceding hemiparesis, headache, trauma, fit, recreational drug or alcohol intake, or a history of cancer, diabetes, liver or renal disease. Examination should include a full body inspection for features of trauma, fundoscopy, cranial nerves and motor function (including power, tone and reflexes). The power, sensory, cerebellar and visual assessments may not be possible due to lack of cooperation. One should attempt to examine for meningism by assessing nuchal rigidity (diminished neck flexion with otherwise retained neck movements) and knee extension with the patient supine, with the hip and knee preflexed (pain on knee extension is Kernig's sign).

Table 9.11 Logical thinking in the poorly conscious patient

Primary cranial diffuse or multifocal disease, where structural lesions will be obvious on imaging	**Primary cranial diffuse disease where no structural lesions will be obvious on imaging**
Vascular Infection Inflammation Tumours Trauma	Infection Inflammation Trauma ('concussion') Non-convulsive status epilepticus or postictal state Psychiatric (conversion, stupor)
Secondary cranial disease: systemic	**Secondary cranial disease: metabolic**
Hypoxia/anoxia Hypotension Hypothermia	Alcohol Drugs Hypoglycaemia Endocrine disturbance (sodium balance, thyroid disturbance) Liver Renal Non-cranial infection

A very brief description may be made here of common pathologies leading to changes in conscious level:

- Vascular lesions include cerebral arterial or venous thromboses leading to infarcts. Intracranial haemorrhages may be subarachnoid or intracerebral. Relevant cases should be referred early to stroke units or neurosurgeons.
- Primary cranial infections may manifest as meningitis, encephalitis or meningoencephalitis. One may also become acutely encephalopathic from widespread non-infective inflammatory vascular lesions. With infective and inflammatory pathologies, changes may or may not be evident on cranial imaging. Treatment with antibiotics and/or antiviral agents will initially be empirical, and should not be withheld in favour of preceding lumbar puncture, especially if the patient is critically unwell.
- After trauma, extradural and subdural haematomata may be suspected, as may subarachnoid and intracerebral haemorrhages. The condition known as 'diffuse axonal injury' (DAI) refers to extensive lesions in white matter tracts, and is one of the major causes of unconsciousness after head trauma. 'Concussion' is the most common type of traumatic brain injury, where there is temporary loss of brain function with a variety of subsequent physical, cognitive and emotional symptoms. There are usually no changes visible on imaging, and symptoms usually resolve spontaneously over days or weeks. Relevant cases should be referred early to the neurosurgical unit.
- Non-convulsive status epilepticus as a cause of altered consciousness is often overlooked. There will often be no obvious clinical clues other than eye deviation or involuntary eye movements. Often, the unconscious patient who has been intensely investigated in the emergency department, and who spontaneously becomes more alert over the subsequent hours, will have had an unwitnessed seizure.
- If opioid overdose is suspected, one may consider administering the opioid antagonist naloxone. This may be essential if the unconscious state is affecting the airway. If the vital observations are stable, however, the benefit of rapid opioid reversal should be weighed against the disadvantages (e.g. disorientation, aggression, vomiting, removal of analgesia).
- The psychiatric patient (with or without a known past history) may have a poor

Table 9.12 Relationship of pupillary changes to site of anatomical damage

Unilateral pathological dilatation (mydriasis)	Unilateral pathological constriction (miosis)	Mid-point pupil
Pupillary fibres close to the origin of the third cranial nerve are especially susceptible when uncal herniation or a posterior communicating aneurysm compresses the nerve This mydriasis is usually accompanied with sparing of oculomotor function When pupillary fibres more distal in the third cranial nerve are affected, the mydriasis usually occurs together with oculomotor dysfunction	Hypothalamic damage may lead to ipsilateral Horner's syndrome Pontine damage may lead to bilateral miosis Lateral medullary and ventrolateral cervical cord lesions may lead to ipsilateral Horner's syndrome	Mid-brain damage: the mid-point pupil shows no reaction to light

consciousness level from conversion disorder, or stupor secondary to depression or schizophrenia. Often, the diagnosis will be made after preceding exhaustive negative tests, and will need an expert assessment by the psychiatrist.

Pupillary examination deserves special mention. As pupillary pathways are resistant to metabolic insult, the identification of absent pupillary reflexes usually implies structural pathology. The brainstem areas governing conscious level are anatomically close to the areas controlling the pupils and so pupillary changes help to identify brainstem pathology causing altered conscious level (Table 9.12).

Investigations, as always, should be targeted to the index of suspicion from clinical assessment. Those pertaining to resuscitation, including chest X-ray, electrocardiogram (ECG) and blood sugar, should be performed on initial encounter. Cranial imaging (usually a cranial CT scan) will be indicated if there is a significant possibility of structural lesions. It should be remembered, however, that the displacement of the patient to the radiology department may carry major risk, particularly if the patient requires general anaesthesia for intubation. Therefore, the advantages of performing neuroradiology should always be measured against risk. A lumbar puncture may be required; contraindications according to existing national and local guidelines should be referred to and, if present, the procedure should be deferred. An electroencephalogram (EEG) may reveal abnormalities consistent with a seizure disorder. Plasma alcohol may easily be measured, and may lend support to a clinical diagnosis of alcohol toxicity. Some, though not all, hospitals are able to perform urine toxicology analyses for recreational and other drugs. Plasma levels for paracetamol, salicylates and anticonvulsant medications are also easily available. These may be relevant in cases of deliberate or inadvertent self-harm. Some plasma levels for drugs are only available in specialist 'poisons' units. It is therefore often good practice to have a saved sample of serum, which may subsequently be transported if required. Tests of renal function and liver function (including blood clotting) should be included in the context of altered conscious level.

Table 9.13 Logical thinking for conditions causing syncope

Mechanism	Common or important examples
Cardiac structural disease	Valvular heart disease Obstructive cardiomyopathy Atrial myxoma Severe systolic dysfunction
Cardiac dysrhythmia	Any dysrhythmia
Pulmonary hypertension (poor left atrial filling)	Acute pulmonary embolism Any cause of chronic pulmonary hypertension
'Steal' syndromes	Subclavian 'steal'
Nervous system mediated	'Vasovagal' Carotid sinus disease Autonomic nerve dysfunction (e.g. secondary to alcohol, antihypertensive drugs, hypoglycaemia and diabetes mellitus)
Hypovolaemia	Blood loss Diarrhoea Vomiting

The syncopal patient

Syncope is a frequent cause of presentation to hospital and the emergency department. It may be defined as temporary loss of consciousness with rapid onset and spontaneous recovery. The implication is that there is temporary, global hypoperfusion to the brain. The brevity of the event is mostly limited to a few minutes. Although the causes of syncope are often not sinister (the most common cause is a vasovagal episode), the consequences may be catastrophic if, for instance, the onset occurs while driving. The condition should therefore always be taken seriously (Table 9.13).

It is likely from the above definition that the doctor will meet a patient who has fully preserved brain function and a history (or collateral history from witnesses) of recent syncope, thereby excluding patients with ongoing brain dysfunction and altered conscious level (discussed elsewhere in this chapter).

When the duration of the period of loss of consciousness is unknown or thought to be prolonged, the possibility of seizures should be considered. This impression may be reinforced by the presence of tongue biting, urinary incontinence, preceding aura or unusual behaviour, ongoing drowsiness, confusion or headache or a collateral history of involuntary movements during the episode. The approach to patients with seizures is discussed elsewhere in this chapter.

The history of the syncopal event will not be complete when told by the patient, though events preceding and following it may be recounted. It is important, therefore, that any witnesses of the event are available to give a collateral history. Dramatic sequelae such as motor vehicle accidents or personal injury will prompt urgent investigations. The history should explore any relationship between syncope and exertion, chest pain, palpitations, dyspnoea, posture changes, body fluid losses and overt bleeding. A careful drug and alcohol history should be taken and a past history of heart and lung disease or diabetes noted. A family history of sudden death should be taken very seriously.

One should examine for an implanted cardiac device (such as a pacemaker), irregular or rapid heart rate and heart murmurs. Measurement of lying and standing blood pressure is mandatory unless there is a clear alternative cause. Investigations could initially include full blood count, ECG, echocardiography and 24-hour ECG monitoring. Formal autonomic function testing may be needed.

Table 9.14 Simple terminology for seizures

Term	Description
Generalized seizure	Involvement of the whole cerebral cortex and therefore abnormalities (e.g. convulsions) may be seen in the whole of the body Consciousness is always impaired
Focal (partial) seizure	Involvement of a focus in the cerebral cortex and therefore abnormalities (e.g. convulsions) may be seen in one part of the body Consciousness may be retained (simple partial seizure) or impaired (complex partial seizure) There may be secondary generalization (i.e. a focal seizure leading on to a generalized seizure)
Convulsive seizure	For example tonic-clonic, tonic and clonic
Non-convulsive seizure	The term 'absence seizure' should generally be avoided unless a specific syndromic diagnosis is being made by a clinician experienced in epilepsy
Status epilepticus	Historically, one definition has been 'prolonged seizures for more than 30 minutes', although in modern times it is more sensible to accept that 'any prolonged seizure' may be classified as status epilepticus

The patient with seizures

One definition of 'seizure' is the 'uncontrolled electrical activity in the brain, which may produce a physical convulsion, minor physical signs, thought disturbances or a combination of symptoms'. 'Epilepsy' is a pattern of repeated seizures. The occurrence of a seizure or 'fit' is a common mode of presentation to the emergency department. In most cases, the final diagnosis will not be epilepsy.

If the patient is actively having a seizure, the 'ABC' of resuscitation should be meticulously followed. Intravenous anticonvulsant agents should be administered promptly, within the constraints of formulary guidelines. The aim should be to suppress the seizure as quickly as possible. If there is no success with standard anticonvulsants, the administration of a general anaesthetic (together with intubation, ventilation and admission to intensive care) should be considered. The definition of 'status epilepticus' is under continuous scrutiny (Table 9.14).

If the patient is not actively having a seizure at the time of clinical assessment, the task is to identify whether the episode preceding admission was a seizure or not. It should be remembered that a diagnosis of seizures may lead to social and employment consequences (including the ability to drive), so it is crucial to establish a credible collateral history together with a detailed history from the patient. Tongue biting and post-event drowsiness, headache or confusion may help lend support to a diagnosis of seizures. Although urinary and faecal incontinence is often quoted, it is not a strong differentiating feature between seizures and non-seizures.

The diagnosis of non-convulsive status epilepticus may be missed unless specifically thought of. The patient may present with non-specific features, such as prolonged confusion or drowsiness. On occasions there may be clinical features to arouse suspicion such as nystagmoid eye movements or repetitive (often stereotypic for the patient) movements of the tongue, jaw or limbs.

Some conditions are commonly misdiagnosed as seizures. Severe exacerbation of extrapyramidal disease may mimic myoclonus. Vasovagal episodes may, on occasions, be followed by jerking of the limbs. Pseudoseizures (seizures simulated by patients for psychological and other complex reasons) are often difficult to differentiate from genuine seizures, even for many experienced neurologists (Table 9.15).

Table 9.15 Awareness of conditions commonly misdiagnosed as seizures

Condition	Awareness
Pseudoseizure	The reasons for patients presenting with contrived movements mimicking seizures are complex. They often occur in known epileptics. The risk of death is significantly higher in epileptic patients with pseudoseizures, and so the latter needs to be taken seriously and not merely dismissed as a non-organic event. Many epilepsy experts maintain that with increasing clinical experience, there is increased awareness of the difficulty in the differentiation of seizures from pseudoseizures. There are, however, some features which may lend support to the diagnosis of pseudoseizures: resistance to attempted eye opening by the clinician, limb thrashing and pelvic thrusting, full alertness immediately after the event (i.e. lack of postictal drowsiness) and down-going plantar responses during attack
Vasovagal episode	Prolonged vasovagal episodes may lead to cerebral hypoperfusion and brief, self-limiting convulsive-type movements
Cranial trauma	This is particularly seen in sports events, where cranial trauma may lead to brief, self-limiting convulsive-type movements, similar to those seen in vasovagal episodes
Extrapyramidal disease	Patients may present with worsening or poorly controlled Parkinson's disease, manifested as severe coarse tremor which, to the untrained eye, may resemble myoclonus

In history taking, there is considerable overlap with the principles described for the patient with syncope. It is essential that witnesses are available to give a collateral history, as the seizure itself will not be recalled by the patient. However, on recovery, the events preceding and following the seizure may be recounted by the patient. As with syncope, dramatic sequelae such as motor vehicle accidents or personal injury should be taken seriously. It should be established whether there is a known history of epilepsy. In patients with known epilepsy, a history should be taken for compliance, anticonvulsant changes, concurrent illnesses, alcohol intake and lifestyle issues. In other cases, specifically ask about alcohol intake, recreational drug usage, diabetes, head injury, foreign travel and pregnancy.

General examination will include the assessment of features of infection. Mild, transient, fever is a common phenomenon after seizures from muscle contractions. Persistent fever together with other abnormal observation such as tachycardia and raised respiratory rate may suggest the presence of an infection. If there is genuine doubt as to whether the fever is related to the seizure or an infection, one should look vigorously for a source of infection (including performing a lumbar puncture) and consider administering empirical intravenous antibiotics while awaiting investigations. One should examine for evidence of cranial trauma, alcoholic foetor and severe hypertension.

In the drowsy postictal patient, some aspects of neurological examination such as visual fields, voluntary eye movements, cerebellar function, power and sensory deficits will be difficult or impossible to ascertain. However, the following should be performed to a high standard: fundoscopy; pupillary, corneal and gag reflexes; limb tone; limb reflexes; and spontaneous limb movement. Any asymmetry should be noted and it may prompt urgent investigations.

Blood sugar should be performed urgently, as hypoglycaemia may be quickly reversed and brain injury prevented. Plasma biochemistry and liver function tests will identify reversible electrolyte deficiencies and features of liver disease. Possible infections should be identified with the help of white cell count, blood culture and urinalysis. Toxicology tests may include blood alcohol and urine drug analysis. Women of childbearing age should have a pregnancy test. Patients with unexplained seizures and a history of travel abroad should have parasite analysis. If the patient has no known identity and therefore no known past history, plasma anticonvulsant analysis may lend support to recent ingestion and therefore the possibility of previously diagnosed epilepsy.

A cranial CT scan will be required if one or more of the following are present: the seizure is unexplained, there are features of cranial trauma, there are focal or lateralizing features, there are fundoscopic features of raised intracranial pressure and there are features of infection. The gross features uncovered by a cranial CT may include intracranial haemorrhage or space-occupying lesions. Although it is a misconception that a CT scan is always required prior to lumbar puncture, it is overwhelmingly recognized that lumbar puncture for the investigation of meningitis in the patient with seizures should always be preceded by a cranial CT. The cerebrospinal fluid from the lumbar puncture should be analysed for meningitis and for subarachnoid haemorrhage. An EEG may be performed acutely to lend support to the diagnosis of a postictal state and occasionally to identify features of herpes encephalitis.

Once a seizure is diagnosed, the clinician should advise the patient of his duty to contact the driving licensing authority, who in turn will issue guidelines for cessation of driving for a defined period. The diagnosis of epilepsy should be made by an expert in epilepsy, as this diagnosis will have social and drug-therapy implications. The epilepsy expert will also decide, together with the patient, on the clinical value of prescription of anticonvulsants after a first seizure.

The patient with acute confusion

Patients with acute confusion are often seen in the emergency setting. Often, the patient will have pre-existing cognitive dysfunction, which may have been present for weeks, months or years. It is important in this scenario to investigate both the acute confusion and the pre-existing pathology. Remember that those with longer-standing cognitive dysfunction (e.g. consequent upon cerebrovascular pathology) will be more susceptible to episodes of acute confusion when affected by minor pathology such as infection and metabolic derangement. In elderly patients, particularly, systemic problems such as infections or cardiac disease may not lead to any symptoms other than acute confusion.

The causes and mechanisms of confusion should be logically arranged in the mind of the clinician (Table 9.16). Toxaemia from infections, inflammation and drugs will lead to varying degrees of cerebral dysfunction, as will metabolic derangements. Any episode of acute pain or anxiety affects intellectual function. Poor cerebral oxygenation will occur with episodes of hypoxia and diminished cerebral perfusion from circulatory impairment. Any brain pathology may cause cerebral dysfunction; one should be aware that in these cases, confusion may progress to diminished consciousness level. The possibility of underlying psychiatric disorder should be borne in mind, particularly in the younger patient.

The history, as in cases of altered conscious level, syncope and seizures, will often not be meaningful when given by the patient. The collateral history from relatives and other sources is therefore paramount. The presence of any long-standing cognitive issues should be established. Specific, directed questioning should deal with the presence of head injury, pain (including chest pain), breathlessness, light-headedness, headache and features of infection. A meticulous history should be taken for drugs and alcohol. Nutritional history should be explored and the presence of established chronic diseases such as diabetes, seizure disorders, liver, kidney or thyroid disease documented. Previous psychiatric illness and long-standing mood changes should be noted.

The examination should be targeted, as the patient will most likely not be able to comply with complicated directions which are required in neurological and other assessments. Start with the 'vital' observations: oxygen saturation, respiratory rate, blood pressure (erect and supine) and heart rate. Pyrexia, features of head injury, smell of alcohol, cachexia and features of jaundice or uraemia should be looked for. There may be obvious features of a thyroid disorder. The presence of pain on palpation and abnormalities on chest examination should be identified. Neurological examination will elicit any gross focal or lateralizing features and also features of meningism. The examination should also include an abbreviated mental test (see Ch. 7 on elderly medicine). The latter will objectively document the confusion and help track any progress.

Table 9.16 Logical thinking for conditions causing acute confusion

Mechanism	Common or important examples
Infection	Urine, chest
Inflammatory	Acute pancreatitis, vasculitis, ischaemic bowel, myocardial ischaemia
Drugs and external toxins	Prescription drugs, recreational drug usage, alcohol (toxicity or withdrawal) The most severe form of alcohol withdrawal is 'delirium tremens', a condition which traditionally starts up to 3 days after cessation of heavy alcohol consumption
Metabolic derangement	Hypoglycaemia, hyperglycaemia, hyponatraemia, hypernatraemia, hypercalcaemia, liver dysfunction (synthetic or cholestasis), uraemia, thyroid dysfunction, nutritional deficiency (particularly vitamin B_{12}, thiamine and niacin)
Acute pain or anxiety	Urinary retention, severe constipation
Psychiatric issues	Depression, schizophrenia
Hypoxaemia	Chest infection, pulmonary oedema, pulmonary embolism
Circulatory impairment	Cardiac disease (dysrhythmia, systolic dysfunction), sepsis, haemorrhage, prolonged vagal episode
Brain pathology	Haemorrhage, ischaemia, seizure disorder, infection (encephalitis and meningoencephalitis), head injury, cerebral vasculitis

Unless the diagnosis is absolutely clear, investigations may commence with full blood count, C-reactive protein, standard electrolytes, liver function, thyroid function, vitamin B_{12}, urinalysis, urine and blood cultures, chest X-ray, toxicology, blood alcohol (to help differentiate alcohol withdrawal from toxicity), ECG and arterial blood gases (if low oxygen saturation is identified). If there is evidence of focal or lateralizing features, meningism, altered conscious level or unexplained headache, a cranial CT scan should be considered. A lumbar puncture should be performed if meningitis remains a consideration.

The patient with acute headache

Many patients present to the emergency department with severe acute headache. This will either be a 'worst ever' exacerbation in the context of chronic, long-term headache or a first presentation of headache.

On initial presentation, it should be established whether there have been any additional features which may suggest sinister pathology. One should specifically enquire about severity (is this the 'worst ever'?); rapidity of onset (implying vascular pathology such as subarachnoid haemorrhage); recent head injury; loss of consciousness; altered intellect; features of sepsis; features of meningism (photophobia and neck stiffness); features of raised intracranial pressure (headache exacerbated by straining, coughing and lying flat); asymmetry (consistent with temporal arteritis and glaucoma, as well as migraine and sinusitis); and blurred visual disturbance (consistent with raised intracranial pressure, glaucoma and temporal arteritis).

There are additional features that need clarification. A past history and temporal patterns of long-standing headache need to be established, as does the presence of coexisting illness. Viral infections and pneumonia are not uncommonly associated with headache. Foreign travel may be relevant as well as the drug history.

It is important to be aware of some distinctive features of the more common causes of headache (Table 9.17). Distinctive features in the history of a patient with a subarachnoid haemorrhage include a sudden-onset, occipital 'worst ever' headache (classically described as like being kicked on the back of the head). There may have been an episode of loss of consciousness (this may be seen in up to half of all patients presenting with subarachnoid haemorrhage). Features of meningism and raised intracranial pressure are not uncommon. Urgent investigations (cranial CT scan, with targeted lumbar puncture) and specialist referral are paramount. Bacterial meningitis may be rapidly fatal, and treatment with intravenous antibiotics must commence as soon as the diagnosis is suspected. Viral meningitis is usually less dramatic, although this is not inevitably the case. The headache of meningitis is of acute onset and severe. There are accompanying features of photophobia and neck stiffness. In severe cases, there may be features of raised intracranial pressure. Although pure encephalitis does not produce features of meningism, meningoencephalitis does. Temporal arteritis is a form of vasculitis in which the temporal arteries are inflamed and tender. The headache is usually asymmetrical. There may be pain in the jaw with chewing ('jaw claudication'). Vision changes (blurred vision) should prompt urgent treatment with steroids (to prevent complete loss of vision), followed by specialist referral and confirmation of the diagnosis with a temporal artery biopsy. The migrainous headache is typically unilateral and pulsating. The acute period often lasts between 4 and 72 hours, and there may be accompanying nausea, vomiting, photophobia, phonophobia (increased sensitivity to sound) or osmophobia (sensitivity to pungent smells).

Table 9.17 Logical thinking for conditions causing acute headache

Mechanism	Common or important examples
Vascular – haemorrhage	Subarachnoid, intracerebral, subdural, extradural
Vascular – occlusive	Migraine, temporal arteritis, carotid artery dissection
Muscular	Tension-type headache
Meningeal irritation	Meningitis (bacterial, viral), subarachnoid haemorrhage
Raised intracranial pressure	Space-occupying lesion (tumour, abscess, localized haemorrhage), malignant hypertension, benign intracranial hypertension
Drugs and toxins	Oral or sublingual nitrates, carbon monoxide
Carbon dioxide retention from respiratory failure	Obstructive sleep apnoea, obesity hypoventilation syndrome
Tropical disease	Malaria, any one of the tropical endemic encephalitides
Upper respiratory tract infections	Influenza, sinusitis
Intraocular pressure	Glaucoma
Neuralgia	Trigeminal neuralgia, cluster headache

The examination should include identification of general and specific features of sepsis, such as pyrexia, tachycardia and signs of lung consolidation. Altered consciousness level should have been detected on initial encounter and immediately acted upon. Altered intellectual function and disorientation, though, may only be apparent later in more detailed conversation. A history of neck stiffness should prompt an examination of nuchal rigidity in which there is a painful deficit of neck flexion with relative preservation of all other neck movements. When meningism is suspected, both legs should also be examined where each leg in turn is bent at the hip and knee at 90° angles; if subsequent further extension in the knee is painful (leading to resistance), this should be described as a 'Kernig's positive' sign, which in turn suggests that there is significant inflammation of the meninges. Positive features of meningism should prompt the clinician to search for a non-blanching purpuric rash, which may lend support to a diagnosis of meningococcal meningitis. A full neurological examination should identify any focal or lateralizing motor or sensory abnormalities, and also any cranial nerve or cerebellar deficits. One should look for papilloedema on fundoscopy. Additional areas of clinical examination may include palpation of the temporal arteries or the sinuses, looking for tenderness in these areas; examination of the scalp, looking for herpetic lesions; and inspection of the sclerae, looking for the acute red eye of glaucoma.

In cases of suspected subarachnoid haemorrhage, a cranial CT is not diagnostic in all cases, particularly more than 24 hours after the acute event. If the diagnosis is suspected and the CT scan is normal, a lumbar puncture is mandatory to exclude the diagnosis and is best done more than 12 hours after the onset of symptoms. If encephalitis is suspected, a magnetic resonance image (MRI) should be considered. Lumbar puncture for cerebrospinal fluid analysis should be performed when meningitis is suspected. Antibiotics should never be withheld while waiting for the lumbar puncture. Other investigations which may help identify or support a diagnosis are chest X-ray, white cell count, blood culture, parasite analysis for malaria and viral serology. In unexplained headache, particularly in the presence of drowsiness, plasma carboxyhaemoglobin may support a diagnosis of carbon monoxide poisoning.

The acutely weak patient

The term 'weakness' will often be used by patients for a variety of complaints. Although the term should be reserved for the original definition of 'reduced motor power', many patients will confess to 'weakness' when in fact they are 'fatigued' or 'lethargic'. It is reasonable to infer reduced motor power when weakness is present without significant tiredness. This should be contrasted with fatigue and lethargy, where the diminished power is generalized, commensurate with and caused by significant tiredness. This should form the basis of initial questioning. ('Do you feel weak because you are tired, or do you think that you have specifically lost muscle power?') Sometimes, even with an experienced history taker and a cooperative patient it may not be possible to differentiate between weakness, fatigue and lethargy. The term 'fatigue', which is used here synonymously with the term 'lethargy', should not be confused with the neurological term 'fatiguability' (Table 9.18).

When assessing the patient, it is also helpful to differentiate between lesions of the 'upper motor neuron' (lesions of the motor cortex or pyramidal tracts) from the 'lower motor neuron' (lesions of the 'motor unit', that is the anterior horn cell, axon, neuromuscular junction or muscle). This differentiation is important in order to help direct investigations.

Acute quadriparesis and paraparesis deserve special mention. It should be assumed that the cause is external cord compression until proven otherwise. As recovery from the latter depends on speedy decompression, one should urgently organize imaging

Table 9.18 Logical thinking for conditions causing acute weakness

Scenario	Common or important examples
Fatigue or lethargy leading to generalized weakness	Chronic heart failure, chronic lung disease, sleep disorders, anaemia, chronic kidney disease, diabetes mellitus, chronic infection, malignancy, depression
Loss of motor power leading to generalized weakness	Myasthenia gravis (crisis), post-infectious inflammatory polyneuropathy ('Guillain-Barré syndrome'), acute myopathy (myositis, rhabdomyolysis)
Hemiparesis or hemiplegia (weakness or total paralysis of one side of body)	Lesion in contralateral cerebral motor cortex or contralateral brainstem Lesion in ipsilateral high cervical cord (often with ipsilateral dorsal column, i.e. proprioception deficit, and contralateral spinothalamic tract deficit, i.e. pain and temperature)
Monoparesis or monoplegia (weakness or total paralysis of single limb)	Lesion in contralateral cerebral motor cortex, contralateral brainstem Lesion in ipsilateral spinal cord (often with ipsilateral dorsal column, i.e. proprioception deficit, and contralateral spinothalamic tract deficit, i.e. pain and temperature) Lesion of nerve roots Mononeuropathy or mononeuritis multiplex
Paraparesis or paraplegia (weakness or total paralysis of both legs)	Lesion in parasagittal cerebral motor cortex Lesion in spinal cord (external compression, ischaemia, inflammation, e.g. transverse myelitis, infection, intramedullary space-occupying lesion) Post-infectious inflammatory polyneuropathy ('Guillain-Barré syndrome'), acute myopathy (myositis, rhabdomyolysis) Lesion of nerve roots and cauda equina lesions – usually affects one leg more than the other Mononeuropathy or mononeuritis multiplex – usually affects one leg more than the other
Quadriparesis and quadriplegia (weakness or total paralysis of both arms and both legs)	Lesion in brainstem Lesion in upper cervical cord (external compression, ischaemia, inflammation, e.g. transverse myelitis, infection, intramedullary space-occupying lesion) Post-infectious inflammatory polyneuropathy ('Guillain-Barré syndrome'), acute myopathy (myositis, rhabdomyolysis)

and specialty assessment. Any delay in imaging should not lead to a delay in specialty assessment.

The history should establish the speed of onset and distribution of weakness. Rapid onset of weakness over minutes suggests a vascular pathology, whereas an onset over hours or days is more indicative of an infective or inflammatory condition. Associated pain is most often a consequence of nerve root or peripheral nerve involvement and also occurs with acute myopathy, in which there may be muscle tenderness. A careful drug history should be taken to identify agents such as chemotherapy drugs which may cause peripheral neuropathy, and a family history enquiry may uncover inherited muscle disorders. Risk factors for stroke, such as hypertension, hyperlipidaemia, diabetes mellitus, alcohol intake and smoking history, should be documented.

On general inspection, look for gait disturbance, facial palsy, muscle wasting and fasciculation. Test for tone and reflexes before testing power, as muscle tone may be affected by pre-existing muscle contraction. Diminished tone and diminished reflexes are seen in lower motor neuron conditions. In addition to formally testing power, a quick functional test for power is to ask the patient to stand from a sitting position, testing hip and knee extension; walk on his heels, to test ankle dorsiflexion; and walk on his toes, to test ankle plantarflexion. Coordination should be tested in the upper limbs (finger-to-nose tests) and lower limbs (heel-to-knee-to-toe), although one should be aware that weakness in itself will affect coordination. Sensory examination, testing for sensory loss, paraesthesiae, hyperaesthesiae and pain, will be meaningful only in cooperative and coherent patients. This should not prevent the clinician from attempting to establish sensory deficits consistent with nerve, nerve root or central pathology.

Timely cranial CT scans are essential in stroke, while MR scans are useful in a variety of cranial and spinal cord lesions. The spinal cord MR scan should be booked as an emergency when cord compression is suspected. Nerve conduction studies and electromyography (EMG) are useful to confirm the diagnosis of Guillain-Barré syndrome and on occasion will help differentiate peripheral nerve from nerve-root pathology.

The patient with acute abdominal pain

It is important to be familiar with some principles governing the location of pain. Oesophageal, gastric or duodenal pain may be evident over the lower chest or epigastrium (and oesophageal pain may radiate to the arms); gallbladder pain usually commences in the right upper quadrant and often radiates around the right chest wall to the right dorsal area; pancreatic pain usually localizes over the epigastrium and radiates through to the back; pain from the small bowel is often manifested diffusely or over the periumbilical area, whereas large bowel pain is usually found over the site of the pathology or lesion (e.g. splenic flexure); pain from the distal colon may be referred to the lumbar area; any pathology affecting or irritating the diaphragm (e.g. a subphrenic abscess) may present with referred pain in the shoulder; ureteric colic usually radiates from the flank to the inguinal area on the affected side ('loin to groin'). (See Table 9.19.)

Table 9.19 Logical thinking for conditions causing acute abdominal pain

Mechanism	Common or important examples
Enteral visceral pain (usually colicky pain)	Oesophageal spasm or oesophagitis, duodenal ulcer, small bowel enteritis or ischaemia, colitis, colonic obstruction or ischaemia, complex gut perfusion deficit (diabetic ketoacidosis, sickle crisis)
Non-enteral visceral pain	Gallbladder pain from cholecystitis, pancreatic pain from pancreatitis or malignancy
Peritoneal pain (exacerbated by any changes in intra-abdominal pressure such as coughing, moving)	Perforated enteral viscus (gastric, duodenal, small bowel, appendix, large bowel), perforated non-enteral viscus (gallbladder, spleen, ruptured ectopic pregnancy), inflamed organ (pancreatitis), spontaneous bacterial peritonitis, malignant infiltration, bleeding vessel
Non-visceral pain	Aortic aneurysm, renal colic, referred pain

In contrast, pathology in areas distant to the abdomen may present with referred or radiated pain in the abdomen. For example, pneumonia, pleuritis and pleural effusions may manifest as upper quadrant pain on the affected side, and pain due to myocardial ischaemia may be felt most in the epigastrium. When taking a history, establishing the abdominal location of pain will help identify the affected organ, using the principles outlined above. The speed of onset of pain is also relevant; rapid onset may be associated with vascular catastrophes and rupture. The timing of the last menstrual period and the possibility of pregnancy should be considered in younger women. There may be an association between eating and abdominal pain: exacerbation by food may indicate gastritis, intestinal obstruction or gut ischaemia, whereas rapid relief upon eating may be suggestive of peptic ulceration. The presence of diarrhoea with or without blood may be suggestive of gut infection, inflammatory bowel disease or gut ischaemia.

The examination should initially focus on general features, such as hydration and cachexia, and vital parameters including respiratory rate, peripheral pulses, heart rate and blood pressure. Peritonitis may

Table 9.20 Logical thinking for conditions causing haematemesis or melaena

Mechanism	Common or important examples
Peptic ulcer disease	Gastric or duodenal (with or without *Helicobacter pylori* colonization)
Inflammation of upper gastrointestinal tract	Reflux oesophagitis, gastritis, duodenitis (the latter two often occur secondary to excess alcohol intake or usage of non-steroidal anti-inflammatory drugs)
Oesophageal and/or gastric varices, or portal hypertensive gastropathy	Portal hypertension from chronic liver disease
Coagulopathy or increased bleeding tendency	Liver synthetic dysfunction, altered warfarin metabolism (infection, antibiotics), clotting factor deficiencies, thrombocytopenia, anti-platelet drug usage (aspirin, clopidogrel), recent thrombolytic therapy – note: over-anticoagulation may reveal bleeding from specific pathology previously unknown
Upper gastrointestinal malignancy or malformation	Oesophageal carcinoma, gastric carcinoma, upper gastrointestinal angiodysplasia (vascular malformation)
Mallory–Weiss tear	Tear of lower oesophagus or upper stomach from recurrent vomiting
Nose bleeds (epistaxis)	A large amount of swallowed blood may lead to melaena

particularly be associated with severe hypotension or shock. Abdominal distension consistent with intestinal obstruction should be noted. Initial palpation may reveal diffuse, severe tenderness consistent with peritoneal inflammation, or localized tenderness. Rectal examination should be performed as a matter of routine; rectal masses and evidence of bleeding per rectum should be identified. If there is any suspicion of pelvic pathology in women, a gynaecological assessment is necessary.

General investigations which may help include full white cell count, haemoglobin, urea and electrolytes, liver function tests, amylase and pregnancy test (for the appropriate age group). Samples of diarrhoea should be sent for *Clostridium difficile* toxin analysis and also culture. A chest X-ray may demonstrate a perforated viscus or primary chest pathology. Erect and supine abdominal films may show features of obstruction. Abdominal ultrasound may demonstrate biliary tract dilatation or ureteric stones. Abdominal CT scans may reveal free fluid, the site of intestinal obstruction, pancreatic structure, evidence of ruptured aortic aneurysm or some detail with regard to intra-abdominal masses. Sigmoidoscopy may be useful if inflammatory bowel disease is suspected.

The patient with haematemesis and/or melaena

Haematemesis and melaena are common causes of presentation to the emergency department. The term 'haematemesis' describes the vomiting of blood, which may be bright red and fresh or altered (commonly described as 'coffee grounds'). The presence of haematemesis usually means acute bleeding from a source above the duodenojejunal flexure. 'Melaena' is faeces containing digested blood; they have a black (often described as 'jet black') tarry appearance and a characteristic and offensive smell. Although its presence may suggest acute bleeding from any source proximal to the ascending colon, the most common source is in the upper gastrointestinal tract (Table 9.20).

The passing of fresh blood per rectum (as opposed to melaena) usually means that the source of bleeding is in the large or small bowel. However, it is possible for very rapid upper gastrointestinal bleeding to lead to fresh blood per rectum as there is insufficient time for melaena to develop. Patients who incidentally describe dark stools without the characteristic appearance and smell of melaena do not usually have gastrointestinal bleeding. Iron-stained stool is black but usually solid and formed.

The history should enquire about epistaxis, alcohol intake, pre-existing liver disease and both prescription and over-the-counter drugs. One severe or several episodes of vomiting before the onset of haematemesis may suggest a Mallory-Weiss tear. Epigastric pain may suggest peptic ulcer disease, and unexplained weight loss and anorexia is suggestive of malignancy.

The initial examination should focus on identifying if the patient is in shock and acting accordingly (see above). Young, otherwise fit hypovolaemic individuals may compensate with raised cardiac output and remain normotensive for some considerable time but exhibit a fall in blood pressure on sitting or standing up. Features of malignancy (cachexia, supraclavicular lymphadenopathy, abdominal mass) and chronic liver disease (spider naevi, palmar erythema, jaundice, splenomegaly, ascites) should be noted. The clinical features of anaemia could suggest that there has been a period of occult bleeding before the acute bleed. Rectal examination is mandatory to see if there is objective evidence of melaena or fresh blood.

The initial investigations should include full blood count, clotting screen, urea, electrolytes and liver function tests. Blood should be 'grouped and saved', unless the patient is in shock, in which case, for example, four units of blood should be 'cross-matched' immediately. Blood is the best replacement fluid for a patient in shock with gastrointestinal bleeding but should not necessarily be given immediately for the stable patient who is anaemic. The availability of urgent upper gastrointestinal endoscopy varies widely among hospitals and different healthcare systems. Whatever the local provision, it follows, rather than replaces, prompt and effective resuscitation in the patient in shock.

Patients with a fever 10

Caryn Rosmarin and Ali Jawad

Introduction

Fever is one of the most common presenting features in any doctor's practice. It is the hallmark of the body's response to infection or inflammation. Before looking at the causes of fevers it is important to understand what we mean by the term and how the reaction is generated in the body.

Fever is an increase in the core body temperature (the temperature within the deep tissues of the body) above the daily range for an individual. The daily range of core body temperature is between 35.6°C and 37.8°C (97.0°F and 100.4°F). The closest to core body temperature we can measure is rectal temperature. As this is usually not easily performed and is less acceptable to patients, the next best is ear (tympanic) temperature. This requires a specific device that can be inserted into the ear using disposable covers. Oral temperature is about 0.5°C less than ear temperature and axillary temperature a further 0.5°C lower than oral temperature.

The normal core temperature of any individual does not remain static but varies according to certain rhythms and characteristics. It is affected by time of the day (known as diurnal variation), age, gender, height, time in the menstrual cycle, as well as with exercise and meals.

The diurnal variation of core body temperature is usually up to 0.6°C but can be exaggerated with a variation of 2-3°C. Core body temperature is at its highest in the late afternoon and evening, with lowest point in the early hours of the morning (Fig. 10.1).

How is normal core body temperature regulated?

Control of body temperature is termed thermoregulation, and under normal circumstances the body temperature will be in a state of stable internal temperature, or in homeostasis.

The temperature of the body depends on the balance between heat production and heat loss. Core body temperature is regulated by a system of control mechanisms affecting heat generation and heat loss. These include the autonomic nervous system, the endocrine system, musculoskeletal system and behavioural responses. The centre of this mechanism is called the thermoregulatory centre. It lies in the hypothalamus and acts like a thermostat in controlling the systems to produce the right balance of heat production and loss. The thermoregulatory centre has heat-sensitive receptors which respond to changes in body temperature by switching on and off systems to keep the balance within normal range. The range of temperature considered normal by the hypothalamus is termed the set point (Fig. 10.2). Damage to the hypothalamus can lead to loss of its thermostat control and result in very high or low core body temperatures.

Heat is gained and lost by the body through normal body functioning. Heat is produced all the time in the tissues of the body as a product of their metabolic processes. Heat is also produced by increased activity of skeletal muscles, such as during exercise or when shivering.

Normally this heat is lost to the environment through transfer from deep tissues, via the blood stream, to body areas in contact with the outside. This is mostly through the skin but also occurs through the lungs. Heat loss occurs through four main mechanisms called evaporation, convection, conduction and radiation as described in Box 10.1.

The amount of heat lost from the skin via the above mechanisms depends on environmental conditions with more heat loss occurring in cold, dry and windy environments. When the temperature of the environment is higher than body temperature or when there is a lot of humidity, heat cannot easily be lost, leading to a rise in body temperature (Fig. 10.3).

What effects on thermoregulation lead to fever?

Despite fever being an indicator of an abnormal clinical finding, it is a normal physiological response. While fever is an increase above normal in the core body temperature, it is not an indicator that the thermoregulatory system has lost control of its thermostatic function. It is rather a function of the up-regulating or resetting of the set point of the thermoregulatory centre to a higher level, much like

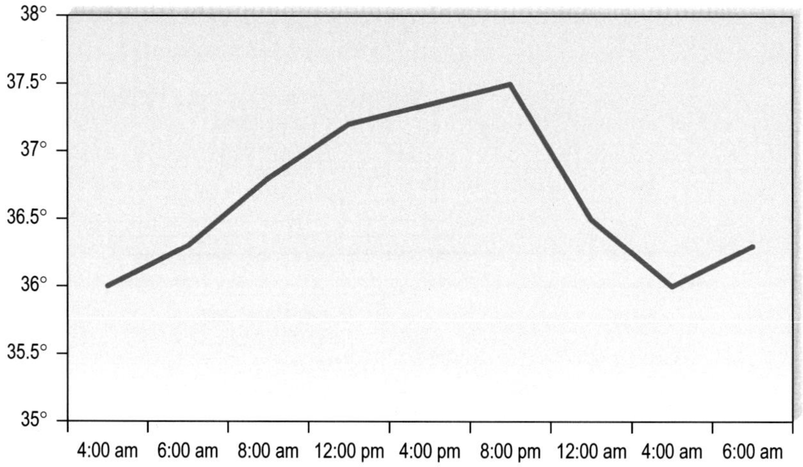

Figure 10.1 Diurnal variation of core body temperature.

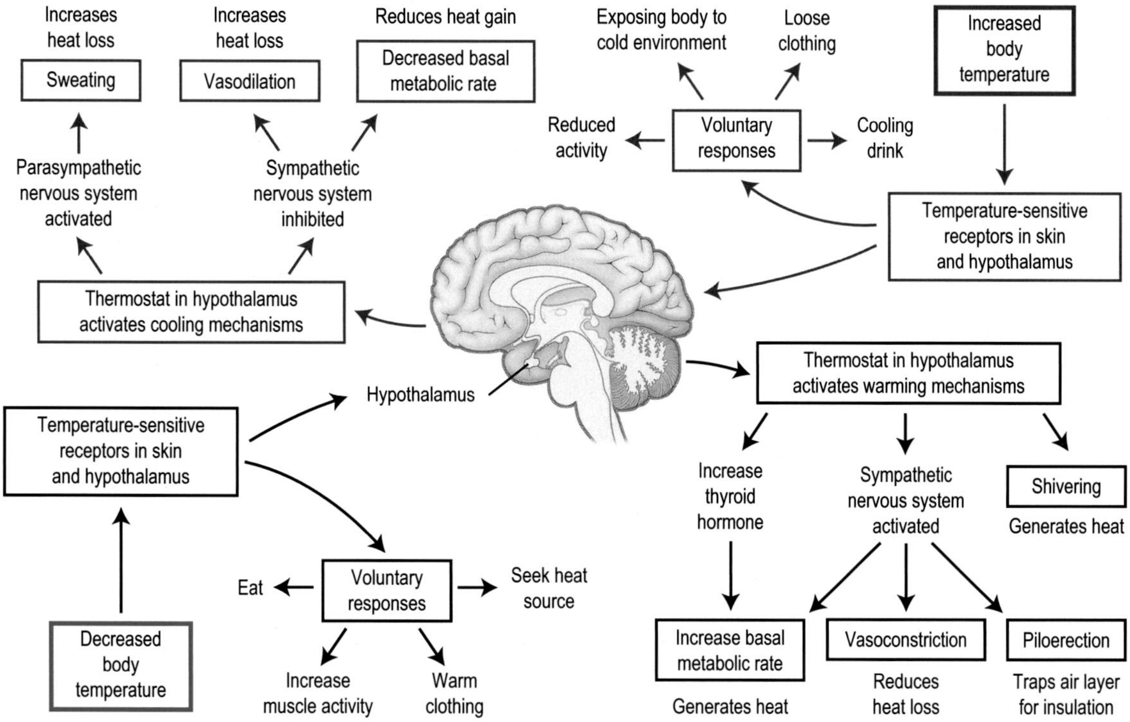

Figure 10.2 Regulation of core body temperature.

Box 10.1 Mechanisms of bodily heat loss

Evaporation: Sweating and panting cool by increasing heat loss

Convection: Increasing blood flow to body surfaces leads to heat loss

Conduction: Losing heat by being in contact with a colder surface, e.g. swimming in cold water or lying on a cold floor

Radiation: Increased exposure of the body surface will lead to increased heat loss

turning up the thermostat to a higher temperature. So long as the reset temperature remains below the range of the normal function of the thermoregulatory centre (<41.5°C) it will function to keep the body at this higher temperature. Above this temperature, the centre can no longer function to control body temperature and the fever is termed hyperpyrexia, a medical emergency requiring immediate and rapid cooling of the body.

Hyperthermia, on the other hand, is an example of a high temperature that is not a fever. It differs from a fever in that it is not associated with a change in the set point of the thermoregulatory centre but occurs due to raising the body temperature above

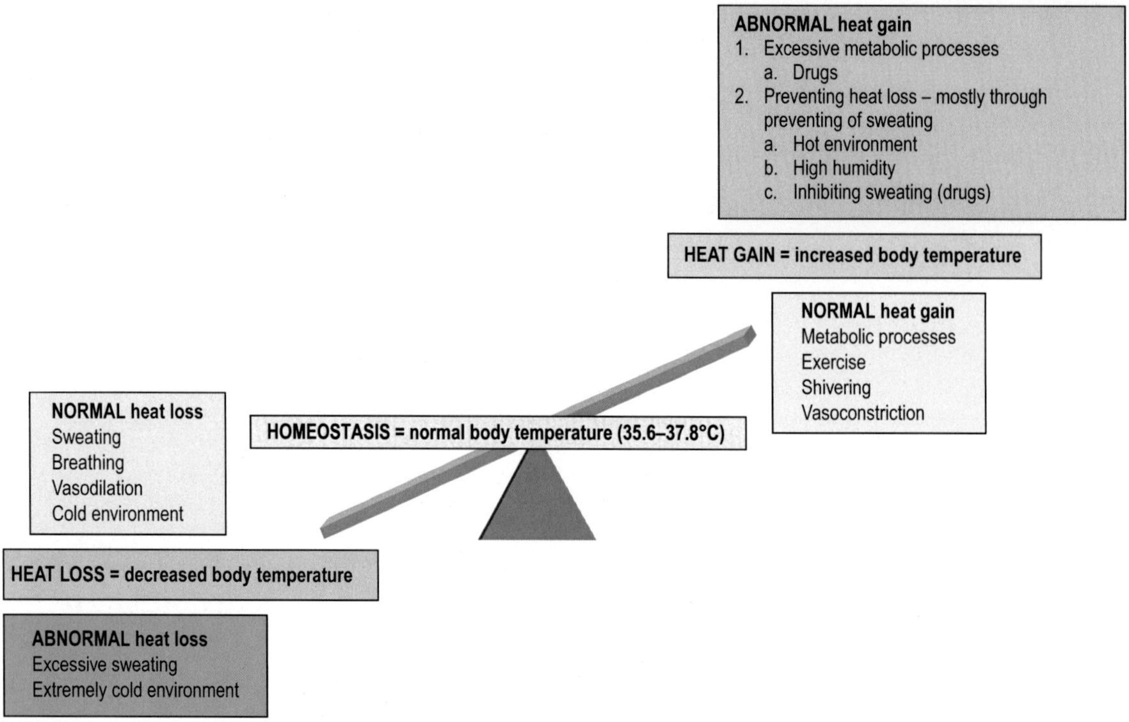

Figure 10.3 Mechanisms of thermoregulation and disregulation.

the normal set point. It can be caused by heatstroke, neuroleptic malignant syndrome, malignant hyperthermia, and stimulants such as amphetamines and cocaine.

Fever is produced when a stimulus from either outside (external) or inside (internal) the body is detected by the body's immune system as foreign, and a host of immune responses occur. External stimuli are usually in the form of infectious agents or drugs, while internal stimuli may be in the form of antibodies or damaged tissue. These (perceived) foreign objects activate the cells of the immune system to release chemical mediators called cytokines, including TNF-α, interferon, IL-1 and IL-6. These cytokines act on the hypothalamus to reset the set point to a higher temperature, or to 'turn up the thermostat'. Some bacterial proteins can act directly on the thermoregulatory centre in the hypothalamus to cause the same effect.

Elevation of the internal set point results in a higher core body temperature and causes the individual to feel cold. This leads to increased generation of heat and reduction of heat loss in the form of peripheral vasoconstriction and shivering. Rigors are a form of severe shivering.

Should you always treat a fever?

As fever is a physiological response of the body, it must have some inherent value, so is there a need to always be so quick to reduce it? Benefits of having a high temperature include an increase in the phagocytic and bactericidal activity of neutrophils and the cytotoxic effects of lymphocytes, impairment of the growth and virulence of bacteria and evidence of survival benefit for individuals with an elevated body temperature in response to infection.

On the other hand, there are negative effects of a raised body temperature. Oxygen consumption and fluid and calorie requirements increase; increased metabolic activity can increase stress if organs are failing; inflammatory cytokines increase muscle breakdown; and fever can reduce mental acuity, cause delirium and can trigger convulsions, especially in children.

Therefore there is indication to treat fever in those who are pregnant, in children, in those with impaired organ function, or those with a very high temperature of >41.5°C.

Fever can be treated by increasing heat loss through physical cooling or by resetting the upregulated hypothalamic set point using antipyretics.

The patterns of fever

Fever can reveal a characteristic pattern in some diseases and this pattern of rise and fall of temperature may be a clue for diagnosis (Fig. 10.4).

Approach to a patient with a fever – causes of fever

Fever is one of the commonest presenting features at medical facilities around the world. Although it is a characteristic sign of infection, not all fever is

Sustained/continuous: Persistent rise in temperature with minimal (<1°C) diurnal variation.
Causes: Pneumonia, meningitis, urinary tract infection, brucella

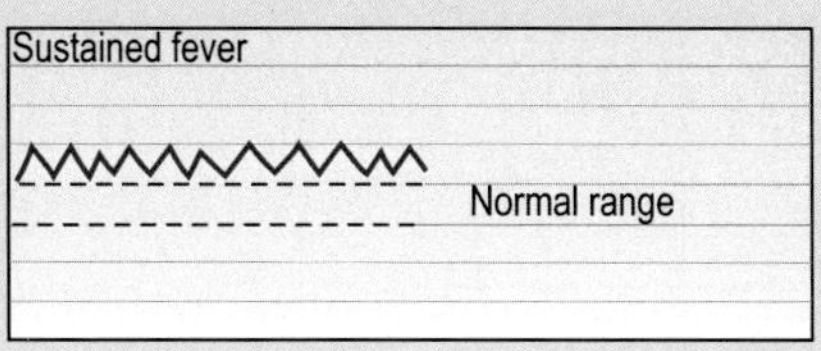

1

Step-ladder fever: A type of sustained fever where the temperature rises gradually to a higher level with every spike.
Causes: Typhoid, typhus

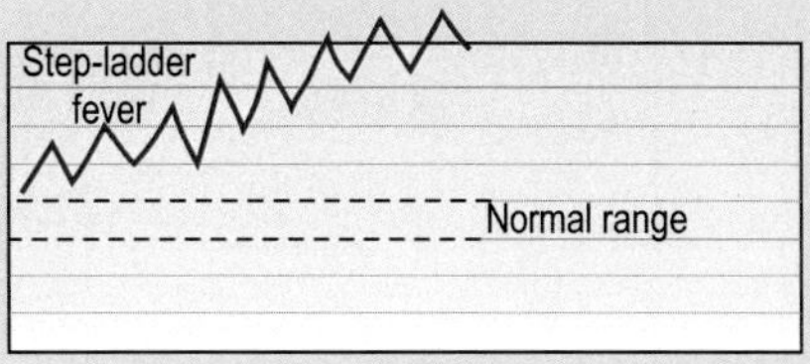

2

Intermittent: Exaggeration of the normal circadian rhythm. If the variation between high and low is extremely large it is called ***hectic***.
Causes: Deep seated infection, abscesses, kala-azar, malignancy, drug fever

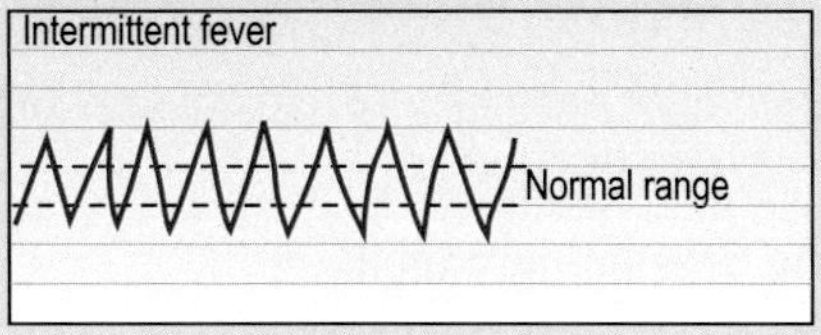

3

Remittent: Temperature spikes fall daily with diurnal variation of >2°C, but don't go down to normal.
Causes: Tuberculosis, infective endocarditis, many viral and bacterial infections

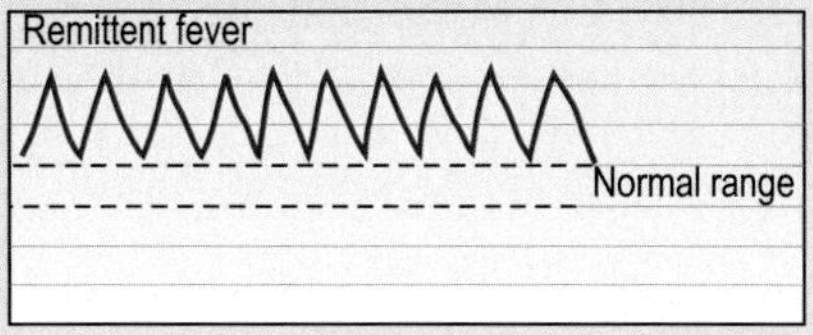

4

Relapsing: Febrile episodes are separated by intervals of normal temperature.
Causes: Malaria, borrelia (relapsing fever), tuberculosis, lymphoma

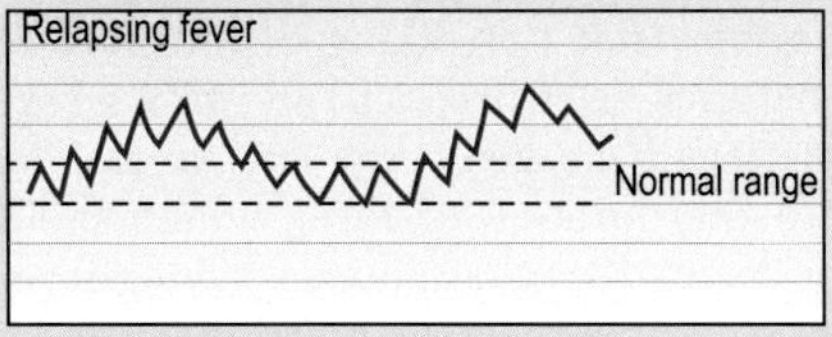

If this occurs daily, it is called ***quotidian*** fever.
Causes: *Plasmodium falciparum*

A ***double quotidian*** fever occurs when there are two spikes of fever every day, generally once in the morning and once in the evening.
Causes: Miliary tuberculosis

If it occurs every 48 hours it is called ***tertian*** fever.
Causes: *Plasmodium falciparum, Plasmodium vivax, Plasmodium ovale*

If it occurs every 72 hours it is called ***quartan*** fever.
Causes: *Plasmodium malariae*

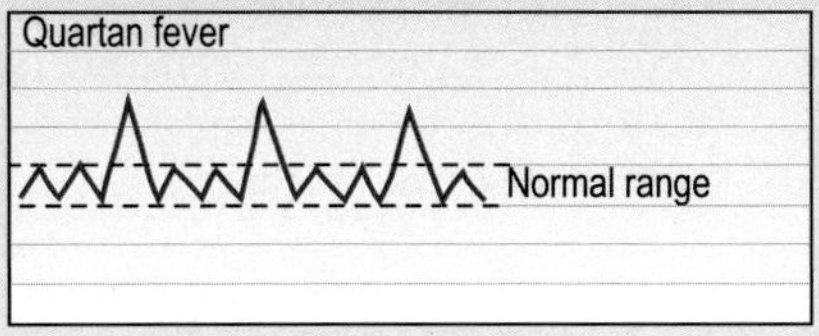

5

Inverse fever: The temperature rises in the early hours of morning rather than in the evening
Causes: Some cases of miliary tuberculosis

6

Night sweats: In some diseases, the rise in body temperature is evident only in the evening or late at night when the patient is woken up sweating. This pattern is seen when the mild rise in temperature is added to the normal diurnal evening rise leading to the body temperature rising beyond the normal level.
Causes: Tuberculosis, leukaemia, lymphoma, autoimmune disorders

7

Temperature-pulse disparity: This is the counter-intuitive response of a slower pulse associated with a high fever, commonly associate with typhoid fever.

8

Figure 10.4 The patterns of fever.

associated with an infectious cause. It is also a feature of a number of non-infectious inflammatory diseases (autoimmune connective tissue and autoinflammatory disease and vasculitis) and neoplasms. It may also occur as a drug reaction. In a significant number of cases, the temperature subsides spontaneously and no cause is identified (Box 10.2).

The likelihood that fever is due to an infection differs from one area of the world to another and reflects the burden of disease in the particular country

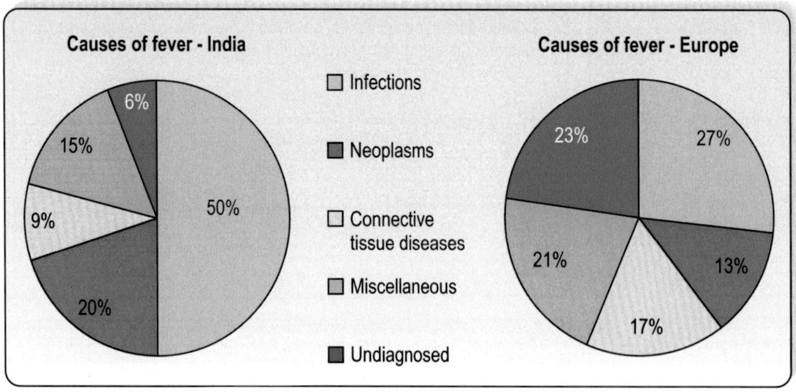

Figure 10.5 Causes of fever in India and Europe.

Box 10.2 Causes of fever

- Infections
- Non-infectious inflammatory diseases
  - Autoimmune inflammatory
  - Autoinflammatory
  - Vasculitis
- Malignancy
- Miscellaneous causes such as drug reactions
- Undiagnosed

(Fig. 10.5). It is also important to remember that the very young and the very old may have a serious infection without producing a fever.

History

As with any medical condition, the starting point of diagnosis is a detailed and meticulous history. The history taking should follow a logical scheme to ensure important questions are not missed, as causes of fever have a broad aetiology and can present as multisystem diseases. Taking a 'Fever History' is unlike any other, as it does not focus on a particular body system. Aspects of the personal, general and specific histories of all other systems need to be explored.

All histories should begin with an introduction, stating clearly your designation as a trainee, student or observer. Ensure you have the correct patient and that the patient understands the language. If the patient is a minor or a guardian or parent is present, be aware that certain sensitive questions may have to be asked at a later time when you are alone with the patient.

Main presenting complaint

Patients presenting with fever will often have a raft of associated complaints, many or all of which may be perceived as the main problem to the patient. It is therefore prudent to refer to the fever as the main presenting complaint and the associated complaints as part of the systematic history.

History of the presenting complaint

Details of the fever itself should be taken and the pattern described as continuous, intermittent or recurrent as noted above. Ask whether the fever is worse in the morning or at night. Some open-ended questions should be followed by direct questions to elicit the finer distinguishing characteristics of the fever. Remember that the taking of antipyretics, anti-inflammatories or antibiotics can mask a fever, so ask the patient if he has taken any medication. Enquire as to the duration of fever, which should reflect when the patient first noticed having fevers. This differs from the onset of fever that may be sudden or gradual; the former more likely to represent a more virulent disease, while the latter suggests a more indolent one. A description of the fever should include the presence or absence of *rigors* (profound chills associated with exaggerated shivering and chattering of teeth), which usually indicates a rapidly rising temperature found in malaria or severe bacterial sepsis.

High fever of more than 39°C is the initial symptom in most patients with adult onset Still's disease (AOSD). The classic fever pattern is one or two daily febrile spikes exceeding 39°C, usually occurring late during the day. At times the fever is continuous or, less commonly, there is an early morning spike.

Personal history

While the patients name, age and date of birth are used as identifiers, the country of birth and countries of residence are the first questions of the infection history. These are important both in respect to disease exposures and disease protection in the form of childhood and other vaccinations. Rates of diseases such as tuberculosis are higher in people who were born or resided in a country with a high incidence of tuberculosis, even if they have left the country. Vaccination schedules differ among countries and following this, immunity to certain childhood diseases may vary.

History of associated and constitutional symptoms

These include the presence of any of the following:

- **Headache** is a non-specific symptom and does not differentiate the cause of the fever. A severe headache associated with photophobia or vomiting could indicate meningitis. Vasculitides affecting the head and neck vessels may present with headache.
- **Muscle aches** (myalgia) is again a non-specific finding present in all causes of fever. If infectious, myalgia is more suggestive of infection with intracellular pathogens, particularly viral infections and malaria.
- **Joint pain** (arthralgia) is an additional non-specific symptom and may be caused by multiple infectious and non-infectious aetiologies. In a patient complaining of arthralgia, one should distinguish between mono-arthralgia (single joint) and poly-arthralgia (multiple joint) involvement.
- Presence or absence of a **rash** is particularly important to enquire about, as many infections and autoimmune disorders are associated with a typical rash both in pattern and evolution. The rash may not be present at the time of consultation or may have changed over the course of the illness. Ask details about the rash history, finding out where on the body it began, its associations, where it spread, whether the lesions changed over time and, if no longer present, how it resolved. Further details to help the diagnosis include details on the colour, type of lesion (e.g. vesicle, pustule, lacey) and whether it was pruritic, painful or neither.
- **Weight loss** in a patient with a fever suggests a more chronic process and is a classic feature of tuberculosis (consumption) or malignancy.
- A full systematic history should be included looking for a pattern of disease in systemic infectious or non-infectious disease, or a specific organ source of infection – e.g. cough, abdominal pain, dysuria, diarrhoea and redness or pain of skin or soft tissue.

History of behaviours and exposures are important in infectious diseases

- Contact with anyone having similar symptoms or living with someone who has been treated for an infection.
- Living arrangements including access to clean water and sanitation, proximity to animals or rodents. A history of insect or animal bite or scratches.
- Occupation, hobbies and sports, especially those involving exposure to water, animals or healthcare.
- Recreational habits, especially illicit drug use or tattoos.
- Sexual habits are vitally important and patients may need some encouragement to be open and honest about these risks. Unprotected sexual practices increase the risk of both sexually transmitted diseases and blood-borne viruses.
- Food habits including ingestion of unpasteurised milk or cheese.
- Taking of appropriate prophylaxis, including vaccinations, either when travelling or at home.
- Travel is one of the most important histories to explore. Detail of the destinations include whether the stay was in an urban or rural setting, stay was with family or friends, in a hotel or without facilities (Box 10.3).

Past medical and surgical history

While all past history is important to obtain, certain aspects play a more important role as risks for infections.

- Infections are more frequent and more serious in patients with diabetes. A past history of rheumatic heart disease increases the risk for infective endocarditis. Previous TB assumes a risk of recurrence.
- Immune compromise increases the risk, severity and scope of infections. The patient's immune status should be determined, specifically by asking about underlying diseases such as HIV, medications such as steroids or chemotherapy or a history of a splenectomy.
- Recent hospitalisation is associated with hospital-acquired multiresistant pathogens.
- Surgery, invasive procedures, medical devices, implants and transfusions all provide means for introduction of infectious agents.
- Antibiotic use may select for more resistant pathogens and increases the risk of antibiotic-associated diarrhoea. Antibiotics may also

Box 10.3 Infections to consider if there is a history of travel

Sub-Saharan Africa – malaria, reproductive tract infection (RTI), diarrhoeal illness, HIV, rickettsia, haemorrhagic fevers, TB, hepatitis

South East Asia – dengue, malaria, diarrhoeal illness

Sub-Continent Asia/India – enteric fever, dengue, malaria, diarrhoeal illness, hepatitis

South America – diarrhoeal illness, RTI, dengue, malaria, mosquito-borne viruses

Central America/Caribbean - diarrhoeal illness, RTI, dengue, malaria, mosquito-borne viruses

North America/Europe – influenza, HIV, Lyme, tick-borne viruses, TB (eastern Europe)

provide protection against infection in certain groups of immune compromised patients.

- A history of immune compromise, radiation, toxin exposure or certain chronic infections may increase the risk of certain malignancies.
- A family history of non-infectious inflammatory diseases can indicate a genetic predisposition that may increase the risk of developing a non-infectious inflammatory disease.

Systematic history

Symptoms focussing on specific organ systems will provide direction towards the likely diagnosis when considering infectious causes of fever. Malignancies may also be found in any organ system. Non-infectious inflammatory diseases tend to affect multiple systems together, although a single system may predominate. The following detail focuses on infectious causes of fever.

Respiratory tract

- **Upper respiratory tract infection** is suggested by rhinorrhoea, nasal stuffiness, sneezing, sore throat, cough and a hoarse voice.
- **Sinusitis** is likely to cause facial pain and headache.
- **Otitis** is associated with ear pain, ear discharge with or without auditory symptoms such as deafness.
- **Lower respiratory tract infections** present with a cough, productive of purulent sputum, shortness of breath, wheeze or chest pain. Haemoptysis (coughing blood) suggests invasion of or damage to the blood vessels of the lung. This is present in tuberculosis, invasive fungal infection or non-infectious causes such as lung cancer or vasculitis.

Genitourinary tract

- **Lower urinary tract infection** classically presents with a combination of dysuria, frequency, urgency, change in smell and colour of urine.
- **Upper urinary tract infection** may have the above (or a history of the above) with additional loin or back pain.
- **Sexually transmitted infections and pelvic inflammatory disease** can present with the same symptoms as a lower or upper urinary tract infection but may have the additional symptoms of a vaginal or urethral discharge, dyspareunia (pain during intercourse), anogenital ulcers, genital warts, painful swelling of the scrotum, pubic itch or swelling of lymph glands in the groin.
- **Vaginal candidiasis** is not uncommon in women, particularly those who use vaginal douches or after a course of antibiotics. It may present as urinary tract infections do with a whitish vaginal discharge and vaginal itching.
- **Bacterial vaginosis** is not considered a true infection but rather an imbalance of normal vaginal flora and overgrowth of anaerobes. It presents with watery, foul-smelling vaginal discharge.

Gastrointestinal tract

Abdominal pain is central to almost all gastrointestinal causes of infections. It is important to characterise the pain including the site and radiation, associated abdominal symptoms and relieving and aggravating factors.

- **Gastroenteritis** is the commonest gastrointestinal infection and is associated with abdominal pain and diarrhoea, with or without vomiting. Characterising the diarrhoea may help in narrowing the aetiology due to the characteristic pathogenesis of some of the gastrointestinal pathogens. Determining whether the diarrhoea is acute or chronic can distinguish infective from non-infective causes. Direct questions to ask about diarrhoea include: frequency, colour and consistency, presence of mucous and/or blood in the stool (rather than just on the paper).
- **Hepatitis** is usually caused by viral agents but can also occur as a complication of medications or other toxins. Jaundice is the classic sign of hepatitis, along with a history of exposure to risk factors involving contact with body fluids or excretions.
- **Cholecystitis and cholangitis** classically present with pain in the right upper quadrant of the abdomen associated with nausea with or without jaundice.
- **Other forms of intra-abdominal infection** including bowel perforation and peritonitis present with varying abdominal symptoms including generalised or localised abdominal pain, bowel distension, diarrhoea, constipation or vomiting.

Nervous system

Headache, photophobia, vomiting, altered consciousness, fits, fainting, muscle weakness, numbness, paralysis, tremor, abnormal sensation and change of behaviour can all suggest an infection of the central nervous system. In neonates and young children the symptoms of infection are mostly non-specific.

Patients with multisystem non-infectious inflammatory diseases can have central and peripheral nervous system symptoms. A variety of neurological complications can be present including spinal cord involvement in rheumatoid arthritis, neuropsychiatric involvement in systemic lupus erythematosus and neurological sequelae in vasculitic disorders.

Certain predisposing factors play a role in various forms of nervous system infection. A history of immune suppression, head injury and neurosurgery should be elicited.

- **Meningitis** is an inflammation of the subarachnoid space and meninges (membranes covering the brain and spinal cord) most often secondary to an infection. It classically presents with headache, vomiting, neck stiffness and fever. Depending on the duration of onset, meningitis can be classed as acute, subacute or chronic. Acute meningitis develops over hours to days, chronic meningitis over weeks or longer, and may last for months to years; while subacute meningitis is in between the two, usually over weeks.
- Acute meningitis is most often bacterial, with the frequency of pathogens differing according to age group and immune status. Some forms of acute bacterial meningitis (meningococcal disease) can present with a typical purpuric non-blanching rash and may be associated with severe sepsis and shock. Viral meningitis is usually less severe and self-limiting and often begins with symptoms of a viral infection such as fever, malaise, headache and muscle aches.
- Head injury increases the risk of meningitis by damaging the protective layer of meninges and allowing respiratory or skin flora into the protected subarachnoid space. Neurosurgery predisposes to infection with the above and also hospital-acquired pathogens.
- Chronic meningitis presents with the same symptoms as acute, only over a more prolonged period. Associated features should be sought for the more common causes of chronic meningitis including tuberculosis, cryptococcus and Lyme disease.
- **Encephalitis** is inflammation of the brain tissue resulting in altered level of consciousness, headache and fever. Additional symptoms may be present depending on the site of infection and include seizures, tremors, stroke, hallucinations and abnormal behaviours. Encephalitis is usually viral in aetiology but may also be bacterial (e.g. syphilis) or parasitic (e.g. toxoplasmosis).
- **Intracranial abscesses** are bacterial infections of the CNS and include brain abscess, subdural or extradural empyema, classified according to their anatomic location. These abscesses occur secondary to seeding from a primary site, either from a contiguous one such as in otitis media, sinusitis, mastoiditis or dental infection; secondary to haematogenous spread from a remote site such as endocarditis; after a head injury or neurosurgery and, rarely, following meningitis.

Not all patients with nervous system symptoms and fever have a primary nervous system infection. Some systemic infections can cause neurological symptoms such as severe or cerebral malaria, neurologic signs in severe typhoid fever and meningeal signs in HIV seroconversion illness.

Skin and soft tissue

A detailed history of any skin conditions should be sought, even if this is not present at the time of consultation. Many skin conditions and rashes have a characteristic course, may fluctuate or change over time and therefore a full 'progress report' of the condition can help to guide the diagnosis. The presence of a rash is more likely to suggest a systemic than localised condition. Many multisystem non-infectious inflammatory diseases have an associated rash, such as the typical butterfly facial rash of systemic lupus erythematosus and petechial rash in vasculitic disorders.

Remember to ask about any insect or tick bites, as rashes following a bite (including an eschar at the bite site) could indicate a vector-borne disease.

It is important to distinguish a generalised rash illness from a localised skin or soft tissue lesion. The latter is more likely to be asymmetrical or unilateral, involve tissues deeper than the skin, affect surrounding structures and be associated with localised enlarged lymph nodes.

Some examples of localised infections include:

- **Impetigo** is a contagious infection caused by staphylococci or occasionally streptococci, found mainly in preschool children or in other ages associated with playing contact sports. It usually starts as a small pustule around the nose or mouth which bursts, oozes fluid and leaves a golden crust. It characteristically occurs in groups of lesions.
- **Cellulitis** is a bacterial infection of the skin involving deeper structures most commonly affecting the leg. There are other causes of a red or swollen leg and these should be excluded before the diagnosis is made. Cellulitis is rarely bilateral. Certain groups of people are at increased risk, including diabetics. It can affect any area of the body and facial cellulitis should be managed as a medical emergency.
- **Necrotising fasciitis** is a severe and rapidly spreading form of cellulitis. It is a medical emergency and requires urgent surgical as well as antibiotic management.
- **A history of human or animal bite or scratch** preceding the infection is important to elicit as specific pathogens are associated with these, including blood-borne virus transmission.

Musculoskeletal system

Bone, joint and muscle pain can form part of the constitutional symptoms of infectious and non-infectious diseases.

- **Joint infections** occur in both native and prosthetic joints. A history of joint replacement or joint procedure such as arthroscopy increases the risk of infection developing in the joint. In a patient complaining of arthralgia, one should distinguish between monoarthralgia (single joint) and polyarthralgia (multiple joint) involvement. Monoarthralgia is more likely to be a septic arthritis in the affected joint while polyarthralgia suggests a more systemic disease. Many viral infections and collagen vascular diseases present with polyarthralgia.

- **Bone infection** (osteomyelitis) can occur in any bone in the body either as a primary infection or secondary to an overlying skin or soft tissue infection or previous surgical procedure. Bone pain, swelling, deformities or pus draining through the skin overlying a bone should alert you to the possibility of this diagnosis.
- **Adult onset Still's disease** (AOSD) presents with a classic triad of persistent high spiking fevers, joint pain and a distinctive evanescent salmon pink, macular or maculopapular rash that peaks with the rise in the temperature. The rash occurs mainly on the trunk and extremities but rarely involves the palms of the hands, the soles of the feet or the face. Joint pains may range from arthralgia to a severe arthritis. Other features include lymphadenopathy, hepatomegaly and splenomegaly, sore throat and constitutional symptoms such as anorexia, arthralgia, myalgia, fatigue and weight loss. The classic fever pattern is one or two daily febrile spikes exceeding 39°C, usually occurring late during the day. At times the fever is continuous or less commonly spikes in the early morning.
- Although fever and constitutional symptoms occur in around half the patients with **polymyalgia rheumatica,** they are rarely the dominating features.

Cardiovascular system

- **Infective endocarditis** is an infection of the endocardium or lining of the heart. The most common form of this infection is infection of the heart valves. Symptoms are usually non-specific and the diagnosis should be considered in patients with damaged or prosthetic heart valves or those patients with risk factors for recurrent bacteraemias, e.g. poor dentition, intravenous drug use, long-term use of a intravascular device or underlying bowel cancer.
- **Myocarditis** is an inflammation of the muscle of the heart and is usually caused by viral infections. Symptoms are non-specific and may include chest pain, shortness of breath or palpitations.
- **Vascular infection** can occur as primary vascular infection of the endothelium or secondary to damage caused by catheters or cannulas, trauma or surgery.

Examination

General assessment

Examination should begin when you first make visual contact with the patient. Get a general impression of whether the patient looks well, unwell or severely ill.

Summaries of the pertinent features are described in Table 10.1.

Systematic assessment

A systematic and thorough examination of all organ systems may be necessary to elicit the cause of the fever. Both autoimmune disorders and systemic infections may produce clinical findings in multiple organ systems, and the pattern and collection of signs should be able to be collated into a single cause most of the time. It is not unusual for those with compromised immune systems or those who have travelled to have more than one infection at a time.

Skin and mucous membranes

Rashes are of particular importance and many infectious diseases present with a rash. Describe the location of the rash. Is it generalised, localised, symmetrical or asymmetrical? Rashes may indicate either a localised or generalised infection. Some rashes are typical of the causative infection; a few examples given in Table 10.2.

Fever and constitutional symptoms although common in patients with antineutrophil cytoplasmic antibodies (ANCA)-associated vasculitis (AAV) rarely occur in isolation. Palpable (non-thrombocytopenic) purpura is present in half the patients. Erythematous cutaneous nodules with or without superficial crusting may occur on the scalp, elbows, hands and feet (cutaneous extravascular necrotizing granulomas or Churg-Strauss granulomas) in patients with granulocytosis with polyangiitis (GPA) and eosinophilic granulocytosis with polyangiitis (EGPA). Subcutaneous nodules, skin ulcers, subungual splinter haemorrhages, digital gangrene and livedo reticularis may be seen and, mainly in EGPA, urticarial rash (Box 10.4).

Mild fever may accompany around a fifth of patients with Behçet's syndrome (BS) with active lesions. Febrile attacks seem to be associated strongly with vascular, neurological or joint involvement. Other features of BS include mouth and genital ulcers,

Box 10.4 ANCA-associated vasculitis

- Granulomatosis with polyangiitis (GPA)(Wegener's granulomatosis)
- Eosinophilic granulomatosis with polyangiitis (EGPA) (Churg-Strauss syndrome)
- Microscopic polyangiitis (PA)

Table 10.1 General examination in patients with fever

Temperature	Oral or ear temperature is preferred to axillary to give a closer indication of core temperature. Ear temperature is 0.5°C higher and axillary temperature is 0.5°C lower than oral temperature. Fever is defined as a core temperature above normal. In clinical practice this translates to an oral temperature of ≥38.3°C.
Pulse	Tachycardia is characteristic during fever. For every 1°C rise in temperature the pulse increases by 10 beats per minute. A pulse-temperature dissociation is characteristically seen in typhoid, brucellosis, leptospirosis and diphtheria.
Respiratory rate	For every 1°C rise in temperature the respiratory rate rises by 4 breaths per minute. Higher respiratory rates signify additional lung pathology such as pneumonia.
Blood pressure	Hypotension may signify severe sepsis or septic shock.
Lymph nodes	Note the pattern and groups involved. Check cervical, axillary and inguinal areas. Describe the consistency of the nodes. Are they firm, hard, regular, irregular, mobile or fixed? Are enlarged lymph nodes unilateral, bilateral, above and/or below the diaphragm? Note the size of the lymph nodes and whether there is a single or multiple lymph nodes present. Significant lymphadenopathy is found in tuberculosis, brucellosis, toxoplasmosis, viral infections such as HIV or infectious mononucleosis. They are also a predominant feature of lymphoma and metastatic spread of malignancies.
Jaundice	Examine the conjunctivae, nail beds and skin for evidence of jaundice. This may indicate underlying either haemolysis such as in malaria and haemorrhagic fevers, or liver disease as in viral hepatitis, cholangitis or liver abscess.
Eyes	Conjunctivitis may indicate a localised eye infection or be associated with a systemic infection such as measles. Roth's spots on the retina may be found in infective endocarditis. Tubercles of miliary TB may be found on the choroid.
Ears	Inflammation and redness of the external ear canal indicates otitis externa, while a bulging red eardrum suggests otitis media. If the eardrum has perforated, fluid or pus may be found in the external ear canal.
Mouth	Examination of the mouth may yield a host of information and should include visualisation of the inner cheeks, palate, tongue, pharynx, tonsils, gums and teeth. General oral and dental hygiene should be noted. Lesions on the wall of the mouth or palate should be characterised as described for skin rashes below. White lesions may indicate oral thrush; the throat and tonsils should be examined for erythema and exudates; ulcers in or around the mouth may indicate oral herpes. Dry mouth is a feature of some non-infectious inflammatory diseases.
Skin	The entire surface of the skin should be examined, as a lesion or rash may be present only in an area hidden to view in a clothed individual. Describe and characterise any rash, petechiae, and areas of redness or swelling. Determine if there are any open wounds, ulcers or bite marks, including an eschar. The presence of open wounds, intravascular devices or injection sites should be noted and closely examined for signs of erythema, swelling or tenderness. Intravascular devices may be the source of either localised skin or disseminated infections.
Hands and nails	Splinter haemorrhages on the palms and nail beds require further investigation for infective endocarditis. Scaly, itchy lesions between the fingers suggest the presence of scabies mites. Typical nail deformities of non-infectious inflammatory diseases, such as psoriasis, should be noticed.

erythema nodosum-like lesions, pyoderma gangrenosum, folliculitis and uveitis.

Respiratory tract

Perform a full respiratory examination looking for signs of upper respiratory tract infection such as pharyngitis, tonsillitis, tonsilar abscess (quinsy) or otitis.

Use palpation, percussion and auscultation to determine whether there is any suggestion of a lower respiratory tract infection such as bronchitis, pneumonia, pleural effusion or empyema, cavitation or lung abscess.

Palpate for tenderness over the sinuses or mastoids.

Harshening of normal breath sounds may indicate inflammation of the bronchi in bronchitis. The presence of consolidation in the lung indicating pneumonia can be determined by finding dullness to percussion along with increased vocal resonance of crepitation and/or bronchial breathing. Pleural effusion or empyema is suggested by dullness to percussion and decreased or absent vocal resonance. Cavitation or abscess formation suggesting tuberculosis produces an increase in resonance.

The presence of rhinorrhoea, nasal congestion, sneezing, cough and a hoarse voice suggest a viral upper respiratory tract infection.

Cardiovascular system

The diagnosis of infective endocarditis is based on the modified Duke's criteria. While relying mainly on investigations for confirmation, certain clinical signs are suggestive and should be looked for in patients with risk factors. These include new valvular

Table 10.2 Examples of rashes in patients with fever	
Maculopapular	Scarlet fever, measles (look for conjunctivitis and white lesions in the mouth – Koplik's spots), rubella, erythema infectiosum, roseola, typhus, typhoid (rose spots), dengue, rickettsial infection
Vesicular	Herpes simplex, chicken pox, shingles, coxackie virus, allergy
Petechial, purpuric, haemorrhagic, vasculitic	Meningococcal (non-blanching), viral haemorrhagic fevers, dengue, splinter haemorrhages of infective endocarditis, non-infective vasculitis
Erythematous	Cellulitis, erysipelas, drug allergy
Pustular	Staphylococcal, disseminated gonococcal infection
Rash on palm and soles	Enteroviral infections, meningococcal infection, spotted fever, typhus, infective endocarditis, secondary syphilis, scabies (burrows between fingers and toes)
Nodular	Erythema nodosum, TB, leprosy, non-infective vasculitis, Behçet's syndrome

regurgitation, temperature >38°C, splinter and conjunctival haemorrhages, Janeway lesions (small, non-tender red lesions on the palms or soles) and Osler's nodes (painful, red raised lesions on hands and feet). (See also Box 13.25.)

Infected thrombophlebitis or vasculitis may occur secondary to a cannula or catheter insertion into a vein or as a primary infection of the vessels by certain pathogens (*Campylobacter fetus*, non-typhi *Salmonellae*), usually in immunocompromised patients.

Genitourinary tract

Examine for suprapubic and renal angle tenderness in suspected cases of urinary tract infection. Note the presence or absence of a urinary catheter.

Genital examination should be performed with a chaperone present if requested or when a male clinician is examining a female patient.

Female genital examination is best performed in lithotomy position to enable ease of examination. External examination should note any evidence of redness, swelling, vaginal, urethral or anal discharge, vesicles, ulcers, warts or foreign bodies. Unilateral swelling of the labia may indicate an abscess of the Bartholin's gland, which can be palpated only when enlarged.

The groin should be examined for evidence of lymphadenopathy or diseases such as tinea, candida or pubic lice.

Speculum examination allows examination of the cervix as well as the vaginal vault. If a discharge is present, describe its consistency. Candidiasis is white and cheesy, while trichomonas infection gives a frothy greenish fish-smelling discharge. A purulent discharge coming from the cervix is suggestive of gonococcal infection, while chlamydia causes a more mucoid or mucopurulent discharge. Cervical warts may appear as flat or raised.

If anal lesions or symptoms are present, a proctoscope can be used to examine the rectal mucosa.

A bimanual examination is required for palpation of cervical excitation tenderness, fallopian or uterine tenderness in suspected pelvic inflammatory disease.

Male genital examination includes examination of the penis, scrotum, testes, epididymis, spermatic cord and anorectum. External examination should note the presence of any ulcers, warts, excoriations or rashes. Examine the urethral meatus for any discharge or ulcer not visible on external examination. Examine the scrotum for redness, swelling, ulcers or other lesions. Tenderness on palpation of the testes and/or epididymis may suggest epididymo-orchitis.

Gastrointestinal tract

Abdominal examination begins by inspection of the patient with an exposed abdomen between the xiphisternum and symphysis pubis (allowing for patient privacy).

Determine if ascites or abdominal swelling is present and whether the abdomen is tender. Palpate for the presence of hepatomegaly, splenomegaly or a distended gall bladder and whether any of these organs are tender.

Splenomegaly may be present in many diseases, caused by either increase in its function or by direct infiltration. Infectious causes of increased function are due to immune stimulation in response to the infection and include Infectious mononucleosis, viral hepatitis, AIDS, typhoid, brucellosis, tuberculosis, histoplasmosis, infective endocarditis, leptospirosis, leishmaniasis and malaria.

Infective causes of hepatomegaly include infectious mononucleosis, liver abscess, amoebic infection, hydatid cyst, malaria, leptospirosis and actinomycosis. Viral hepatitis rarely causes an enlarged liver.

Nervous system

Global examination of the nervous system includes cognitive as well as physical function. The level of consciousness can be determined using the Glasgow coma score. Reduced, altered or fluctuating levels of consciousness may be present in any infection of the central nervous system but is more likely in encephalitis and brain abscess than in meningitis.

The characteristic triad signs of meningitis include nuchal rigidity (neck stiffness), photophobia and headache. To detect neck stiffness, passively bend the patient's chin towards the chest. This will elicit pain by stretching the inflamed meninges leading to resistance in movement. Other signs caused by pain on stretching the inflamed meninges include Brudzinski's and Kernig's signs.

Kernig's sign is positive when the thigh is bent 90 degrees at both the hip and knee, and the knee is then straightened leading to pain and resistance. Brudzinski's sign is positive if the patient involuntary lifts their legs when the clinician lifts the patient's head off the examination bed.

Focal neurological signs could be suggestive of a space-occupying lesion such as a brain abscess, tuberculoma or toxoplasmosis. Focal signs may also be present due to cranial nerve involvement caused by meningitis.

Some forms of NS infection have associated features which should be noted. Meningococcal meningitis may occur with a typical purpuric non-blanching rash.

Musculoskeletal system

Joint infections occur in both native and prosthetic joints. A history of joint replacement or joint procedure such as arthroscopy increases the risk of infection developing in the joint. In a patient complaining of arthralgia one should distinguish between monoarthralgia (single joint) and polyarthralgia (multiple joint) involvement. Monoarthralgia is more likely to be a septic arthritis in the affected joint while polyarthralgia suggests a more systemic disease. Many viral infections and collagen vascular diseases present with polyarthralgia.

Bone infection (osteomyelitis) can occur in any bone in the body either as a primary infection or secondary to on overlying skin or soft tissue infection or previous surgical procedure. Bone pain, swelling, deformities or pus draining through the skin overlying a bone should alert you to the possibility of this diagnosis. Spinal infection can affect the bone itself as in Pott's disease caused by tuberculosis or the intervertebral disc, most often caused by staphylococcal infection, when spinal percussion is often tender.

Rheumatic fever can occur in any age group but is rare under the age of 3 and above 15 years. In Western countries, acute rheumatic fever is generally preceded 2 to 4 weeks by group A streptococcal (GAS) tonsillopharyngitis but not by GAS skin infections. Fever is one of the four minor manifestations of rheumatic fever and may be high or low. The period between the GAS infection and the onset of rheumatic fever is free of clinical features and C-reactive protein is normal. The most common major manifestation of rheumatic fever is arthritis followed by pancarditis, chorea (Sydenham's), erythema marginatum and subcutaneous nodules.

Although fatigue is a prominent complaint in idiopathic inflammatory myositis, fever occurs mainly in patients with **juvenile dermatomyositis** and antisynthetase syndrome. Other features include Raynaud's phenomenon, hyperkeratosis especially of the radial side of the index fingers (mechanic's hands), polyarthritis and interstitial lung disease. These patients have positive antiaminoacyl-tRNA synthetase antibodies such as Jo-1.

About one fifth of patients with relapsing **polychondritis** present with fever and in the absence of chondritis of the external ear and the nose, the diagnosis may be difficult to make.

Multisystem diseases

Fever in autoinflammatory periodic syndromes

Apart from familial Mediterranean fever (FMF), the autoinflammatory periodic syndromes are rarely encountered in routine clinical practice (Box 10.5). Nearly 90% of patients with FMF become symptomatic before the age of 20 years. However, genetic testing has helped diagnose mild disease in adults. More males are affected than females. A typical acute attack, usually lasting 1 to 3 days, is characterized by fever, serositis, and arthritis or skin rash. The attacks may recur every few weeks but may be as infrequent as every few years. Acute abdominal pain, due to acute sterile peritonitis, occurs in 90% of patients. Pleurisy is another clinical feature but mainly occurs in patients of Armenian origin. The term FMF is confusing as in a significant number of cases, there is no family history, no Mediterranean roots (Arabs, Armenians, Italians and Jews), and fever may be absent. The patient may present with acute arthritis or an erysipelas-like erythema (neutrophilic dermatosis) with mild or even absent fever. The arthritis may last up to a week.

Nearly two thirds of patients with polyarteritis nodosa develop fever and constitutional symptoms (arthralgia, myalgia, malaise and weight loss). Hypertension, usually mild, is present in up to half the patients, particularly in those with hepatitis B viral infection. Cutaneous lesions include livedo reticularis (Fig. 10.6), ischemic changes in the digits (Fig. 10.7), subcutaneous nodules and ulcerations.

Fever and constitutional symptoms may be the main clinical features in patients with **Takayasu's arteritis**. In more than half the patients there is decreased or absent peripheral pulse. In a small number of patients, the inflammation of the wall of the carotid artery may cause local tenderness (carotidynia).

Fever in patients with systemic lupus erythematosus (SLE) can prove a challenging clinical problem. Fever may be a major feature in about two fifths of patients with active SLE. Infection is not easy to exclude and the fever may be drug induced. Very rarely the fever may be caused by lymphoma complicating lupus. The most challenging situation is when the patient with lupus presents with high fever, respiratory symptoms and radiographic changes. The difficulty

Box 10.5 The classic periodic fever syndromes (monogenic autoinflammatory diseases)

- Familial Mediterranean fever (FMF)
- TNF receptor-associated periodic syndrome (TRAPS)
- Hyperimmunoglobulinemia D with periodic fever syndrome (HIDS)

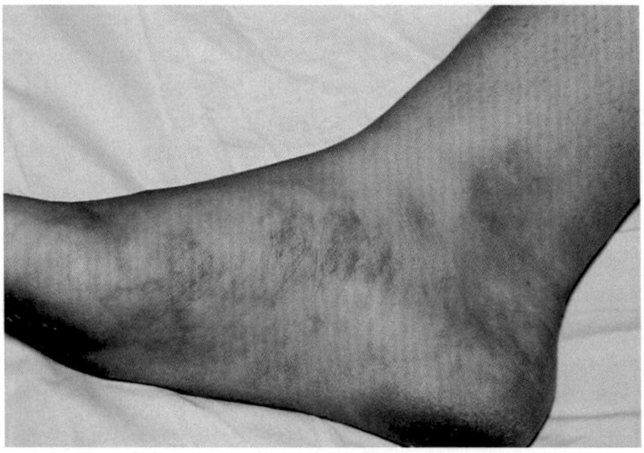

Figure 10.6 Livedo reticularis in a 39-year-old woman with polyarteritis nodosa.

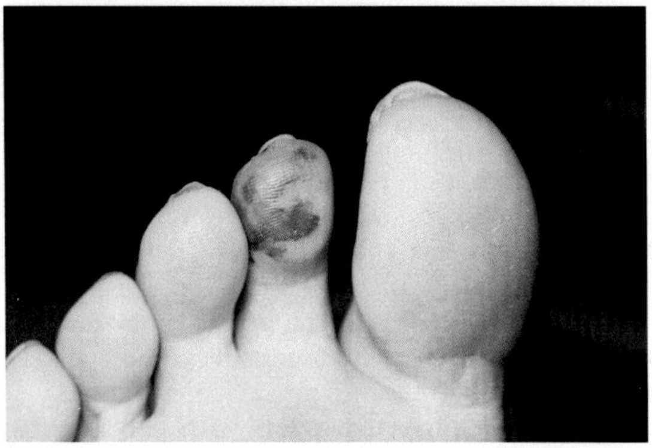

Figure 10.7 Ischemic changes in the right second digit in a 39-year-old woman with polyarteritis nodosa.

is whether the radiographic changes are caused by complicating infection or organizing pneumonia.

Fever is not a feature in patients with uncomplicated scleroderma.

Drug fever

Drugs can cause fever via several mechanisms (Table 10.3). This is a diagnosis by exclusion. A rash is not always present nor eosinophilia. By definition the fever coincides with administration of the drug and disappears when the drug is discontinued. The risk of developing drug fever increases with the number of drugs prescribed especially in elderly patients, patients with active HIV infection and patients with cystic fibrosis.

Table 10.3 Mechanisms of drug fever

Mechanism	Examples
Hypersensitivity	Anticonvulsants, penicillin, minocycline, sulfonamide, allopurinol
Altered thermoregulatory mechanisms	Thyroxine, drugs with anticholinergic activity, amphetamine, cocaine
Directly related to administration of the drug	Paraldehyde, pentazocine, amphotericin B, bleomycin
Direct extension of the pharmacologic action of the drug	Chemotherapy
Idiosyncrasy	Succinylcholine, haloperidol, serotonin syndrome

Investigations for infectious causes of fever

Testing for infectious disease should include both laboratory and radiological investigations.

Laboratory

Both routine and specialist tests should be performed in the haematology, chemistry, microbiology and virology laboratory where appropriate.

Full blood count with differential and film

White blood cell count is often raised in infection although a low count may indicate specific pathogens or overwhelming infection. In patients on immune suppression or chemotherapy the white cell count should not be used as a marker of infection as it may be falsely raised or suppressed.

- **Neutrophilia** with band forms and toxic granulation suggest bacterial infection.
- **Neutropenia** may be seen post chemotherapy or with typhoid fever, brucellosis, severe sepsis or viral infection.
- A reactive **lymphocytosis** may be seen in acute viral illnesses, particularly infectious mononucleosis when atypical lymphocytes may be present. It may also occur in tuberculosis, brucellosis, or in leukaemias and lymphomas.
- **Lymphopaenia** is common in viral infection (influenza, dengue, HIV) and typhoid fever.
- **Eosinophilia** is seen in hypersensitivity reactions as well as invasive parasitic infections.

Platelets

- **Thrombocytopaenia** may be seen in malaria, haemorrhagic fevers, meningococcal sepsis or disseminated intravascular coagulation (DIC) associated with overwhelming infection.
- **Thrombocytosis** may occur as an acute response to inflammation or can occur in chronic infections such as TB.

A **blood film** or smear is used to look for parasites that may be present in the blood. The commonest of this is malaria, but can also be used to detect babesia, trypanosomiasis or microfilaria. It may suggest Epstein-Barr virus (EBV) if atypical lymphocytes are seen.

Inflammatory markers

Acute-phase reactants (APRs) are a heterogeneous group of plasma proteins that increase or decrease in response to inflammatory stimuli such as infections, trauma, arthritis, autoimmune disorders and malignancies. The levels of APRs rise and fall in response to the rise and fall of the inflammatory process. Common tests used for this purpose include C-reactive protein (CRP) and erythrocyte sedimentation rate (ESR) and more recently procalcitonin (PCT). ESR is an indirect APR as it measures the rate of movement of red blood cells, which is increased by binding of an APR. Most APRs are produced in the liver.

The ESR rises fairly rapidly (within 24-48 hours) from the onset of inflammation and is slow to fall once the cause of inflammation resolves. It has a low sensitivity for infection and is affected by many factors including age, gender, weight and renal function. Despite this, an ESR over 100 mm/hour warrants further investigation.

CRP is a more sensitive marker of inflammation than ESR and is less affected by external factors such as age and gender. It rises more rapidly (within 6-24 hours) and is quicker to fall than ESR. Very high levels of CRP are more likely to be associated with bacterial infection than other causes of inflammation.

Procalcitonin has several advantages over both ESR and CRP. It rises within 3-4 hours, quicker than either ESR or CRP, and a result can be obtained in 30 minutes or less using a semiquantitative point-of-care test. It is more sensitive a marker of bacterial infection as raised PCT levels are not seen in other non-infectious inflammatory conditions, and viral infections tend to inhibit PCT rather than raise it. It can, however, be raised in invasive fungal infection, malaria, by massive trauma such as severe burns or major surgery, any therapy that stimulates cytokines such as T-cell antibody therapy, granulocyte transfusion or graft-versus-host disease.

The usefulness of the above tests may differ depending on the situation and site of infection.

Basic biochemistry tests

Renal and liver function tests are useful in determining the presence of any renal or hepatic impairment, which may assist in determining severity of disease and affect antimicrobial dosing. Abnormal liver function tests may also assist in diagnosis of gastrointestinal infections such as hepatitis or cholecystitis.

Microbiology and virology tests

The type of samples sent will depend on the site of infection identified. A few examples are listed below.

Blood cultures should be taken if you suspect the patient may have bacteraemia from any source. The signs of sepsis, severe sepsis or septic shock should be used to indicate the need to take these cultures. If possible, two sets should be taken aseptically prior to any antibiotic therapy.

Bone marrow cultures may be more useful than blood cultures for some intracellular pathogens.

Sample any fluid that represents the possible site of infection as follows:

1. **Urine**
   - Dip, culture and microscopy for lower or upper urinary tract infection and urogenital infections
   - Molecular tests for urogenital infections
   - Urine antigen testing for Legionella and *Streptococcus pneumoniae* in cases of community-acquired pneumonia
2. **Urethral, vaginal and cervical swabs for urogenital infections**
   - Culture and microscopy for lower or upper urinary tract infection and urogenital infections
   - Molecular tests for urogenital infections
3. **Cerebrospinal, peritoneal, joint and pleural fluid, biopsy tissue, sputum and bronchoalvelolar lavage**
   - Microscopy, culture and sensitivity for bacterial and fungal infection
   - Ziehl-Neelsen (ZN) staining and culture for acid-fast bacilli for diagnosis of TB
   - Molecular tests for viral pathogens
4. **Stool**
   - Culture and sensitivity for bacterial infection
   - Microscopy for parasites
   - Molecular tests for viral pathogens
5. **Pus and tissue samples from abscesses, surgical debridement, biopsies and wound infections**
   - Microscopy, culture and sensitivity for bacterial and fungal infection
   - ZN staining and culture for acid-fast bacilli for diagnosis of TB

Serology

This is used mainly in the diagnosis of viral infections. A positive IgM usually indicates current or recent infection and a positive IgG indicates a previous infection or vaccination. The following are common serology tests used in the diagnosis of infectious diseases:

Rash diseases: Measles, rubella, parvovirus, varicella, rickettsia, typhus, syphilis

Gastrointestinal infection: Viral hepatitis, cytomegalovirus (CMV), amoebic liver abscess

Systemic infections: HIV, Lyme, dengue, brucellosis, leptospirosis

Molecular diagnostics

This diagnostic platform is used mainly in the diagnosis of viral infections but is increasingly used for bacterial, fungal and parasitic infections. It is a rapid and sensitive technique and is not affected by previous antibiotic treatment or the inability to culture the pathogen. Most sample types can be used for molecular diagnostics. It is used routinely to diagnose viral infections such as gastroenteritis, respiratory tract infections, central nervous system infections and viral haemorrhagic fevers. Bacterial infections commonly

Box 10.6 Common disease presenting atypically

Bacterial

Abscesses (dental, subphrenic, liver, ovarian, prostate)
Vascular infections
Extrapulmonary TB, atypical mycobacteria
Protected sites
- Sinuses/Ears
- Heart
- Prostate/Ovaries
- Bone, joint, intervertebral disc
- Thyroid

Partially treated infections

Viral

Immune compromised host
Partial immunity

Fungal

Immune compromised host

Protozoal and rickettsial

Travel history

Box 10.7 Uncommon disease presenting typically

Bacterial	
Brucella	Bartonella
Atypical mycobacteria	Borrelia
HACEK organisms*	Leptospirosis
Nocardia	Actinomycosis
Viral	
HIV	Hepatitis D & E
EBV, CMV	Viral haemorrhagic fever
Fungal	
Cryptococcus	Histoplasmosis
Protozoal	
Malaria	Amoebiasis
Trypanosomiasis	Leishmaniasis
Schistosomiasis	Toxoplasmosis
Rickettsial	
Q fever	
Mycoplasmas	

*HACEK includes *Haemophilus parainfluenzae, Haemophilus aphrophilus, Actinobacillus, actinomycetemcomitans, Cardiobacterium hominis, Eikenella corrodens*, and *Kingella kingae*

diagnosed in this way include pertussis, meningococcal disease and tuberculosis.

Immunological tests

Systemic lupus erythematosus is defined by the presence of autoantibodies. Antinuclear and double-stranded antibodies, antibodies to the extractable nuclear antigens and complement 3 and 4 need to be tested. The predictive value of ANCA testing depends on the clinical presentation of the patient and the laboratory performing the test. It is best that all reasonable attempts to confirm clinical suspicions of systemic vasculitis with histopathological proof should be undertaken before treating the patient with potentially toxic medications.

Histopathology

Biopsy and staining of lymph nodes, tissue, fluid or bone marrow may reveal infectious structures such as caseating granulomas, acid-fast bacilli, protozoal cysts, fungal hyphae or spores.

Radiology

Imaging studies may help to elucidate the source and extent of infection in those with a fever and localised site. All modalities of imaging have a role in diagnosis with the indications for X-rays, ultrasound, CT scan, MRI, radionucleotide or PET scan, depending on the site of infection being investigated.

Pyrexia of unknown origin

Despite an adequate history, examination and set of investigations, the cause of some fevers remains unknown. This is termed a PUO or pyrexia of unknown origin. The classic definition of a PUO is a fever of >38.3°C for >2 weeks during which time there has been at least:

- Three separate outpatient appointments, OR
- 3 days in hospital, OR
- 1 weeks' worth of appropriate and thorough investigation

Infections account for 40% of cases of PUO. Causes of a PUO often fall into one of two categories:

1. A common disease presenting in an atypical way
2. An uncommon disease presenting typically

A common disease presenting in an atypical way requires more thought about the less common sites of infection, acquiring samples from more protected sites, consideration of testing in the immune compromised and the possibility of partially treated infections. (See Boxes 10.6 and 10.7 for examples.)

An uncommon disease presenting in a typical manner requires thought about travel, occupation, pets, hobbies, habits and any other unusual activity that may present an infection risk.

Non-infectious causes of a PUO need to be considered and include neoplasms, autoimmune syndromes, granulomatous diseases, drug fevers and other miscellaneous causes such as haematomas, brain lesions, hyperthyroidism, tissue ischaemia or infarction.

A thorough history, examination and investigations, as described above, should be performed on all patients with pyrexia of unknown origin, and the examination repeated from time to time.

Patients in pain 11

Richard M. Langford and Shankar Ramaswamy

Introduction

Pain is a familiar phenomenon which is part of our everyday life and is a feature of various diseases. It most commonly accompanies an injury, where it serves its most important purpose, namely, to protect us, alert us and make us remove ourselves from danger. It can possibly trigger a spinal withdrawal reflex (Fig. 11.1). Both congenital insensitivity to pain and extreme sensitivity to pain (paroxysmal extreme pain disorder and erythromelalgia) are rare genetic conditions which are disabling and shorten life span, highlighting the importance of pain to our welfare and survival. The severity of pain, and its impact on an individual, ranges from a trivial occurrence such as a needle-prick injury to a sensation of such intensity that it induces thoughts of suicide.

Definition

The International Association for the Study of Pain (IASP) proposed the following definition (1979): 'Pain is an unpleasant sensory and emotional experience associated with actual or potential tissue damage or described in terms of damage'. This definition has important implications: pain is not necessarily or always associated with ongoing tissue damage; it is a subjective experience and has an emotional as well as a sensory component and is always unpleasant.

Pain is notoriously difficult to describe. It is difficult to assess and even harder to quantify. Nevertheless, pain assessment is crucial in order to evaluate its impact on the sufferer and also to plan a treatment strategy. It has been termed 'the 5th vital sign' and is mandated as part of routine assessment of patients in hospital. In 2004 the IASP declared that the relief of pain should be a human right.

Classification of pain

There are many ways in which pain can be classified in order to formulate an optimal treatment strategy. Despite this, classifying a particular pain state can be challenging because the pain syndrome may be of mixed aetiology rather than fit a single category.

Pain is commonly classified according to the following:

- Aetiology and underlying condition
- Mechanism
- Duration

Aetiology/underlying condition

- Trauma – an acute response to an injury
- Surgery
- Medical illness such as myocardial infarction or appendicitis
- Physiological conditions such as menstruation and labour

Mechanism

- Inflammatory/Nociceptive – pain generated and maintained by inflammatory mediators (such as prostaglandin E_2), secondary to an ongoing disease process. Examples include inflammatory arthritis or mechanical back pain.
- Neuropathic – Neuropathic pain is generated in malfunctioning nerves and is defined as 'pain arising as a direct consequence of a lesion or disease affecting the somatosensory system'. This type of pain has special clinical features as described below and may arise from injury or dysfunction of the central or peripheral nervous system. Examples include painful diabetic neuropathy and post-stroke pain.
- Mixed pain – This includes features of both nociceptive and neuropathic pain, such as back pain with radiculopathy (radiating leg pain due to nerve irritation or compression).
- Psychosomatic – Purely psychosomatic pain is rare. However, pain, especially chronic pain, almost invariably has an emotional and behavioural component.

Duration

- Acute – most commonly a physiological response to an injury. It resolves with the

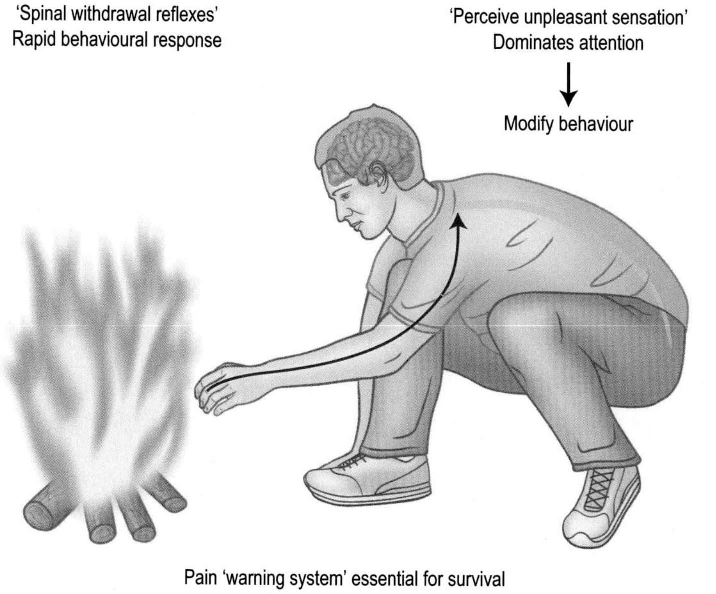
'Spinal withdrawal reflexes'
Rapid behavioural response
'Perceive unpleasant sensation'
Dominates attention
Modify behaviour
Pain 'warning system' essential for survival

Figure 11.1 Spinal withdrawal reflex with pain.

disappearance of a noxious stimulus or within the time frame of a normal healing process.

- Chronic – it can either be associated with an ongoing pathological process, such as rheumatoid arthritis or malignancy, or be present for longer than is consistent with a normal healing time. Pain is arbitrarily described as chronic if it persists for longer than 3 months. Chronic pain is often associated with disability, mood and sleep disturbance and a significant behavioural response. It is sometimes subdivided into pain associated with cancer and pain associated with non-malignant conditions.

Mechanisms of pain

At its simplest, pain is generated by a noxious stimulus that excites the central nervous system. This mechanism was first proposed by Descartes in the 16th century and conceptually still holds true, but it is crucial to appreciate that the final subjective experience of pain is shaped by various modulatory factors (Fig. 11.2).

A stimulus (which can be thermal, pressure or chemical) excites nociceptors and the resulting impulse is then transmitted to the spinal cord by two different classes of nerve fibres, via the first-order neurons located in the dorsal root ganglion (Fig. 11.3): (i) faster, myelinated Aδ fibres and (ii) smaller, slower unmyelinated C fibres transmit the sensation to the dorsal horn of the spinal cord, where these primary afferents synapse in lamina I, lamina II (substantia gelatinosa), lamina IV and some in lamina V. All these afferent sensory fibres are excitatory. Second-order fibres are then carried in the spinothalamic and spinoreticular tracts to the thalamus, where they synapse. From the thalamus, third-order neurons project to the somatosensory cortex, anterior cingulate gyrus and the insular cortex, where they terminate. It is at this cortical level that a stimulus is perceived as pain (Fig. 11.3).

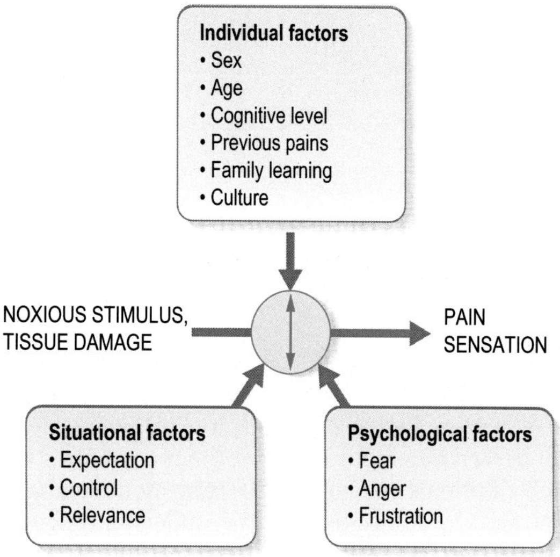
Individual factors
• Sex
• Age
• Cognitive level
• Previous pains
• Family learning
• Culture
NOXIOUS STIMULUS, TISSUE DAMAGE
PAIN SENSATION
Situational factors
• Expectation
• Control
• Relevance
Psychological factors
• Fear
• Anger
• Frustration

Figure 11.2 Biopsychosocial model of pain.

However, we now know that the noxious sensory input may be modulated at several levels in the spinal cord and brain, thus altering the final pain experience. At the spinal level, the gate theory proposed by Melzack and Wall in 1965 states that non-noxious stimulation of the large Aβ fibres inhibits the response to painful stimuli of neurons with wide dynamic range (WDR neurons, located primarily in lamina V), reducing the input of small fibres mediating the sensation of pain. A good example of this effect is 'rubbing it better'. In addition, descending input from

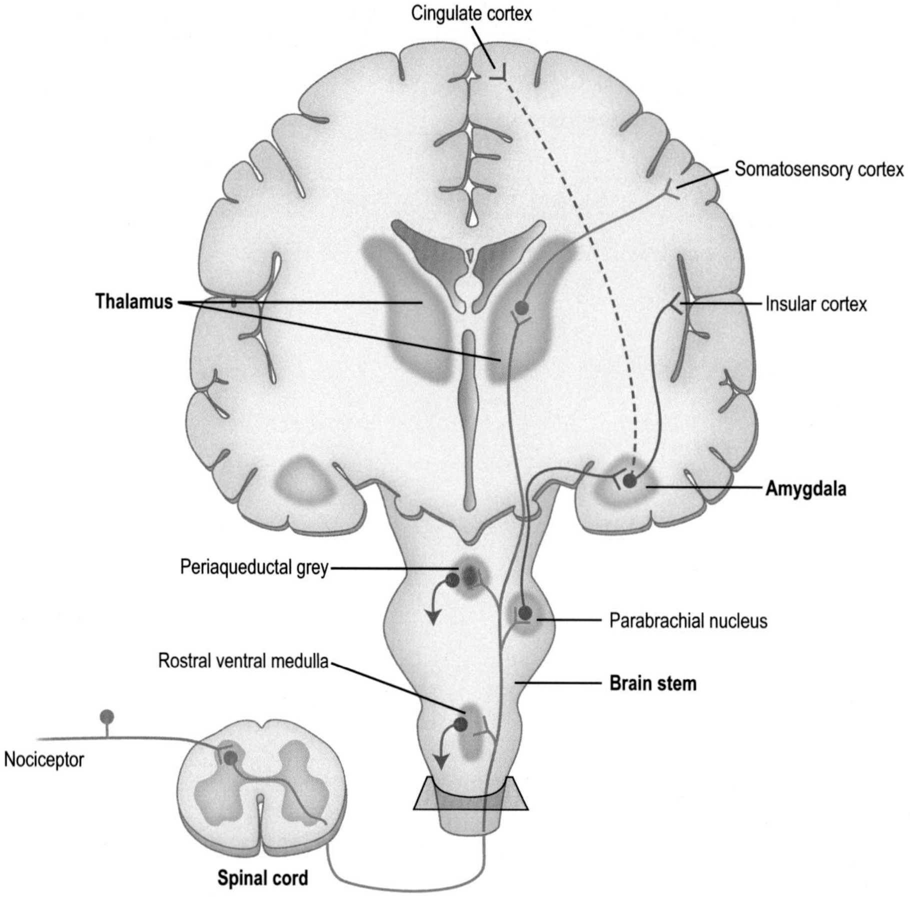

Figure 11.3 Pain pathway.

higher centres (periaqueductal grey matter and rostral ventral medulla) also modulate neural activity in the spinal cord, reducing or enhancing pain sensation. Such descending input is one of the mechanisms by which emotional and cognitive factors modulate pain perception. Much remains to be understood about the central pathophysiology of pain.

In recent years, pain management has increasingly adopted a biopsychosocial model. This has highlighted the need to take into account the interactions between biological, psychological and social factors leading to an individual's emergent pain experience.

The patient in pain

As with any other branch of medicine, careful and meticulous assessment of a patient's symptoms and signs is fundamental. Two key questions should be considered when dealing with a patient in pain:

- Is the pain a symptom of ongoing tissue damage or of another condition that needs to be dealt with by another medical professional?
- What is the optimal treatment strategy: to either abolish the pain altogether or reduce it to a more bearable level?

Unfortunately, no single standardized approach will allow assessment of pain in every situation. Pain is essentially a subjective experience. Therefore, what the patient describes as his experience is of paramount importance. As in most areas of medicine, the history is the most useful tool in assessment and diagnosis.

History

Taking a history from a patient in pain is more complex than recording symptoms and making a diagnosis. Even in acute pain states, where pain represents a protective function and is a symptom of an injury, approaching the patient as a whole and bearing in mind the overall context, emotional, cognitive and behavioural aspects is crucial for optimising the treatment strategy.

The first step is to evaluate the pain and thereby try to understand its underlying mechanisms. This process is described in Boxes 11.1 and 11.2 and Tables 11.1 and 11.2.

Examination

The purpose of examination as part of pain evaluation is described in Box 11.3.

Box 11.1 Scheme for evaluating history associated with pain

- The site of pain – this may give a clue to the underlying pathology.
- Distribution – pain may follow a dermatomal or peripheral nerve distribution or have no relation to anatomical patterns.
- Character of pain – nociceptive (somatic or visceral) versus neuropathic (Table 11.1).
- Duration of pain – this may have a bearing on the level of disability and psychosocial cost of the pain.
- Rapidity of onset and any precipitating factors – a rapid or relatively recent-onset pain syndrome is more likely to follow a conventional medical model, whereby it is appropriate to search for an underlying cause. Chronic pain requires a more biopsychosocial approach.
- Severity of pain and its change over time – this requires a consistent method for measuring pain (see below).
- Alleviating and exacerbating/aggravating factors – these may support a better understanding of mechanisms that sustain the pain.
- Exclusion of more sinister pathology – 'red flags'. Important conditions not to be missed include pain related to underlying (or undiagnosed) cancer, pain related to inflammation (such as rheumatoid arthritis) and pain related to other serious medical/surgical conditions requiring emergency treatment such as cauda equina syndrome due to spinal cord compression.
- Evaluation of psychosocial elements also known as 'yellow flags' (Box 11.2) – These are not life-threatening symptoms, but their presence means that the psychosocial history has special relevance. Major psychological illness should be addressed, along with symptomatic relief of the pain, in the interim.
- Previous and current treatments and their impact
- Past medical history – Taking a full medical history must not be overlooked. It may give invaluable clues as to the aetiology and pathogenesis of pain. For instance: history of recent herpes zoster (shingles) infection along with a dermatomal distribution of neuropathic-type pain (confirmed on examination with a residual, typical rash, allodynia and hypoalgesia/hyperalgesia) will suggest a diagnosis of postherpetic neuralgia. Certain common illnesses associated with neuropathic pain are listed in Table 11.2.
- Impact of pain – consider the effect of pain on the patient's activity, ability to work, mood, sleep, relationships etc.
- Psychosocial history – The psychosocial assessment of pain should be directed at finding out the psychological setting of the pain, particularly mood. It should explore the patient's beliefs and expectations. Generally speaking this is more relevant in chronic pain states, because acute pain usually resolves quickly.

Box 11.2 Psychosocial aspects of pain

Pain is described as having at least five dimensions, each of which should be addressed:

- The sensation of pain – the subjective experience
- Suffering and distress – the emotional component
- Expectations and beliefs – the cognitive component
- Verbal (complaints) or non-verbal communication – the behavioural component (illness behaviour) is the way in which the patient responds to and expresses the sensation of pain which is influenced by various cultural and social factors
- Impact of social environment

Box 11.3 The purpose of examination as part of pain evaluation

- To elucidate and evaluate any physical signs associated with a particular painful condition
- To reassure the patient that pain does not imply any ongoing damage
- To define baseline parameters and monitor their change over time
- To understand the mechanisms which generate and sustain the pain, in particular to identify neuropathic elements

Table 11.1 Nociceptive versus neuropathic pain

	Nociceptive	**Neuropathic**
Description of pain	Aching, localized, toothache-like, sharp, squeezing	Shooting, radiating, stabbing, burning, electric shock-like
Movement impact	Associated with movement	Independent
Physical examination	Normal response	Allodynia, hyperalgesia, vasomotor changes
Examples	Injury, postoperative pain	Peripheral neuropathies, shingles, cancer pain
Treatment strategies	More classical approach, conventional analgesics	More biopsychological approach, conventional analgesics +/– non-conventional (antidepressants, anticonvulsants etc.)

Table 11.2 Common illnesses associated with chronic pain

Illness	Nature of pain disorder
Diabetes	Diabetic neuropathy – Commonly glove and stocking peripheral neuropathic pain
Connective tissue disorder	Variable presentation of accompanying neuropathy
HIV	Neuropathy due to disease as well as due to antiretroviral drugs
Trauma	Multifactorial aethiology – Associated nerve injury causing neuropathy and or complex regional pain syndrome
Herpes zoster infection	Post-herpetic neuralgia – Neuropathic pain with dermatomal distribution
Multiple sclerosis	Central neuropathic pain including trigeminal neuralgia
Cerebrovascular accident	Post-stroke central neuropathic pain
Fibromyalgia	Neuropathic type musculoskeletal pain, usually primary but could be secondary to other disorders such connective tissue disease
Complex regional pain syndrome	Most likely due to previous injury – Usually neuropathic pain of the extremities
Chronic post surgical pain	Variable incidence following variety of surgeries causing neuropathic pain
Degenerative bone and joint disease	Variable sites – Mostly nociceptive but with possible neuropathic component
Phantom limb pain	Neuropathic pain following amputation most commonly of extremities
Cancer	Cancer and its treatment such as radiotherapy and chemotherapy cause chronic pain with neuropathic and/or nociceptive features.

Detailed examination will focus on different systems according to a particular pain condition. It may involve basic orthopaedic, neurological or surgical examination. Regardless of the approach, it should follow conventional basic methods: inspection, palpation and range of movement where appropriate. For example, a patient who presents with back pain will require at least inspection to check for muscle spasm, posture, deformity, gait and use of aids such as crutches and evidence of previous surgery; palpation of paravertebral and bony areas; and range of movement to evaluate any restriction. The examination will also need to include a neurological examination looking at dermatomal sensory dysfunction (suggesting radiculopathy) and particular tests (depending on the region of the spine) to detect signs of nerve root irritation using stretch tests such as Lasègue's test (or straight leg raising test) for low back pain; and for the neck, the Spurling test (turning the patient's head to the affected side while extending and applying downward pressure to the top of the patient's head – a positive test is indicated by pain arising in the neck radiating in the direction of the ipsilateral corresponding dermatome). The examination should also assess glove and stocking sensory loss (characteristic of peripheral neuropathy), reflexes and plantar response, muscle power, sensation and reflexes.

As part of the clinical examination it is important to elicit features of neuropathic pain such as allodynia (pain due to a stimulus that does not usually provoke pain, for example a light touch using cotton wool eliciting pain) and hyperalgesia or hypoalgesia (increased or decreased pain, respectively, from a stimulus such as pressure or pinprick that usually provokes pain).

Investigation

Investigation of a patient in pain is tailored to the individual's presentation. It serves three important goals:

- To exclude more sinister pathology
- To provide diagnostic clues
- To arrive at an optimal management strategy

The commonest investigation employed by pain specialists is imaging, for example using simple X-rays to exclude a pathological fracture, MRI to demonstrate changes within the central nervous system or an ultrasound examination of the abdomen. Neurophysiological (EMG) studies are helpful to determine the presence and extent of any nerve damage, and various blood tests may be used to determine, for example, the activity of rheumatoid arthritis. Any test used must be considered only as a part of a more global approach, never in isolation. Some tests such as Quantitative Sensory Testing and functional imaging using PET-CT or fMRI are used in the research setting to understand more about the underlying pain mechanisms.

By the end of the assessment, any pathology that needs to be dealt with by the relevant medical professional should be identified, either for urgent management, if 'red flags' are elicited, or electively.

Difficult cases

As the history is the key to pain assessment and treatment, it is clear that communication is paramount. Difficulty arises if there is a language barrier between the physician and the patient, if the patient is a young child or has learning difficulties, confusion or dementia.

It is important as a physician to understand that the pain a patient perceives could be influenced by social and cultural factors as well as past experience. The pain may prove refractory to treatment, with all treatment options already exhausted, which again can pose a challenging situation, necessitating a change in goal setting.

Measuring pain

Pain is a subjective experience and therefore difficult to quantify. However, being able to quantify pain will aid management by assessing severity and allowing the measurement of treatment or intervention effect and is crucial in research studies looking at new treatment modalities. Measurement tools may be unidimensional or multidimensional, with the latter being more useful in chronic pain conditions.

Unidimensional scales

Unidimensional scales are very commonly used particularly in acute pain. They are simple, sensitive, reproducible and quickly applied and give a numerical value to the pain severity. They can be either analogue or discrete. The latter may be numerical or verbal.

The most common of these scales is the Visual Analogue Scale (VAS): the patient is given a horizontal line 10 cm long with 'no pain' on the left-hand side and 'worst possible pain' on the right and is asked to mark the line according to the severity of the pain.

I. Pain Rating Index (PRI):

The words below describe average pain. Place a check mark (✓) in the column that represents the degree to which you feel that type of pain. Please limit yourself to a description of the pain in your pelvic area only:

			None		Mild		Moderate		Severe
	Throbbing	0		1		2		3	
	Shooting	0		1		2		3	
	Stabbing	0		1		2		3	
	Sharp	0		1		2		3	
	Cramping	0		1		2		3	
a	Gnawing	0		1		2		3	
	Hot-Burning	0		1		2		3	
	Aching	0		1		2		3	
	Heavy	0		1		2		3	
	Tender	0		1		2		3	
	Splitting	0		1		2		3	
	Tiring-Exhausting	0		1		2		3	
b	Sickening	0		1		2		3	
	Fearful	0		1		2		3	
	Punishing-Cruel	0		1		2		3	

II. Present Pain Intensity (PPI)–Visual Analog Scale (VAS). Tick along scale below for pelvic pain:

No Pain — Worst possible pain

III. Evaluative overall intensity of total pain experience. Please limit yourself to a description of the pain in your pelvic area only. Place a check mark (✓) in the appropriate column:

Evaluation		
0	No pain	
1	Mild	
2	Discomforting	
3	Distressing	
4	Horrible	
5	Excruciating	

IV. Scoring

		Score
I-a	S-PRI (Sensory Pain Rating Index)	
I-b	A-PRI (Affective Pain Rating Index)	
I-a+b	T-PRI (Total Pain Rating Index)	
II	PPI-VAS (Present Pain Intensity-Visual Analog Scale)	
III	Evaluative overall intensity of total pain experience	

Figure 11.4 Short form McGill Pain Questionnaire.

The numerical rating scale: the patient is asked to assign a number from 0 to 10 to his pain, 0 being no pain at all and 10 being the worst imaginable pain. In the verbal rating scale the patient rates his pain into one of the following categories: none, mild, moderate or severe.

Multidimensional (complex) scales

The development of multidimensional scales acknowledges the multidimensional impacts of pain on a sufferer's life. Common scales used include the McGill Questionnaire and Brief Pain Inventory. The original McGill Questionnaire assesses various aspects of pain, including sensory qualities of pain, affective qualities (tension, fear etc.) and has evaluative words that describe the subjective intensity of the total pain experienced. There are various measurements derived from the data, but a short form of the McGill Questionnaire is most often used (Fig. 11.4). It is easy to apply and reproducible.

To build up a complete assessment of a patient with longstanding disabling pain, a battery of measurement tools may be required which may include anxiety and depression measurement scales, catastrophising scales and disability index.

To assess for neuropathic pain, recently introduced and validated tools such as the 'painDETECT' and 'LANSS' questionnaires are used to look for specific features pertaining to neuropathic pain.

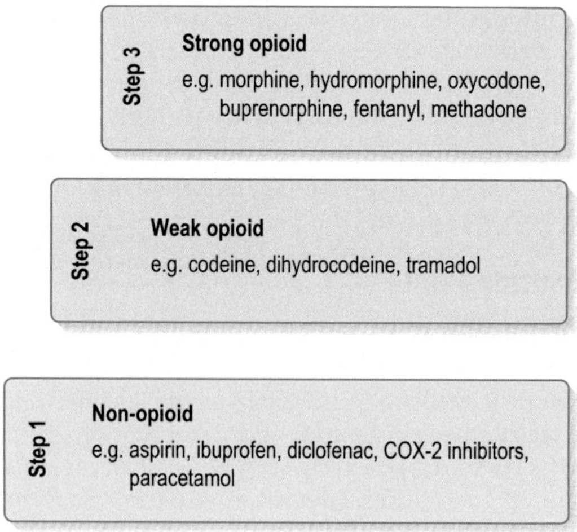

- The World Health Organization (WHO) guidelines advocate that when pain occurs, there should be prompt oral administration of drugs, administered in accordance with steps 1–3.
- To maintain freedom from pain, drugs should be taken 'by the clock' every 3–6 hours, rather than 'on demand' and each patient should receive tailored pain management.
- This 3-step approach of administering the right drug in the right dose at the right time is inexpensive and 80–90% effective.

Figure 11.5 WHO pain ladder.

Treatment strategies

Acute pain

Acute pain management should be directed to the treatment of the underlying cause as well as symptomatic pain relief itself. For example fractures should be reduced and immobilized and infections treated with antibiotics. Pain in the acute setting as well as that due to cancer is then treated symptomatically with analgesic drugs in accordance with the World Health Organization (WHO) pain ladder (Fig. 11.5). Pharmacological options include simple analgesics such as paracetamol, non-steroidal anti-inflammatory drugs and opioids. There is also an option for considering local anaesthetic nerve blocks especially for pain following surgery and trauma. It is increasingly recognized that poorly treated acute pain can result in a chronic pain state which can become quite refractory to treatment.

Chronic pain

In chronic pain the emphasis shifts from management of the pain itself to addressing its psychosocial sequelae as well as improving the patient's function. This often involves a multimodal treatment approach under the umbrella of a biopsychosocial model. The pharmacological options include the same as that for acute pain, but medications can be less effective. In particular there should be less emphasis on the use of strong opioids in chronic pain, as they become less effective and are associated with significant short-term as well as long-term side effects. The British Pain Society guidelines on the use of opioids for persistent pain recommend a maximum dose of 120 mg morphine-equivalent dosage per 24 hours in the non-specialist setting. Chronic pain often has a neuropathic component, which is treated with antineuropathic agents including antidepressants such as amitriptyline and anticonvulsants such as gabapentin and pregabalin.

Non-pharmacological options

The non-pharmacological management of chronic pain is multidisciplinary and is usually available only through specialized pain clinics. A detailed discussion is beyond the scope of this chapter but pain management may include interventional techniques such as spinal injections (such as with steroids), radiofrequency therapy and neuromodulation, acupuncture and transcutaneous nerve stimulation and also involve physiotherapy, occupational therapy and psychological techniques. The aim is to provide physical and psychological rehabilitation leading, where possible, to patient self-management. As the presence of chronic pain can be considered a long-term illness or a disease, the goal for treatment is to attain a good functional outcome rather than being pain free.

Conclusions

Pain is complex and essentially a patient-reported, subjective phenomenon. Pain assessment includes unidimensional and also multidimensional tools looking at its social and psychological consequences as well as its sensory characteristics. With wide inter-patient variability, perhaps more than with any other symptom, management must be individualized to the context and needs of each patient.

SECTION 3

Basic systems

Respiratory system 12

Veronica L.C. White

Introduction

Diseases of the respiratory system account for up to a third of deaths in most countries and for a major proportion of visits to the doctor and time away from work or school. As with every aspect of diagnosis in medicine, the key to success is a clear and carefully recorded history; symptoms may be trivial or extremely distressing, but either may indicate serious and life-threatening disease.

The history

Most patients with respiratory disease will present with breathlessness, cough, excess sputum, haemoptysis, wheeze or chest pain.

Breathlessness

Everyone becomes breathless on strenuous exertion. Breathlessness inappropriate to the level of physical exertion, or even occurring at rest, is called dyspnoea. Its mechanisms are complex and not fully understood. It is not due simply to a lowered blood oxygen tension (hypoxia) or to a raised blood carbon dioxide tension (hypercapnia), although these may play a significant part. People with cardiac disease (see Ch. 13) and even non-cardiorespiratory conditions such as anaemia, thyrotoxicosis or metabolic acidosis may become dyspnoeic as well as those with primarily respiratory problems (Box 12.1).

An important assessment is whether the dyspnoea is related only to exertion and how far the patient can walk at a normal pace on the level (exercise tolerance). This may take some skill to elicit, as few people note their symptoms in this form, but a brief discussion about what they can do in their daily lives usually gives a good estimate of their mobility (Box 12.2).

Other clarifications will include whether there is variability in the symptoms, whether there are good days and bad days and, very importantly, whether there are any times of day or night that are usually worse than others. Variable airways obstruction due to asthma is very often worse at night and in the early morning. By contrast, people with predominantly irreversible airways obstruction due to chronic obstructive pulmonary disease (COPD) will often say that as long as they are sitting in bed, they feel quite normal; it is exercise that troubles them.

Cough

The symptom of cough can be short lived or last years; cough can be defined as acute (lasting less than 3 weeks) or chronic (lasting more than 8 weeks) (Box 12.3). A cough may be dry or it may be productive with sputum. Acute cough is most commonly caused by recent infection, either viral or bacterial; however, any cough that is associated with haemoptysis should be a cause for concern, prompt appropriate assessment and a baseline chest X-ray (CXR) at the very least. Any patient with a chronic cough, i.e. one that lasts more than 8 weeks, should be sent for a CXR and spirometry as baseline investigations (Box 12.4). Discussion about cough should include:

- How long has the cough been present? A cough lasting a few days following a cold has less significance than one lasting several weeks in a middle-aged smoker, which may be the first sign of a malignancy.
- Is the cough worse at any time of day or night? A dry cough at night may be an early symptom of asthma, as may a cough that comes in spasms lasting several minutes.
- Is the cough aggravated by anything, for example allergic triggers such as dust, animals or pollen, or non-specific triggers such as exercise or cold air? The increased reactivity of the airways seen in asthma and in some normal people for several weeks after viral respiratory infections may present in this way. Severe coughing, whatever its cause, may be followed by vomiting (Box 12.5).

Sputum

- Is sputum produced?
- What does it look like? Children and some adults swallow sputum, but it is always worth

Box 12.1 Causes of breathlessness

Acute	Subacute	Chronic
Airways obstruction	Pneumonia	COPD
Anaphylaxis	Exacerbation of COPD	Pleural effusion
Asthma	Angina	Malignancy
Pneumothorax	Cardiac tamponade	Chronic pulmonary emboli
Pulmonary embolus	Metabolic acidosis	Restrictive lung disorders, including interstitial lung disease
Myocardial infarction	Pain	Congestive cardiac failure
Pulmonary oedema	Pontine haemorrhage	Valvular dysfunction
Arrhythmias		Cardiomyopathy
Anxiety		Diastolic dysfunction Pulmonary hypertension Anaemia Neuromuscular disorders Deconditioning Obesity

COPD, chronic obstructive pulmonary disease.

Box 12.2 Medical Research Council grading of dyspnoea (breathlessness scale)

1 Not troubled by breathlessness except on strenuous exercise.
2 Short of breath when hurrying or walking up a slight hill.
3 Walks slower than contemporaries on the level because of breathlessness, or has to stop for breath when walking at own pace.
4 Stops for breath after about 100 m or after a few minutes on the level.
5 Too breathless to leave the house, or breathless when dressing or undressing.

asking for a description of its colour and consistency. Yellow or green sputum is usually purulent. People with asthma may produce small amounts of very thick or jelly-like sputum, sometimes in the shape of a cast of the airways. Eosinophils may accumulate in the sputum in asthma, causing a purulent appearance even when no infection is present.

- How much is produced? When severe lung damage in infancy and childhood was common, bronchiectasis was often found in adults. The amount of sputum produced daily often exceeded a cupful. Bronchiectasis is now rare, and chronic bronchitis causes the production of smaller amounts of sputum.

Box 12.3 Causes of cough

Causes of cough	Examples
Respiratory	Viral or bacterial infection, bronchospasm, COPD, non asthmatic eosinophilic asthma, bronchiolitis, malignancy, parenchymal disease e.g. ILD, bronchiectasis, cystic fibrosis, sarcoidosis, pleural disease, aspiration
Upper airways disease	Post nasal drip, sinusitis, inhaled foreign body, tonsillar enlargement
Cardiovascular disease	LVF, mitral stenosis
Gastro-oesophageal disease	GORD
Neurological disease	Aspiration
Drugs and irritants	ACE inhibitors, cigarette smoke

ACE, angiotensin converting enzyme; COPD, chronic obstructive pulmonary disease; ILD, interstitial lung disease; LVF, left ventricular failure; GORD, gastro-oesophageal reflux disease – also associated with laryngopharyngeal reflux (LPR)

Box 12.4 Five most common causes of chronic cough with a normal CXR

- Post viral upper respiratory tract infection (URTI)
- Smoking
- Asthma – including cough variant asthma and non-asthmatic eosinophilic asthma
- Post nasal drip (hay fever)
- Gastro-oesophageal reflux disease (GORD)

Box 12.5 Important questions in the history of chronic cough

- Have you had a recent cold, sore throat or viral infection?
- Do you have a history of asthma, nocturnal cough or wheeze?
- Do you experience nasal discharge or sinusitis?
- Do you suffer from acid reflux, indigestion or coughing after meals?
- What time of day is the cough worse?
- Do you smoke?
- Are you breathless?
- Have you coughed up blood?
- Do you have a hoarse voice?
- Have you had fevers or night sweats?
- Have you lost weight?
- Are you getting chest pain?

Haemoptysis

Haemoptysis means the coughing up of blood in the sputum. It should never be dismissed without very careful evaluation of the patient. The potentially

Box 12.6 Causes of haemoptysis

- Malignancy and benign lung tumours, including lung metastasis
- Pulmonary infection including bacterial pneumonia, tuberculosis (TB), lung abscesses and fungal infection
- Bronchiectasis including cystic fibrosis
- Pulmonary emboli
- Congestive heart failure
- Pulmonary fibrosis
- Pulmonary vasculitis
- Severe pulmonary hypertension
- AV malformation
- Chest trauma and foreign bodies
- Endometriosis
- Anticoagulation or coagulopathy
- Drugs, e.g. cocaine, thrombolytics

serious significance of blood in the sputum is well known, and fear often leads patients not to mention it: a specific question is always necessary, as well as an attempt to decide if it is fresh or altered blood, how much is produced, when it started and how often it happens (Box 12.6).

Blood may be coughed up alone, or sputum may be bloodstained. It is sometimes difficult for the patient to describe whether or not the blood has originated from the chest or whether it comes from the gums or nose or even from the stomach. Patients should always be asked about associated conditions such as epistaxis (nose bleeds) or the subsequent development of melaena (altered blood in the stool), which occurs in the case of upper gastrointestinal bleeding. Usually, however, it is clear that the blood originates from the chest, and this is an indication for further investigation.

Wheezing

Always ask whether the patient hears any noises coming from the chest. Even if a wheeze is not present when you examine the patient, it is useful to know that he has noticed it on occasions. Sometimes wheezing will have been noticed by others (especially by a partner at night, when asthma is worse) but not by the patient.

Sometimes stridor (see Ch. 21) may be mistaken for wheezing by both patient and doctor. This serious finding usually indicates narrowing of the larynx, trachea or main bronchi. It is also not unusual for patients with a pneumothorax to describe 'rubbing' or 'gurgling' sounds in their chest which may well be due to the displaced lung.

Pain in the chest

Apart from musculoskeletal aches and pains consequent upon prolonged bouts of coughing, chest pain caused by lung disease usually arises from the pleura. Pleuritic pain is sharp and stabbing and is made worse by deep breathing or coughing. It occurs when the pleura is inflamed, most commonly by infection in the underlying lung. More constant pain, unrelated to breathing, may be caused by local invasion of the chest wall by a lung or pleural tumour.

A spontaneous pneumothorax causes pain which is worse on breathing but which may have more of an aching character than the stabbing pain of pleurisy. If a pulmonary embolus causes infarction of the lung, pleurisy and hence pleuritic pain may occur, but an acute pulmonary embolus can also cause pain which is not stabbing in nature. A large pulmonary embolus causing haemodynamic disturbance may cause cardiac-type chest pain.

Other symptoms

Quite apart from the common symptoms of respiratory disease, there are some other aspects of the history that are particularly relevant to the respiratory system.

Upper airway

Questions related to the ear, nose and throat are relevant. Rhinosinusitis often coexists with asthma or less commonly, bronchiectasis, and can be an aggravating factor. A common cause of chronic cough is postnasal drip secondary to rhinitis. A change in the voice may indicate involvement of the left recurrent laryngeal nerve by a carcinoma of the lung. Sometimes patients using inhaled corticosteroids for asthma develop oropharyngeal candidiasis or even hoarseness or weakness of the voice, which improves on changing the treatment. Do not ascribe hoarseness to this cause in older patients, as carcinoma of the vocal cords can also be present with hoarseness or a change in the quality of the voice. Laryngoscopy is always indicated if hoarseness persists for more than 4 weeks.

The smoking and recreational drug history

Always take a full smoking and recreational drug history. Do so in a sympathetic and non-judgemental way, or the detail is unlikely to be accurate. The time for advice about smoking cessation is after completion of your assessment, not at the outset. Simply asking 'Do you smoke?' is not enough. Novices will be astonished at how often closer probing of the answer 'no' reveals that the patient gave it up yesterday or that he states his intention of doing so from the time of your consultation. Age of starting and stopping if an ex-smoker and average consumption for both current and ex-smokers are the bare minimum information needed.

Identification of an individual as a current or ex-smoker will greatly influence the interpretation you place on your findings upon history and examination. Almost all cases of lung cancer and chronic obstructive

Box 12.7 List of common occupations that may be associated with asthma

- Car paint sprayers – isocyanates
- Electricians – colophony
- Woodworkers
- Rubber and plastic industries
- Bakers – flour dust and enzymes, e.g. amylase
- Working with animals – vets, zoo keepers, laboratory worker – rodent urinary proteins
- Working with agriculture – farmers, fish worker – salmon proteins
- Healthcare professionals – latex and diathermy
- Hairdressing – persulphate, henna
- Tea sifters and packers

Box 12.8 List of activities that may lead to asbestos exposure

- Mining and manufacture of asbestos
- Shipbuilding and aircraft manufacturing
- Dock and rail workers – unloading asbestos from ships/trains
- Thermal and fire insulation – lagging
- Construction, building repair and demolition
- Plumbers and gas fitters
- Car mechanics (brake linings)
- Electricians, carpenters, upholsterers
- Manufacture of gas masks in World War II
- Family member of one of the above, and/or working or living near an asbestos source (particularly if asbestos fibres taken home on workers' clothing)

pulmonary disease (COPD) occur in those who have smoked.

Recreational drug use tends to be commoner in younger people, but do not assume that this is the case and ask all patients from all walks of life. Again, sounding sympathetic rather than judgemental is crucial and a good opening line can be, 'If you don't mind me asking…'. Heroin, crack, cannabis and other drugs are smoked and in some cases cause more damage to the lungs than tobacco. Cannabis can cause severe emphysema in younger patients, who are often unaware of effects. Use the consultation to discuss its long-term sequelae.

The family history

There is a strong inherited susceptibility to asthma. Associated atopic conditions such as eczema and hay fever may also be present in relatives of those with asthma, particularly in those who develop the condition when young.

The occupational history

No other organ is as susceptible to the working environment as much as the lungs. Several hundred different substances have now been recognized as causing occupational asthma. Paint sprayers, workers in the electronics, rubber or plastics industries and woodworkers are relatively commonly affected (Box 12.7). Always ask about a relationship between symptoms and work.

Damage from inhalation of asbestos may take decades to become manifest, most seriously as malignant mesothelioma. In industrialized countries, this once extremely rare tumour of the pleura has become more common and will become even more common in the next 20 years. In middle-aged individuals who present with a pleural effusion, often the first sign of a mesothelioma, always ask about possible asbestos exposure in jobs back to the time of first employment (Box 12.8).

As far as the occupational history is concerned, the best way to proceed is chronologically. Most people cannot randomly remember, for example, what they might have been doing 20 years ago or indeed, if asked in isolation, when they worked in a particular job. But if you start at the beginning of their life and work forward they find it much easier to remember (try it yourself starting with your school exams!)

Start by asking the patient how old he was when he left school, then what job or further education he had; then ask him to continue through his life to the present day. Particularly for those who went on to further education, ask about holiday jobs (you might be surprised at their responses!) and it might be worth asking if they travelled overseas with their employment, especially if they were in the armed forces. Don't assume that all 80-year-olds are retired or indeed that all young patients are employed.

The examination

General assessment

An examination of the respiratory system is incomplete without a simultaneous general assessment (Box 12.9). Watch the patient as he comes into the room, during your history taking and while he is undressing and climbing on to the couch. If this is a hospital inpatient, is there breathlessness just on moving in bed? A breathless patient may be using the accessory muscles of respiration (e.g. sternomastoid) and, in the presence of severe COPD, many patients find it easier to breathe out through pursed lips (Fig. 12.1).

- Is there an audible wheeze or stridor?
- Is the voice hoarse?
- Is the patient continually coughing? Dry or productive?
- Is the patient capable of producing a normal, explosive cough, or is the voice weak or non-existent even when he is asked to cough?

Box 12.9 Points to note in a general assessment

- Physique and gait
- Voice
- Breathlessness
- Clubbing of the fingers
- Tobacco staining of fingers
- Bruising and/or thinness of skin
- Venous pulses
- Cyanosis or pallor
- Ptosis
- Swollen face
- Collateral vessels across anterior chest wall
- Intercostal recession
- Use of accessory respiratory muscles
- Lymph nodes

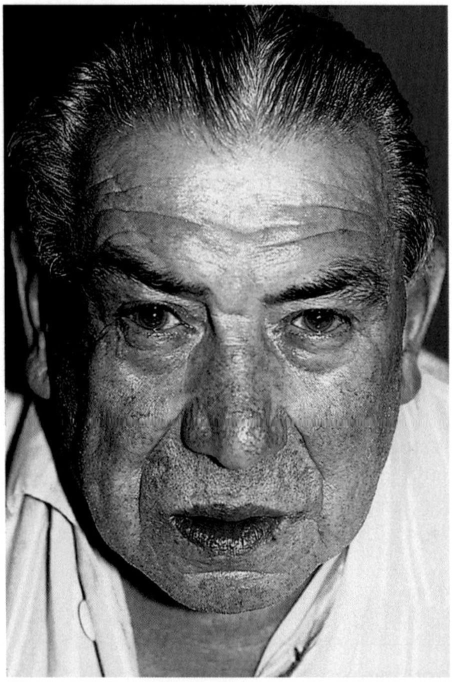

Figure 12.1 Respiratory failure. The patient is breathless at rest and there is central cyanosis with blueness of the lips and face. The lips are pursed during expiration, a characteristic feature of COPD. This facial appearance is often accompanied by heart failure with peripheral oedema (cor pulmonale).

- Is the wheezing audible, usually loudest in expiration, or is there stridor, a high-pitched inspiratory noise?
- What is on the bedside table (e.g. inhalers, a peak flow meter, tissues, a sputum pot, an oxygen mask, nebulizer, CPAP machine)?
- What is the physique and state of general nourishment of the patient?

For the examination, the patient should be resting comfortably on a bed or couch, supported by pillows so that he can lean back comfortably at an angle of 45° (this is often more upright than patients choose for themselves).

Box 12.10 Signs to look for in the hands

Clubbing
Pallor
Warm, well-perfused palms (CO_2 retention)
Cyanosis
Flap
Tremor
Tobacco staining
Bruising and/or thin skin
Pulse rate and character

Box 12.11 Observing the chest

- Rate of respiration
- Rhythm of respiration
- Chest expansion
- Symmetry
- Surgical scars

Hands

The hands should be inspected for clubbing, pallor or cyanosis (Box 12.10). Tobacco-stained fingers may indicate a heavy smoker. Respiratory causes of clubbing include carcinoma of the bronchus, pulmonary fibrosis, bronchiectasis, lung abscess and pleural empyema. A fine tremor may indicate the use of inhaled β_2 agonists, such as salbutamol. A flap may indicate carbon dioxide retention or hypercapnia. Such patients are often drowsy, with warm hands and a bounding pulse. In a significant asthma attack, the pulse rate is usually raised. The systolic blood pressure also falls during the severe inspiratory effort of acute asthma, and the degree of this fall (the degree of pulsus paradoxus) can be used as a measure of asthma severity.

Respiratory rate and rhythm

The respiratory rate and pattern of respiration should be noted. The normal rate of respiration in a relaxed adult is about 14-16 breaths per minute (Box 12.11). Tachypnoea is an increased respiratory rate observed by the doctor, whereas dyspnoea is the symptom of breathlessness experienced by the patient. Apnoea means cessation of respiration.

Cheyne-Stokes breathing is the name given to a disturbance of respiratory rhythm in which there is cyclical deepening and quickening of respiration, followed by diminishing respiratory effort and rate, sometimes associated with a short period of complete apnoea, the cycle then being repeated. This is often observed in severely ill patients and particularly in severe cardiac failure, narcotic drug poisoning and neurological disorders. It is occasionally seen, especially during sleep, in elderly patients without any obvious serious disease.

Some patients may have apnoeic episodes during sleep owing to complete cessation of respiratory effort (central apnoea) or, much more commonly, apnoea despite continuation of respiratory effort. This is known as obstructive sleep apnoea, is due to obstruction of the upper airways by soft tissues in the region of the pharynx and is commoner in obese patients.

Venous pulses

The venous pulses in the neck (see Ch. 13) should be inspected. A raised jugular venous pressure (JVP) may be a sign of cor pulmonale, right heart failure caused by chronic pulmonary hypertension in severe lung disease, commonly COPD. Pitting oedema of the ankles and sacrum is usually present. However, engorged neck veins can be due to superior vena cava obstruction (SVCO), usually because of malignancy in the upper mediastinum. SVCO can also be associated with facial swelling and plethora (redness) and collateral circulation across the anterior chest wall.

Head

Examination of the eyes may reveal anaemia or, rarely, Horner's syndrome, secondary to a cancer at the lung apex (Pancoast tumour) invading the cervical sympathetic chain. The lips and tongue should be inspected for central cyanosis, which almost always indicates poor oxygenation of the blood by the lungs, whereas peripheral cyanosis alone is usually due to poor peripheral perfusion. Oral candida may indicate use of inhaled steroids or be a sign of debilitation or underlying immune suppression in the patient.

Examination of the chest

Relevant anatomy

The interpretation of signs in the chest often causes problems for the beginner. A review of the relevant anatomy may help.

The bifurcation of the trachea corresponds on the anterior chest wall with the sternal angle, the transverse bony ridge at the junction of the body of the sternum and the manubrium sterni. Posteriorly, the level is at the disc between the fourth and fifth thoracic vertebrae. The ribs are most easily counted downwards from the second costal cartilage, which articulates with the sternum at the extremity of the sternal angle.

A line from the second thoracic spine to the sixth rib, in line with the nipple, corresponds to the upper border of the lower lobe (oblique or major interlobar fissure). On the right side, a horizontal line from the sternum at the level of the fourth costal cartilage, drawn to meet the line of the major interlobar fissure, marks the boundary between the upper and middle lobes (the horizontal or minor interlobar fissure). The greater part of each lung, as seen from behind, is composed of the lower lobe; only the apex belongs to the upper lobe. The middle and upper lobes on the right side and the upper lobe on the left occupy most of the area in front (Fig. 12.2). This is most easily visualized if the lobes are thought of as two wedges fitting together, not as two cubes piled one on top of the other (Fig. 12.3).

The stethoscope is so much a part of the 'image' of a doctor that it is very easy for the student to forget that listening is only one part of the examination of the chest. Obtaining the maximum possible

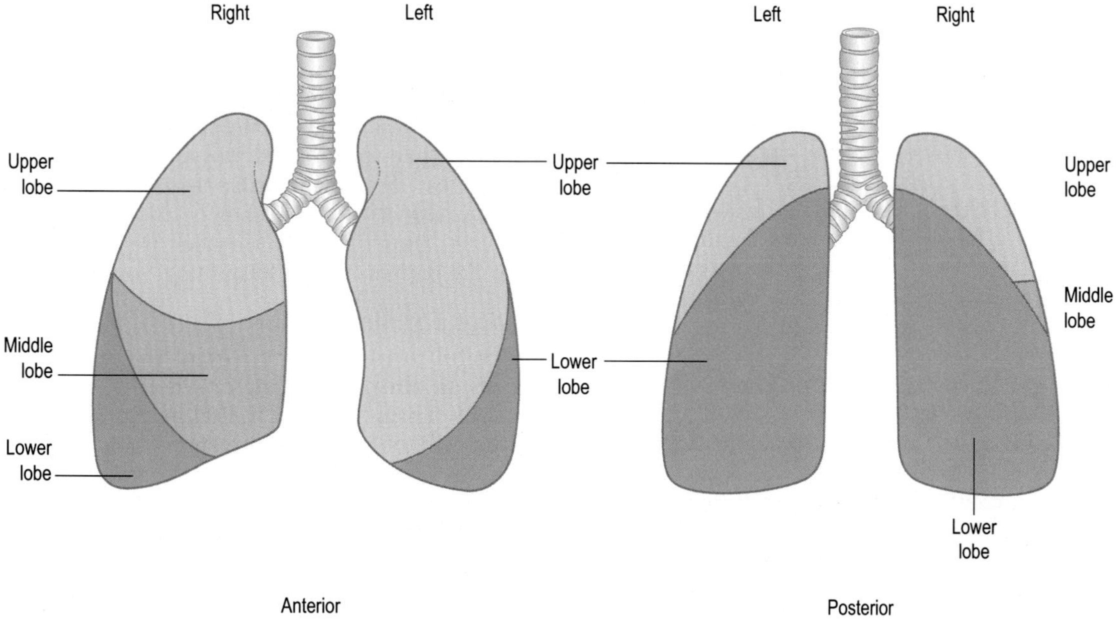

Figure 12.2 Anterior and posterior aspects of the lungs.

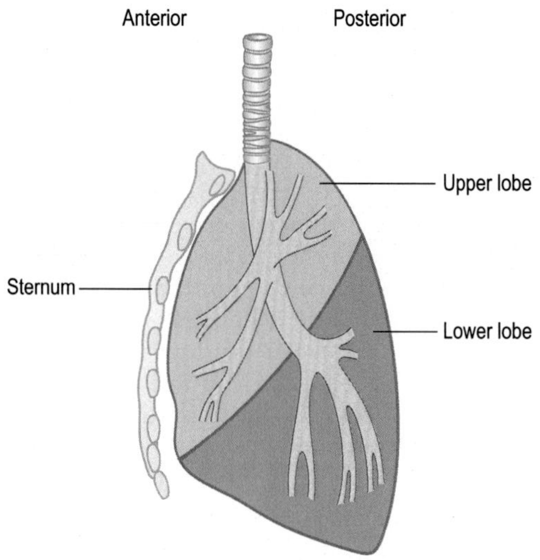

Figure 12.3 Lateral aspect of the left lung.

information from your examination requires you to look, then to feel and, only then, to listen.

Looking: inspection of the chest

Appearance of the chest

First, look for any obvious scars from previous surgery. Thoracotomy scars (from lobectomy or pneumonectomy (removal of the whole lung)) are usually visible running from below the scapula posteriorly, sweeping round the axilla to the anterior chest wall. Pleural procedures such as intercostal drain insertion, biopsy or VATS (video-assisted thoracoscopic surgery) may be associated with small scars, often in the axilla or posteriorly. A small scar above the sternal notch indicates a previous tracheostomy. Older patients may have small scars in the midline below the clavicle indicative of a phrenic nerve crush (a previous treatment for TB). Look for any lumps visible beneath the skin or any lesions on the skin itself. If you are examining from the right of the patient, ensure that you thoroughly inspect the left side. It is easy to miss a lateral thoracotomy scar or one that is hidden in a skinfold.

Next, inspect the shape of the chest itself. The normal chest is bilaterally symmetrical and elliptical in horizontal cross-section, with the narrower diameter being anteroposterior. The chest may be distorted by disease of the ribs or spinal vertebrae as well as by underlying lung disease (Box 12.12). Lobar collapse produces characteristic changes on chest X-ray and they are shown in Fig. 12.4.

Kyphosis (forward bending) or scoliosis (lateral bending) of the vertebral column will lead to asymmetry of the chest and, if severe, may significantly restrict lung movement. A normal chest X-ray is seen in Fig. 12.5. Severe airways obstruction, particularly long-term as in COPD (Fig. 12.6), may lead to overinflated lungs. On examination, the chest may be 'barrel shaped', most easily appreciated as an increased anteroposterior diameter, making the horizontal cross-section more circular. On X-ray, the hemidiaphragms appear lower than usual, and flattened.

Box 12.12 Features to note in assessing the shape of the chest

- Kyphosis
- Scoliosis
- Flattening
- Overinflation
- Previous surgery causing asymmetry such as thoracoplasty

Box 12.13 Points to note on palpation of the chest

- Swelling
- Surgical emphysema
- Pain and tenderness
- Tracheal position
- Cardiac impulse
- Asymmetry
- Tactile vocal fremitus

Movement of the chest

Look to see if the chest movements are symmetrical. If they seem to be diminished on one side, that is likely to be the side on which there is an abnormality. Intercostal recession, a drawing-in of the intercostal spaces with inspiration, may indicate severe upper airways obstruction, as in laryngeal disease or tumours of the trachea. In COPD, the lower ribs often move paradoxically inwards on inspiration instead of the normal outwards movement.

Feeling: palpation of the chest

Lymph nodes

The lymph nodes in the supraclavicular fossae, cervical regions and axillary regions should be palpated; don't forget to feel gently behind the sternocleidomastoid muscles. If they are enlarged, this may be secondary to the spread of malignant disease from the chest, and such findings will influence decisions regarding treatment. Lymph nodes in the neck are best felt by sitting the patient up and examining from behind.

Swellings and tenderness

It is useful to palpate any part of the chest that presents an obvious swelling or where the patient complains of pain (Box 12.13). Feel gently, as pressure may increase the pain. It is often important, particularly in the case of musculoskeletal pain, to identify a site of tenderness (Box 12.14). Surgical emphysema (air in the tissues), which feels like popcorn or bubble paper underneath the skin, is caused by trauma, pneumothorax, pneumomediastinum and infection, as well as chest instrumentation following surgery or a chest drain.

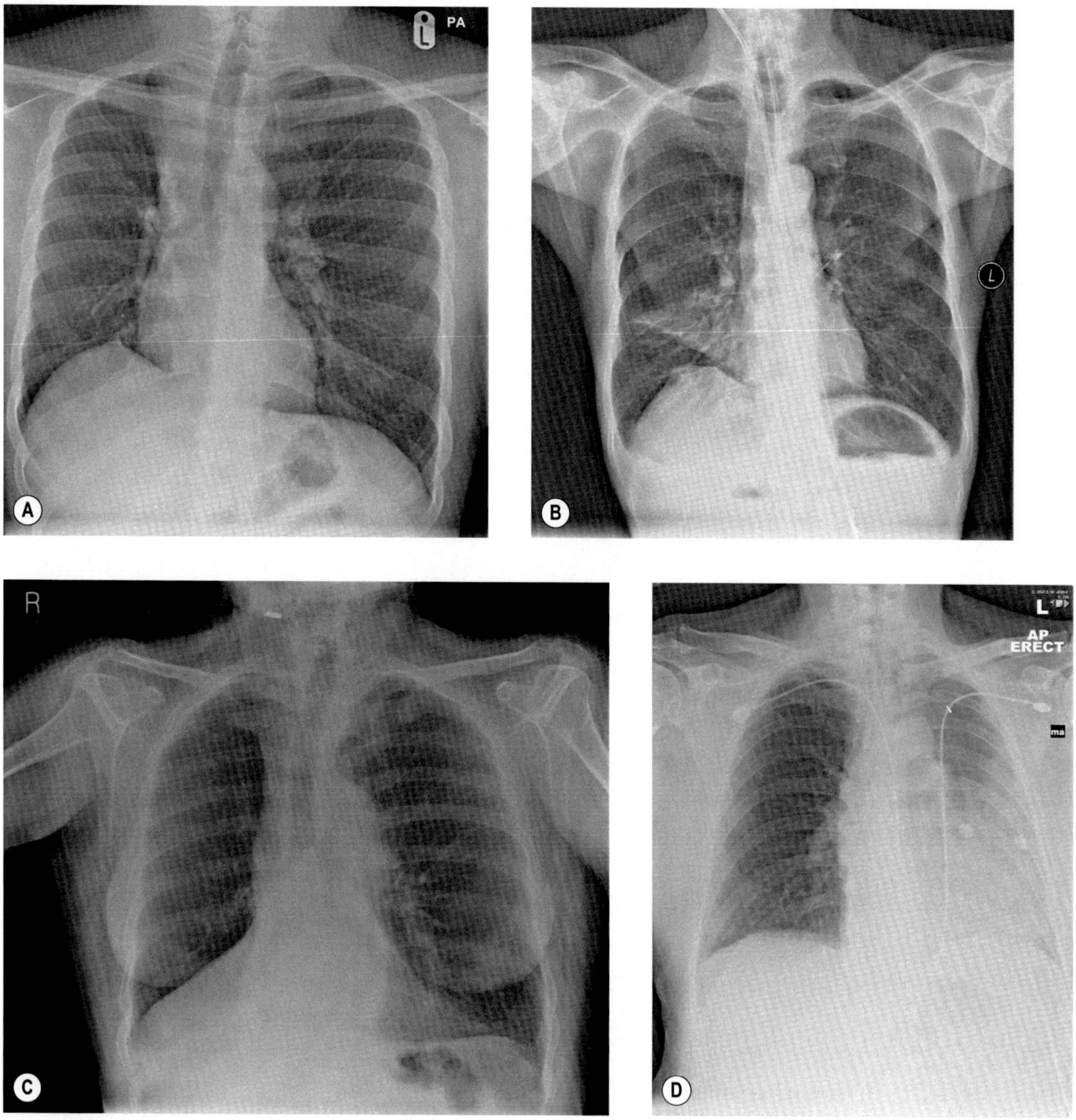

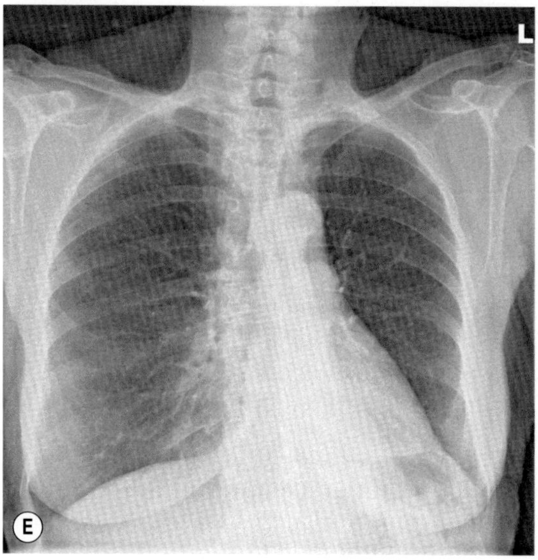

Figure 12.4 Chest X-rays (CXR) showing lobar collapses. (Courtesy of Dr Stephen Ellis.) **(A)** CXR showing right upper lobe collapse; note the raised 'tented' right hemidiaphragm. **(B)** CXR showing right middle lobe collapse; the right heart border has become obscured. **(C)** CXR showing right lower lobe collapse, note the right hilum is lowered and now behind the right heart. **(D)** CXR showing left upper lobe collapse; note the 'veil-like' appearance over the left hemithorax with loss of the left heart border silhouette. **(E)** CXR showing left upper lobe collapse; also known as 'sail-sign' because the lobe collapses and sits behind the left side of the cardiac silhouette and obscures the medial hemidiaphragmatic silhouette.

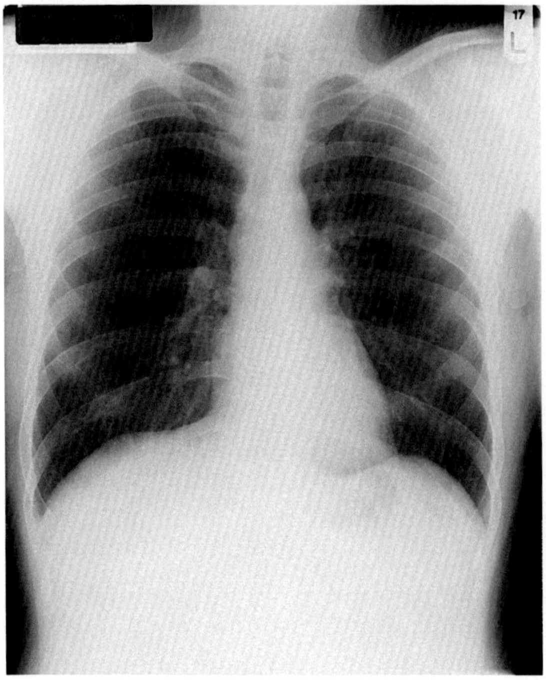

Figure 12.5 Normal chest X-ray.

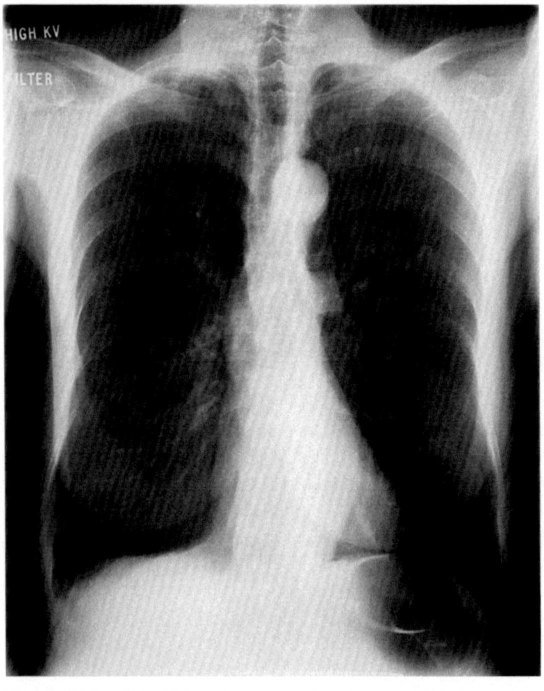

Figure 12.6 Chest X-ray in severe chronic obstructive pulmonary disease.

Trachea and heart

The positions of the cardiac impulse and trachea should then be determined. Feel for the trachea by putting the second and fourth fingers of the examining hand on each edge of the sternal notch and use the third finger to assess whether the trachea is central or deviated to one side. Warn the patient in advance what you are about to do and avoid heavy-handedness in this situation. Rough technique is uncomfortable for the patient who may feel like he is being choked. A slight deviation of the trachea to the right may be found in healthy people.

Displacement of the cardiac impulse without displacement of the trachea may be due to scoliosis, to a congenital funnel depression of the sternum or to enlargement of the left ventricle. In the absence of these conditions, a significant displacement of the cardiac impulse or trachea or of both together suggests that the position of the mediastinum has been altered by disease of the lungs or pleura. The mediastinum may be pushed away from the affected side (contralateral deviation) by a pleural effusion or pneumothorax. Fibrosis or collapse of the lung will pull the mediastinum towards the affected side (ipsilateral deviation).

Box 12.14 Causes of pain and tenderness in the chest

- A recent injury of the chest wall or inflammatory conditions
- Intercostal muscular pain – as a rule, localized painful spots can be discovered on pressure
- A painful costochondral junction
- Secondary malignant deposits in the rib
- Herpes zoster before the appearance of the rash

Chest expansion

As well as by simple inspection, possible asymmetrical expansion of the chest may be explored further by palpation. Face the patient and place the fingertips of both hands on either side of the lower ribcage so that the tips of the thumbs meet in the midline in front of the chest but are not touching the skin. A deep breath by the patient will increase the distance between the thumbs and indicate the degree of expansion. If one thumb remains closer to the midline, this suggests diminished expansion on that side. Essentially the hands are being used like a pair of calipers to measure expansion in the lateral bases of the lungs where maximum expansion occurs.

Tactile vocal fremitus is detected by palpation, but this is not a commonly used routine examination technique. It is discussed further under auscultation, below.

Feeling: percussion of the chest

The technique of percussion was probably developed as a way of ascertaining how much fluid remained in barrels of wine or other liquids. Auenbrugger applied percussion to the chest, having learned this method in his father's wine cellar. Effective percussion is a knack that requires consistent practice; do so upon yourself or on willing colleagues, as percussion can be uncomfortable for patients if performed repeatedly and inexpertly.

The middle finger of the left hand is placed on the part to be percussed and pressed firmly against it, with slight hyperextension of the distal interphalangeal joint. The back of this joint is then struck with the tip of the middle finger of the right hand (vice versa if you are left-handed). The movement should be at your wrist rather than at your elbow. The percussing finger is bent so that its terminal phalanx is at right angles and it strikes the other finger perpendicularly. As soon as the blow has been given, the striking finger is raised: the action is a tapping movement.

The two most common mistakes made by the beginner are first, failing to ensure that the finger of the left hand is applied flatly and firmly to the chest wall and second, striking the percussion blow from the elbow rather than from the wrist. The character of the sound produced varies both qualitatively and quantitatively (Box 12.15). When the air in a cavity of sufficient size and appropriate shape is set vibrating, a resonant sound is produced, and there is also a characteristic sensation felt by the finger placed on the chest. Try tapping a hollow cupboard and then a solid wall. The feeling is different as well as the sound. The sound and feel of resonance over a healthy lung has to be learned by practice, and it is against this standard that possible abnormalities of percussion must be judged.

The normal degree of resonance varies between individuals and in different parts of the chest in the same individual, being most resonant below the clavicles anteriorly and the scapulae posteriorly where the muscles are relatively thin and least resonant over the scapulae. On the right side, there is loss of resonance inferiorly as the liver is encountered. On the left side, the lower border overlaps the stomach, so there is a transition from lung resonance to tympanitic stomach resonance.

Always systematically compare the percussion note on the two sides of the chest, moving backwards and forwards from one side to the other, not all the way down one side and then down the other. Percuss over the clavicles; traditionally, this is done without an intervening finger on the chest, but there is no reason for this and it is more comfortable for the patient if the finger of the left hand is used in the usual way. Percuss three or four areas on the anterior chest wall, comparing left with right. Percuss the axillae, then three or four areas on the back of the chest.

Reduction of resonance (i.e. the percussion note is said to be dull) occurs in two important circumstances:

1 When the underlying lung is more solid than usual, usually because of consolidation or collapse.

2 When the pleural cavity contains fluid, i.e. a pleural effusion is present.

Less commonly, a dull percussion note may be due to thickened pleura. The percussion note is most dull when there is underlying fluid, as in a pleural effusion. Pleural effusion causes the sensation in the percussed finger to be similar to that felt when a solid wall is percussed. This is often called 'stony dullness'. By comparing side with side, it is usually easy to detect a unilateral pleural effusion. Pleural effusion usually leads to decreased chest wall movement. Effusions may occur bilaterally in some patients, and this may be more difficult to detect clinically.

An increase in resonance, or hyper-resonance, is more difficult to detect than dullness, and there is no absolute level of normal percussion against which extra resonance can be judged. It may be noticeable when the pleural cavity contains air, as in pneumothorax. Sometimes, however, in this situation one is tempted to think that the slightly duller side is the abnormal side. Further examination and chest X-ray will reveal the true situation.

Box 12.15 Points to note on percussion of the chest

- Resonance
- Dullness
- Pain and tenderness

Listening: auscultation of the chest

Listen to the chest with the diaphragm, not the bell, of the stethoscope (chest sounds are relatively high pitched, and therefore the diaphragm is more sensitive than the bell). Ask the patient to take deep breaths in and out through the mouth. Demonstrate what you would like the patient to do, and then check visually that he is doing it while you listen to the chest. If the patient has a tendency to cough, ask him to breathe more deeply than usual but not so much as to induce a cough with each breath. As with percussion, you should listen in comparable positions to each side alternately, switching back and forth from one side to the other to compare (Box 12.16).

The breath sounds

Breath sounds have intensity and quality. The intensity (or loudness) of the sounds may be normal, reduced or increased. The quality of normal breath sounds is described as vesicular.

Breath sounds will be normal in intensity when the lung is inflating normally but may be reduced if there is localized airway narrowing, if the lung is extensively damaged by a process such as emphysema

Box 12.16 Points to note on auscultation of the chest

- Vesicular breath sounds – normal breath sounds
- Bronchial breath sounds – consolidation
- Vocal fremitus and resonance:
  - whispering pectoriloquy – consolidation
  - aegophony – top of pleural effusion, consolidation
- Added sounds:
  - pleural rub – associated with infection
  - wheezes – asthma, COPD, infection, cardiac failure
  - crackles – pulmonary fibrosis, cardiac failure, COPD

or if there is intervening pleural thickening or pleural fluid. Breath sounds may be of increased intensity in very thin subjects.

Breath sounds probably originate from turbulent airflow in the larger airways. When you place your stethoscope upon the chest, you are listening to how those sounds have been changed on their journey from their site of origin to the position of your stethoscope diaphragm. Normal lung tissue makes the sound quieter and selectively filters out some of the higher frequencies. The resulting sound that you hear is called a vesicular breath sound. There is usually no distinct pause between the end of inspiration and the beginning of expiration.

When the area underlying the stethoscope is airless, as in consolidation, the sounds generated in the large airways are transmitted more efficiently, so they are louder and there is less filtering of the high frequencies. The resulting sounds heard by the stethoscope are termed bronchial breathing, classically heard over an area of consolidated lung in cases of pneumonia. The sound resembles that obtained by listening over the trachea, although the noise there is much louder. The quality of the sound is rather harsh, the higher frequencies being heard more clearly. The expiratory sound has a more sibilant (hissing) character than the inspiratory one and lasts for most of the expiratory phase.

The intensity and quality of all breath sounds is so variable from patient to patient and in different situations that it is only by repeated auscultation of the chests of many patients that one becomes familiar with the normal variations and learns to recognize the abnormalities.

Added sounds

Added sounds are abnormal sounds that arise in the lung itself or in the pleura. The added sounds most commonly arising in the lung are best referred to as wheezes and crackles. Older terms such as râles to describe coarse crackles, crepitations to describe fine crackles and rhonchi to describe wheezes are poorly defined, have led to confusion and are best avoided.

Wheezes are musical sounds associated with airway narrowing. Widespread polyphonic wheezes, particularly heard in expiration, are the most common and are characteristic of diffuse airflow obstruction, especially in asthma and COPD. These wheezes are probably related to dynamic compression of the bronchi, which is accentuated in expiration when airway narrowing is present. A fixed monophonic wheeze can be generated by localized narrowing of a single bronchus, as may occur in the presence of a tumour or foreign body. It may be inspiratory or expiratory or both and may change its intensity in different positions.

Wheezing generated in smaller airways should not be mistaken for stridor associated with laryngeal disease or localized narrowing of the trachea or the large airways. Stridor almost always indicates a serious condition requiring urgent investigation and management. The noise is often both inspiratory and expiratory. It may be heard at the open mouth without the aid of the stethoscope. On auscultation of the chest, stridor is usually loudest over the trachea.

Crackles are short, explosive sounds often described as bubbling or clicking. When the large airways are full of sputum, a coarse rattling sound may be heard even without the stethoscope. However, crackles are not usually produced by moistness in the lungs. It is more likely that they are produced by sudden changes in gas pressure related to the sudden opening of previously closed small airways. Crackles at the beginning of inspiration are common in patients with chronic obstructive pulmonary disease. Localized loud and coarse crackles may indicate an area of bronchiectasis. Crackles are also heard in pulmonary oedema. In diffuse interstitial fibrosis, crackles are characteristically fine in character and late inspiratory in timing (and said to sound like rolling your fingers through your hair near your ear).

The pleural rub is characteristic of pleural inflammation and usually occurs in association with pleuritic pain. It has a creaking or rubbing character (said to sound like a foot crunching through fresh-fallen snow) and, in some instances, can be felt with the palpating hand as well as being audible with the stethoscope.

Take care to exclude false added sounds. Sounds resembling pleural rubs may be produced by movement of the stethoscope on the patient's skin or of clothes against the stethoscope tubing. Sounds arising in the patient's muscles may resemble added sounds: in particular, the shivering of a cold patient makes any attempt at auscultation almost useless. The stethoscope rubbing over hairy skin may produce sounds that resemble fine crackles.

Vocal resonance

When listening to the breath sounds, you are detecting with the stethoscope vibrations that have been made in the large airways. Vocal resonance is the resonance within the chest of sounds made by the voice. Vocal resonance is the detection of vibrations transmitted to the chest from the vocal cords as the patient repeats a phrase, usually the words 'ninety-nine'. The ear perceives not the distinct syllables but a resonant sound, the intensity of which depends on the loudness and depth of the patient's voice and the conductivity of the lungs. As always in examining the chest, each point examined on one side should be compared at once with the corresponding point on the other side.

Not surprisingly, conditions that increase or reduce conduction of breath sounds to the stethoscope have similar effects on vocal resonance. Consolidated lung conducts sounds better than air-containing lung, so in consolidation the vocal resonance is increased and the sounds are louder and often clearer. In such circumstances, even when the patient whispers a phrase (e.g. 'one, two, three'), the sounds may be heard clearly; this is known as whispering pectoriloquy.

Above the level of a pleural effusion, or in some cases over an area of consolidation, the voice may sound nasal or bleating; this is known as aegophony, but is an unusual physical finding.

Vocal fremitus

Vocal fremitus is detected with the hand on the chest wall. It should, therefore, perhaps be regarded as part of palpation, but it is usually carried out after auscultation (see below). As with vocal resonance, the patient is asked to repeat a phrase such as 'ninety-nine'. The examining hand feels distinct vibrations when this is done. Some examiners use the ulnar border of the hand, but there is no good reason for this; the flat of the hand, including the fingertips, is far more sensitive.

From the above, it should be clear that listening to the breath sounds, listening to the vocal resonance and eliciting vocal fremitus are all doing essentially the same thing: they are investigating how vibrations generated in the larynx or large airways are transmitted to the examining instrument, the stethoscope in the first two cases and the fingers in the third. It follows that in the various pathological situations, all three physical signs should behave in similar ways. Where there is consolidation, the breath sounds are better transmitted to the stethoscope, so they are louder and there is less attenuation of the higher frequencies, that is, 'bronchial breathing' is heard. Similarly, the vocal resonance and the vocal fremitus are increased. Where there is a pleural effusion, the breath sounds are quieter or absent and the vocal resonance and vocal fremitus are reduced or absent.

The intelligent student should now ask: 'Why try to elicit all three signs?' The experienced physician will answer: 'Because it is often difficult to interpret the signs that have been elicited, and three pieces of information are more reliable than one.'

Putting it together: an examination of the chest

There is no single perfect way of examining the chest, and most doctors develop their own minor variations of order and procedure. The following is one scheme that combines efficiency with thoroughness:

- Observe the patient generally and the surroundings. Look for any medicine, sputum pots, inhalers, nebulizers or, for example, CPAP machine around the patient's bed. Is the patient using oxygen – if so, how much, what is the rate?
- Ask the patient's permission for the examination and ensure he is lying comfortably at 45°.
- Examine the hands and take the pulse.
- Count the respiratory rate.
- Assess the jugular venous pressure (JVP).
- Check the face for signs of anaemia or cyanosis as well as evidence of ptosis and miosis.
- Inspect the chest movements and the anterior chest wall.
- Feel the position of the trachea and check for axillary lymphadenopathy.
- Feel the position of the apex beat.
- Check the symmetry of the chest movements by palpation.
- Percuss the anterior chest and axillae.

Sit the patient forward:

- Inspect the posterior chest wall.
- Check for cervical and supraclavicular lymphadenopathy.
- Percuss the back of the chest.
- Listen to the breath sounds.
- Check the vocal resonance.
- Check the tactile vocal fremitus.
- Check for sacral oedema.

If you are examining a hospital inpatient, always take the opportunity to turn the pillow over before lying the patient back again; a cool, freshened pillow is a great comfort to an ill person.

- Listen to the breath sounds on the front of the chest.
- Check the vocal resonance.
- Check the tactile vocal fremitus.
- Check for pitting oedema of the ankles.

Stand back for a moment and reflect upon whether you have omitted anything or whether you need to check or repeat anything. Thank the patient and ensure he is dressed or appropriately covered.

Putting it together: interpreting the signs

Developing an appropriate differential diagnosis on the basis of the signs you have elicited requires thought and practice. Keeping the following in mind will help:

- If movements are diminished on one side, there is likely to be an abnormality on that side.
- The percussion note is dull over a pleural effusion and over an area of consolidation – the duller the note, the more likely it is to be a pleural effusion.
- The breath sounds, the vocal resonance and the tactile vocal fremitus are quieter or less obvious over a pleural effusion, and louder or more obvious over an area of consolidation.
- Over a pneumothorax, the percussion note is more resonant than normal but the breath sounds, vocal resonance and tactile vocal fremitus are quieter or reduced. Pneumothorax is easily missed.

Other investigations

Sputum examination

At the bedside

Hospital inpatients should have a sputum pot which must be inspected (Box 12.17). Mucoid sputum is characteristic in patients with chronic bronchitis

Box 12.17 Characteristics to note when assessing sputum

- Mucoid
- Purulent
- Frothy
- Bloodstained
- Rusty
- Frank haemoptysis
- Casts

when there is no active infection. It is clear and sticky and not necessarily produced in a large volume. Sputum may become mucopurulent or purulent when bacterial infection is present in patients with bronchitis, pneumonia, bronchiectasis or a lung abscess. In these last two conditions, the quantities may be large and the sputum is often foul smelling.

Occasionally asthmatics have a yellow tinge to the sputum, owing to the presence of many eosinophils. People with asthma may also produce a particularly tenacious form of mucoid sputum, and sometimes they cough up casts of the bronchial tree, particularly after an attack. Patients with bronchopulmonary aspergillosis may bring up black sputum or sputum with black parts in it, which is the fungal element of the *Aspergillus*.

When sputum is particularly foul smelling, the presence of anaerobic organisms should be suspected. Very ill patients with pulmonary oedema may bring up pink or white frothy sputum. Rusty-coloured sputum is characteristic of pneumococcal lobar pneumonia. Blood may be coughed up alone or bloodstained sputum produced in bronchogenic carcinoma, pulmonary tuberculosis, pulmonary embolism, bronchiectasis or pulmonary hypertension (e.g. with mitral stenosis) being possible causes.

In the laboratory

Sputum may be examined under the microscope in the laboratory for the presence of pus cells and organisms and may be cultured in an attempt to identify the causative agent of an infection and antibiotic resistance patterns. It is seldom practical to wait for the results of such examinations, and most clinical decisions have to be based on the clinical probability of a particular infection being present.

Do not forget to ask for sputum to be examined for acid-fast bacilli when appropriate; tuberculosis (TB) requires specialized techniques of laboratory microscopy and culture to identify the responsible organisms, and if the diagnosis is suspected, these tests must be specifically requested. Non-tuberculous mycobacteria (NTN) can occur in patients with chronic underlying lung pathology such as COPD and bronchiectasis.

Lung function tests

Measurements of respiratory function may provide valuable information. First, in conjunction with the clinical assessment and other investigations, they may help establish a diagnosis. Second, they will help indicate the severity of the condition. Third, serial measurements over time will show changes indicating disease progression or, alternatively, a favourable response to treatment. Finally, regular monitoring of lung function in chronic diseases such as idiopathic pulmonary fibrosis, cystic fibrosis or obstructive airways disease may warn of deterioration.

Simple respiratory function tests fall into three main groups:

1. Measuring the size of the lungs.
2. Measuring how easily air flows into and out of the airways.
3. Measuring how efficient the lungs are in the process of gas exchange.

A spirometer will measure how much air can be exhaled after a maximal inspiration: the patient breathes in as much as he can, then blows out into the spirometer until no more air at all can be breathed out. This volume is called the vital capacity (VC). The amount of air in the lungs at full inspiration is a measure of the total lung capacity and that still remaining after a full expiration is called the residual volume.

The actual value of total lung capacity cannot be measured with a spirometer. The simplest way of determining it is to get the patient to inspire a known volume of air containing a known concentration of helium. Measuring the new concentration of helium that exists after mixing with the air already in the lungs enables the total lung capacity to be calculated. Subtraction of the vital capacity from this value gives the residual volume.

Usually, vital capacity is measured after the patient has blown as hard and fast as possible into the spirometer, when the measurement is known as the forced vital capacity, or FVC. In normal lungs, VC and FVC are almost identical, but in COPD, compression of the airways during a forced expiration leads to closure of the airways earlier than usual, and FVC may be less than VC.

Fig. 12.7A shows the trace produced by a spirometer. Time in seconds is on the x-axis and volume in litres is on the y-axis. Thus, the trace moves up during expiration assessing FVC and along the x-axis as time passes during expiration.

The volume of air breathed out in the first second of a forced expiration is known as the forced expiratory volume in the first second – almost always abbreviated to FEV_1. In normal lungs, the FEV_1 is >70% of FVC. When there is obstruction to airflow, as in COPD, the time taken to expire fully is prolonged and the ratio of FEV_1 to FVC is reduced. An example is shown in Fig. 12.7B. A trace like this is described as showing an obstructive ventilatory defect. As noted above, the FVC may be reduced in severe airways obstruction but, in such cases, the FEV_1 is reduced even more and the FEV_1/FVC ratio remains low.

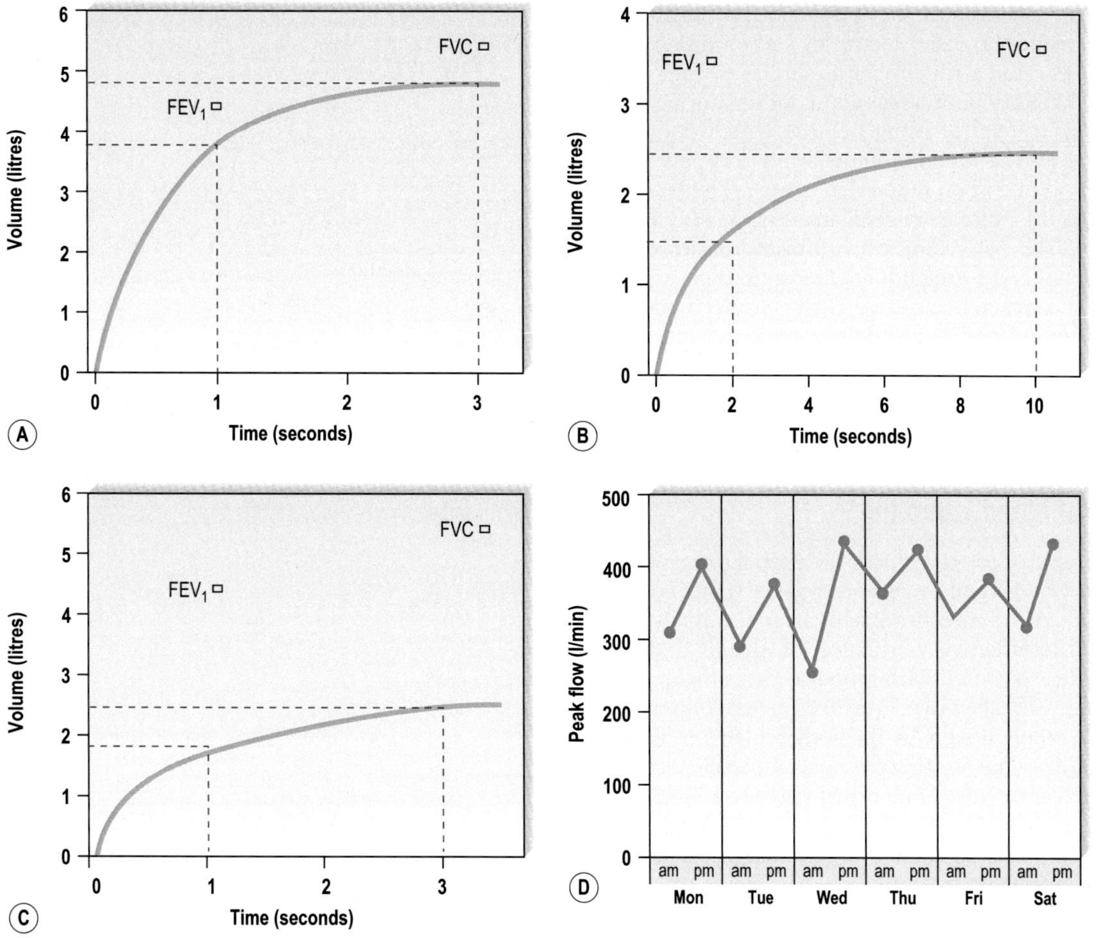

Figure 12.7 **(A)** Normal expiratory spirometer trace. **(B)** Spirometer trace showing an obstructive defect. Note the very prolonged (10-second) expiration. **(C)** Spirometer trace showing a restrictive defect. **(D)** Typical diurnal variation of peak flow, worse in the mornings, seen in a young asthmatic, during an exacerbation.

Some lung conditions restrict expansion of the lungs but do not interfere with the airways. In such individuals, both FEV_1 and FVC are reduced in proportion to each other, so the ratio remains normal even though the absolute values are reduced. Fig. 12.7C shows a trace of this kind, a restrictive ventilatory defect in a patient with diffuse pulmonary fibrosis.

Look again at the normal expiratory spirogram (Fig. 12.7A). The slope of the trace is steepest at the onset of expiration. The trace thus shows that the rate of change of volume with time is greatest in early expiration; in other words, the rate of airflow is greatest then. This measurement, the peak expiratory flow rate (PEFR), can be easily measured with a peak flow meter. A simplified version of this device is shown in Fig. 12.8. This mini-peak flow meter is light and inexpensive, and people with asthma can use it to monitor themselves and alter their medication, as suggested by their doctor, at the first signs of any fall in peak flow measurement, which indicates a deterioration in their condition (Fig. 12.7D).

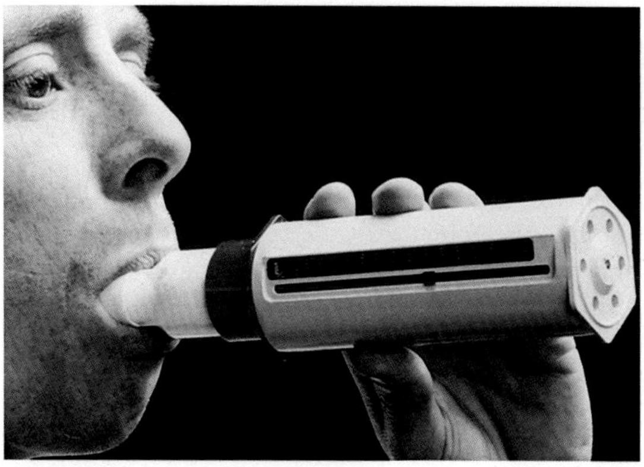

Figure 12.8 A mini-peak flow meter.

Normal gas exchange consists of the uptake of oxygen into the pulmonary capillary blood and the release of carbon dioxide into the alveoli. For this to be achieved, the ventilation of the lungs by air and their perfusion by blood need to be anatomically matched. An approximation of the efficiency of the process of gas exchange may be obtained by measuring the pulmonary transfer factor for carbon monoxide. This is assessed with apparatus similar to that used for the helium-dilution technique for measuring lung volumes. Instead of using helium, which does not easily enter the blood, a known and very low concentration of carbon monoxide is used. The haemoglobin in the pulmonary capillaries very readily binds this gas. The patient inspires to total lung capacity (TLC), holds the breath for 10 seconds, then expires fully. The difference between the inspired carbon monoxide concentration and the expired concentration is a measure of the efficiency of gas exchange and can be expressed per unit lung volume if TLC is simultaneously measured by the helium-dilution technique.

Arterial blood sampling

In a sample of arterial blood, the partial pressures of oxygen (PaO_2) and of carbon dioxide ($PaCO_2$) and the pH can be measured. The arterial $PaCO_2$ will reflect the effective ventilation of alveoli that are adequately perfused with blood so that efficient gas exchange can take place. Provided the rate of production of carbon dioxide by the body remains constant, the $PaCO_2$ will be directly related to the level of alveolar ventilation. The normal range is 4.7-6.0 kPa (36-45 mmHg). When alveolar ventilation is reduced, the $PaCO_2$ will rise. A number of different conditions may reduce alveolar ventilation. Alveolar ventilation rises and $PaCO_2$ may fall in response to metabolic acidosis, in very anxious individuals who hyperventilate and in many lung conditions that tend to reduce the oxygenation of the blood. The PaO_2 is normally in the range 11.3-14.0 kPa (80-100 mmHg). Any lung disease that interferes with gas exchange may reduce arterial PaO_2 (Box 12.18).

Box 12.18 Arterial blood gases

Type 1 Respiratory failure (on air)
pH – 7.43
PCO_2 – 3.8
PO_2 – 7.5
HCO_3 – 22.0
O_2 Sats – 91%
Type 2 Decompensated respiratory failure (on air)
pH – 7.25
PCO_2 – 9.3
PO_2 – 7.5
HCO_3 – 31.2
O_2 Sats – 92%
Type 2 Compensated respiratory failure (1 L O_2 and overnight bilevel positive airway pressure (BIPAP))
pH – 7.41
PCO_2 – 6.3
PO_2 – 8.3
HCO_3 – 30.0
O_2 Sats – 94%

Imaging the lung and chest

The chest X-ray

The chest X-ray is an important extension of the clinical examination (Box 12.19). This is particularly so in patients with respiratory symptoms, and a normal X-ray taken some time before the development of symptoms should therefore not be accepted as a reason for not taking an up-to-date film. In many instances, it is of great value to have previous X-rays for comparison but, if these are lacking, then careful follow up with subsequent films may provide the necessary information.

The standard chest X-ray is a posteroanterior (PA) view taken with the film against the front of the patient's chest and the X-ray source 2 m behind the patient (see Fig. 12.5). The X-ray is examined systematically on a viewing box or computer screen, according to the following plan and referring to the thoracic anatomy described at the beginning of this chapter. (See Figs 12.14-12.18 for more X-rays.)

Box 12.19 Points to note when assessing the chest X-ray

- Name of patient and date (and time) of X-ray
- Bony skeleton
- Position of the patient
- Position of the trachea
- Outline of heart
- Outline of mediastinum
- Diaphragm
- Lung fields

The position of the patient

Is the patient straight or rotated? If straight, the inner ends of the clavicles will be equidistant from the midline of the vertebral body. This is important because any rotation will usually tend to alter the appearance of the mediastinum and the hilar shadows.

The outline of the heart and the mediastinum

Is this normal in size, shape and position?

The position of the trachea

This is seen as a dark column representing the air within the trachea. Is the trachea centrally placed or deviated to either side?

The diaphragm

Can the diaphragm be seen on each side? Is it normal in shape and position? Normally, the anterior end of the sixth or seventh rib crosses the midpart of the diaphragm on each side, although the diaphragm on the right is usually a little higher than on the left. Are the cardiophrenic angles clearly seen?

The lung fields

For radiological purposes, the lung fields are divided into three zones:

1 The upper zone extends from the apex to a line drawn through the lower borders of the anterior ends of the second costal cartilages.
2 The mid-zone extends from this line to one drawn through the lower borders of the fourth costal cartilages.
3 The lower zone extends from this line to the bases of the lungs.

Each zone is systematically examined on both sides, and any area that appears abnormal is carefully compared with the corresponding area on the opposite side. The horizontal fissure, which separates the right upper and middle lobes, may sometimes be seen running horizontally in the third and fourth interspaces on the right side.

The bony skeleton

- Is the chest symmetrical?
- Is scoliosis present?
- Are the ribs unduly crowded or widely spaced in any area?
- Are cervical ribs present?
- Are any ribs eroded or absent?

As well as the standard PA view, lateral views are sometimes carried out to help localize any lesion that is seen. In examining a lateral view, as in Fig. 12.9, follow this plan:

- Identify the sternum anteriorly and the vertebral bodies posteriorly. The cardiac shadow lies anteriorly and inferiorly.
- There should be a lucent (dark) area retrosternally which has approximately the same density as the area posterior to the heart and anterior to the vertebral bodies. Check for any difference between the two or for any discrete lesion in either area.
- Check for any collapsed vertebrae.
- The lowest vertebrae should appear darkest, becoming whiter as they progress superiorly. Interruption of this smooth gradation suggests an abnormality overlying the vertebral bodies involved.

The computed tomography scan

The routine chest X-ray consists of shadows at all depths in the chest superimposed on one another. In computed tomography (CT) scanning, X-rays are passed through the body at different angles and the resulting information is processed by computer to generate a series of cross-sectional images. A thoracic CT scan thus comprises a series of cross-sectional 'slices' through the thorax at various levels.

The CT scan is a vital part of the staging of lung cancer, and inoperability may be demonstrated by

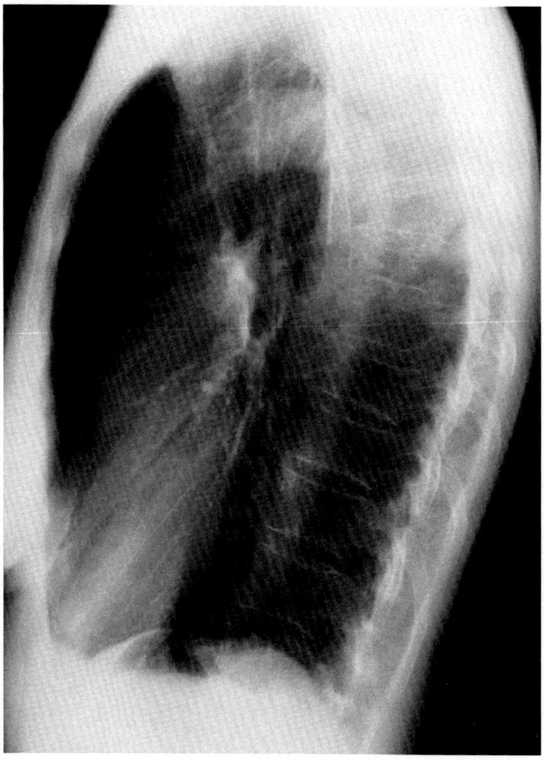

Figure 12.9 A lateral chest X-ray.

evidence on CT of mediastinal involvement. CT scanning will demonstrate the presence of dilated and distorted bronchi, as in bronchiectasis. Diffuse pulmonary fibrosis will be shown by a modified high-resolution/thin-section scan technique. Emboli in the pulmonary arteries can be demonstrated by a rapid data acquisition spiral CT technique and has advantages over isotope lung scanning (see below) in diagnosing pulmonary embolism in patients with pre-existing lung disease. Many scanners can now generate three-dimensional representations of the thoracic structures (Fig. 12.10).

Radioisotope imaging

In the lungs, the most widely used radioisotope technique is combined ventilation and perfusion scanning, used to aid the diagnosis of pulmonary embolism.

The perfusion scan is performed by injecting intravenously a small dose of macroaggregated human albumin particles labelled with technetium-99m (^{99m}Tc). A gamma-camera image is then built up of the radioactive particles impacted in the pulmonary vasculature; the distribution of perfusion in the lung can then be seen. The ventilation scan is obtained by inhalation of a radioactive gas such as krypton-81m (^{81m}Kr), again using scanning to identify the distribution of the radioactivity.

Blood is usually diverted away from areas of the lung that are unventilated, so a matched defect on both the ventilation and perfusion scans usually indicates parenchymal lung disease. If there are areas of ventilated lung which are not perfused (i.e. an unmatched defect), this is evidence in support of an embolism to the unperfused area. Fig. 12.11 shows a ventilation-perfusion isotope scan. The unmatched defects (areas ventilated by the inspired air but not perfused by blood) suggest a high probability of pulmonary embolism.

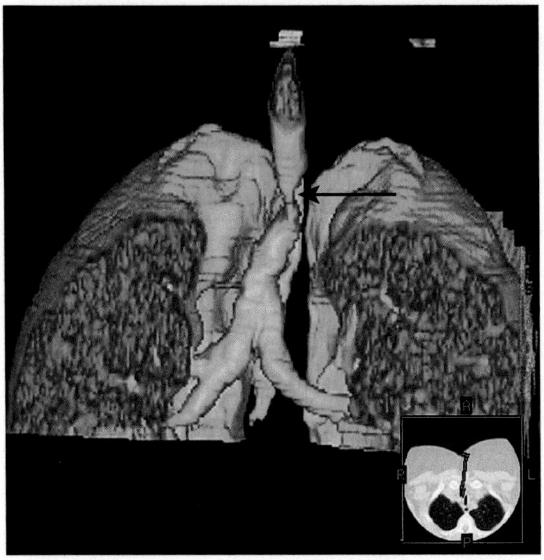

Figure 12.10 A CT-generated 3D reconstruction demonstrating that the patient has a tracheal stenosis (arrow). (Courtesy of Professor R.H. Reznek.)

Magnetic resonance imaging

Magnetic resonance imaging (MRI) is useful in demonstrating mediastinal abnormalities and can help evaluate invasion of the mediastinum and chest wall by tumour. Apart from the fact that it does not use ionizing radiation, currently it has few other advantages over CT in imaging the thorax. MRI is particularly degraded by movement artefact in imaging the chest because of the relatively long data acquisition time and therefore is not used for assessing the lung parenchyma, but faster scanners are beginning to overcome this drawback.

Ultrasound

Ultrasound reveals much less detail than CT scanning but has the advantages that it does not involve radiation and, as it gives 'real-time' images, the operator can visualize what is happening as it happens. It is used for examining diaphragmatic movement and, when available, it is recommended that ward-based pleural procedures, such as chest drain insertion and pleural aspiration or biopsy, be undertaken under ultrasound guidance.

A paralysed hemidiaphragm usually results from damage to the phrenic nerve by a mediastinal tumour. If the patient is asked to make a sudden inspiratory effort, as in sniffing, the non-paralysed side of the

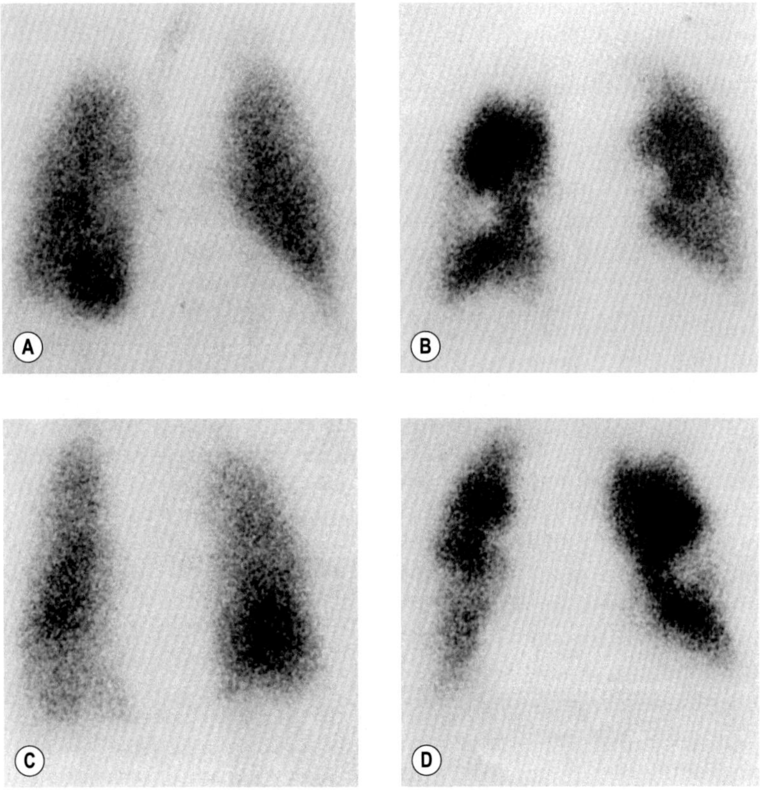

Figure 12.11 Ventilation/perfusion isotope scan of the lungs. Segmental and subsegmental loss of perfusion **(B and D)** can be seen with relatively normal ventilation **(A and C)**. The clear punched-out areas in the perfusion **(B and D)** scans indicate areas of reduced isotope concentration during the perfusion scan. Thus these are areas of reduced blood flow. The ventilation scans show normal aeration of the lungs as depicted by the isotope distribution in the pulmonary airways. These sequences of scans are suggestive of pulmonary embolism because they show impaired perfusion with normal ventilation.

diaphragm moves down, so intrathoracic pressure drops, and the paralysed side moves up.

Ultrasound is also valuable in distinguishing pleural thickening from pleural fluid. With real-time imaging, the latter can be seen to move with changes in posture. When such fluid is present, ultrasound may be used to aid placement of a catheter to drain the collection and also to steer a draining catheter accurately into an intrapulmonary abscess.

Positron emission tomography (PET) scanning

In this technique, a radiolabelled 18-flurodeoxyglucose (FDG) molecule is administered, which is taken up by metabolically active tissues such as cancers, showing as 'hot spots' on the image. It is useful in detecting regional and mediastinal lymphadenopathy and is now widely used in the staging of lung cancers and to assess suitability for surgery in patients with lung cancer.

Flexible bronchoscopy and endobronchial ultrasound (EBUS)

Bronchoscopy is an essential tool in the investigation of many forms of respiratory disease. For discrete abnormalities, such as a mass seen on chest X-ray and suspected to be a lung cancer, bronchoscopy is usually indicated to investigate its nature. Under local anaesthesia, the flexible bronchoscope is passed through the nose, pharynx and larynx, down the trachea, and the bronchial tree is then inspected. Figs 12.12 and 12.16 shows a lung cancer seen down the bronchoscope. Flexible biopsy forceps are passed down a channel inside the bronchoscope and are used to obtain tissue samples for histological examination. Similarly, aspirated bronchial secretions and brushings of any endobronchial abnormality can be sent to the laboratory for cytological examination.

At bronchoscopy, specimens are also taken for microbiological examination in order to determine the nature of any infecting organisms and should include samples for AFB. In diffuse interstitial lung disease, such as sarcoidosis or pulmonary fibrosis, the technique of transbronchial biopsy can be used to obtain small specimens of lung parenchyma for histological examination to help confirm the diagnosis.

Endobronchial ultrasound (EBUS) is gradually becoming more available. It involves a modified bronchoscope fitted with an ultrasound probe and a fine-gauge aspiration needle and is used to biopsy thoracic lymph nodes. The procedure is normally undertaken as a day case and under sedation. The scope is thicker than the average bronchoscope and is passed into the patient's airways via a plastic mouth guard rather than the nose. The ultrasound processor is able to image lymph nodes on the other side of the bronchial airways; the operator can then use the aspiration needle to puncture that bronchial wall and biopsy the lymph nodes. A similar procedure, endoscopic ultrasound (EUS), can be used via the oesophagus, and combining these two techniques allows all of the mediastinal lymph nodes to be biopsied. In the majority of cases, they have replaced mediastinoscopy as the biopsy technique of choice and are particularly useful in the diagnosis and staging of lung cancer, sarcoidosis and tuberculosis.

Pleural aspiration and biopsy

A pleural effusion (Fig. 12.17) can give rise to diagnostic problems and, sometimes, management

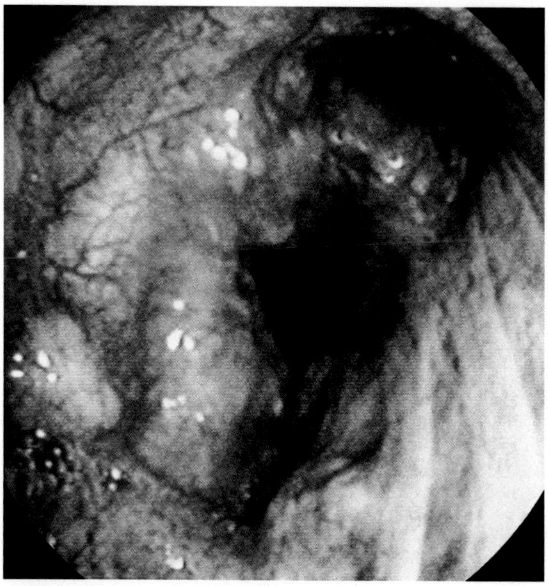

Figure 12.12 A lung cancer, seen down the bronchoscope.

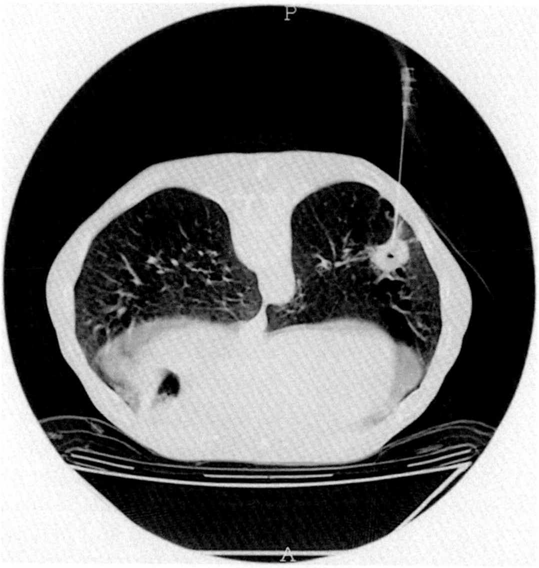

Figure 12.13 A CT-guided percutaneous biopsy in progress. The radiodense (white) structure penetrating the chest wall is the biopsy needle.

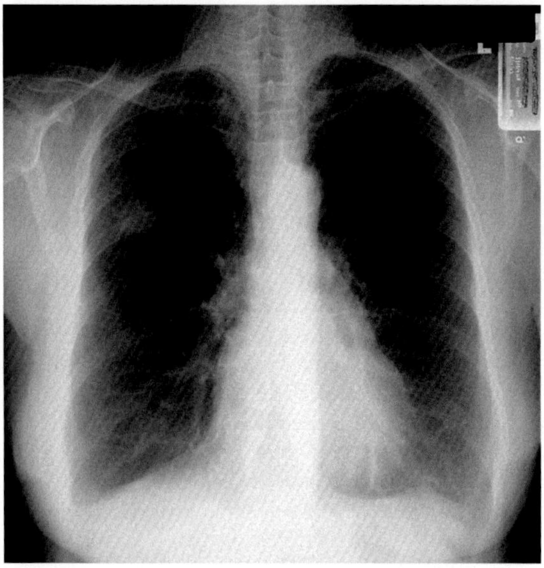

Figure 12.14 Chest X-ray showing a right upper lobe mass in a 70-year-old smoker presenting with haemoptysis.

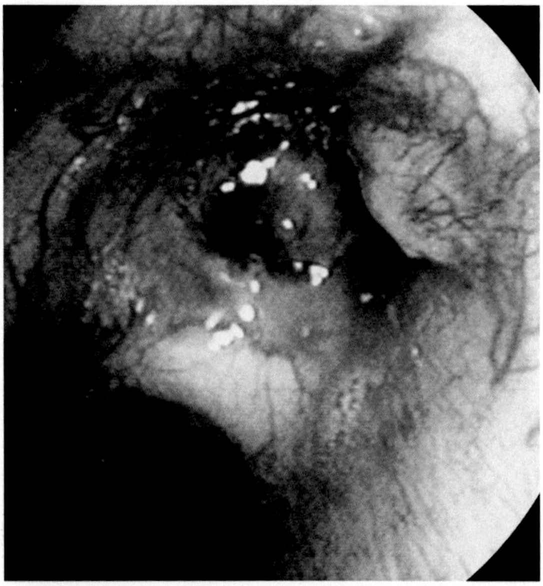

Figure 12.15 Bronchoscopic view of the tumour seen radiologically in Fig. 12.14 – histology showed a squamous carcinoma.

problems when the amount of fluid causes respiratory embarrassment. When a pleural effusion is seen as a presenting feature in a middle-aged or older patient, the most likely cause is a malignancy. Less commonly, particularly in younger patients, it may be due to tuberculosis. In either case, the diagnosis is best obtained by both aspiration of the fluid and pleural biopsy. Aspiration alone has a lower diagnostic yield.

After anaesthetizing the skin, subcutaneous tissues and pleura, pleural fluid may be aspirated by syringe and needle for microbiological and cytological

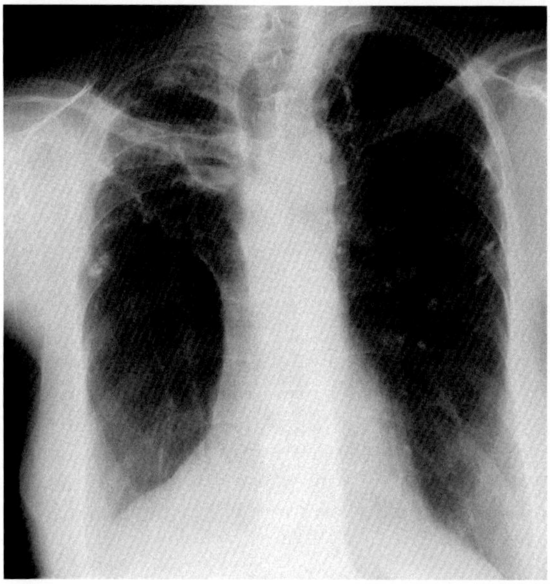

Figure 12.16 Chest X-ray showing right apical scarring and tracheal deviation (detectable clinically) from previous tuberculosis and hyperinflation of the lungs due to chronic obstructive pulmonary disease in a 66-year-old long-term smoker with 5 years of increasing breathlessness.

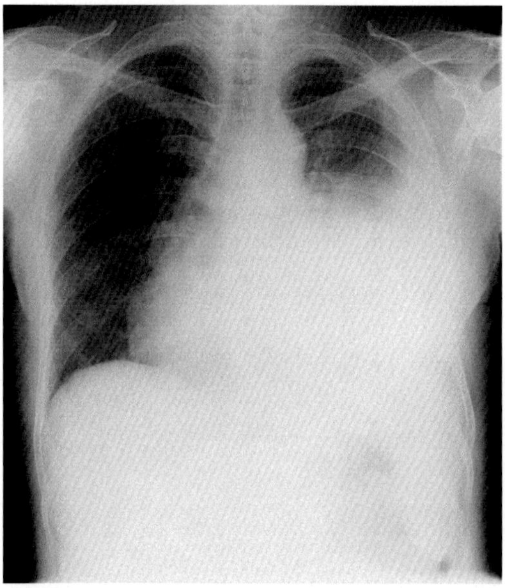

Figure 12.17 Chest X-ray showing a large left pleural effusion in a young man with a 4-month history of malaise, fever, night sweats and weight loss. The diagnosis of tuberculosis was confirmed on histology of a pleural biopsy and culture of the pleural fluid.

examination. Large pleural effusions may need to be drained by an indwelling catheter, left *in situ* until the fluid has been fully removed. As noted above, ultrasound guidance can be helpful, particularly if the fluid is loculated in various pockets, and should be used whenever equipment and trained personnel are available.

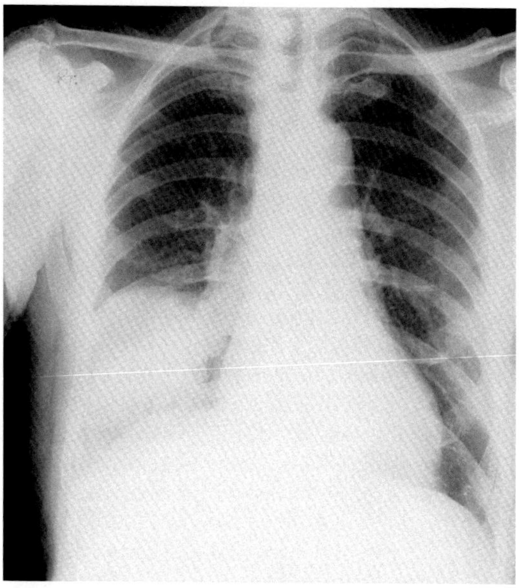

Figure 12.18 Chest X-ray showing a right basal pneumonia in a previously fit 40-year-old man with fever, breathlessness, central cyanosis and pleuritic pain. Chest signs included bronchial breathing and a pleural rub in the right lower zone. The cyanosis was due to the shunting of deoxygenated blood through the consolidated lung, the increased respiratory rate leading to a low $PaCO_2$ because of increased clearance of carbon dioxide by the unaffected alveoli. *Streptococcus pneumoniae* was grown on blood cultures.

Box 12.20 Light's criteria for diagnosing a pleural effusion

An effusion is exudative if it meets one of the following criteria:

- Pleural fluid protein/serum protein >0.5
- Pleural fluid lactate dehydrogenase (LDH)/serum LDH ratio >0.6
- Pleural fluid LDH > two-thirds the upper limit of normal serum LDH

Cytological examination of pleural fluid may demonstrate the presence of malignant cells. Many polymorphs may be seen if the effusion is secondary to an underlying pneumonic infection. With tuberculosis, the fluid usually contains many lymphocytes, although tubercle bacilli are rarely seen. Therefore, all pleural fluid samples should be cultured for possible tuberculosis, because this infection can coexist with other pathologies and it is so important not to miss it. In empyema, pus is present in the pleural cavity. It has a characteristic appearance and is full of white cells and organisms.

The pleural fluid should also be examined for protein content. A transudate (resulting from cardiac or renal failure) can be distinguished from an exudate (from pleural inflammation or malignancy) by its lower protein content (<30 g/l). Light's criteria may also be applied (Box 12.20). When infection is suspected, pleural fluid pH should be measured in non-purulent effusions and, if not available, pleural fluid glucose should be assessed. A pH <7.2 strongly suggests the need for pleural drainage (pleural fluid glucose <3.4 mmol/l). Pleural fluid LDH is also raised in the presence of infection.

Biopsies of the pleura can be obtained percutaneously and under local anaesthesia using an Abram's pleural biopsy needle. This technique can be used when there is pleural fluid present to obtain pleural tissue for histological examination and, whenever tuberculosis is a possibility, for microbiological culture. If ultrasound or CT examination shows the pleura to be thickened, biopsies may be obtained under image guidance by Abram's needle, a Tru-cut needle and similar techniques.

Ridge thoracoscopy and video-assisted thoracoscopic surgery (VATS)

These techniques enable the pleural cavity to be examined directly and biopsies taken; VATS is now becoming the procedure of choice. The ridge method is normally performed under a general anaesthetic by a surgeon who uses direct vision down a rigid thoracoscope after the lung has been deflated. Increasingly, however, more minimally invasive procedures using flexible thoracoscopes attached to cameras are being used (video-assisted thoracoscopic surgery, or VATS) and are not only able to biopsy the pleura but also biopsy the lung, mediastinal nodes and tumours, decortication of empyemas, lobectomy and pneumonectomy, pleurodesis and endoscopic stapled bullectomy (lung volume reduction surgery).

Lung biopsy

As noted above, the technique of transbronchial biopsy can be used to obtain samples of lung parenchyma, but often samples are too small for diagnosis. In this circumstance, biopsies of the lung taken at thoracoscopy may be of value. Occasionally, a formal open lung biopsy obtained at thoracotomy may be necessary.

When there is a discrete, localized lesion, it may be possible to obtain a biopsy percutaneously with the aid of CT scanning to direct the insertion of the biopsy needle (Fig. 12.13). All samples should be sent for histology, microbiology and TB culture.

Immunological tests

Asthma attacks may be due to type I immediate hypersensitivity reactions on exposure to common environmental proteins known as allergens. In such individuals, an inherited tendency to produce exaggerated levels of immunoglobulin E (IgE) against these allergens is responsible. Part of the assessment of such allergic patients might include skin-prick tests (see Ch. 19). Alternatively, serum levels of specific (individual) IgEs against allergens may be measured by blood tests (formerly known as RAST tests) to demonstrate sensitization. The total IgE level is often raised in patients with asthma, rhinitis or eczema. Delayed (type IV, cell-mediated) hypersensitivity is shown by the Mantoux and Heaf skin tests, used to detect the presence of sensitivity to tuberculin protein. Precipitating immunoglobulin G (IgG) antibodies in the circulating blood are present in patients with some fungal diseases, such as bronchopulmonary aspergillosis or aspergilloma. In patients suspected of having an allergic alveolitis, IgG antibodies may be demonstrated to the relevant antigens.

Tests for Tuberculosis (TB)

Tuberculosis (TB) continues to be a worldwide problem, occurring most frequently as a pulmonary infection but also commonly in the lymph nodes, as well as being able to affect any organ of the body. As outlined above, sending relevant samples for smear and culture is essential and often forgotten in hospitals where TB is less common. Sputum can easily be tested by light microscopy using a Zeihl-Neelsen or auramine stain to look for the acid-fast bacilli (AFB). Where available, culture should be undertaken as drug monoresistance and multidrug-resistant TB (MDR TB) continue to be a major problem in the flight against the infection. Newer techniques help to diagnose active infection and drug resistance using molecular methods to detect *Mycobacterium tuberculosis* (MTB) complex DNA, e.g. the polymerase chain reaction (PCR) assay Xpert® MTB/RIF (Cepheid, California, United States) and the line probe assay MTBDRplus® (Hain Lifescience, Nehren, Germany).

Tests for latent TB and Heaf and Mantoux skin tests are still widely used to look for evidence of previous TB exposure. In many centres, they are being superseded by blood tests that use the interferon gamma-releasing assay (IGRA) which measures interferon gamma released from T-cells activated by the presence of *Mycobacterium tuberculosis*. At the present time, the IGRA blood test does not differentiate between active and latent TB and should be used only to diagnosis latent disease. False negatives can occur in disseminated and non-pulmonary active disease and can therefore be misleading when diagnosing active infection.

Cardiovascular system 13

Ceri Davies

Introduction

The recent decades have seen major changes in patterns of cardiovascular disease. In the developed world, syphilitic and tuberculous involvement of the cardiovascular system has become rare, and the incidence of rheumatic disease has declined considerably. Myocardial and conducting tissue disease are diagnosed with increasing frequency and the importance of arterial hypertension has become recognized. Coronary artery disease has emerged as the major cardiovascular disorder of the era, becoming the most common cause of premature death throughout Europe, North America and Australasia. In the last 30 years, there has been a steady fall in age-specific death rates from coronary artery disease in Western societies, but elsewhere its prevalence is increasing and in the underdeveloped world it now threatens to overtake malnutrition and infectious disease as the major cause of death.

As patterns of cardiovascular disease have changed, so have the cardiologist's diagnostic tools, although a good history and thorough clinical examination remain cornerstones of the assessment of patients with cardiovascular disease. A century that started with the stethoscope, the sphygmomanometer, the chest X-ray and a very rudimentary electrocardiogram saw the development of a variety of new imaging modalities, using ultrasound, radioisotopes, X-rays and magnetic resonance. This non-invasive capability was complemented by introduction of the catheterization laboratory, permitting angiographic imaging, electrophysiological recording and tissue biopsy of the heart. Add to this the resources of the chemical pathology, bacteriology and molecular biology laboratories, and the array of diagnostic technology available to the modern cardiologist becomes almost overwhelming.

The cardiac history

The history should record details of presenting symptoms, of which the most common are chest pain, fatigue and dyspnoea, palpitations, and presyncope or syncope (see below and Box 13.1). Previous illness should also be recorded, as it may provide important clues about the cardiac diagnosis – thyroid, connective tissue and neoplastic disorders, for example, can all affect the heart. Rheumatic fever in childhood is important because of its association with valvular heart disease and diabetes and dyslipidaemias because of their association with coronary artery disease. Smoking is a major risk factor for coronary artery disease. Alcohol abuse predisposes to cardiac arrhythmias and cardiomyopathy. The cardiac history should quantify both habits in terms of pack-years smoked and units of alcohol consumed. The use of other recreational drugs (in particular cocaine) can be associated with acute presentations of chest pain, and intravenous drug use is an increasingly important cause of infective endocarditis. The family history should always be documented because coronary artery disease and hypertension often run in families, as do some of the less common cardiovascular disorders, such as hypertrophic cardiomyopathy. Indeed, in patients with hypertrophic cardiomyopathy, a family history of sudden death is probably the single most important indicator of risk. Finally, the drug history should be recorded, as many commonly prescribed drugs are potentially cardiotoxic. β-blockers and some calcium channel blockers (diltiazem, verapamil), for example, can cause symptomatic bradycardias, and tricyclic antidepressants and β-agonists can cause tachyarrhythmias. Vasodilators cause variable reductions in blood pressure, which can lead to syncopal attacks, particularly in patients with aortic stenosis. The myocardial toxicity of certain cytotoxic drugs (notably doxorubicin and related compounds) is an important cause of cardiomyopathy.

Chest pain

Myocardial ischaemia, pericarditis, aortic dissection and pulmonary embolism are the most common causes of acute, severe chest pain. Chronic, recurrent chest pain is usually caused by angina, oesophageal reflux or musculoskeletal pain.

Box 13.1 Structure for the cardiac history

Presenting complaint (PC)

- The symptom that prompts the patient to seek medical attention – commonly chest pain, breathlessness (dyspnoea), palpitation, dizziness or blackouts (syncope)

History of presenting complaint (HPC)

- This should define the nature of the symptoms, initially through open questioning. Closed questions are used to elicit the presence or absence of features which help to differentiate between diagnoses:
  - Chest pain: site, radiation, character, duration, provoking and relieving factors, associated symptoms?
  - Breathlessness: orthopnoea, paroxysmal nocturnal dyspnoea, ankle swelling, cough, wheeze, haemoptysis?
  - Palpitation: sudden onset and offset, 'thumps' or 'pauses', presyncope or syncope?
  - Dizziness/syncope: provoking factors, warning, duration, recovery?

Risk factors for cardiovascular disease

- Smoking, hypertension, hypercholesterolaemia, diabetes, family history of premature vascular disease

Past medical history (PMH)

- Stroke or transient ischaemic attack (TIA), renal impairment, rheumatic fever, peripheral vascular disease, other
- Operations, hospital clinic attendances

Family history

- Cardiac disease, sudden death

Drug history

- Include quantification of alcohol intake
- If a patient with known cardiovascular disease is not taking the recognized standard treatment, the reason for this should be established. For example, why no statin treatment in a patient with previous myocardial infarction? – 'Because it caused muscle pains'

Myocardial ischaemia

Ischaemia of the heart results from an imbalance between myocardial oxygen supply and demand, producing pain called angina (Boxes 13.2 and 13.3). Angina is usually a symptom of atherosclerotic coronary artery disease, which impedes myocardial oxygen supply. Other causes of coronary artery disease (Box 13.4) are rare. However, it is important to be vigilant for causes of angina due to increased myocardial oxygen demand, such as aortic stenosis. The history is diagnostic for angina if the location of the pain, its character, its relation to exertion and its duration are typical. The patient describes retrosternal pain that may radiate into the arms, the throat or the jaw. It has a constricting character, is provoked by exertion and relieved within minutes by rest. The patient's

Box 13.2 Angina

Typical patient

- Middle-aged or elderly man or woman often with a family history of coronary heart disease and one or more of the major reversible risk factors (smoking, hypertension, hypercholesterolaemia, diabetes)

Major symptoms

- Exertional chest pain and shortness of breath. Pain often described as 'heaviness' or 'tightness' and may radiate into arms, neck or jaw

Major signs

- None, although hypertension and signs of hyperlipidaemia (xanthelasmata, xanthomas) may be present
- Peripheral vascular disease, evidenced by absent pulses or arterial bruits, is commonly associated with coronary heart disease

Diagnosis

- Typical history is most important diagnostic tool
- Electrocardiogram (ECG): often normal; may show Q waves in patients with previous myocardial infarction
- Exercise ECG test: exertional ST depression
- Isotope or magnetic resonance perfusion scan: stress-induced perfusion defects
- Coronary angiogram: confirms coronary artery disease

Additional investigations

- Blood sugar and lipids to rule out diabetes and dyslipidaemia

Comments

- A careful history is the single most important means of diagnosing angina

Box 13.3 Causes of angina

Impaired myocardial oxygen supply

- Coronary artery disease:
  - atherosclerosis
  - arteritis in connective tissue disorders
  - diabetes mellitus
- Coronary artery spasm
- Congenital coronary artery disease:
  - arteriovenous fistula
  - anomalous origin from pulmonary artery
- Severe anaemia or hypoxia

Increased myocardial oxygen demand

- Left ventricular hypertrophy:
  - hypertension
  - aortic valve disease
  - hypertrophic cardiomyopathy
- Tachyarrhythmias

Box 13.4 Causes of coronary artery disease

- Atherosclerosis
- Arteritis
  - systemic lupus erythematosus
  - polyarteritis nodosa
  - rheumatoid arthritis
  - ankylosing spondylitis
  - syphilis
  - Takayasu's disease
- Coronary dissection
  - spontaneous
  - catheter or angioplasty induced
- Embolism
  - infective endocarditis
  - left atrial/ventricular thrombus
  - left atrial/ventricular tumour
  - prosthetic valve thrombus
  - paradoxical embolism
  - complication of cardiac catheterization
- Coronary mural thickening
  - amyloidosis
  - radiation therapy
  - Hurler's disease
  - pseudoxanthoma elasticum
- Other causes of coronary luminal narrowing
  - aortic dissection
  - coronary spasm
- Congenital coronary artery disease
  - anomalous origin from pulmonary artery
  - arteriovenous fistula

threshold for angina is typically reduced after eating or in cold weather due to the diversion of blood to the gut and the increased myocardial work consequent upon peripheral vasoconstriction, respectively. Occasionally angina is provoked only by the first significant activity of the day, a phenomenon known as the 'warm-up effect' due to myocardial preconditioning. Less commonly, myocardial ischaemia may manifest as breathlessness, fatigue or symptoms that the patient finds difficult to describe – 'I just have to stop' – in which case the clues to the diagnosis are the relation of symptoms to exertion, the presence of risk factors for coronary artery disease and the absence of an alternative explanation for the symptoms, such as heart failure.

Box 13.5 Acute coronary syndromes

Typical patient

- Middle-aged (male) or elderly (either sex) patient, often with a family history of coronary heart disease and one or more of the major reversible risk factors (smoking, hypertension, hypercholesterolaemia, diabetes)
- In many patients, there is no preceding history of angina

Major symptoms

- Chest pain and shortness of breath. Pain usually prolonged and often described as 'heaviness' or 'tightness', with radiation into arms, neck or jaw. Alternative descriptions include 'congestion' or 'burning', which may be confused with indigestion

Major signs

- Frequently none
- Autonomic disturbance, sweating, vomiting implies myocardial infarction
- Tachycardia (anterior myocardial infarction), bradycardia (inferior myocardial infarction)
- Fourth heart sound, dyskinetic precordial impulse, pulmonary oedema with large infarcts

Diagnosis

(STEMI = ST elevation myocardial infarction)

	STEMI	Non-STEMI	Unstable angina
ECG	ST elevation	Normal, ST depression, T-wave inversion	Normal, ST depression, T-wave inversion
Cardiac biomarkers, e.g. troponin I or T	Raised	Raised	Normal

Additional investigations

- Biochemistry: blood sugar and lipids to rule out diabetes and dyslipidaemia
- Risk stratification: echocardiogram (left ventricular function), coronary angiogram in high-risk patients, perfusion imaging in low-risk patients

Comments

- History and troponin testing most useful diagnostic tools in non-ST elevation acute coronary syndromes

Acute coronary syndromes

In these life-threatening cardiac emergencies, the pain is similar in location and character to angina but is usually more severe, more prolonged and unrelieved by rest (Box 13.5).

Pericarditis

Pericarditis causes central chest pain, which is sharp in character and aggravated by deep inspiration, cough or postural changes. Characteristically, the pain is exacerbated by lying recumbent and reduced by sitting forward. Pericarditis is usually idiopathic or caused by Coxsackie B infection. It may also occur as a complication of myocardial infarction, but other causes are seen less commonly (Box 13.6).

Aortic dissection

Aortic dissection produces severe tearing pain in either the front or the back of the chest. The onset

Box 13.6 Causes of acute pericarditis

- Idiopathic
- Infective:
  - viral (Coxsackie B, influenza, herpes simplex)
  - bacterial (*Staphylococcus aureus*, *Mycobacterium tuberculosis*)
- Connective tissue disease:
  - systemic lupus erythematosus
  - rheumatoid arthritis
  - polyarteritis nodosa
- Uraemia
- Malignancy (e.g. breast, lung, lymphoma, leukaemia)
- Radiation therapy
- Acute myocardial infarction
- Post-myocardial infarction/cardiotomy (Dressler's syndrome)

Box 13.7 Aortic dissection

Typical patient

- Middle-aged or elderly patient with a history of hypertension or arteriosclerotic disease
- Occasionally younger patient with aortic root disease (e.g. Marfan syndrome)

Major symptoms

- Chest pain, typically interscapular

Major signs

- Often none
- Sometimes regional arterial insufficiency (e.g. occlusions of coronary artery causing myocardial infarction, carotid or vertebral artery causing stroke, spinal artery causing hemi- or quadriplegia, renal artery causing renal failure); subclavian artery occlusion may cause differential blood pressure in either arm; aortic regurgitation; cardiac tamponade; sudden death

Diagnosis

- Chest X-ray: widened mediastinum, occasionally with left pleural effusion
- Transoesophageal echocardiogram, computed tomography (CT) scan, or magnetic resonance imaging (MRI) scan confirms dissection

Comments

- Type A dissections involve the ascending aorta and are usually treated surgically. Type B dissections involve the arch and/or descending aorta and are usually managed medically or with an endovascular stent

is abrupt, unlike the crescendo quality of ischaemic cardiac pain (Box 13.7).

Pulmonary embolism

Peripheral pulmonary embolism causes sudden-onset sharp, pleuritic chest pain, breathlessness and haemoptysis. Major, central pulmonary embolism presents with breathlessness and chest pain that can be indistinguishable from ischaemic chest pains and syncope. Risk factors for pulmonary embolism should be sought in the history (Box 13.8).

Box 13.8 Pulmonary embolism

Typical patient

- Recent surgery, lower limb fracture or long-distance air travel; obese; sedentary; heart failure; malignancy

Major symptoms

- Chest pain, dyspnoea, haemoptysis, syncope

Major signs

- Peripheral emboli, pleural rub
- Large, central emboli, tachycardia, hypotension, cyanosis, raised jugular venous pressure (JVP)

Diagnosis

- D-Dimer: a negative D-dimer in a low-risk patient makes pulmonary embolism very unlikely
- ECG: sinus tachycardia, right bundle branch block (RBBB), classical 'S1, Q3, T3' pattern uncommon
- Chest X-ray: normal, wedge-shaped peripheral opacification, absent pulmonary vascular markings
- Echocardiogram: dilated right heart in some cases of large central pulmonary embolism
- CT pulmonary angiogram: has superseded V/Q scanning as the diagnostic test of choice

Comments

- Suspect pulmonary embolism in patients with unexplained hypoxia. Thrombolytic therapy should be considered for patients with pulmonary embolism associated with shock and/or a dilated right heart on echo. Patients with no risk factors for pulmonary embolism should be investigated for prothrombotic states.

Rare cardiovascular causes of chest pain include mitral valve disease associated with massive left atrial dilatation. This causes discomfort in the back, sometimes associated with dysphagia due to oesophageal compression. Aortic aneurysms can also cause pain in the chest owing to local compression.

Dyspnoea

Dyspnoea is an abnormal awareness of breathing occurring either at rest or at an unexpectedly low level of exertion. It is a major symptom of many cardiac disorders, particularly left heart failure (Table 13.1), but its mechanisms are complex. In acute pulmonary oedema and orthopnoea, dyspnoea is due mainly to the elevated left atrial pressure that characterizes left heart failure (Box 13.9). This produces a corresponding elevation of the pulmonary capillary pressure and increases transudation into the lungs, which become oedematous and stiff. Oxygenation of blood in the pulmonary arterioles is reduced, causing hypoxaemia, and this, together with the extra

Box 13.9 Acute left ventricular failure

Typical patient

- Patient with acute myocardial infarction or known left ventricular disease

Major symptoms

- Severe dyspnoea, orthopnoea, frothy sputum

Major signs

- Low-output state (hypotension, oliguria, cold periphery), tachycardia, S3, sweating, crackles at lung bases

Diagnosis

- Chest X-ray: bilateral air space consolidation with typical perihilar distribution
- Echocardiogram: usually confirms left ventricular disease

Additional investigations

- ECG: may show evidence of acute or previous myocardial infarction
- Blood gas analysis: shows variable hypoxaemia

Comments

- Although most cases are caused by acute myocardial infarction or advanced left ventricular disease, it is vital to exclude valvular disease which is potentially correctable by surgery

Table 13.1 Causes of heart failure

Ventricular pathophysiology	Clinical examples
Restricted filling	Mitral stenosis Constrictive pericarditis Restrictive cardiomyopathy Hypertrophic cardiomyopathy
Pressure loading	Hypertension Aortic stenosis Coarctation of the aorta
Volume loading	Mitral regurgitation Aortic regurgitation
Contractile impairment	Coronary artery disease Dilated cardiomyopathy Myocarditis
Arrhythmia	Severe bradycardia Severe tachycardia

Box 13.10 Congestive heart failure

Typical patient

- Middle-aged (male) or elderly (either sex) patient with a history of myocardial infarction or long-standing hypertension
- In cases where there is no clear cause, always enquire about alcohol consumption

Major symptoms

- Exertional fatigue and shortness of breath, with orthopnoea and paroxysmal nocturnal dyspnoea in advanced cases

Major signs

- Fluid retention: basal crackles, raised JVP, peripheral oedema
- Reduced cardiac output: cool skin, peripheral cyanosis
- Other findings: third heart sound

Diagnosis

- ECG: usually abnormal; often shows Q waves (previous myocardial infarction), left ventricular hypertrophy (hypertension), or left bundle branch block (LBBB)
- Chest X-ray: cardiac enlargement, congested lung fields
- Echocardiogram: left ventricular dilatation with regional (coronary heart disease) or global (cardiomyopathy) contractile impairment

Additional investigations

- Raised B-type natriuretic peptide useful in cases of diagnostic uncertainty
- Renal function as prelude to diuretic and angiotensin converting enzyme (ACE) inhibitor therapy
- Blood count to rule out anaemia

Comments

- The echocardiogram is the single most important diagnostic test in the patient with heart failure

Table 13.2 NYHA classification

NYHA class	Description
I	Asymptomatic
II	Symptoms on normal exertion, e.g. walking up a flight of stairs
III	Symptoms on minimal exertion, e.g. getting dressed
IV	Symptoms at rest

effort required to ventilate the stiff lungs, causes dyspnoea.

Exertional dyspnoea

Exertional dyspnoea is the most troublesome symptom in heart failure (Box 13.10). Exercise causes a sharp increase in left atrial pressure and this contributes to the pathogenesis of dyspnoea by causing pulmonary congestion (see above). However, the severity of dyspnoea does not correlate closely with exertional left atrial pressure, and other factors must therefore be important. These include respiratory muscle fatigue and the effects of exertional acidosis on peripheral chemoreceptors. As left heart failure worsens, exercise tolerance deteriorates. In advanced disease, the patient is dyspnoeic at rest.

Breathlessness in heart failure can be simply classified by use of the New York Heart Association Classification (Table 13.2). It is simple to acquire and, despite poor reproducibility and its subjective nature, provides powerful prognostic information. For example, patients with Class IV heart failure have a very poor outlook.

Orthopnoea

In patients with heart failure, lying flat causes a steep rise in left atrial and pulmonary capillary pressure, resulting in pulmonary congestion and severe dyspnoea. To obtain uninterrupted sleep, extra pillows are required, and in advanced disease, the patient may choose to sleep sitting in a chair.

Paroxysmal nocturnal dyspnoea

Frank pulmonary oedema on lying flat wakes the patient from sleep with distressing dyspnoea and fear of imminent death. The symptoms are corrected by standing upright, which allows gravitational pooling of blood to lower the left atrial and pulmonary capillary pressure, the patient often feeling the need to obtain air at an open window.

Fatigue

Exertional fatigue is an important symptom of heart failure and is particularly troublesome towards the end of the day. Its aetiology is complex, but it is caused partly by deconditioning and muscular atrophy.

Palpitation

Awareness of the heartbeat is common during exertion or heightened emotion. Under other circumstances it may be indicative of an abnormal cardiac rhythm. A description of the rate and rhythm of the palpitation is essential as are exacerbating behaviours, such as exercise or caffeine intake. Extrasystoles are common but rarely signify important heart disease. They are usually experienced as 'missed' or 'dropped' beats; the forceful beats that follow may also be noticed. Rapid irregular palpitation is typical of atrial fibrillation. Rapid regular palpitation of abrupt onset occurs in atrial, junctional and ventricular tachyarrhythmias.

Dizziness and syncope

Cardiovascular disorders produce dizziness and syncope by transient hypotension, resulting in abrupt cerebral hypoperfusion. For this reason, patients who experience cardiac syncope usually describe either brief lightheadedness or no warning symptoms at all prior to their syncopal attacks. Recovery is usually rapid, unlike with other common causes of syncope (e.g. stroke, epilepsy, overdose).

Postural hypotension

Syncope on standing upright reflects inadequate baroreceptor-mediated vasoconstriction. It is common in the elderly in whom it is frequently compounded by medication. Abrupt reductions in blood pressure and cerebral perfusion cause the patient to fall to the ground, whereupon the condition corrects itself.

Vasovagal syncope

This is caused by autonomic overactivity, usually provoked by emotional or painful stimuli, less commonly by coughing or micturition ('cough syncope' or 'micturition syncope'). Only rarely are syncopal attacks so frequent as to be significantly disabling ('malignant' vasovagal syndrome). Vasodilatation and inappropriate slowing of the pulse combine to reduce blood pressure and cerebral perfusion. Recovery is rapid if the patient lies down.

Carotid sinus hypersensitivity

Exaggerated vagal discharge following external stimulation of the carotid sinus (e.g. from shaving or a tight shirt collar) causes reflex vasodilatation and slowing of the pulse. These may combine to reduce blood pressure and cerebral perfusion in some elderly patients, causing loss of consciousness.

Valvular obstruction

Fixed valvular obstruction in aortic stenosis may prevent a normal rise in cardiac output during exertion, such that the physiological vasodilatation that occurs in exercising muscle produces an abrupt reduction in blood pressure and cerebral perfusion, resulting in syncope. Vasodilator therapy may cause syncope by a similar mechanism. Intermittent obstruction of the mitral valve by left atrial tumours (usually myxoma or thrombus) may also cause syncopal episodes (Fig. 13.1).

Stokes-Adams attacks

These are caused by self-limiting episodes of asystole (Fig. 13.2) or rapid tachyarrhythmias (including ventricular fibrillation). The loss of cardiac output causes syncope and striking pallor. Following restoration of normal rhythm, recovery is rapid and associated with flushing of the skin as flow through the dilated cutaneous bed is re-established.

The cardiac examination

A methodical approach is recommended, starting with inspection of the patient and proceeding to examination of the radial pulse, measurement of heart rate and blood pressure, examination of the neck (carotid pulse, jugular venous pulse), palpation of the anterior chest wall, auscultation of the heart, percussion and auscultation of the lung bases and, finally, examination of the peripheral pulses and auscultation for carotid and femoral arterial bruits (Box 13.11).

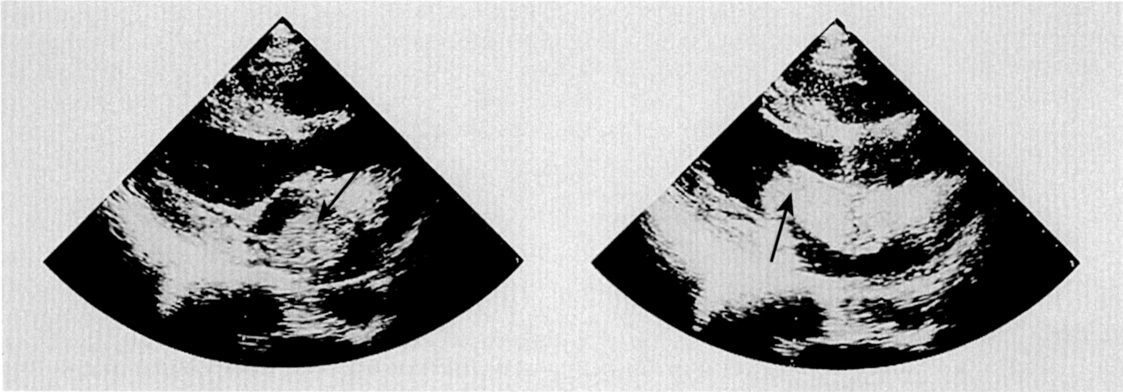

Figure 13.1 Left atrial myxoma. 2D echocardiogram (long-axis view). During diastole, the tumour (arrow) prolapses through the mitral valve and obstructs left ventricular filling.

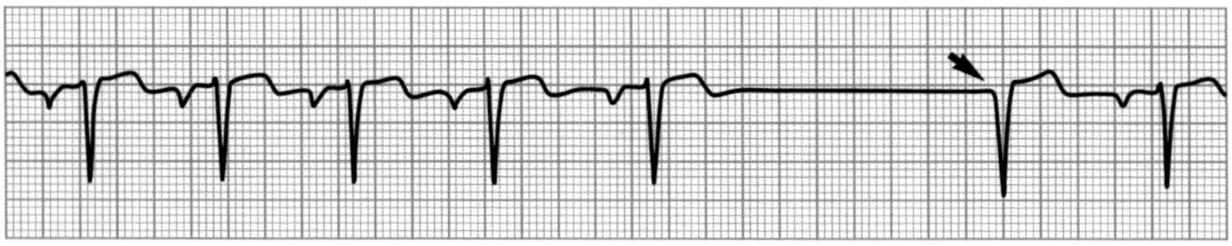

Figure 13.2 Prolonged sinus arrest. After the fifth sinus beat there is a pause of about 1.8 seconds terminated by a nodal escape beat (arrow) before sinus rhythm resumes.

Box 13.11 Routine for the cardiovascular system examination

- Wash hands
- Introduce yourself to patient
- Recline patient at 45°
- Observe general appearance – comfortable, breathless, pale?
- Inspect the hands for clubbing, splinter haemorrhages, nicotine staining
- Examine the radial pulse(s) for symmetry, rate, rhythm, character (collapsing?)
- Measure the blood pressure
- Assess the height and waveform of the JVP
- Examine the carotid pulse character (slow rising?) and volume (Corrigan's sign?)
- Inspect the face, eyes and mucous membranes for xanthelasma, corneal arcus and anaemia, and cyanosis, respectively
- Inspect the chest for scars and pulsations
- Assess the position and character of the apex beat
- Palpate the praecordium for heaves and thrills
- Auscultate the heart
- Auscultate the lungs
- Examine the ankles and sacrum for oedema
- Examine the peripheral pulses

Inspection of the patient

Chest wall deformities such as pectus excavatum should be noted, as these may compress the heart and displace the apex, giving a spurious impression of cardiac enlargement. The presence of a median sternotomy scar usually indicates previous coronary artery bypass graft (CABG) and/or cardiac valve surgery. The long saphenous vein is the standard conduit for vein grafts, so patients with prior CABG often also have a scar along the medial aspect of one or both legs. A lateral thoracotomy scar may indicate previous mitral valvotomy. Large ventricular or aortic aneurysms may cause visible pulsations. Superior vena caval obstruction is associated with prominent venous collaterals on the chest wall. Prominent venous collaterals around the shoulder occur in axillary or subclavian vein obstruction.

Hypercholesterolaemia may be suggested by the presence of tendon and ocular xanthelasma.

Anaemia

Anaemia may exacerbate angina and heart failure. Pallor of the mucous membranes is a useful but sometimes misleading physical sign, and diagnosis requires laboratory measurement of the haemoglobin concentration.

Cyanosis

Cyanosis is a blue discoloration of the skin and mucous membranes caused by increased concentration of reduced haemoglobin in the superficial blood vessels. Peripheral cyanosis may result when cutaneous vasoconstriction slows the blood flow and increases oxygen extraction in the skin and the lips. It is physiological during cold exposure. It also occurs in heart failure, when reduced cardiac output produces reflex cutaneous vasoconstriction. In mitral stenosis, cyanosis over the malar area produces the characteristic mitral facies or malar flush.

Central cyanosis may result from the reduced arterial oxygen saturation caused by cardiac or pulmonary disease. It affects not only the skin and the lips but also the mucous membranes of the mouth. Cardiac causes include pulmonary oedema (which prevents adequate oxygenation of the blood) and congenital heart disease. Congenital defects associated with central cyanosis include those in which desaturated venous blood bypasses the lungs by ('reversed') shunting through septal defects or a patent ductus arteriosus (e.g. Eisenmenger's syndrome, Fallot's tetralogy).

The mouth should also be inspected for signs of poor dental hygiene.

Clubbing of the fingers and toes

In congenital cyanotic heart disease, clubbing is not present at birth but develops during infancy and may become very marked. Infective endocarditis is the only other cardiac cause of clubbing.

Other cutaneous and ocular signs of infective endocarditis

Other signs of infective endocarditis are caused by immune complex deposition in the capillary circulation. A vasculitic rash is common, as are splinter haemorrhages in the nail bed, although these are very non-specific findings. Other 'classic' manifestations of endocarditis including Osler's nodes (tender erythematous nodules in the pulps of the fingers), Janeway lesions (painless erythematous lesions on the palms) and Roth's spots (erythematous lesions in the optic fundi) are now rarely seen.

Coldness of the extremities

In patients hospitalized with severe heart failure, coldness of the extremities is an important sign of reduced cardiac output. It is caused by reflex vasoconstriction of the cutaneous bed.

Pyrexia

Infective endocarditis is invariably associated with pyrexia, which may be low grade or 'swinging' in nature if paravalvular abscess develops. Pyrexia also occurs for the first 3 days after myocardial infarction.

Oedema

Subcutaneous oedema that pits on digital pressure is a cardinal feature of congestive heart failure. Pressure should be applied over a bony prominence (tibia, lateral malleoli, sacrum) to provide effective compression. Oedema is caused by salt and water retention by the kidney. Two mechanisms are responsible:

1. Reduced sodium delivery to the nephron. This is caused by reduced glomerular filtration due to constriction of the preglomerular arterioles in response to sympathetic activation and angiotensin II production.
2. Increased sodium reabsorption from the nephron. This is the more important mechanism. It occurs particularly in the proximal tubule early in heart failure but, as failure worsens, renin-angiotensin activation stimulates aldosterone release, which increases sodium reabsorption in the distal nephron.

Salt and water retention expands plasma volume and increases the capillary hydrostatic pressure. Hydrostatic forces driving fluid out of the capillary exceed the osmotic forces reabsorbing it, so that fluid accumulates in the interstitial space. The effect of gravity on capillary hydrostatic pressure ensures that oedema is most prominent around the ankles in the ambulant patient and over the sacrum in the bedridden patient. In advanced heart failure, oedema may involve the legs, genitalia and trunk. Transudation into the peritoneal cavity (ascites), the pleural and pericardial spaces may also occur.

Arterial pulse

The arterial pulses should be palpated for evaluation of rate, rhythm, character and symmetry.

Rate and rhythm

By convention, both rate and rhythm are assessed by palpating the right radial pulse. Rate, expressed in beats per minute (bpm), is measured by counting the number of beats in a timed period of 15 seconds and multiplying by 4. Normal sinus rhythm is regular, but in young patients may show phasic variation in rate during respiration (sinus arrhythmia). An irregular rhythm usually indicates atrial fibrillation but may also be caused by frequent ectopic beats or self-limiting paroxysmal arrhythmias. In patients with atrial fibrillation, the rate should be measured by auscultation at the cardiac apex, because beats that follow very short diastolic intervals may create a 'pulse deficit' by not generating sufficient pressure to be palpable at the radial artery.

Character

Character is defined by the volume and waveform of the pulse and should be evaluated at the right carotid artery (i.e. the pulse closest to the heart and least subject to damping and distortion in the arterial tree). Pulse volume provides a crude indication of stroke volume, being small in heart failure and large in aortic regurgitation. The waveform of the pulse is of greater diagnostic importance (Fig. 13.3). Severe aortic stenosis produces a slow-rising carotid pulse; the fixed obstruction restricts the rate at which blood can be ejected from the left ventricle. In aortic regurgitation, in diastole, the left ventricle receives

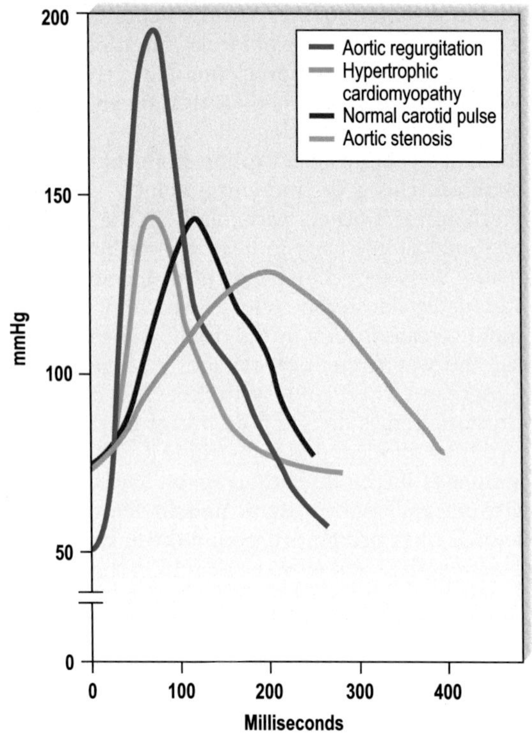

Figure 13.3 The waveform of the pulse is characterized by the rate of rise of the carotid upstroke. Note that in aortic regurgitation, the upstroke is rapid and followed by abrupt diastolic 'collapse'. In hypertrophic cardiomyopathy, the upstroke is also rapid and the pulse has a jerky character. In aortic stenosis, the upstroke is slow with a plateau.

not only its normal pulmonary venous return but also a proportion of the blood ejected into the aorta during the previous systole as it flows back through an incompetent valve. The resultant large stroke volume, vigorously ejected, produces a rapidly rising carotid pulse, which collapses in early diastole owing to backflow through the aortic valve. This collapsing pulse can be exaggerated at the radial artery by lifting the arm. In mixed aortic valve disease, a biphasic pulse with two systolic peaks is occasionally found. Alternating pulse – alternating high and low systolic peaks – occurs in severe left ventricular failure but the mechanism for this is unknown. Paradoxical pulse refers to an inspiratory decline in systolic pressure greater than 10 mmHg (Fig. 13.4). In normal circumstances, inspiration results in an increase in venous return as blood is 'sucked into' the thorax by the decline in intrathoracic pressure. This increases right ventricular stroke volume, but left ventricular stroke volume falls slightly (ventricular interdependence). When the heart is constrained in a 'fixed box' by a pericardial effusion (cardiac tamponade) or by thickened pericardium (pericardial constriction), the increased inspiratory right ventricular blood volume reduces left ventricular compliance, resulting in a more pronounced reduction in left ventricular filling, stroke volume and systolic blood pressure during

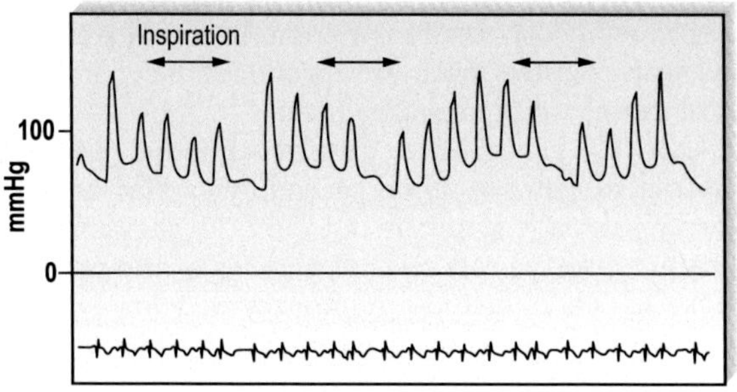

Figure 13.4 Paradoxical pulse (radial artery pressure signal). The patient had severe tamponade. Note the exaggerated (>10 mmHg) decline in arterial pressure during inspiration.

inspiration. 'Pulsus paradoxus' therefore represents an exaggeration of the normal inspiratory decline in systolic pressure and is not truly paradoxical. Pulsus paradoxus in acute severe asthma is thought to be due to negative pleural pressure increasing afterload and thereby impedance to left ventricular emptying.

It is measured by inflating a blood pressure cuff until no sounds are heard. The pressure is then slowly decreased until systolic sounds are first heard during expiration but not during inspiration – note this reading. The pressure is slowly decreased further until sounds are heard throughout the respiratory cycle (inspiration and expiration) – note this second reading. If the pressure difference between the two readings is >10 mmHg, it can be classified as pulsus paradoxus

Symmetry

Symmetry of the radial, brachial, carotid, femoral, popliteal and pedal pulses should be confirmed. A reduced or absent pulse indicates an obstruction more proximally in the arterial tree, usually caused by atherosclerosis or thromboembolism and less commonly by aortic dissection. Coarctation of the aorta causes symmetrical reduction and delay of the femoral pulses compared with the radial pulses ('radiofemoral delay'), a sign that should be looked for in younger patients with hypertension. Bruits from collateral vessels may also be heard over the back of such patients.

Measurement of blood pressure

Blood pressure is measured indirectly, traditionally by sphygmomanometry, but automated blood pressure monitors are being used increasingly in clinical practice. The principle of manual blood pressure measurement is that turbulent flow through a partially compressed artery (typically the brachial) creates noises that can be auscultated with a stethoscope and the points at which these noises (called Korotkoff sounds) change in intensity correlate with systemic arterial pressures. Accurate blood pressure measurement requires careful technique; patients should be sitting or lying at ease as significant changes in arterial pressure occur with exertion, anxiety and changes in posture. The manometer should be at the same level of the cuff on the patient's arm and the observer's eye. For most adult patients, a standard cuff (12 cm width) is appropriate, but obese subjects require use of a wider (thigh) cuff of 15 cm or the blood pressure will be overestimated. For children, various sized cuffs are available; select the one which covers most of the upper arm leaving a gap of 1 cm or so below the axilla and above the antecubital fossa.

Palpate the radial pulse as the cuff is inflated to a pressure of 20 mmHg above the level at which radial pulsation can no longer be felt. Place the stethoscope lightly over the brachial artery and reduce the pressure in the cuff at a rate of 2-3 mmHg/s until the first sounds are heard. This is the first Korotkoff sound and correlates with systolic blood pressure as flow is just possible through the pressure applied by the compressive cuff. As the pressure is lowered further, subtle changes in pitch and volume occur; these are the second and third Korotkoff sounds and are not important clinically. With further lowering of the pressure in the cuff, the artery becomes less compressed, flow becomes less turbulent and the sounds over the brachial artery become muffled. This is the fourth Korotkoff sound. Shortly after this (usually 1-10 mmHg lower), the sounds die away completely as flow is unimpeded by the cuff; this is the fifth Korotkoff sound and correlates most accurately with diastolic blood pressure. Its identification is also less subjective than the fourth, but in some conditions (aortic regurgitation, arteriovenous fistula, pregnancy), the Korotkoff sounds remain audible despite complete deflation of the cuff. In such situations, phase four must be used for the diastolic measurement. Both systolic and diastolic values are recorded; the difference between these two values is called the pulse pressure. Certain conditions of the aortic valve may cause important abnormalities of pulse pressure. Supine and erect blood pressure measurements provide an assessment of baroreceptor function, a postural drop being defined by a fall in systolic blood pressure on standing. It is essential to work swiftly as well as accurately, as compression of a limb will, by itself, cause a rise in blood pressure. If several successive measurements are made, the air pressure in the cuff should be allowed to fall to zero between readings.

Jugular venous pulse

Fluctuations in right atrial pressure during the cardiac cycle generate a pulse that is transmitted backwards into the jugular veins. It is best examined in good light while the patient reclines at 45°. If the right atrial pressure is very low, however, visualization of the jugular venous pulse may require a smaller reclining angle. Alternatively, manual pressure over the upper right side of the abdomen may be used to produce a transient increase in venous return to the heart which elevates the jugular venous pulse (hepatojugular reflux).

Jugular venous pressure

The jugular venous pressure (JVP) should be assessed from the waveform of the internal jugular vein which lies adjacent to the medial border of the sternocleidomastoid muscle. Distention of the external jugular vein is a useful clue to an elevated JVP but, strictly speaking, it should not be used because it can be compressed as it passes under the clavicle. The JVP is measured in centimetres vertically from the sternal angle to the top of the venous waveform. The normal upper limit is 4 cm. This is about 9 cm above the right atrium and corresponds to a pressure of 6 mmHg. Elevation of the JVP indicates a raised right atrial pressure unless the superior vena cava is obstructed, producing engorgement of the neck veins (Box 13.12). During inspiration, the pressure within the chest decreases and there is a fall in the JVP. In constrictive pericarditis, and less commonly in tamponade, inspiration produces a paradoxical rise in the JVP (Kussmaul's sign) because the increased venous return that occurs during inspiration cannot be accommodated within the constrained right side of the heart (Fig. 13.5).

Box 13.12 Causes of elevated jugular venous pressure

- Congestive heart failure
- Cor pulmonale
- Pulmonary embolism
- Right ventricular infarction
- Tricuspid valve disease
- Tamponade
- Constrictive pericarditis
- Hypertrophic/restrictive cardiomyopathy
- Superior vena cava obstruction
- Iatrogenic fluid overload, particularly in surgical and renal patients

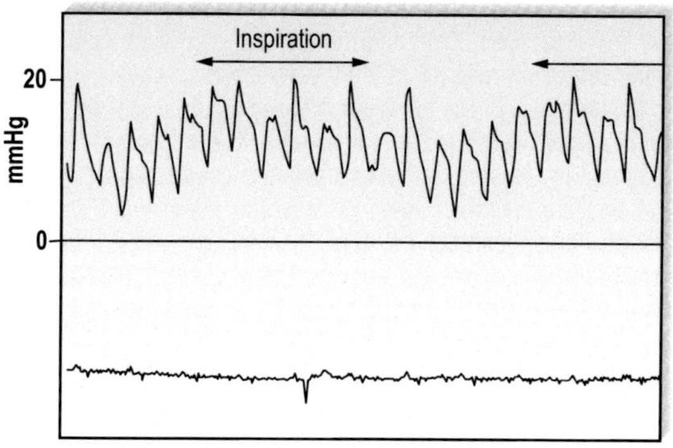

Figure 13.5 Kussmaul's sign. Jugular venous pressure recording in a patient with tamponade. The venous pressure is raised and there is a particularly prominent systolic 'x' descent, giving the waveform of the JVP an unusually dynamic appearance. Note the inspiratory rise in atrial pressure (Kussmaul's sign) reflecting the inability of the tamponaded right heart to accommodate the inspiratory increase in venous return.

Waveform of jugular venous pulses

In sinus rhythm, the jugular venous pulse has a double waveform attributable to the 'a' and 'v' waves separated by the 'x' and 'y' descents. The 'a' wave is produced by atrial systole. It is followed by the 'x' descent (marking descent of the tricuspid valve ring), which is interrupted by the diminutive 'c' wave caused by tricuspid valve closure. Atrial pressure then rises again, producing the 'v' wave as the atrium fills passively during ventricular systole. The decline in atrial pressure as the tricuspid valve opens to allow ventricular filling produces the 'y' descent. Important abnormalities of the pattern of deflections are shown in Fig. 13.6.

In atrial fibrillation, there is no atrial contraction. Consequently, there is no 'a' wave and the jugular venous pulse loses its double waveform. It is not always easy to differentiate venous from arterial pulsations in the neck, but several features help to distinguish the jugular venous pulse from the carotid arterial pulse (Box 13.13).

Box 13.13 Characteristics of the jugular venous pulse

- Double waveform (in sinus rhythm)
- Varies with respiration
- Varies with posture
- Impalpable
- Obliterated by pressure at base of waveform
- Transient increase in volume and height with hepatojugular reflux

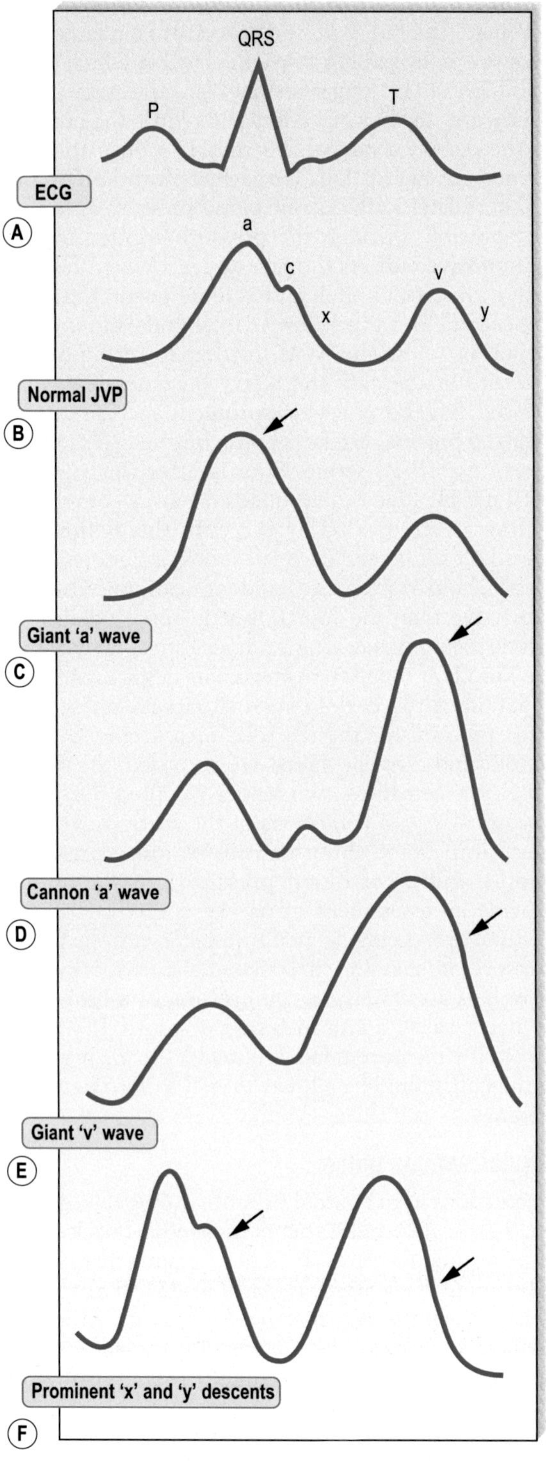

Figure 13.6 Waveform of the jugular venous pulse. **(A)** The ECG is portrayed at the top of the illustration. Note how electrical events precede mechanical events in the cardiac cycle. Thus the P wave (atrial depolarization) and the QRS complex (ventricular depolarization) precede the 'a' and 'v' waves, respectively, of the JVP. **(B)** Normal JVP. The 'a' wave produced by atrial systole is the most prominent deflection. It is followed by the 'x' descent, interrupted by the small 'c' wave marking tricuspid valve closure. Atrial pressure then rises again ('v' wave) as the atrium fills passively during ventricular systole. The decline in atrial pressure as the tricuspid valve opens produces the 'y' descent. **(C)** Giant 'a' wave. Forceful atrial contraction against a stenosed tricuspid valve or a non-compliant hypertrophied right ventricle produces an unusually prominent 'a' wave. **(D)** Cannon 'a' wave. This is caused by atrial systole against a closed tricuspid valve. It occurs when atrial and ventricular rhythms are dissociated (complete heart block, ventricular tachycardia) and marks coincident atrial and ventricular systole. **(E)** Giant 'v' wave. This is an important sign of tricuspid regurgitation. The regurgitant jet produces pulsatile systolic waves in the JVP. **(F)** Prominent 'x' and 'y' descents. These occur in constrictive pericarditis and give the JVP an unusually dynamic appearance. In tamponade, only the 'x' descent is usually exaggerated.

Palpation of the chest wall

The apex beat is defined as the lowest and most lateral point at which the cardiac impulse can be palpated. Inferior or lateral displacement from its normal location in the fifth intercostal space in the mid-clavicular line usually indicates cardiac enlargement. Chronic volume loading of the left ventricle (mitral regurgitation, aortic regurgitation) causes left ventricular dilatation, which can be appreciated clinically. In contrast, isolated pressure loading of the left ventricle (hypertension, aortic stenosis) causes left ventricular hypertrophy, which does not cause displacement of the apex beat. Palpable third and fourth heart sounds give the apical impulse a double thrust. In the past, considerable importance was attached to the character of the apical impulse ('thrusting' in aortic valve disease, 'tapping' in mitral stenosis), but this is of very limited practical value in the modern era.

Left ventricular aneurysms can sometimes be palpated medial to the cardiac apex. Right ventricular enlargement produces a systolic thrust (heave) in the left parasternal area. The turbulent flow responsible for murmurs may produce palpable vibrations (thrills) on the chest wall, particularly in aortic stenosis, ventricular septal defect and patent ductus arteriosus.

Auscultation of the heart

The diaphragm and bell of the stethoscope permit appreciation of high- and low-pitched auscultatory events, respectively. The apex, lower left sternal edge, upper left sternal edge and upper right sternal edge should be auscultated in turn. These locations correspond respectively to the mitral, tricuspid, pulmonary and aortic areas, and loosely identify sites at which sounds and murmurs arising from the four valves are best heard (Box 13.14).

First sound (S1)

This corresponds to mitral and tricuspid valve closure at the onset of systole. It is accentuated in mitral stenosis because prolonged diastolic filling through the narrowed valve ensures that the thickened leaflets are widely separated at the onset of systole. Thus valve closure generates unusually vigorous vibrations. In advanced mitral stenosis, the valve is rigid and immobile and S1 becomes soft again.

Box 13.14 Routine for auscultation of the heart

- Auscultate at apex with diaphragm
- Reposition patient on left side – 'Please turn onto your left side'
- Listen with diaphragm (mitral regurgitation) and then bell (mitral stenosis)
- Return patient to original position, reclining at 45°
- Auscultate with diaphragm at lower left sternal edge (tricuspid regurgitation, tricuspid stenosis, ventricular septal defect)
- Auscultate with diaphragm at upper left sternal edge (pulmonary stenosis, pulmonary regurgitation, patent ductus arteriosus)
- Auscultate with diaphragm at upper right sternal edge (aortic stenosis, hypertrophic cardiomyopathy)
- Sit patient forward. Auscultate with diaphragm at lower left sternal edge in held expiration (aortic regurgitation) – 'breathe in … breathe out … stop'
- Auscultate over the carotid arteries (radiation of murmur of aortic stenosis, carotid artery bruits)

Second sound (S2)

The second sound corresponds to aortic and pulmonary valve closure following ventricular ejection. S2 is single during expiration. Inspiration, however, causes physiological splitting into aortic followed by pulmonary components because increased venous return to the right side of the heart delays pulmonary valve closure. Important abnormalities of S2 are illustrated in Fig. 13.7.

Third and fourth sounds (S3, S4)

The third and fourth are low-frequency sounds that occur early and late in diastole, respectively. When present, they give a characteristic 'gallop' to the cardiac rhythm. Both sounds are best heard with the bell of the stethoscope at the cardiac apex. They are caused by abrupt tensing of the ventricular walls following rapid diastolic filling. Rapid filling occurs early in diastole (S3) following atrioventricular valve opening and again late in diastole (S4) due to atrial contraction. S3 is physiological in children and young

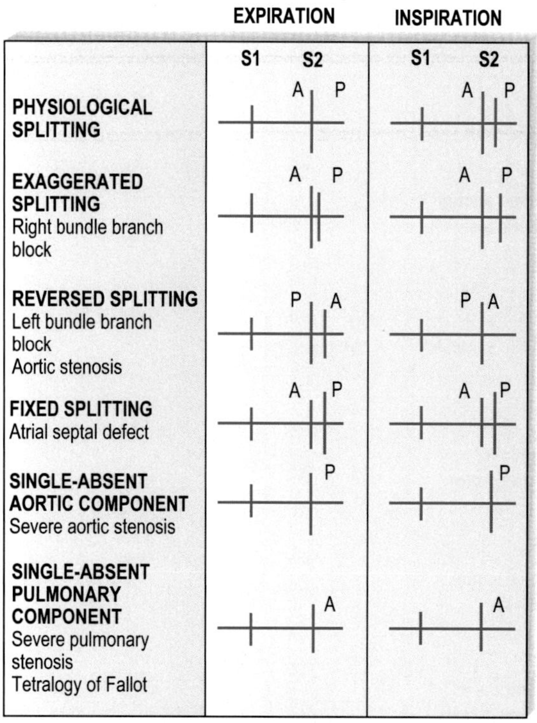

Figure 13.7 Splitting of the second heart sound. The first sound, representing mitral and tricuspid closure, is usually single, but the aortic and pulmonary components of the second sound normally split during inspiration as increased venous return delays right ventricular emptying. Abnormal splitting of the second heart sound is an important sign of heart disease.

adults but usually disappears after the age of 40. It also occurs in high-output states caused by anaemia, fever, pregnancy and thyrotoxicosis. After the age of 40, S3 is nearly always pathological, usually indicating left ventricular failure or, less commonly, mitral regurgitation or constrictive pericarditis. In the elderly, S4 is sometimes physiological. More commonly, however, it is pathological, and occurs when vigorous atrial contraction late in diastole is required to augment filling of a hypertrophied, non-compliant ventricle (e.g. hypertension, aortic stenosis, hypertrophic cardiomyopathy).

Systolic clicks and opening snaps

Valve opening, unlike valve closure, is normally silent. In aortic stenosis, however, valve opening produces a click in early systole that precedes the ejection murmur. The click is audible only if the valve cusps are pliant and non-calcified, and is particularly prominent in the congenitally bicuspid valve. A click later in systole suggests mitral valve prolapse, particularly when followed by a murmur. In mitral stenosis, elevated left atrial pressure causes forceful opening of the thickened valve leaflets. This generates a snap early in diastole that precedes the mid-diastolic murmur.

Heart murmurs

Heart murmurs are caused by turbulent flow within the heart and great vessels (Fig. 13.8). Occasionally the turbulence is caused by increased flow through a normal valve – usually aortic or pulmonary – producing an 'innocent' murmur. However, murmurs may also indicate valve disease or abnormal communications between the left and right sides of the heart (e.g. septal defects).

Rheumatic heart disease has become much less common in developed countries, although it remains common elsewhere and is the cause of many of the classic heart murmurs (Box 13.15). Degenerative valve disease (calcific aortic stenosis, mitral regurgitation due to chordal rupture) is increasingly common. Heart murmurs are defined by four characteristics: loudness, quality, location and timing.

The loudness of a murmur reflects the degree of turbulence. This relates to the volume and velocity of flow and not the severity of the cardiac lesion. Loudness is graded on a scale of 1 (barely audible) to 6 (audible even without application of the stethoscope to the chest wall). The quality of a murmur relates to its frequency and is best described as low, medium or high-pitched. The location of a murmur on the chest wall depends on its site of origin and has led to the description of four valve areas (see above). Some murmurs radiate, depending on the velocity and direction of blood flow. The sound of the high-velocity systolic flow in aortic stenosis and mitral regurgitation, for example, is directed towards the neck and the axilla, respectively; that of the high-velocity diastolic flow in aortic regurgitation is directed towards the left sternal edge. Murmurs are

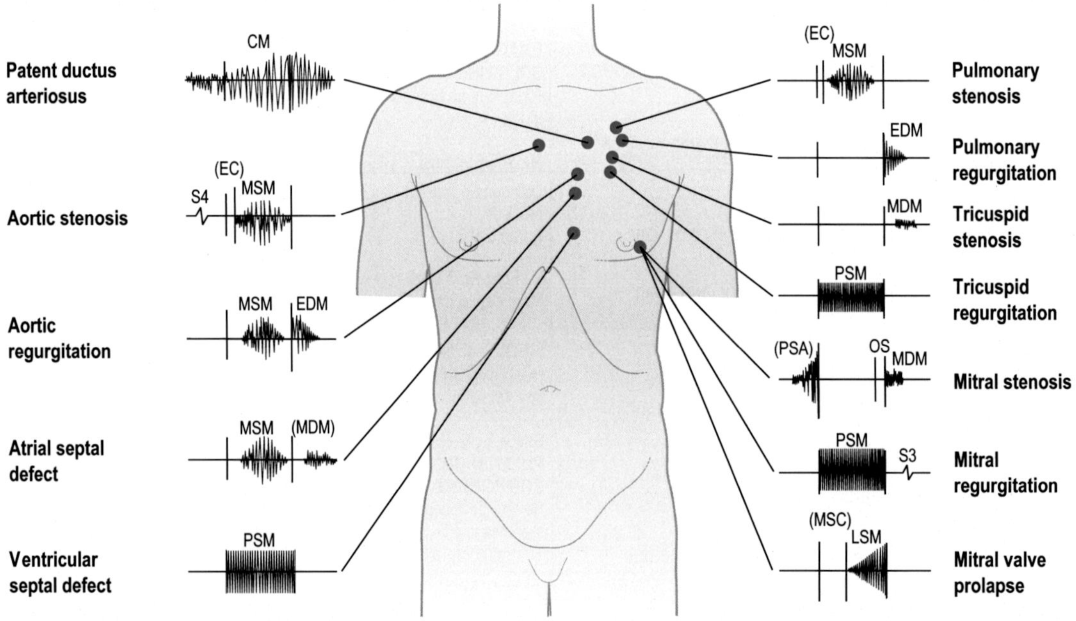

Figure 13.8 Heart murmurs. These are caused by turbulent flow within the heart and great vessels and may indicate valve disease. Heart murmurs may be depicted graphically as shown in this illustration. CM, continuous murmur; EC, ejection click; EDM, early diastolic murmur; LSM, late systolic murmur; MDM, mid-diastolic murmur; MSC, mid-systolic click; MSM, mid-systolic murmur; OS, opening snap; PSA, presystolic accentuation of murmur; PSM, pansystolic murmur; S3, third heart sound; S4, fourth heart sound. Parentheses indicate those auscultatory findings that are not constant.

Box 13.15 Rheumatic heart disease

Typical patient

- Middle-aged woman, less commonly man, with a history of childhood rheumatic fever (often not recognized or dismissed as trivial feverish illness). The mitral valve is almost invariably affected, commonly with associated aortic valve involvement. Right-sided valves less commonly affected. Presentation is usually with exertional dyspnoea, less commonly with unexplained atrial fibrillation or unheralded stroke
- Pregnant woman presenting abruptly with atrial fibrillation and pulmonary oedema

Major symptoms

- Mitral valve disease: dyspnoea or symptoms of frank congestive failure
- Aortic valve disease: dyspnoea, sometimes angina or syncope

Major signs

- Mitral stenosis: atrial fibrillation, signs of fluid retention (raised JVP ± peripheral oedema and basal crackles in lung fields), loud S1, opening snap in early diastole followed by low-pitched mid-diastolic murmur best heard at cardiac apex. With increasing calcification, the valve gets more rigid and the loud S1 and opening snap disappear
- Mitral regurgitation: atrial fibrillation, signs of fluid retention, pansystolic murmur best heard at cardiac apex, often with third heart sound
- Aortic stenosis: slow-rising carotid pulse, ejection systolic murmur best heard at base of heart
- Aortic regurgitation: fast-rising carotid pulse, ejection systolic murmur with early diastolic murmur best heard at left sternal edge

Diagnosis

- Echocardiogram: diagnostic of rheumatic heart disease, Doppler studies providing additional information about the severity of valvular stenosis or regurgitation

Treatment

- Diuretics for fluid retention and vasodilators to increase forward flow through regurgitant left-sided valves. Digoxin or β-blockers for rate control in atrial fibrillation plus warfarin to protect against embolism. Symptomatic mitral valve disease that fails to respond to treatment requires valve surgery (repair or replacement) or, in selected cases of mitral stenosis, percutaneous valvuloplasty. Symptomatic aortic valve disease always requires consideration for valve replacement

timed according to the phase of systole or diastole during which they are audible. It is inadequate to describe the timing of a murmur as systolic or diastolic without more specific reference to the length of the murmur and the phase of systole or diastole during which it is heard: systolic murmurs are mid-systolic, pansystolic or late systolic; diastolic murmurs are early diastolic, mid-diastolic or presystolic in timing. Continuous murmurs are audible in both phases of the cardiac cycle.

A mid-systolic ('ejection') murmur is caused by turbulence in the left or right ventricular outflow tract during ejection. It starts following opening of the aortic or pulmonary valve, reaches a crescendo in mid-systole and disappears before the second heart sound. The murmur is loudest in the aortic area (with radiation to the neck) when it arises from the left ventricular outflow tract and in the pulmonary area when it arises from the right ventricular outflow tract. It is best heard with the diaphragm of the stethoscope while the patient sits forward. Important causes of aortic ejection murmurs are aortic stenosis and hypertrophic cardiomyopathy.

Aortic regurgitation also produces an ejection murmur due to increased stroke volume and velocity of ejection. Pulmonary ejection murmurs may be caused by pulmonary stenosis or infundibular stenosis (as in Fallot's tetralogy).

In atrial septal defect, the pulmonary ejection murmur results from right ventricular volume loading and consequent increased blood flow through the pulmonary valve and does not indicate organic valvular disease. 'Innocent' murmurs unrelated to heart disease are always mid-systolic in timing and are caused by turbulent flow in the left (sometimes right) ventricular outflow tract. In most cases, there is no clear cause, but they may reflect a hyperkinetic circulation in conditions such as anaemia, pregnancy, thyrotoxicosis or fever. They are rarely louder than grade 3, often vary with posture, may disappear on exertion and are not associated with other signs of heart disease.

Pansystolic murmurs are audible throughout systole from the first to the second heart sounds. They are caused by regurgitation through incompetent atrioventricular valves and by ventricular septal defects. The pansystolic murmur of mitral regurgitation is loudest at the cardiac apex and radiates into the left axilla. It is best heard using the diaphragm of the stethoscope with the patient lying on the left side. The murmurs of tricuspid regurgitation and ventricular septal defect are loudest at the lower left sternal edge. Inspiration accentuates the murmur of tricuspid regurgitation because the increased venous return to the right side of the heart increases the regurgitant volume. Mitral valve prolapse may also produce a pansystolic murmur but, more commonly, prolapse occurs in mid-systole, producing a click followed by a late-systolic murmur.

Early diastolic murmurs are high pitched and start immediately after the second heart sound, fading away in mid-diastole. They are caused by regurgitation through incompetent aortic and pulmonary valves and are best heard using the diaphragm of the stethoscope while the patient leans forward. The early diastolic murmur of aortic regurgitation radiates from the aortic area to the left sternal edge, where it is usually easier to hear, in maintained expiration with the patient leaning forward. Pulmonary regurgitation is loudest at the pulmonary area. Mid-diastolic murmurs are caused by turbulent flow through the atrioventricular valves. They start after valve opening, relatively late after the second sound, and continue for a variable period during mid-diastole. Mitral stenosis is the principal cause of a mid-diastolic murmur and is best heard at the cardiac apex using the bell of the stethoscope while the patient lies on the left side. Increased flow across a non-stenotic mitral valve occurs in ventricular septal defect and mitral regurgitation and may produce a mid-diastolic murmur. In severe aortic regurgitation, preclosure of the anterior leaflet of the mitral valve by the regurgitant jet may produce mitral turbulence associated with a mid-diastolic murmur (Austin Flint murmur). A mid-diastolic murmur at the lower left sternal edge, accentuated by inspiration, is caused by tricuspid stenosis and also by conditions that increase tricuspid flow (e.g. atrial septal defect, tricuspid regurgitation).

In mitral or tricuspid stenosis, atrial systole produces a presystolic murmur immediately before the first heart sound. The murmur is perceived as an accentuation of the mid-diastolic murmur associated with these conditions. Because presystolic murmurs are generated by atrial systole, they do not occur in patients with atrial fibrillation.

Continuous murmurs are heard during systole and diastole and are uninterrupted by valve closure. The commonest cardiac cause is patent ductus arteriosus, in which flow from the high-pressure aorta to the low-pressure pulmonary artery continues throughout the cardiac cycle, producing a murmur over the base of the heart which, though continuously audible, is loudest at end systole and diminishes during diastole. Ruptured sinus of Valsalva aneurysm also produces a continuous murmur.

Friction rubs and venous hums

A friction rub occurs in pericarditis. It is best heard in maintained expiration with the patient leaning forward as a high-pitched scratching noise audible during any part of the cardiac cycle and over any part of the left precordium. A continuous venous hum at the base of the heart reflects hyperkinetic jugular venous flow. It is particularly common in infants and usually disappears on lying flat.

Finishing the cardiovascular examination

The assessment of the cardiovascular system should be concluded with the examination of the abdomen for organomegaly (hepatomegaly in heart failure, splenomegaly in infective endocarditis and renal abnormalities in hypertension) and abdominal aortic aneurysm, auscultation of the chest bases for crackles related to impaired LV function and urinalysis for proteinuria and haematuria.

The electrocardiogram

The electrocardiogram (ECG) records the electrical activity of the heart at the skin surface. A good-quality 12-lead ECG is essential for the evaluation of almost all cardiac patients.

Electrophysiology

Generation of electrical activity

The stimulus for every normal ventricular contraction (sinus beat) begins with depolarization of an area of specialized conducting tissue high in the right atrium called the sinoatrial (SA) node. The depolarization spreads through the walls of the atria, causing contraction of the atrial muscle before reaching another area of specialized conducting tissue in the lower part of the right atrium called the atrioventricular (AV) node. Conduction through the AV node is relatively slow which allows atrial contraction to be completed and the ventricles to fill before depolarization travels down the bundle of His and then into the left and right bundle branches. The left bundle branch divides further into the left anterior fascicle and the left posterior fascicle. From here, the depolarization spreads through the Purkinje fibres in the ventricular muscle which stimulates ventricular contraction. Once ventricular contraction has occurred, the muscle cells repolarize and the ventricles relax to allow ventricular filling to occur.

The wave of depolarization that spreads through the heart during each cardiac cycle has vector properties defined by its direction and magnitude. The net direction of the wave changes continuously during each cardiac cycle and the ECG deflections change accordingly, being positive as the wave approaches the recording electrode and negative as it moves away. Electrodes orientated along the axis of the wave record larger deflections than those oriented at right angles. Nevertheless, the size of the deflections is determined principally by the magnitude of the wave, which is a function of muscle mass. Thus the ECG deflection produced by depolarization of the atria (P wave) is smaller than that produced by the depolarization of the more muscular ventricles (QRS complex). Ventricular repolarization produces the T wave.

Inscription of the QRS complex

The ventricular depolarization vector can be resolved into two components:

1 Septal depolarization – spreads from left to right across the septum.
2 Ventricular free wall depolarization – spreads from endocardium to epicardium.

Left ventricular depolarization dominates the second vector component, the resultant direction of which is from right to left. Thus electrodes orientated to the left ventricle record a small negative deflection (Q wave) as the septal depolarization vector moves

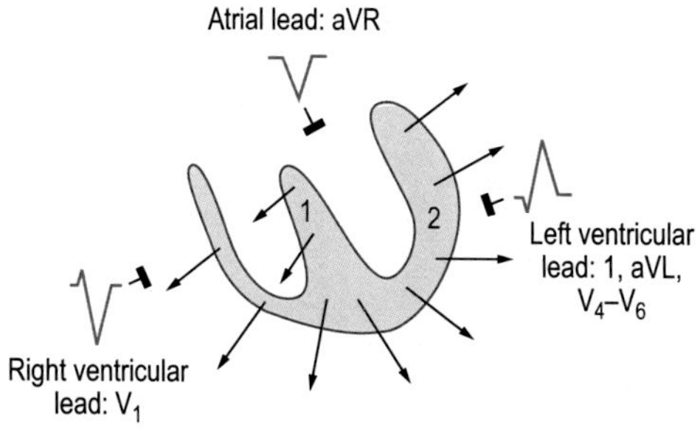

Figure 13.9 Inscription of the QRS complex. The septal depolarization vector **(1)** produces the initial deflection of the QRS complex. The ventricular free-wall depolarization vector **(2)** produces the second deflection, which is usually more pronounced. Lead aVR is orientated towards the cavity of the left ventricle and records an entirely negative deflection.

away, followed by a large positive deflection (R wave) as the ventricular depolarization vector approaches. The sequence of deflections for electrodes orientated towards the right ventricle is in the opposite direction (Fig. 13.9).

Any positive deflection is termed an R wave. A negative deflection before the R wave is termed a Q wave (this must be the first deflection of the complex), whereas a negative deflection following the R wave is termed an S wave.

Electrical axis

Because the mean direction of the ventricular depolarization vector (the electrical axis) shows a wide range of normality, there is corresponding variation in QRS patterns consistent with a normal ECG. Thus correct interpretation of the ECG must take account of the electrical axis. The frontal plane axis is determined by identifying the limb lead in which the net QRS deflection (positive and negative) is least pronounced. This lead must be at right angles to the frontal plane electrical axis, which is defined using an arbitrary hexaxial reference system (Fig. 13.10).

Normal 12-lead ECG

The normal 12-lead ECG is illustrated in Fig. 13.11. Leads I–III are the standard bipolar leads, which each measure the potential difference between two limbs:

- Lead I: left arm to right arm.
- Lead II: left leg to right arm.
- Lead III: left leg to left arm.

The remaining leads are unipolar, connected to a limb (aVR to aVF) or to the chest wall (V_1–V_6). Because the orientation of each lead to the wave of depolarization is different, the direction and magnitude of ECG deflections is also different in each lead. Nevertheless, the sequence of deflections (P wave, QRS complex, T wave) is identical. In some patients, a small U wave can be seen following the T wave. Its orientation (positive or negative) is the same as the T wave but its cause is unknown.

Analysis of the ECG

Heart rate

The ECG is usually recorded at a paper speed of 25 mm/s. Thus each large square (5 mm) represents 0.20 s. The heart rate (bpm) is conveniently calculated by counting the number of large squares between consecutive R waves and dividing this into 300. This method assumes that the heart rate is regular and the distance between successive QRS complexes is constant. An alternative, quick method is to use the 'rhythm strip' that is printed at the bottom of most standard ECG recordings. This is a longer recording of a particular lead and is included in the printout to help with the diagnosis of rhythm disorders. A rhythm strip is a 10-second recording; counting the number of QRS complexes in a 10-second rhythm strip and multiplying by 6 will give the heart rate in beats per minute.

Rhythm

In normal sinus rhythm, P waves precede each QRS complex and the rhythm is regular. Absence of P waves and an irregular rhythm indicate atrial fibrillation.

Electrical axis

Evaluation of the frontal place QRS axis is described above.

P-wave morphology

The duration should not exceed 0.10 s; prolongation indicates left atrial enlargement, often the result of mitral valve disease or left ventricular failure. Tall-peaked 'pulmonary' P waves indicate right atrial enlargement, caused usually by pulmonary hypertension and right ventricular failure.

PR interval

The normal duration of the PR interval is 0.12-0.20 s measured from the onset of the P wave to the first deflection of the QRS complex. Prolongation indicates delayed atrioventricular conduction (first-degree heart block). Shortening indicates rapid conduction through an accessory pathway bypassing the atrioventricular node (Wolff-Parkinson-White (WPW) syndrome).

QRS morphology

The QRS duration should not exceed 0.12 s. Prolongation indicates slow ventricular depolarization due to bundle branch block (Fig. 13.12), pre-excitation (WPW syndrome), ventricular tachycardia or hypokalaemia.

Exaggerated QRS deflections indicate ventricular hypertrophy (Fig. 13.13). The voltage criteria for left ventricular hypertrophy are fulfilled when the sum of the S and R wave deflections in leads V_1 and V_6 exceeds 35 mm (3.5 mV). Right ventricular

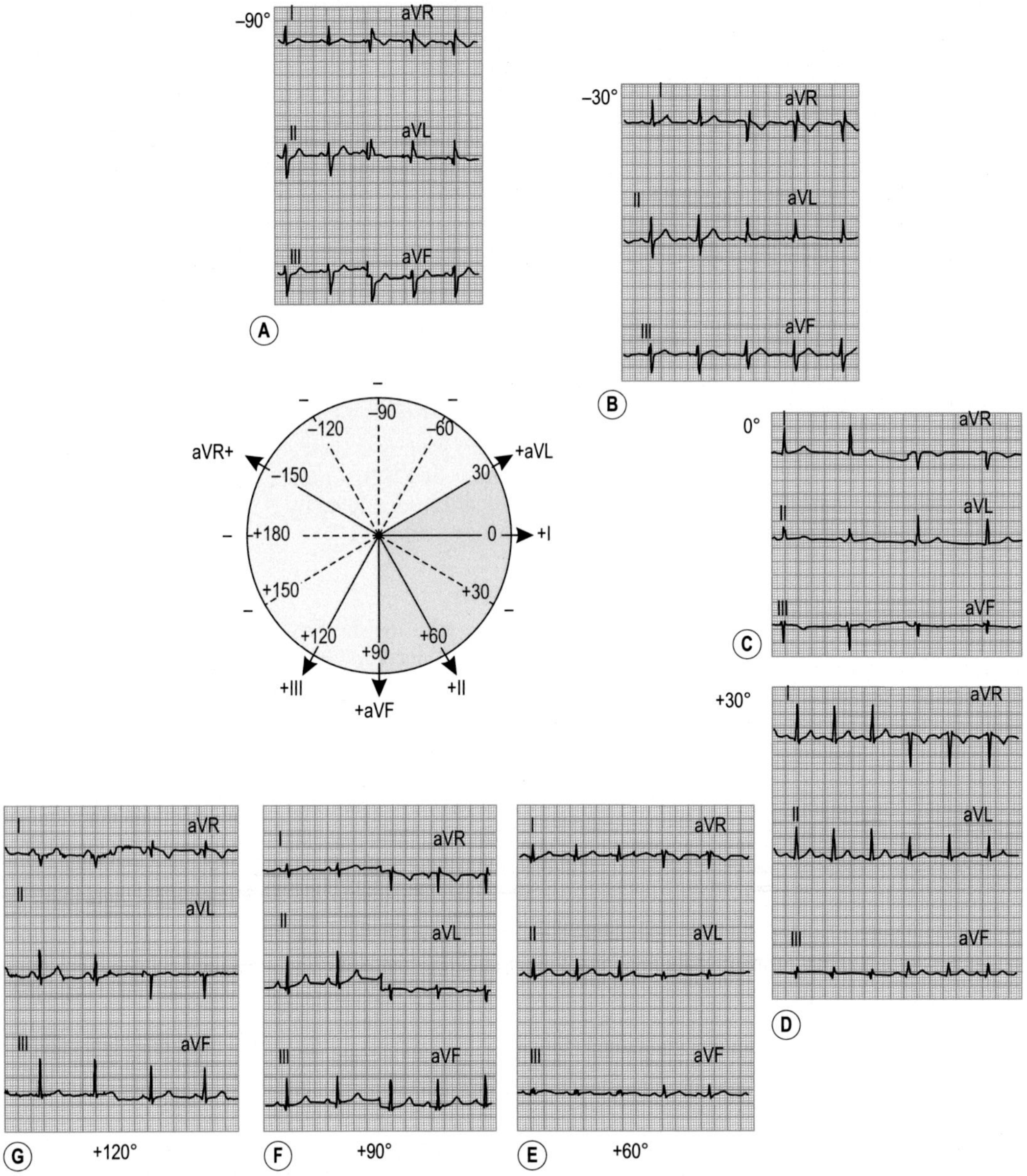

Figure 13.10 Mean frontal QRS axis. This is the mean direction of the left ventricular depolarization vector in those leads (I–aVF) that lie in the frontal plane of the heart. It lies at right angles to the lead in which the net QRS deflexion is least pronounced. It is quantified using a hexaxial reference system. The QRS axis shows a wide range of normality from –30° to 90°. Thus despite the different ECG patterns in this illustration, only recordings **(A)** and **(G)** are abnormal, owing to left and right axis deviation, respectively.

hypertrophy causes tall R waves in the right ventricular leads (V_1 and V_2). A dominant R wave in lead V_1 can also be caused by right bundle branch block, posterior myocardial infarction, WPW syndrome and dextrocardia. Diminished QRS deflections occur in myxoedema and also when pericardial effusion or obesity electrically insulates the heart. The presence of pathological Q waves (duration >0.04 s) usually indicates previous myocardial infarction.

QT interval

The QT interval is measured from the onset of the QRS complex to the end of the T wave and represents the duration of electrical systole (mechanical systole starts between the QRS complex and the T wave). The QT interval (0.35-0.45 s) is very rate sensitive, shortening as heart rate increases. A commonly used way to correct the QT interval (the so-called QTc) involves dividing the measured QT interval by the square root of the RR interval in seconds. As an example, at 60 bpm, the RR interval would be 1 second – the QTc would be equal to $QT/\sqrt{1}$. Abnormal prolongation of the QT interval predisposes to ventricular arrhythmias and may be congenital or occur in response to hypokalaemia, rheumatic fever or drugs (e.g. quinidine, amiodarone, tricyclic

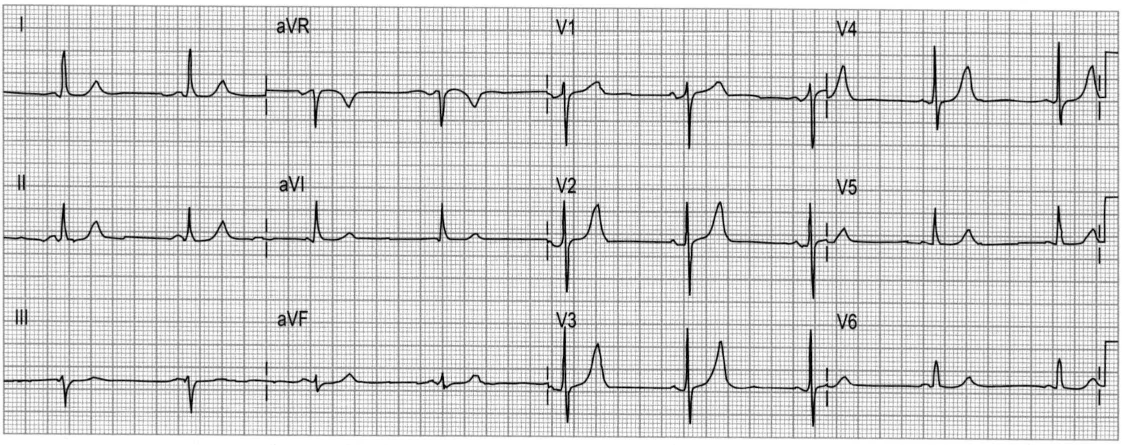

Figure 13.11 Standard 12-lead ECG. This is a normal recording. The QRS deflections are equiphasic in lead aVF. This is at right angles to lead I (see Fig. 13.10), which is dominantly positive. The frontal plane QRS axis is, therefore, 0°. The square wave calibration signal is 1 mV.

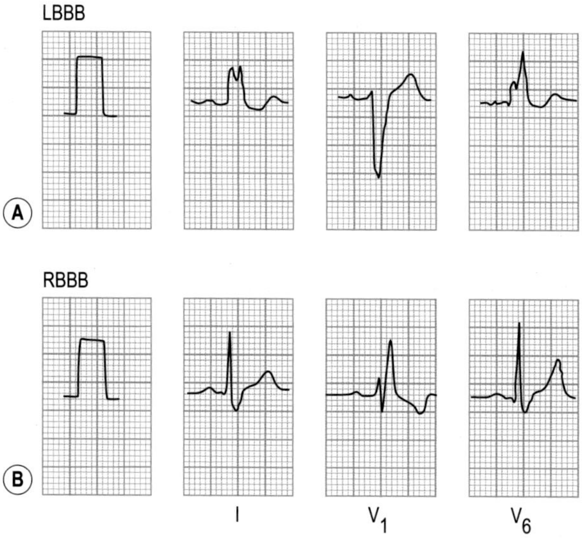

Figure 13.12 Bundle branch block. **(A)** Left bundle branch block (LBBB). The entire sequence of ventricular depolarization is abnormal, resulting in a broad QRS complex with large slurred or notched R waves in I and V_6. **(B)** Right bundle branch block (RBBB). Right ventricular depolarization is delayed, resulting in a broad QRS complex with an 'rSR' pattern in V_1 and prominent S waves in I and V_6.

antidepressants). Shortening of the QT interval is caused by hyperkalaemia and digoxin therapy.

ST segment morphology

Minor ST elevation reflecting early repolarization may occur as a normal variant (Fig. 13.14), particularly in subjects of African or West Indian origin. Pathological elevation (>2.0 mm above the isoelectric line) occurs in acute myocardial infarction, variant angina and pericarditis. Horizontal ST depression indicates myocardial ischaemia. Other important causes of ST depression are digoxin therapy and hypokalaemia

T-wave morphology

The orientation of the T wave should be directionally similar to the QRS complex. Thus T-wave inversion is normal in leads with dominantly negative QRS complexes (aVR, V_1 and sometimes lead III). Pathological T-wave inversion occurs as a non-specific response to various stimuli (e.g. viral infection, hypothermia). More important causes of T-wave inversion are ventricular hypertrophy, myocardial ischaemia and myocardial infarction. Exaggerated peaking of the T wave is the earliest ECG change in ST elevation myocardial infarction. It also occurs in hyperkalaemia.

Clinical applications of ECG

Diagnosis of coronary heart disease

The territories supplied by the three major coronary arteries, although variable, are highly circumscribed, the left anterior descending artery supplying the anterior wall, the circumflex artery the lateral wall and the right coronary artery the inferior wall of the left ventricle. The regional distribution of coronary flow has important implications for electrocardiography (and diagnostic imaging), because patients with coronary heart disease show regional electrocardiographic (or wall motion) abnormalities and patients with diffuse myocardial disease (e.g. cardiomyopathy) show more widespread changes.

Stable angina

The ECG is often normal in patients with stable angina unless there is a history of myocardial infarction, when pathological Q waves or T-wave inversion may be present.

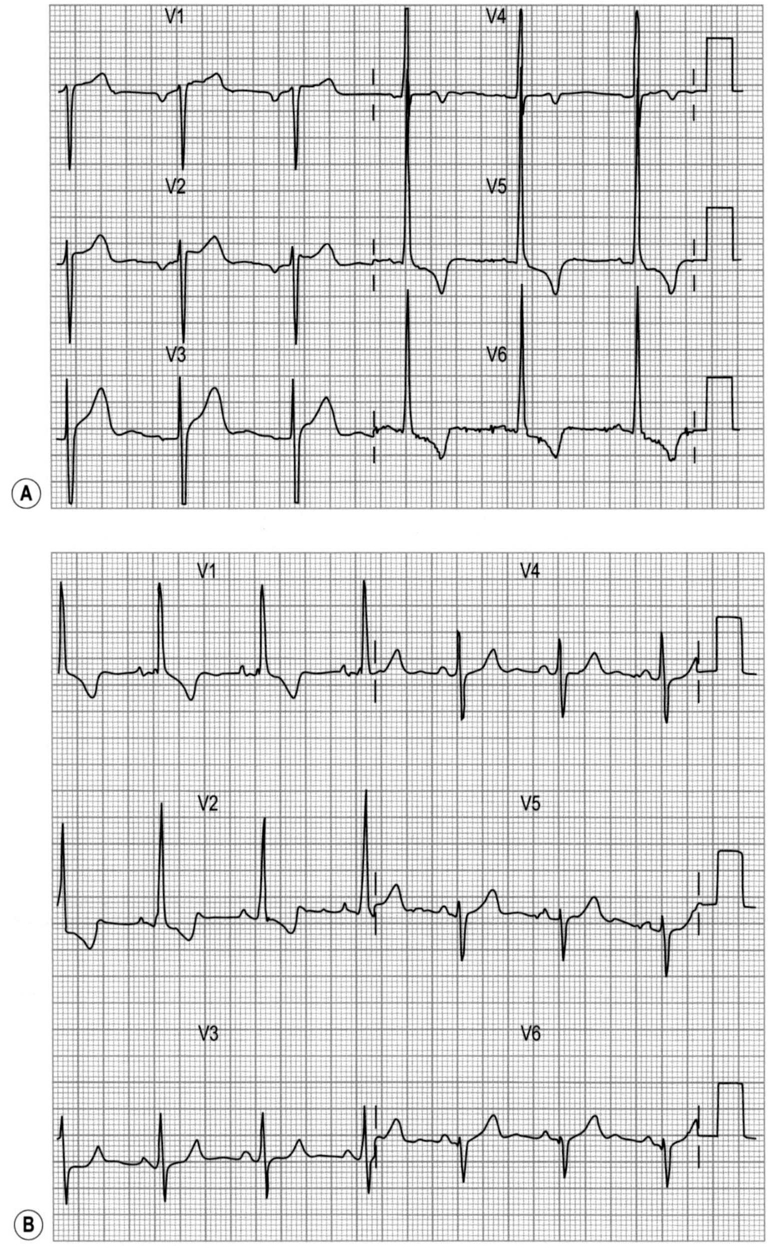

Figure 13.13 Ventricular hypertrophy. **(A)** Left ventricular hypertrophy. The QRS voltage deflections are exaggerated such that the sum of S and R waves in V_1 and V_6, respectively, exceeds 35 mm. T-wave inversion in V_5 and V_6 indicates left ventricular 'strain'. **(B)** Right ventricular hypertrophy. Prominent R waves in V_1 and V_2 associated with T-wave inversion are shown.

Exercise stress testing

The patient is usually exercised on a treadmill, the speed and slope of which can be adjusted to increase the workload gradually. In patients with coronary artery disease, exercise-induced increases in myocardial oxygen demand may outstrip oxygen delivery through the atheromatous arteries, resulting in regional ischaemia. This causes planar or downsloping ST-segment depression, with reversal during recovery (Fig. 13.15). The ready availability of the exercise test means that it is one of the most widely used tests for evaluating the patient with chest pain but its diagnostic accuracy is limited to about 70%, false-positive or false-negative results being common when the pretest probability of coronary disease is very low (as in young women) or very high (as in elderly patients with typical symptoms), respectively. Non-invasive imaging modalities (see later: magnetic resonance perfusion imaging, stress echocardiography, CT coronary angiography) have higher rates of diagnostic accuracy and are now preferred in the assessment of patients with suspected coronary artery disease, where available. The exercise ECG also provides prognostic information in patients who are known to have coronary artery disease: an increased risk of myocardial infarction or sudden death is indicated by ST depression very early during exercise,

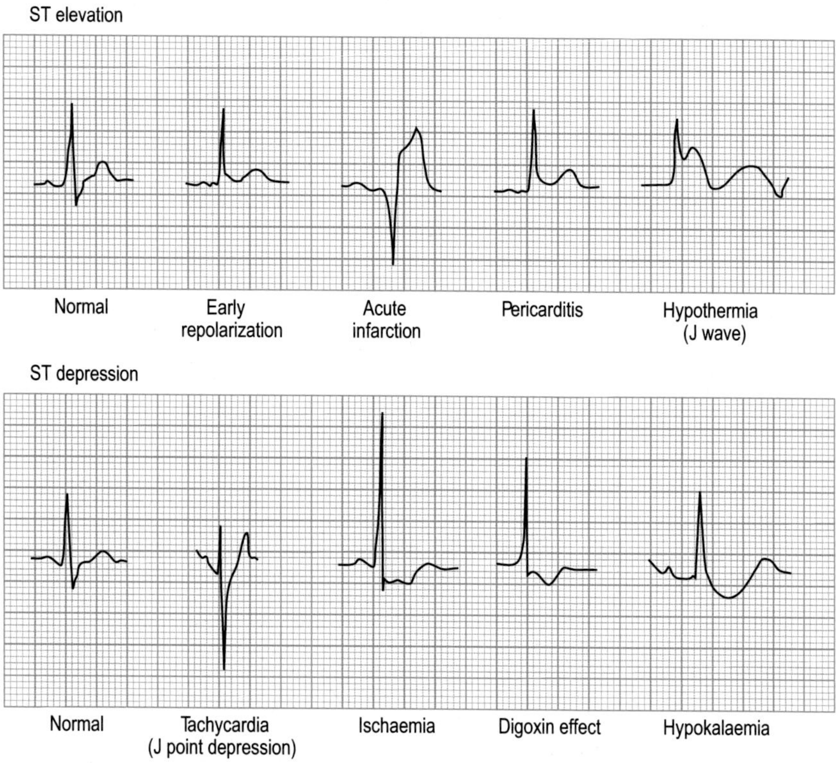

Figure 13.14 ST segment morphology: common causes of ST segment elevation and depression. Note that depression of the J point (junction between the QRS complex and ST segment) is physiological during exertion and does not signify myocardial ischaemia. Planar depression of the ST segment, on the other hand, is strongly suggestive of myocardial ischaemia.

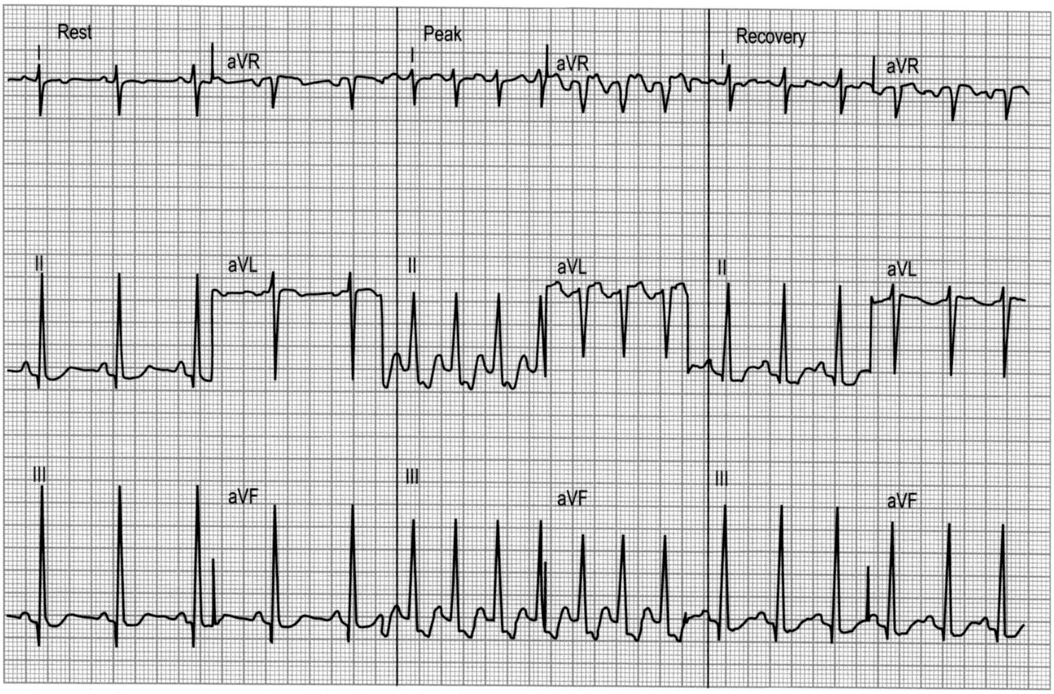

Figure 13.15 Exercise ECG. Ischaemic changes in inferior standard leads (II, III and aVF). At rest, the ST segments are isoelectric. Exercise causes tachycardia and provokes 3 mm of downsloping ST depression in leads II, III and aVF. The changes reverse during recovery. The findings suggest exertional ischaemia affecting the inferior wall of the heart. The probability of coronary artery disease is high.

by an exertional fall in blood pressure or by exercise-induced ventricular arrhythmias. In these cases, urgent coronary angiography is required.

Acute coronary syndromes

Acute myocardial infarction and unstable angina present similarly with unprovoked – often severe – ischaemic cardiac pain. Reliable differentiation between the acute coronary syndromes on clinical grounds cannot be made and requires measurement of cardiac biomarkers, in particular troponin I or T (see below), 12 hours after the onset of symptoms, and observation of the 12-lead ECG. The combination of typical symptoms plus raised troponins is diagnostic of myocardial infarction, which is categorized as ST elevation myocardial infarction (STEMI) or non-ST elevation myocardial infarction (non-STEMI) by the ECG findings. Typical symptoms unassociated with either troponin release or ST elevation are diagnosed as troponin-negative acute coronary syndrome or unstable angina. It therefore follows that acute myocardial infarction and unstable angina may be associated with a completely normal ECG or with ST depression (Fig. 13.16) or T-wave changes, the diagnosis depending on the presence or absence of raised troponins.

In STEMI, the evolution of ECG changes is characteristic, although it may be aborted by timely reperfusion therapy (thrombolysis or primary stenting). Peaking of the T wave followed by ST segment elevation occurs during the first hour of pain (Fig. 13.17). The changes are regional, and reciprocal ST depression may be seen in the opposite ECG leads. Usually a pathological Q wave develops during the following 24 hours and persists indefinitely. The ST segment returns to the isoelectric line within 2-3 days, and T-wave inversion may occur. The ECG is a useful indicator of infarct location. Changes in leads II, III and aVF indicate inferior infarction (Fig. 13.18), whereas changes in leads V_1–V_6 indicate

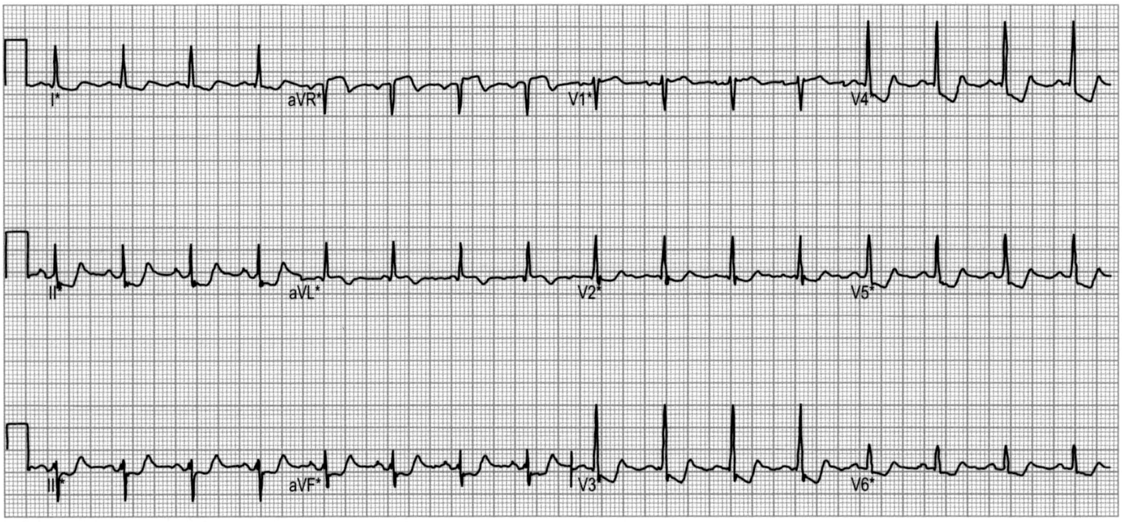

Figure 13.16 Unstable angina or non-ST elevation myocardial infarction (depending on troponin release). 12-lead ECG shows planar/downsloping ST depression in the inferolateral territory.

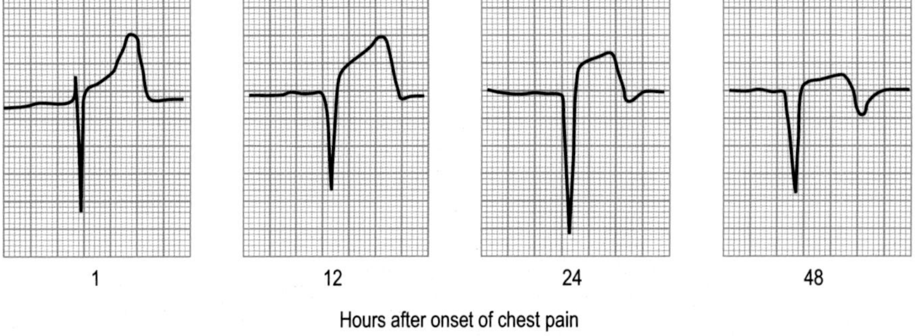

Figure 13.17 Acute myocardial infarction: evolution of ECG changes. Elevation of the ST segment occurs during the first hour of chest pain. The Q wave develops during the subsequent 24 hours and usually persists indefinitely. Within a day of the attack, the ST segment usually returns to the isoelectric line and T-wave inversion may occur.

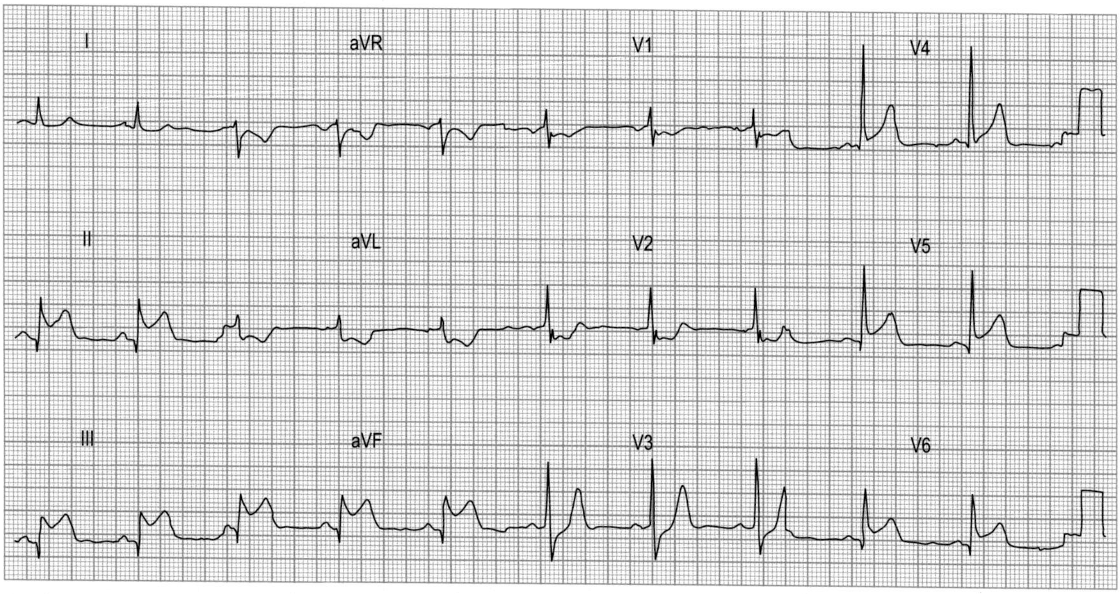

Figure 13.18 Acute inferolateral infarction. ECG 2 hours after the onset of chest pain. Typical ST elevation in leads II, III and aVF is diagnostic of inferior myocardial infarction. ST elevation in leads V_4-V_6 indicates lateral extension. There is reciprocal ST depression in lead aVL. Prominent R waves associated with ST depression in leads V_1 and V_2 indicate posterior wall infarction. This pattern may reflect occlusion of the right coronary artery or a dominant circumflex coronary artery.

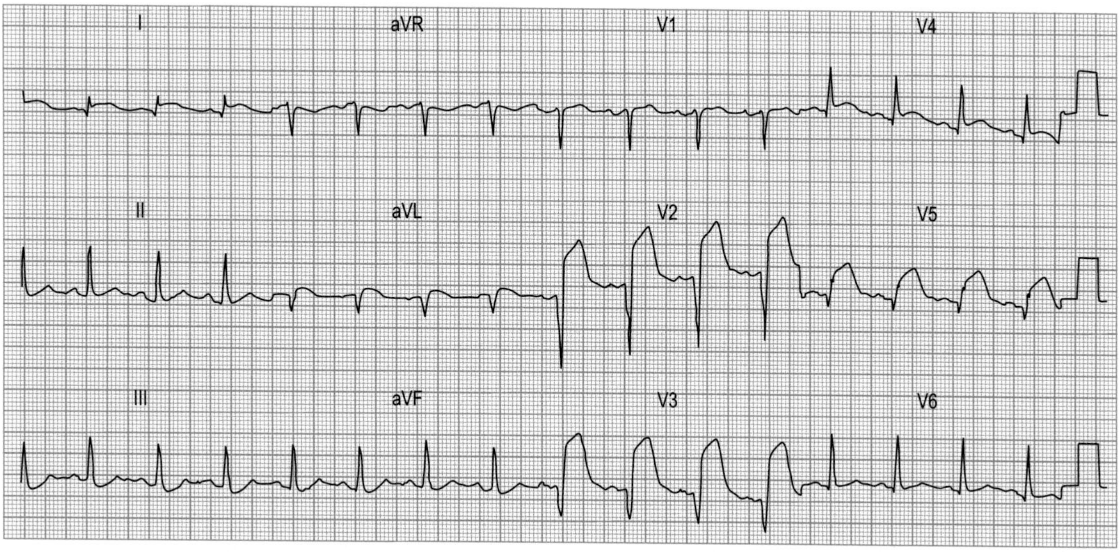

Figure 13.19 Acute anterior infarction. ECG 1 hour after the onset of chest pain. Typical ST elevation in leads V_2–V_5 is diagnostic of anterior myocardial infarction. Additional ST elevation in standard leads I and aVL indicates lateral extension of the infarct. This pattern usually reflects proximal occlusion of the left anterior descending coronary artery.

anteroseptal (V_1–V_3) or anterolateral (V_1–V_6) infarction (Fig. 13.19). When the infarct is located posteriorly, ECG changes may be difficult to detect, but dominant R waves in leads V_1 and V_2 often develop (see Fig. 13.18).

Detection of cardiac arrhythmias

Electrocardiographic documentation of the arrhythmia should be obtained prior to instituting treatment. In patients with sustained arrhythmias, a 12-lead recording at rest is usually diagnostic, but a long continuous recording of the lead showing the clearest P wave (if present) should also be obtained. In patients with paroxysmal arrhythmias, the frequency and severity of symptoms determine which technique is used for electrocardiographic documentation.

In-hospital ECG monitoring

Patients who have had out-of-hospital cardiac arrest or severe, arrhythmia-induced heart failure should undergo continuous ECG monitoring in hospital under the surveillance of staff trained in the recognition and treatment of arrhythmia. Patients with acute myocardial infarction should undergo ECG monitoring

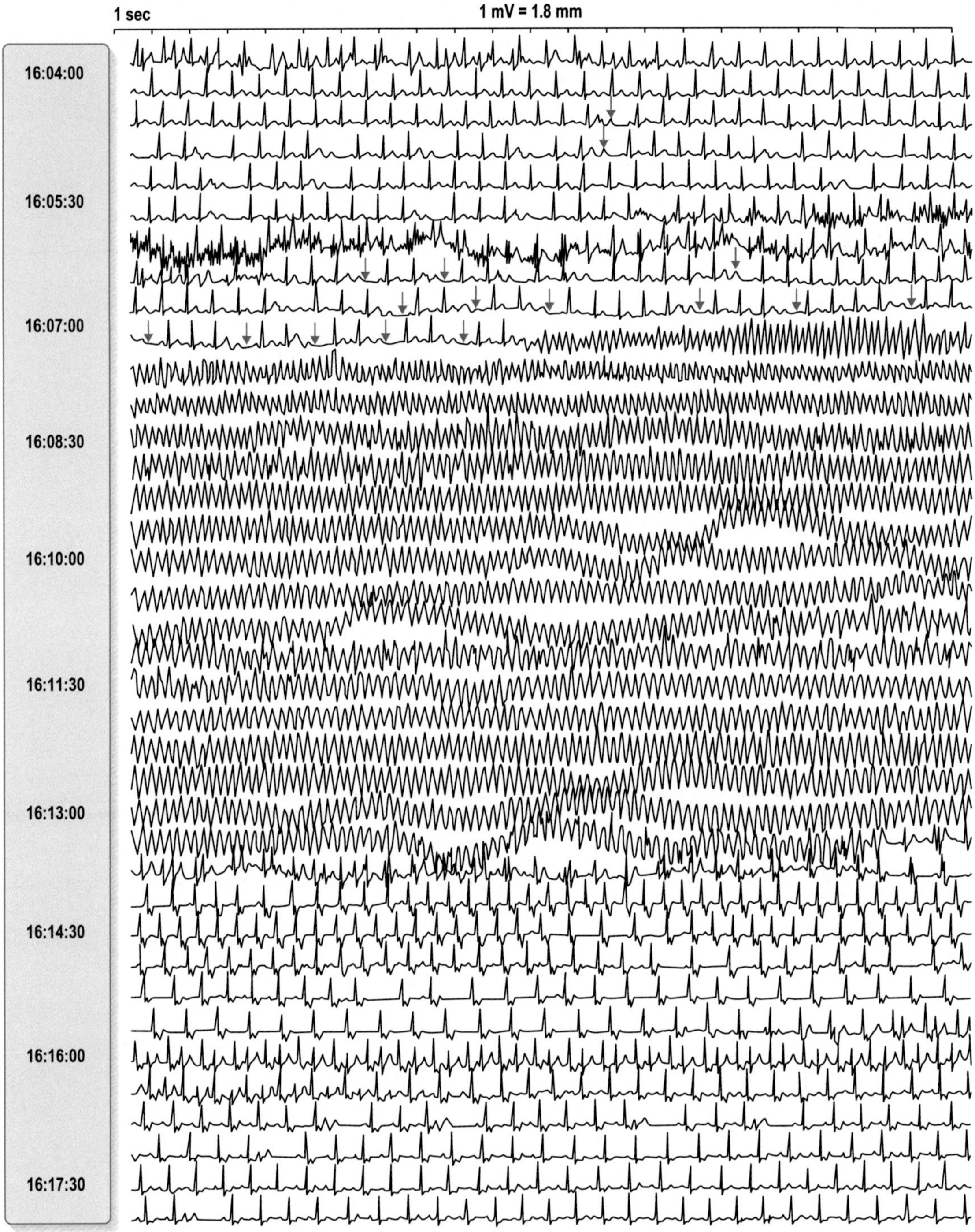

Figure 13.20 Ventricular tachycardia: Holter recording. When tachycardias are paroxysmal in nature, continuous ECG monitoring is often necessary to document the arrhythmia. Here a Holter recording illustrates a long burst of rapid VT lasting a total of 6 minutes. Preceding the VT there is second-degree heart block (arrows).

for 24 hours, after which time the risk of ventricular arrhythmia falls dramatically.

Ambulatory (Holter) ECG monitoring

Patients with frequent palpitation or dizzy attacks are commonly investigated by means of an ambulatory 24-hour ECG. The availability of portable cassette recorders allows this to be performed as an outpatient. Analysis of the tape identifies any cardiac arrhythmias that occurred during the monitoring period (Fig. 13.20). A patient diary allows correlation between symptoms and heart rhythm.

Patient-activated ECG recording

For patients with infrequent symptoms, the detection rate with 24-hour ambulatory monitoring is low and patient-activated recorders are more useful. The patient can keep the recorder for several weeks and activate it when symptoms occur. Rhythm strips are stored for later analysis.

Implantable loop recording

Patients in whom there is clinical suspicion of serious arrhythmia but whose symptoms occur less than once a month pose particular diagnostic difficulty. In this group, a miniaturized recording device can be implanted subcutaneously using local anaesthetic and interrogated electronically through the skin in the event of symptoms.

Exercise testing

The ECG recorded during exercise may be helpful when there is a history of exertional palpitation. Arrhythmias provoked by ischaemia or increased sympathetic activity are more likely to be detected during exercise.

Tilt testing

When malignant vasovagal syndrome is suspected, ECG and blood pressure recordings during tilting from supine to erect posture can be helpful. Abnormal bradycardia or hypotension sufficient to produce presyncope or syncope indicate a 'vasodepressor response' or 'cardioinhibitory response', respectively, and are strongly suggestive of the diagnosis.

Electrophysiological study

Electrophysiological technique requires cardiac catheterization with catheter-mounted electrodes. Premature stimuli are introduced into the atria or ventricles with a view to stimulating re-entry arrhythmias. In the normal heart, sustained arrhythmias are rarely provoked by premature stimuli. Thus arrhythmia provocation is usually diagnostic, particularly when the arrhythmia reproduces symptoms. Electrophysiological study can identify accessory pathways and areas of focal atrial or ventricular ectopy as the prelude to radiofrequency ablation of the arrhythmia substrate.

Diagnosis of atrial arrhythmias

The ECG in atrial arrhythmias (Fig. 13.21) shows a narrow and morphologically normal QRS complex when ventricular depolarization occurs by normal His-Purkinje pathways. Rate-related or pre-existing bundle branch block, however, results in broad ventricular complexes that are difficult to distinguish from ventricular tachycardia.

Atrial ectopic beats

Atrial ectopic beats rarely indicate heart disease. They often occur spontaneously but may be provoked by toxic stimuli such as caffeine, alcohol and cigarette smoking. They are caused by the premature discharge of an atrial ectopic focus; an early and often bizarre P wave is essential for the diagnosis. The premature impulse enters and depolarizes the sinus node such that a partially compensatory pause occurs before the next sinus beat during resetting of the sinus node.

Atrial fibrillation

Prevalence increases with age and it is common in hypertensive heart disease, mitral valve disease, thyrotoxicosis and left ventricular failure. It can be precipitated by pneumonia, major surgery and by various toxic stimuli, particularly alcohol. Atrial activity is chaotic and mechanically ineffective. P waves are therefore absent and replaced by irregular fibrillatory waves (rate 400-600/min). The long refractory period of the atrioventricular node ensures that only some of the atrial impulses are conducted, producing an irregular ventricular rate of 130-200 bpm. If the atrioventricular node is diseased, the ventricular rate is slower, but in the presence of a rapidly conducting accessory pathway in WPW syndrome, dangerous ventricular rates above 300 bpm may occur.

Atrial flutter

Atrial flutter is less common than atrial fibrillation but occurs under identical circumstances. Re-entry mechanisms produce an atrial rate close to 300 bpm. The normal atrioventricular node conducts with 2:1 block, giving a ventricular rate of 150 bpm. Higher degrees of block may reflect intrinsic disease of the atrioventricular node or the effects of nodal blocking drugs. The ECG characteristically shows sawtooth flutter waves, which are most clearly seen when the block is increased by carotid sinus pressure.

Diagnosis of nodal arrhythmias

Nodal arrhythmias are often called supraventricular tachycardias (SVTs) and are usually paroxysmal without obvious cardiac or extrinsic causes. They are re-entry arrhythmias caused either by an abnormal pathway between the atrium and the atrioventricular node (atrionodal pathway) or by an accessory atrioventricular pathway (bundle of Kent), as seen in WPW syndrome. Like atrial arrhythmias, ventricular depolarization usually occurs by normal His-Purkinje pathways, producing a narrow QRS complex which confirms the supraventricular origin of the arrhythmia. Rate-related or pre-existing bundle branch block, however, produces broad ventricular complexes difficult to distinguish from ventricular tachycardia.

Atrioventricular nodal re-entry tachycardia (AVNRT)

The abnormal atrionodal pathway provides the basis for a small re-entry circuit. In sinus rhythm, the electrocardiogram is usually normal, although

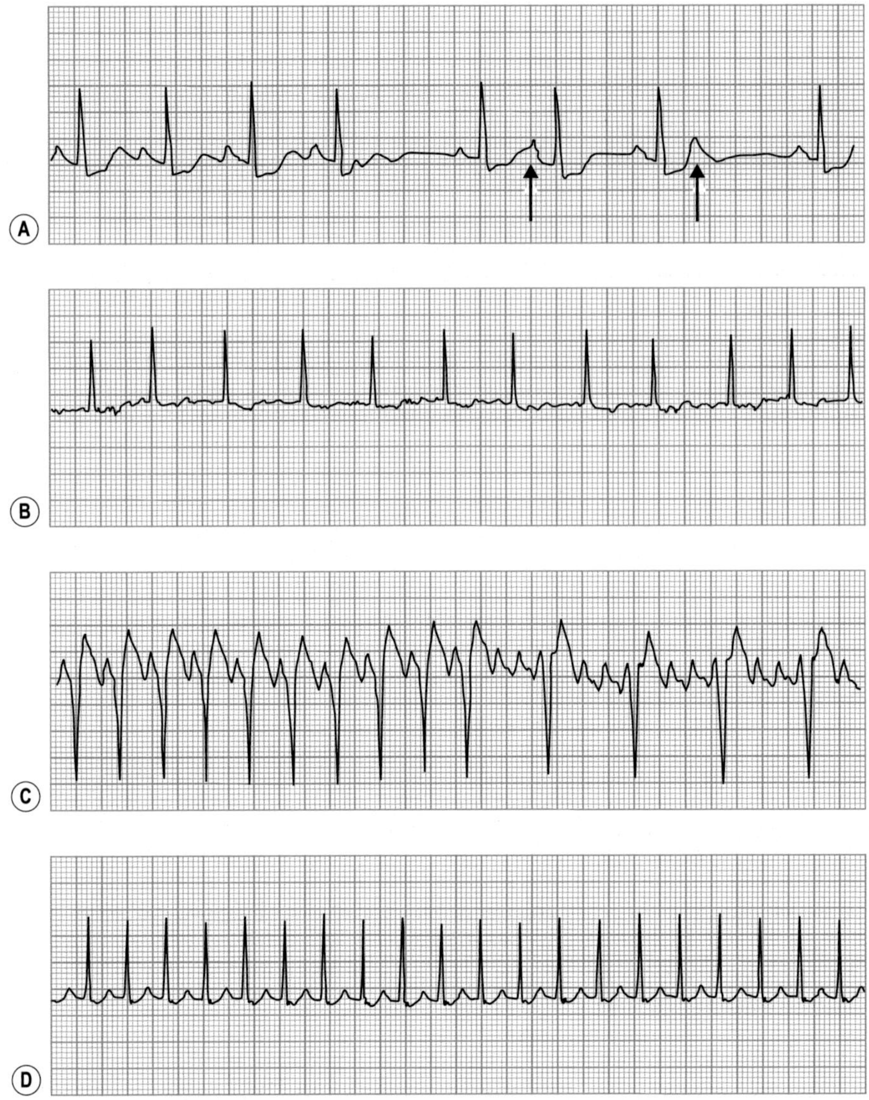

Figure 13.21 Atrial arrhythmias: **(A)** Ectopic beats. After the fourth sinus beat there is a very early P wave which, finding the AV node refractory, is not conducted to the ventricle. This produces a pause before the next sinus beat, which itself is followed by a somewhat later atrial ectopic beat (arrow), which is conducted normally. This is followed by a sinus beat, following which the T wave is distorted by another early atrial ectopic beat (arrow), which is also blocked. **(B)** Atrial fibrillation. Note the irregular fibrillatory waves and the irregular ventricular response. The ventricular rate is fairly slow because the patient was treated with a β-blocker. **(C)** A flutter. AV conduction with 2 : 1 block, giving a ventricular rate of about 150/min, which then gives way to 4 : 1 block. Sawtooth flutter waves at a rate of 300/min are clearly visible. **(D)** AV nodal re-entrant tachycardia (AVNRT). Often called supraventricular tachycardia (SVT), this arrhythmia causes a regular tachycardia, with a ventricular rate of about 180/min.

occasionally the PR interval is short (Lown-Ganong-Levine syndrome). During tachycardia, the rate is 150-250 bpm (see Fig. 13.21). The arrhythmia is usually self-limiting. Sustained AVNRT will sometimes respond to carotid sinus pressure. If this fails, intravenous adenosine or verapamil are usually effective by blocking the re-entry circuit within the atrioventricular node. Antitachycardia pacing or direct current cardioversion may also be used. Many patients are now being treated by catheter ablation to destroy the abnormal atrionodal pathway and avoid the need for long-term drug therapy (see below).

Wolff-Parkinson-White syndrome

Wolff-Parkinson-White syndrome, a congenital disorder which affects 0.12% of the population, is caused by an accessory pathway (bundle of Kent) between the atria and the ventricles. During sinus rhythm, atrial impulses conduct more rapidly through the accessory pathway than the atrioventricular node, such that the initial phase of ventricular depolarization occurs early (pre-excitation) and spreads slowly through the ventricles by abnormal pathways. This produces a short PR interval and slurring of the initial

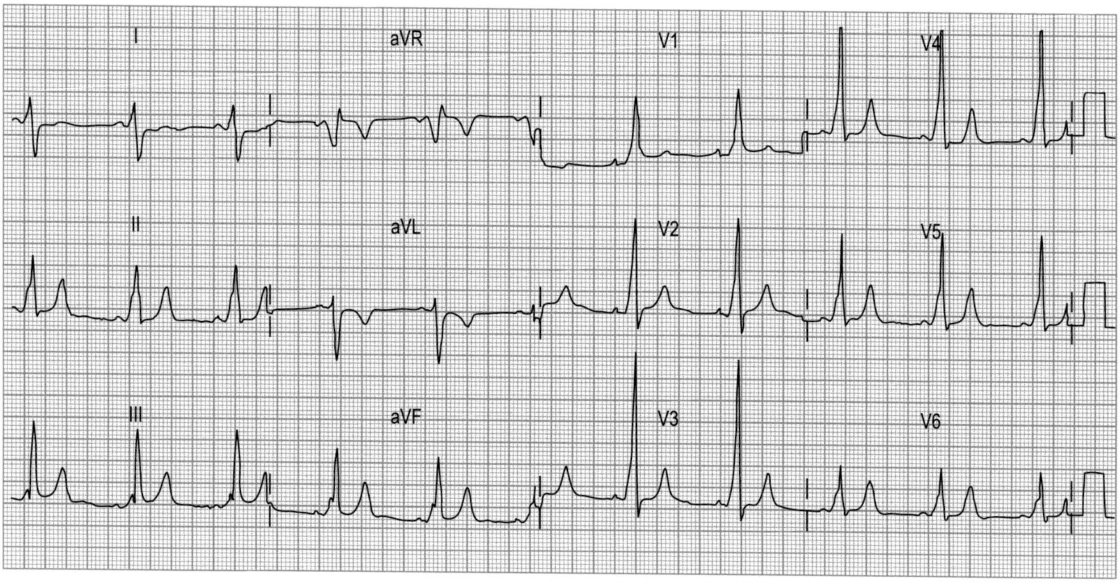

Figure 13.22 WPW syndrome: 12-lead ECG. Ventricular pre-excitation is reflected on the surface ECG by a short PR interval and a slurred upstroke to the QRS complex (δ wave). The remainder of the QRS complex is normal because delayed arrival of the impulse conducted through the AV node rapidly completes ventricular depolarization through normal His-Purkinje pathways.

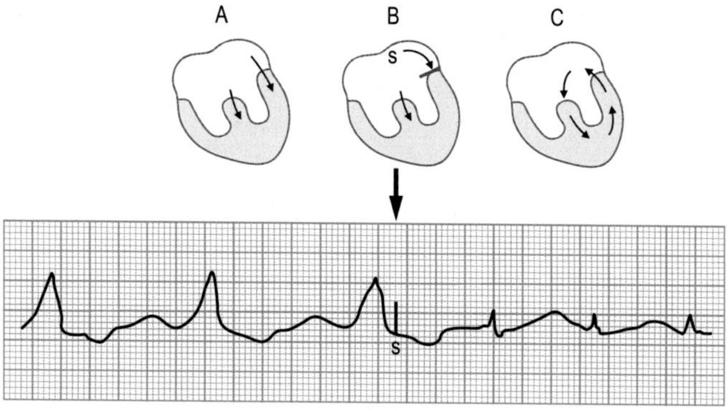

Figure 13.23 WPW syndrome: re-entry tachycardia recorded at fast paper speed. Just after the third pre-excited (broad) complex, a premature atrial pacing stimulus (S) initiates an impulse that is blocked in the bundle of Kent but conducted normally through the AV node, producing ventricular depolarization without pre-excitation. Thus the QRS complex is narrow and lacks a δ wave. The impulse is conducted retrogradely through the bundle of Kent, re-enters the proximal conducting system and completes the re-entry circuit, initiating a self-sustaining orthodromic re-entry tachycardia (last three complexes).

QRS deflection (δ wave). The remainder of ventricular depolarization, however, is rapid because the delayed arrival of the impulse conducted through the atrioventricular node rapidly completes ventricular depolarization by normal His-Purkinje pathways (Fig. 13.22). Cardiac arrhythmias affect about 60% of patients with WPW syndrome and are usually re-entrant (rate 150-250 bpm) triggered by an atrial premature beat. In most patients, the re-entry arrhythmia is 'orthodromic', with anterograde conduction through the atrioventricular node and retrograde conduction through the accessory pathway (atrioventricular re-entry tachycardia (AVRT), Fig. 13.23). This results in a narrow complex tachycardia (without pre-excitation) that is indistinguishable from AVNRT. Occasionally, the re-entry circuit is in the opposite direction ('antidromic'), producing a very broad, pre-excited tachycardia.

Patients with WPW syndrome are more prone than the general population to atrial fibrillation. If the accessory pathway is able to conduct the fibrillatory impulses rapidly to the ventricles, it may result in ventricular fibrillation and sudden death. Digoxin (and to a lesser extent verapamil) should be avoided because it shortens the refractory period of the accessory pathway and can heighten the risk. Patients with dangerous accessory pathways of this type require catheter ablation of the pathway. Ablation therapy also cures AVNRT and is the treatment of choice in patients with frequent attacks.

Diagnosis of ventricular arrhythmias

Ventricular premature beats

Ventricular premature beats may occur in normal individuals, either spontaneously or in response to toxic stimuli such as caffeine or sympathomimetic drugs. They are caused by the premature discharge of a ventricular ectopic focus that produces an early and broad QRS complex (Fig. 13.24). The premature impulse may be conducted backwards into the atria,

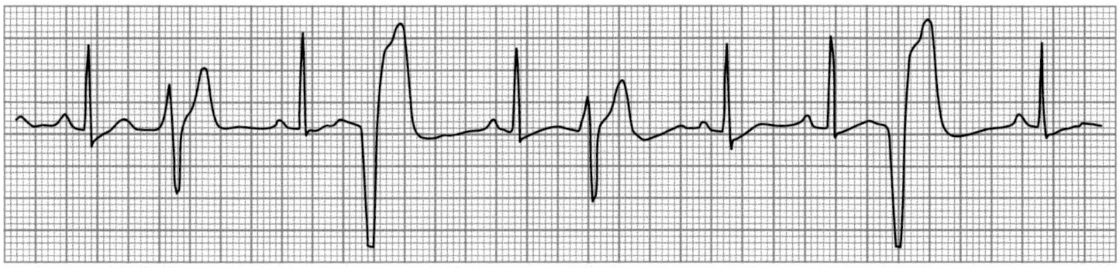

Figure 13.24 Multifocal, ventricular ectopic beats. Frequent broad complex ectopic beats are seen early after the sinus beats. Note, however, that the ectopic beats have two different morphologies, indicating that they arise from different foci. Note also that the coupling interval (interval between QRS complex and ectopic beat) is identical for beats arising from any particular focus.

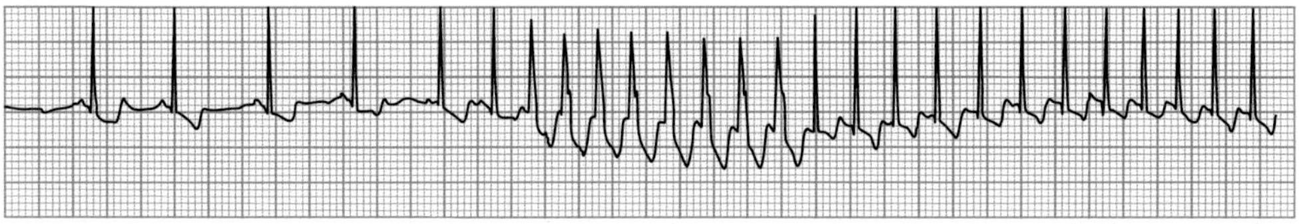

Figure 13.25 Paroxysmal AV nodal re-entrant tachycardia. This Holter recording shows sinus rhythm giving way to a broad complex tachycardia. However, this is clearly the result of temporary bundle branch block because it converts spontaneously to a narrow complex tachycardia, confirming that the arrhythmia is junctional, not ventricular, in origin.

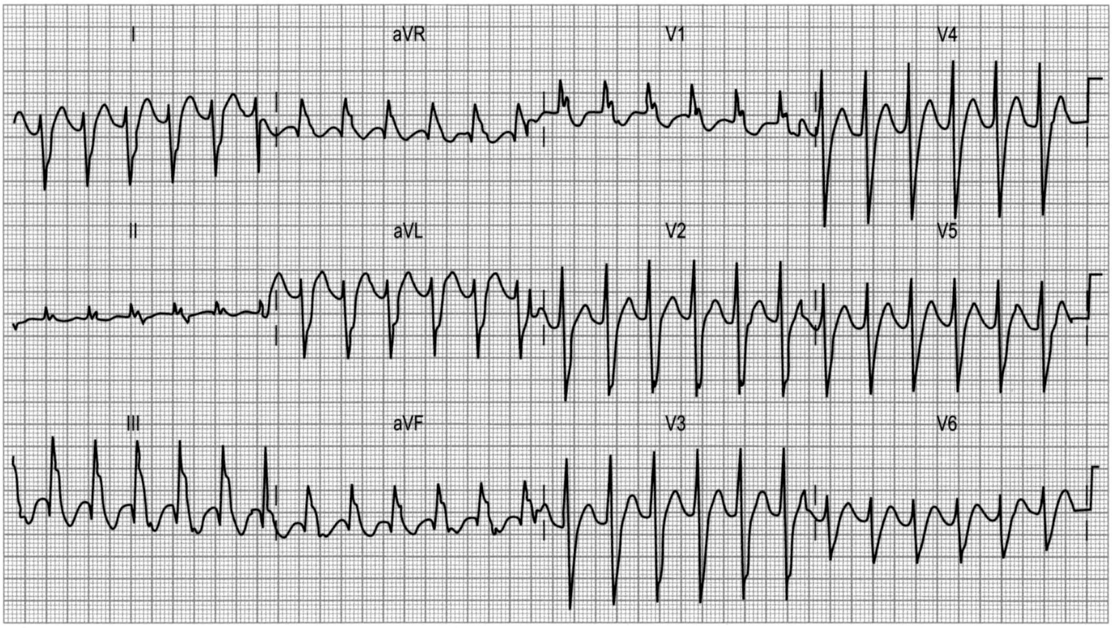

Figure 13.26 Ventricular tachycardia: 12-lead ECG. The recording shows a broad complex tachycardia. The following features suggest or confirm the ventricular origin of the tachycardia: very broad QRS complex (>140 ms); extreme right axis deviation; atrioventricular dissociation – note the dissociated P waves in lead V_1; the 'rSR' complex in V_1.

producing a retrograde P wave, but penetration of the sinus node is rare. Thus, resetting of the sinus node does not usually occur and there is a compensatory pause before the next sinus beat.

Ventricular tachycardia

Ventricular tachycardia is defined as three or more consecutive ventricular beats at a rate above 120 per minute. Ventricular depolarization inevitably occurs slowly by abnormal pathways, producing a broad QRS complex. This distinguishes it from most atrial and junctional tachycardias which have a narrow QRS complex, although differential diagnosis may be more difficult for atrial or junctional tachycardias with a broad QRS complex caused by rate-related or pre-existing bundle branch block (Fig. 13.25). Nevertheless, ventricular tachycardia can usually be identified by careful scrutiny of the 12-lead ECG (Fig. 13.26). Support for the diagnosis is provided by a very broad QRS complex (>140 ms), extreme left or right axis deviation, concordance of the QRS deflections in V_1–V_6 (either all positive or all negative)

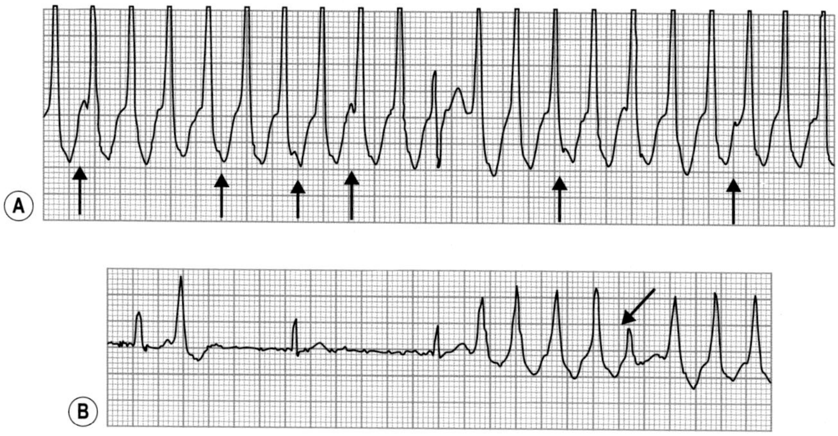

Figure 13.27 **(A)** Ventricular tachycardia: AV dissociation. P waves (arrow) can be seen 'marching through' the tachycardia, confirming its ventricular origin. The tachycardia is interrupted by a narrow capture beat. **(B)** Ventricular tachycardia (VT): fusion. In this example, VT is initiated by a very early ventricular ectopic beat (morphologically similar to the previous isolated ectopic beat) and is interrupted by a fusion beat (arrow), confirming the ventricular origin of the tachycardia.

and configurational features of the QRS complex, including an 'rSR' complex in V_1 and a QS complex in V_6. Confirmation of the diagnosis is provided by any evidence of AV dissociation: either P waves, at a slower rate than the QRS complexes, 'marching through' the tachycardia (Fig. 13.27A), or ventricular capture and/or fusion beats, in which the dissociated atrial rhythm penetrates the ventricle by conduction through the AV node and interrupts the tachycardia, producing a normal ventricular complex (capture, Fig. 13.27A) or, more commonly, a broad hybrid complex (fusion) that is part sinus and part ventricular in origin (Fig. 13.27B). *Torsades de pointes*, a broad complex tachycardia with changing wavefronts, also provides unequivocal evidence of ventricular tachycardia and is particularly characteristic of the arrhythmia that complicates long QT syndrome, often resulting in sudden death. The syndrome may be inherited as an autosomal dominant (Romano-Ward syndrome) or as an autosomal recessive (Lange-Nielsen syndrome) trait when it is associated with congenital deafness. Another important cause of Torsade de pointes is the use of drugs (antiarrhythmics and others such as antipsychotic therapy) that cause prolongation of the QT interval.

Ventricular fibrillation

Ventricular fibrillation occurs most commonly in severe myocardial ischaemia, either with or without frank infarction. It is a completely disorganized arrhythmia characterized by irregular fibrillatory waves with no discernible QRS complexes. There is no effective cardiac output and death is inevitable unless resuscitation with direct current defibrillation is instituted rapidly.

Diagnosis of sinoatrial disease

Sinus node discharge is not itself visible on the surface ECG, but the atrial depolarization it triggers produces the P wave. The spontaneous discharge of the normal sinus node is influenced by a variety of neurohumoral factors, particularly vagal and sympathetic activity, which respectively slow and quicken the heart rate. In sinoatrial disease (Fig. 13.28 and Box 13.16), sinus node discharge may be abnormally slow, blocked (with failure to activate atrial depolarization) or absent altogether. Under these circumstances, the

Box 13.16 Sinoatrial disease

Typical patient

- Elderly, often with no previous cardiac history

Causes

- Acute: myocardial infarction, coronary artery disease, drugs (e.g. β-blockers, digoxin), hypothermia, atrial surgery
- Chronic: idiopathic fibrotic disease, congenital heart disease, ischaemic heart disease, amyloid

Major symptoms

- Intermittent syncopal or presyncopal attacks
- Patients may also complain of exertional fatigue (chronotropic incompetence) or palpitations (tachycardia-bradycardia syndrome)

Major signs

- Often none
- Sometimes sinus bradycardia or slow atrial fibrillation

Diagnosis

- ECG: often normal. May show sinus bradycardia or slow atrial fibrillation
- Ambulatory ECG: 24-hour Holter recording may show pauses diagnostic of sinoatrial disease

Comments

- Documentation of the sinus pauses (or very slow atrial fibrillation) during an attack of symptoms provides the most robust diagnostic information

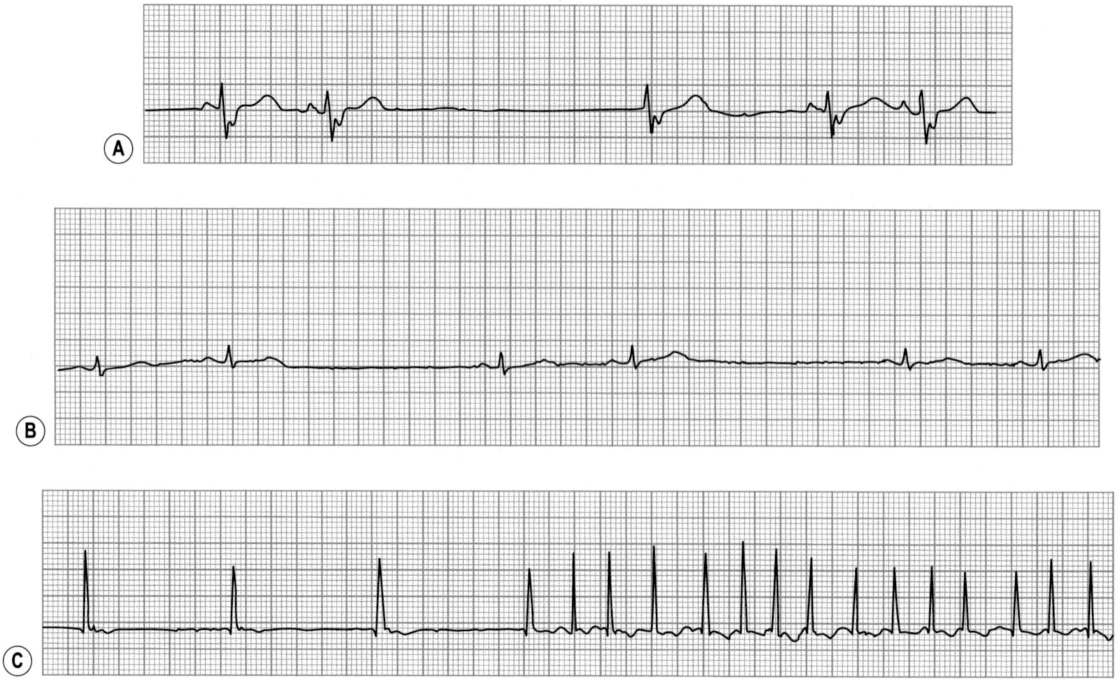

Figure 13.28 Sinoatrial disease. **(A)** Sinus arrest with late junctional escape. After the second sinus beat there is a long pause, interrupted by a single junctional escape beat, before sinus rhythm is re-established. **(B)** Sinoatrial block. Pauses after the second and fourth complexes are the result of sinoatrial block, which has prevented sinus impulses from depolarizing the atrium. No P waves are seen but, because the sinus discharge continues uninterrupted, the pauses are each a precise multiple of the preceding PP interval. Sinoatrial block is probably rare. **(C)** Bradycardia-tachycardia syndrome. A slow junctional rhythm gives way to rapid atrial fibrillation.

sinus rate may be very slow, the atrium may fibrillate, or pacemaker function may be assumed by foci lower in the atrium, the atrioventricular node or the His-Purkinje conducting tissue in the ventricles. The intrinsic rate of these 'escape' pacemaker foci is slower than the normal sinus rate.

Sinus bradycardia (<50 bpm)

Sinus bradycardia is physiological during sleep and in trained athletes but in other circumstances often reflects sinoatrial disease, particularly when the heart rate fails to increase normally with exercise.

Sinoatrial block

If the sinus impulse is blocked and fails to trigger atrial depolarization, a pause occurs in the ECG. No P wave is seen during the pause owing to the absence of atrial depolarization. The electrically 'silent' sinus discharge, however, continues uninterrupted. Thus, the pause is always a precise multiple of preceding PP intervals. Sinoatrial block that cannot be abolished by atropine-induced vagal inhibition usually indicates sinoatrial disease, particularly with pauses longer than 2 seconds.

Sinus arrest

Failure of sinus node discharge produces a pause on the ECG that bears no relation to the preceding PP interval. Pauses longer than 2 seconds are usually pathological. Prolonged pauses are often terminated by an escape beat from a 'junctional' focus in the bundle of His.

Bradycardia-tachycardia syndrome

In bradycardia-tachycardia syndrome, atrial bradycardias are interspersed by paroxysmal tachyarrhythmias, usually atrial fibrillation. Nevertheless, it is the bradycardia that usually causes symptoms, particularly dizzy attacks and blackouts.

Diagnosis of atrioventricular block

In atrioventricular block (Fig. 13.29), conduction is delayed or completely interrupted, either in the atrioventricular node or in the bundle branches (Box 13.17). When conduction is merely delayed (e.g. first-degree atrioventricular block, bundle branch block), the heart rate is unaffected. When conduction is completely interrupted, however, the heart rate may slow sufficiently to produce symptoms. In second-degree atrioventricular block, failure of conduction is by definition intermittent, and if sufficient sinus impulses are conducted to maintain an adequate ventricular rate, symptoms may be avoided. In third-degree atrioventricular block there is complete failure of conduction and continuing ventricular activity depends on the emergence of an escape rhythm. If the block is within the atrioventricular node, the escape rhythm usually arises from a focus just below the node in the bundle of His (junctional escape),

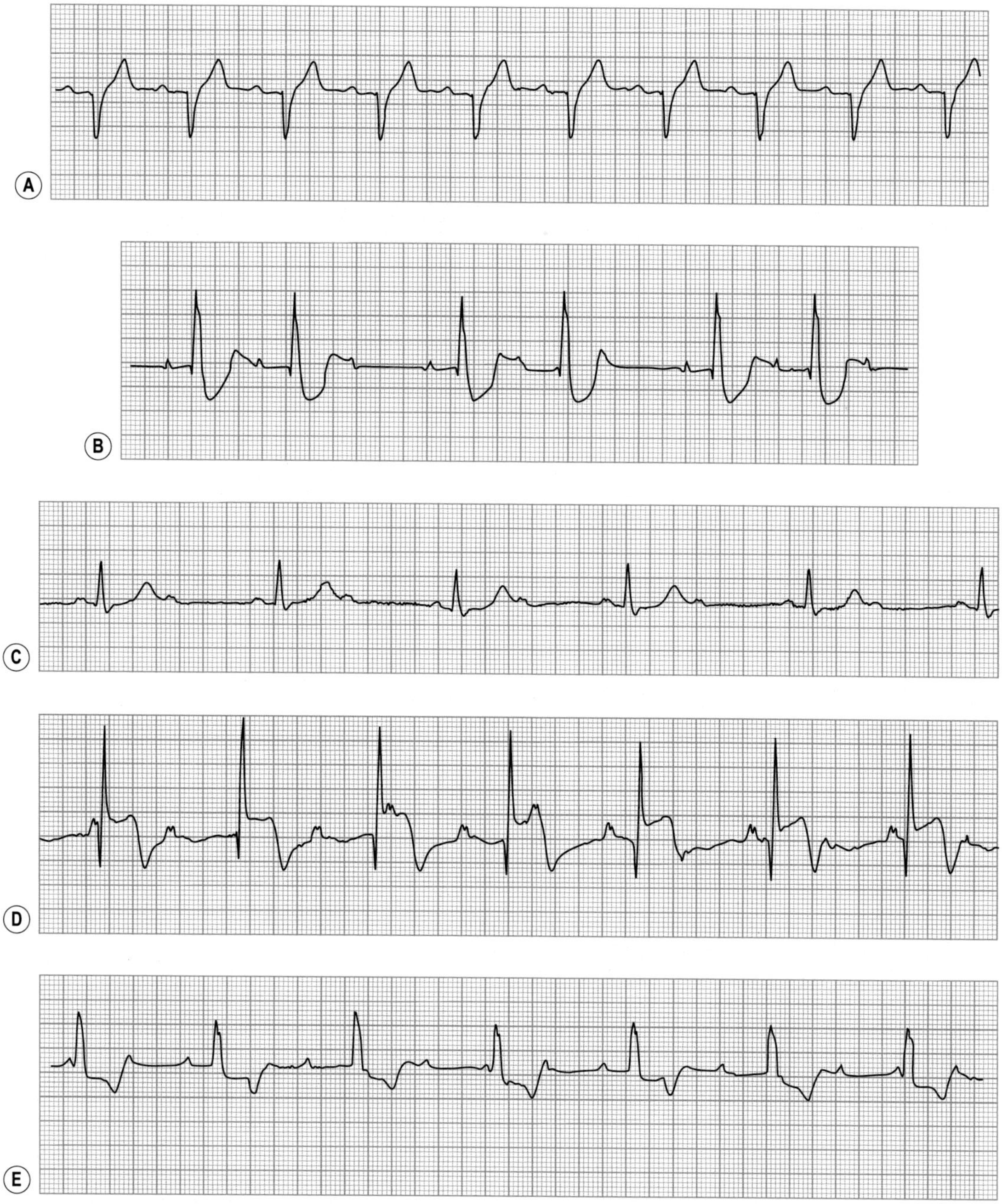

Figure 13.29 Atrioventricular conducting tissue disease. **(A)** 1° AV block. Delayed AV conduction causes a prolonged PR interval (>0.20 s). **(B)** 2° AV block, Wenckebach type. This is also called Mobitz type I block and occurs within the AV node. Three Wenckebach cycles are shown. Successive sinus beats find the AV node increasingly refractory until failure of conduction occurs. This delay permits recovery of nodal function and the process repeats itself. **(C)** 2° AV block at bundle branch level (Mobitz type II). This is standard lead I. Note that the PR interval of conducted beats is normal but the QRS complex shows right bundle branch block. Intermittent block in the left bundle results in failure of conduction of alternate P waves. **(D)** 3° (complete) AV block at level of AV node. In this patient with acute inferior myocardial infarction there is complete failure of AV conduction, as reflected by the dissociated atrial and ventricular rhythms. Note the regular P waves and the regular slower QRS complexes occurring independently of one another. Because block is at the level of the AV node, a junctional escape rhythm has taken over with a narrow QRS complex. **(E)** 3° (complete) AV block at bundle branch level. The atrial and ventricular rhythms are dissociated because none of the atrial impulses is conducted. The ECG shows regular P waves and regular but slower QRS complexes. Because the escape rhythm is ventricular in origin, the QRS complexes are broad and the rate is slow.

Box 13.17 Causes of atrioventricular heart block

Acute

- Myocardial infarction
- Drugs (e.g. β-blockers, verapamil, digoxin, adenosine)
- Surgical or catheter ablation of bundle of His
- Endocarditis complicated by aortic root abscess

Chronic

- Idiopathic fibrosis of both bundle branches
- Ischaemic heart disease
- Congenital heart disease
- Calcific aortic valve disease
- Chagas' disease
- Infiltrative disease (amyloid, haemochromatosis)
- Granulomatous disease (sarcoid, tuberculosis)

and is often fast enough to prevent symptoms. If both bundle branches are blocked, however, the escape rhythm must arise from a focus lower in the ventricles. Ventricular escape rhythms of this type are nearly always associated with symptoms because they are not only very slow but also unreliable and may stop altogether, producing prolonged asystole.

First-degree atrioventricular block

Delayed atrioventricular conduction causes prolongation of the PR interval (>0.20 s). Ventricular depolarization occurs rapidly by normal His-Purkinje pathways and the QRS complex is usually narrow.

Second-degree atrioventricular block: Mobitz type I (Wenckebach)

Mobitz type I second-degree atrioventricular block commonly occurs in inferior myocardial infarction. Successive sinus beats find the atrioventricular node increasingly refractory until failure of conduction occurs. The delay permits recovery of nodal function, and the process may then repeat itself. The ECG shows progressive prolongation of the PR interval, culminating in a dropped beat. Block is within the atrioventricular node itself and ventricular depolarization occurs rapidly by normal pathways. Thus the QRS complex is usually narrow.

Second-degree atrioventricular block: Mobitz type II

Mobitz type II second-degree atrioventricular block indicates advanced conducting tissue disease affecting the bundle branches. The ECG typically shows a normal PR interval with bundle branch block in conducted beats and intermittent block in the other bundle branch, resulting in complete failure of atrioventricular conduction and dropped beats.

Third-degree (complete) atrioventricular block

The atrial and ventricular rhythms are 'dissociated' because none of the atrial impulses are conducted. Thus the ECG shows regular P waves (unless the atrium is fibrillating) and regular but slower QRS complexes occurring independently of each other. When block is within the atrioventricular node (e.g. inferior myocardial infarction, congenital atrioventricular block), a junctional escape rhythm with a reliable rate (40-60 bpm) takes over (see Fig. 13.29). Ventricular depolarization occurs rapidly by normal pathways, producing a narrow QRS complex. However, when block is within the bundle branches (e.g. idiopathic fibrosis), there is always extensive conducting tissue disease. The ventricular escape rhythm is slow and unreliable, with a broad QRS complex (see Fig. 13.29).

Right bundle branch block

Right bundle branch block may be a congenital defect but is more commonly the result of organic conducting tissue disease. Right ventricular depolarization is delayed, resulting in a broad QRS complex with an 'rSR' pattern in lead V_1 and prominent S waves in leads I and V_6.

Left bundle branch block

Left bundle branch block always indicates organic conducting tissue disease. The entire sequence of ventricular depolarization is abnormal, resulting in a broad QRS complex with large slurred or notched R waves in leads I and V_6.

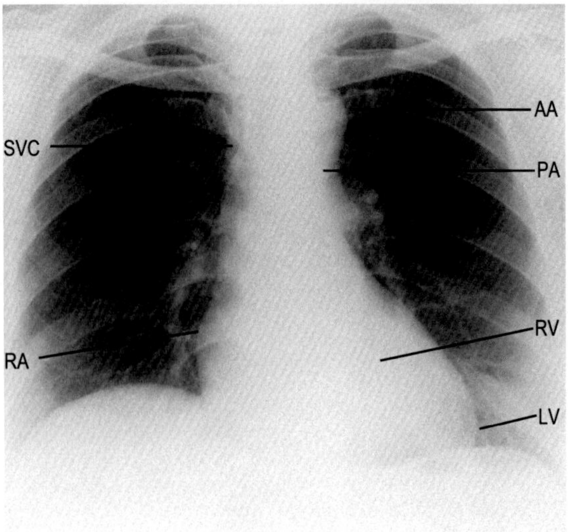

Figure 13.30 Normal chest X-ray: posteroanterior projection. Note the heart is not enlarged (cardiothoracic ratio <50%) and the lung fields are clear. AA, aortic arch; LV, left ventricle; PA, pulmonary artery; RA, right atrium; RV, right ventricle; SVC, superior vena cava.

The chest X-ray

Good-quality posteroanterior (PA) and lateral chest X-rays are always helpful in the assessment of the cardiac patient (Fig. 13.30).

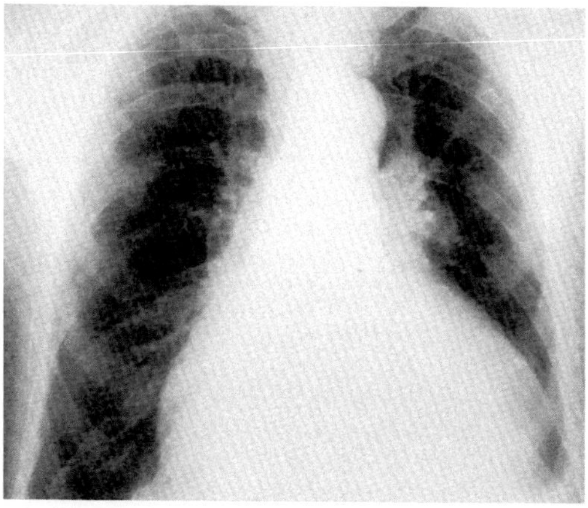

Figure 13.31 Pericardial effusion with tamponade: chest X-ray. There is a left hilar mass caused by carcinoma. Pericardial infiltration has produced effusion and tamponade, evidenced by the severely enlarged and globular cardiac silhouette. Malignant disease is now the most common cause of tamponade in most developed countries.

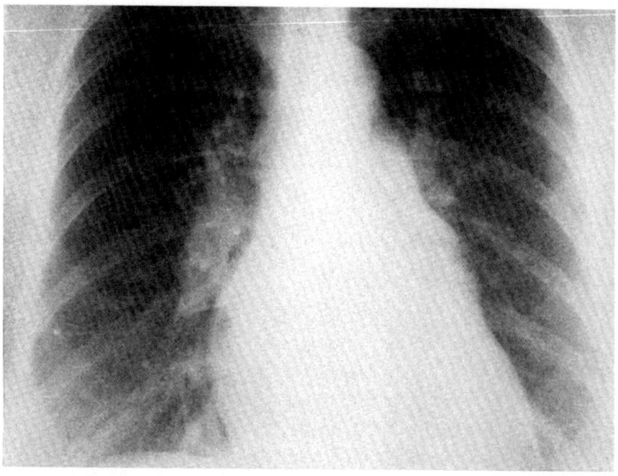

Figure 13.32 Left atrial dilatation. This is a penetrated PA chest X-ray in a patient with mitral stenosis. The dilated left atrium causes a bulge on the left heart border below the pulmonary artery which is also dilated, widening of the carina and the double-density sign at the right heart border.

Cardiac silhouette

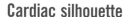

Although the PA chest X-ray exhibits a wide range of normality, the maximum diameter of the heart should not be more than 50% of the widest diameter of the thorax. Cardiac enlargement is caused either by dilatation of the cardiac chambers or by pericardial effusion (Fig. 13.31). Myocardial hypertrophy only affects heart size if very severe.

Ventricular dilatation

The PA chest X-ray does not reliably distinguish left from right ventricular dilatation. For this, the lateral chest X-ray is more helpful. Dilatation of the posteriorly located left ventricle encroaches on the retrocardiac space, whereas dilatation of the anteriorly located right ventricle encroaches on the retrosternal space.

Atrial dilatation

Right atrial dilatation is usually due to right ventricular failure, but occurs as an isolated finding in tricuspid stenosis and Ebstein's anomaly. It produces cardiac enlargement without specific radiographic signs.

Left atrial dilatation occurs in left ventricular failure and mitral valve disease (Fig. 13.32). Radiographic signs are:

- Flattening and later bulging of the left heart border below the main pulmonary artery.
- Elevation of the left main bronchus, with widening of the carina.
- Appearance of the medial border of the left atrium behind the right side of the heart (double-density sign).

Vascular dilatation

Aortic dilatation caused by aneurysm or dissection may produce widening of the entire upper mediastinum.

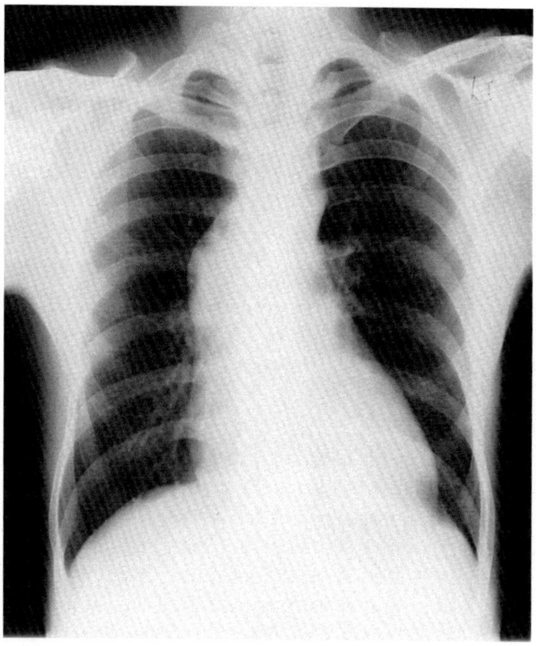

Figure 13.33 Chest X-ray in a patient with Marfan syndrome. Note the dilatation of the ascending aorta.

Localized dilatation of the proximal aorta occurs in aortic valve disease and produces a prominence in the right upper mediastinum (Fig. 13.33). Dilatation of the main pulmonary artery occurs in pulmonary hypertension and pulmonary stenosis and produces a prominence below the aortic knuckle (Fig. 13.34).

Intracardiac calcification

Because the radiodensity of cardiac tissue is similar to that of blood, intracardiac structures can rarely be identified unless they are calcified. Valvular, pericardial or myocardial calcification may occur, and usually indicates important disease of these structures.

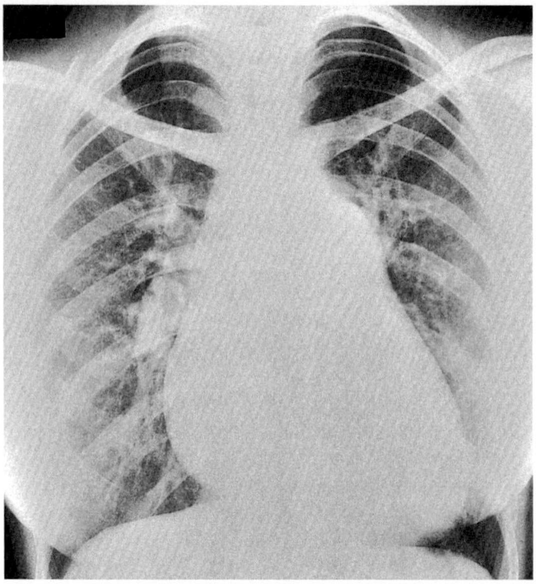

Figure 13.34 Atrial septal defect: chest X-ray. Note the prominent proximal pulmonary arteries and the pulmonary plethora reflecting increased pulmonary flow.

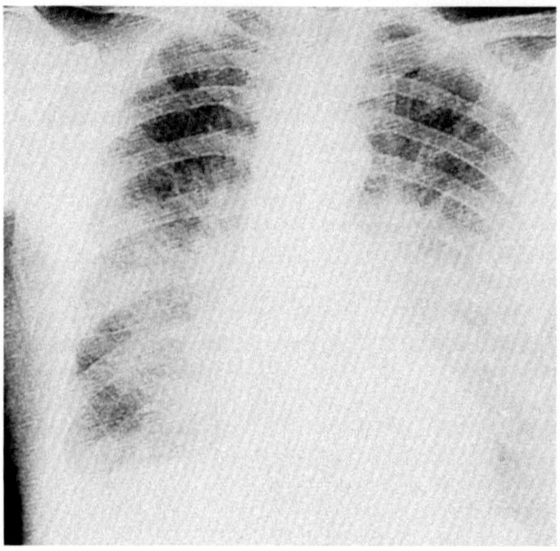

Figure 13.35 Chest X-ray in acute left ventricular failure: the patient had severe pulmonary oedema caused by acute myocardial infarction. The heart is not yet enlarged, but there is prominent alveolar pulmonary oedema in a perihilar ('bat's-wing') distribution. Note the bilateral pleural effusions.

Calcification is best appreciated on the deeply penetrated lateral chest X-ray.

Lung fields

Common lung field abnormalities in cardiovascular disease are caused either by altered pulmonary flow or by increased left atrial pressure.

Altered pulmonary flow

Increments in pulmonary flow sufficient to cause radiographic abnormalities are caused by left-to-right intracardiac shunts (e.g. atrial septal defect; see Fig. 13.34, ventricular septal defect, patent ductus arteriosus). Prominence of the vascular markings gives the lung fields a plethoric appearance. Reductions in pulmonary flow, on the other hand, cause reduced vascular markings. This may be regional (e.g. pulmonary embolism) or global (e.g. severe pulmonary hypertension).

Increased left atrial pressure

Increased left atrial pressure occurs in mitral stenosis and left ventricular failure and produces corresponding rises in pulmonary venous and pulmonary capillary pressures. Prominence of the upper lobe veins is an early radiographic finding. As the left atrial and pulmonary capillary pressures rise above 18 mmHg, transudation into the lung produces interstitial pulmonary oedema, characterized by prominence of the interlobular septa, particularly at the lung bases (Kerley B lines). Further elevation of pressure leads to alveolar pulmonary oedema, characterized by perihilar 'bat's-wing' shadowing (Fig. 13.35).

Other lung field abnormalities

Pulmonary infarction

Localized and typically wedge-shaped areas of consolidation are occasionally seen in pulmonary embolic disease, although more often the bronchial circulation protects against ischaemic damage.

Pneumonic consolidation and abscess

In patients with right-sided endocarditis, infected pulmonary emboli commonly cause septic foci within the lung fields.

Interstitial lung disease

In long-standing pulmonary hypertension complicating rheumatic mitral valve disease, haemosiderosis (stippled shadowing throughout the lung fields) was once a common X-ray finding. It is now rarely seen.

Bony abnormalities

Bony abnormalities are unusual in cardiovascular disease, apart from coarctation of the aorta and thoracic outlet syndromes. In coarctation, dilated bronchial collateral vessels erode the inferior aspect of the ribs to produce notches, although they are rarely present before adolescence. Cervical ribs may compress the neurovascular bundle in the thoracic outlet, and special thoracic outlet views are necessary for radiographic diagnosis.

Echocardiography

Echocardiography is one of the most versatile non-invasive imaging techniques in clinical cardiology. As it does not use ionizing radiation, it is free of risk and can be employed safely throughout pregnancy. Transthoracic imaging with the transducer applied to the chest wall is usually satisfactory, but better quality information is obtained via the transoesophageal approach in which the transducer is mounted on a probe and positioned in the oesophagus, directly behind the heart. This provides higher resolution images because there are no intervening ribs or lung tissue and the probe is closely applied to the posterior aspect of the heart. It is particularly useful for imaging the left atrium, the aorta, the interatrial septum and prosthetic heart valves.

Principles

Physics

A transducer containing a piezoelectric element converts electrical energy into an ultrasound beam that is directed towards the heart. The beam is reflected when it strikes an interface between tissues of different densities. The reflected ultrasound, or echo, is converted back to electrical energy by the piezoelectric element, which permits the construction of an image using two basic units of information:

1. The intensity of the echoes, which defines the density difference at tissue interfaces within the heart.
2. The time taken for echoes to arrive back at the transducer, which defines the distance of the cardiac structures from the transducer.

Density differences within the heart are greatest between the blood-filled chambers and the myocardial and valvular tissues, all of which are clearly visible on the echocardiogram. Because the depth of the myocardial and valvular tissues with respect to the transducer changes constantly throughout the cardiac cycle, the time taken for echo reflection changes accordingly. Thus, real-time imaging throughout the cardiac cycle provides a dynamic record of cardiac function.

M-mode echocardiogram

The M-mode echocardiogram provides a unidimensional view through the heart. Continuous recording on photographic paper provides an additional time dimension, thereby permitting appreciation of the dynamic component of the cardiac image. By convention, cardiac structures closest to the transducer are displayed at the top of the record and more distant structures are displayed below. Thus, on the transthoracic M-mode echocardiogram, anteriorly located ('right-sided') structures lie above the posteriorly located ('left-sided') structures, but on the transoesophageal echocardiogram, the display is reversed. M-mode is particularly useful for measuring chamber dimensions and left ventricular wall thickness and for timing events within the cardiac cycle (Fig. 13.36A).

Two-dimensional echocardiogram

The two-dimensional (2D) echocardiogram provides more detailed information about morphology than the M-mode recording. By projecting a fan of echoes in an arc of up to 80°, a 2D 'slice' through the heart can be obtained, the precise view depending on the location and angulation of the transducer (Fig. 13.36B).

Clinical applications

Congenital heart disease

Echocardiography, particularly the 2D technique, has revolutionized the diagnosis of congenital heart disease, in the majority of cases obviating the need for invasive investigation by cardiac catheterization (Fig. 13.37). The relationships of the cardiac chambers and their connections with the great vessels are readily determined. Valvular abnormalities and septal defects can also be recognized. Recent technology has permitted *in utero* fetal imaging for the antenatal diagnosis of cardiac defects.

Myocardial disease

Echocardiography permits accurate assessment of cardiac dilatation, hypertrophy and contractile function. Dilated cardiomyopathy produces ventricular dilatation with global contractile impairment (Fig. 13.38). This must be distinguished from the regional contractile impairment that follows myocardial infarction in patients with coronary artery disease (Fig. 13.39). Hypertrophic cardiomyopathy is characterized by thickening (hypertrophy) of the left ventricular myocardium, usually with disproportionate involvement of the interventricular septum (asymmetric septal hypertrophy). In aortic and hypertensive heart disease, on the other hand, left ventricular hypertrophy is usually symmetrical (Fig. 13.40).

Valvular disease

Echocardiography is of particular value for identifying both structural and dynamic valvular abnormalities and any associated chamber dilatation or hypertrophy (Boxes 13.18-13.21). The severity of valvular involvement in congenital, rheumatic, degenerative and infective disease may thus be defined; the technique is diagnostic for bicuspid aortic valve and mitral valve prolapse and readily identifies valve thickening and calcification in rheumatic and calcific disease (Figs 13.40 and 13.41). Vegetations in infective endocarditis can usually be visualized if they are large enough (>3 mm, Fig. 13.42). The transoesophageal approach is usually necessary for endocarditis involving prosthetic heart valves.

Pericardial disease

Although the echocardiogram is of little value in constrictive pericarditis, it is the most sensitive technique available for the diagnosis of pericardial effusion (Fig. 13.43). The effusion appears as an echo-free space distributed around the ventricles but

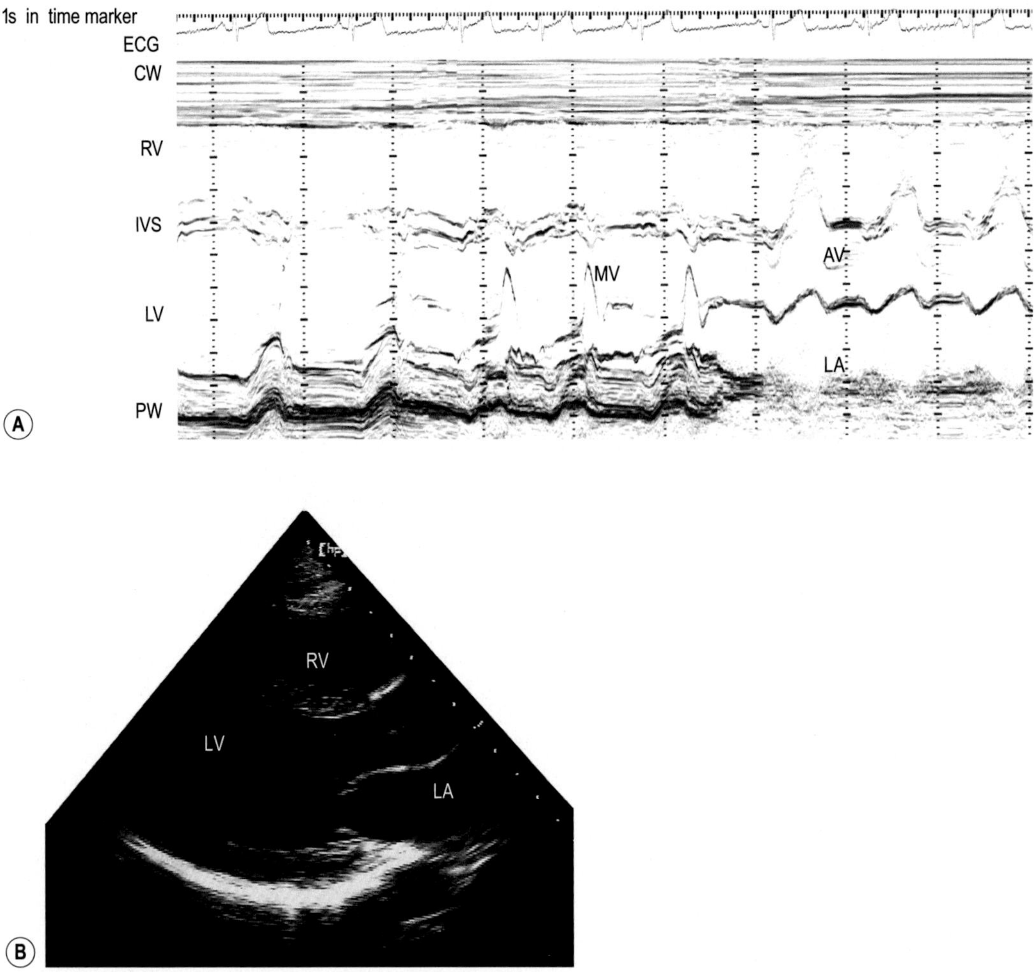

Figure 13.36 **(A)** M-mode echocardiography. The figure shows a sweep as the transducer is angulated from the left ventricle to the aortic root. **(B)** Transthoracic 2D echocardiography. Parasternal long-axis and apical four-chamber views are shown. The dots are a 1-cm scale. AV, aortic valve; CW, chest wall; IVS, interventricular septum; LA, left atrium; LV, left ventricle; MV, mitral valve; PW, posterior LV wall; RV, right ventricle.

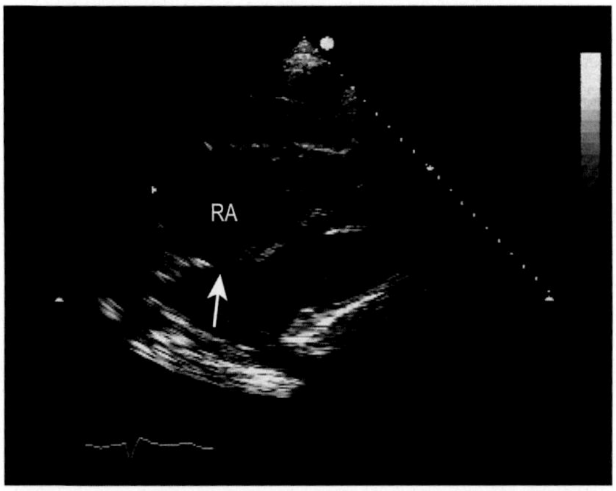

Figure 13.37 Atrial septal defect: 2D echocardiogram (subcostal view). In this view, good views of the interatrial septum can usually be obtained without resorting to transoesophageal echocardiography. Note the atrial septal defect (arrow) and the dilatation of the right atrium (RA).

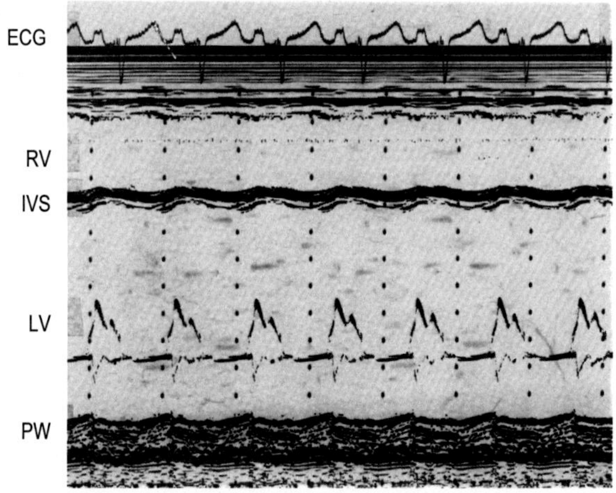

Figure 13.38 Dilated cardiomyopathy: echocardiogram. This M-mode study shows severe dilatation of the left ventricular cavity and severe global contractile impairment. The patient later underwent successful heart transplantation.

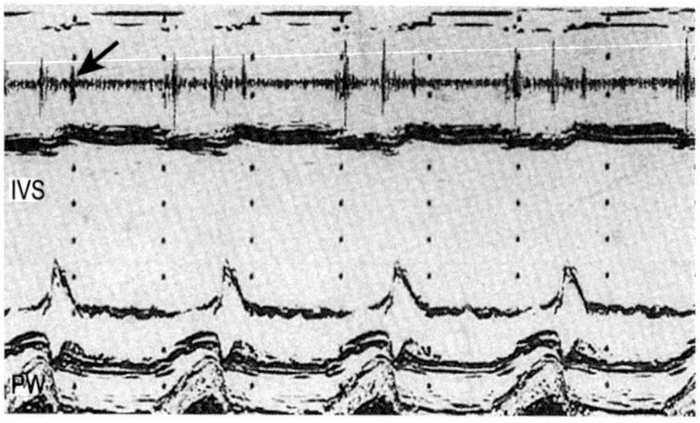

Figure 13.39 Heart failure: echocardiogram. This M-mode study shows considerable dilatation of the left ventricle. Note that the interventricular septum (IVS) is almost akinetic, but the posterior wall (PW) is contracting normally. Regional contractile impairment of this type indicates coronary heart disease. The phonocardiogram recorded simultaneously shows normal first and second heart sounds and also a third heart sound (arrowed).

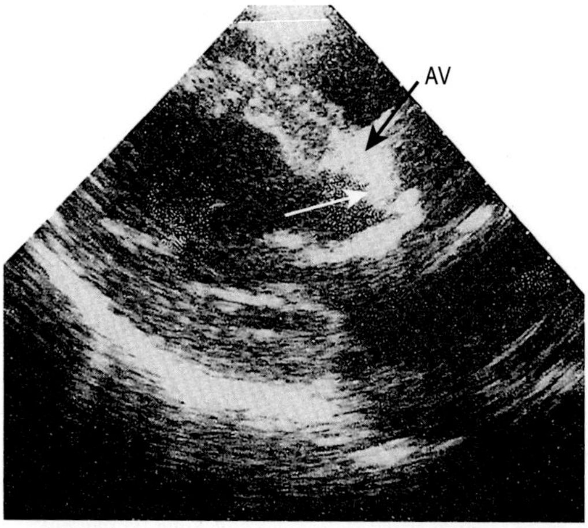

Figure 13.40 Aortic stenosis and left ventricular hypertrophy: 2D echocardiogram (long-axis view). The aortic valve (AV) is grossly thickened and calcified. Concentric left ventricular hypertrophy is present (arrow).

Box 13.18 Aortic stenosis

Typical patient

- Middle-aged (congenitally bicuspid valve) or elderly (degenerative calcific disease) man or woman

Major symptoms

- Exertional shortness of breath is usual presenting symptom
- Angina may also occur and, in advanced cases, syncopal attacks or sudden death

Major signs

- Carotid pulse: slow upstroke with plateau
- Auscultation: fourth heart sound at cardiac apex; ejection systolic murmur at base of heart, radiating to neck. The murmur may be preceded by an ejection click if the valve is mobile and not heavily calcified

Diagnosis

- ECG: left ventricular hypertrophy
- Chest X-ray: dilatation of ascending aorta
- Echocardiogram: calcified immobile aortic valve with left ventricular hypertrophy. Doppler studies permit quantification of the severity of stenosis

Additional investigations

- Cardiac catheterization is necessary to evaluate coronary arteries in patients being considered for aortic valve replacement surgery

Comments

- Aortic stenosis is now the commonest acquired valve lesion in developed countries

Box 13.19 Aortic regurgitation

Typical patient

- Young men (Marfan syndrome, etc.) or older patients (long-standing hypertension) with dilating disease of the aortic root

Major symptoms

- Exertional shortness of breath is usual presenting symptom
- Angina may also occur

Major signs

- Carotid pulse: sharp upstroke with early diastolic collapse
- Blood pressure: systolic hypertension with wide pulse pressure
- Auscultation: early diastolic murmur at left sternal edge. Third heart sound at cardiac apex in severe cases. Mid-diastolic murmur (Austin Flint) may be heard at apex owing to preclosure of mitral valve by regurgitant jet

Diagnosis

- ECG: left ventricular hypertrophy
- Chest X-ray: cardiac enlargement with dilatation of ascending aorta
- Echocardiogram: often normal valve with dilated aortic root. Doppler studies confirm regurgitant jet

Additional investigations

- Cardiac catheterization is necessary to evaluate coronary arteries in older patients (age >50) being considered for aortic valve replacement surgery

Comments

- The timing of valve replacement surgery is difficult but should anticipate irreversible left ventricular contractile failure

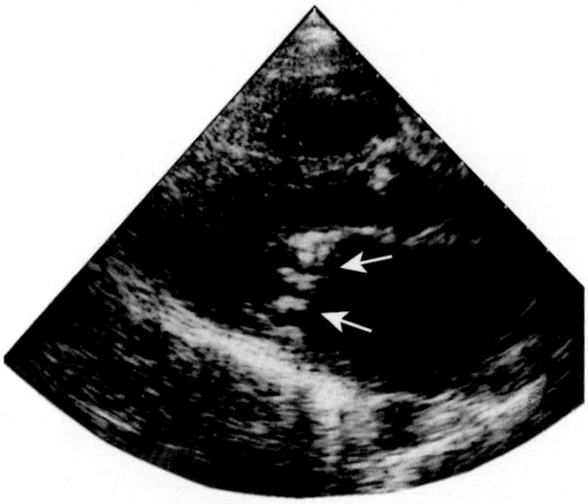

Figure 13.41 Mitral stenosis: 2D echocardiogram (parasternal long-axis view). The mitral valve leaflets are densely thickened (arrow) and the left atrium is severely dilated.

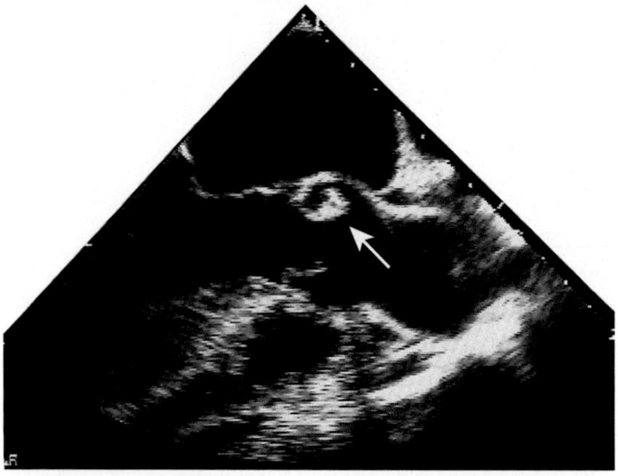

Figure 13.42 Infective endocarditis: transoesophageal echocardiogram. Vegetation (arrow) is adherent to the aortic valve leaflet.

Box 13.20 Mitral stenosis

Typical patient

- Young to middle-aged woman with a history of rheumatic fever in childhood

Major symptoms

- Exertional shortness of breath with orthopnoea in advanced cases
- Palpitations commonly signal the development of atrial fibrillation, which puts the patient at serious risk of peripheral embolism and stroke

Major signs

- Pulse: atrial fibrillation in many cases
- Auscultation: loud S1 with early diastolic opening snap, followed by low-pitched mid-diastolic murmur best heard at cardiac apex. If the patient is in sinus rhythm, there is presystolic accentuation of the murmur

Diagnosis

- ECG: atrial fibrillation usually
- Chest X-ray: signs of left atrial enlargement (flat left heart border, widening of carinal angle, and double-density sign at right heart border). Pulmonary congestion
- Echocardiogram: rheumatic mitral valve and left atrial dilatation. Doppler studies permit quantification of the severity of stenosis

Additional investigations

- Cardiac catheterization is necessary to evaluate coronary arteries in patients aged >50 being considered for mitral valve replacement surgery

Comments

- In patients with atrial fibrillation, anticoagulation with warfarin is mandatory to protect against stroke

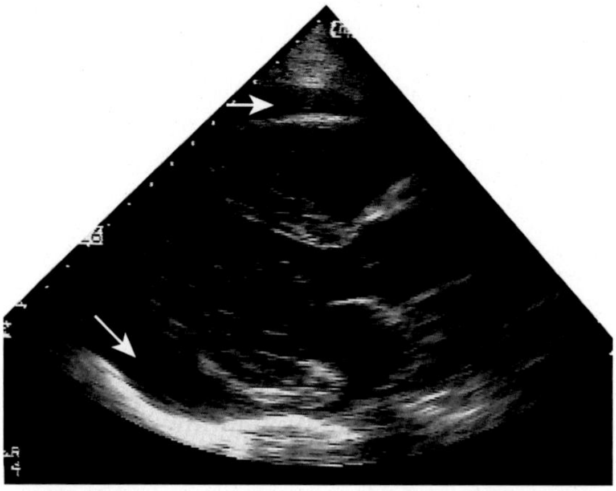

Figure 13.43 Pericardial effusion: 2D echocardiogram (parasternal long-axis view). Note the echo-free space (arrow) around the heart but not behind the left atrium.

usually avoiding the potential space behind the left atrium.

Other clinical applications

Intracardiac tumours, particularly myxomas (see Fig. 13.1) and thrombi (Fig. 13.44), are readily visualized by echocardiography. The transoesophageal technique is more sensitive for identifying thrombus in the left atrial appendage and is also helpful for diagnosing aortic disease, such as aneurysm and dissection, as it provides better views of the thoracic aorta than is possible with conventional 2D echocardiography (Fig. 13.45).

Stress echocardiography

Stress echocardiography is increasingly being used for the diagnosis of myocardial ischaemia in suspected coronary disease. Left ventricular imaging during increasing dobutamine infusion permits assessment

Box 13.21 Mitral regurgitation

Typical patient

- Mitral valve prolapse (floppy mitral valve) causes regurgitation of variable severity and more commonly affects women at almost any age
- Patients with subvalvular disease (papillary muscle dysfunction or chordal rupture) are usually elderly men or women

Major symptoms

- Exertional shortness of breath with orthopnoea in advanced cases
- Palpitations commonly signal the development of atrial fibrillation, which puts the patient at serious risk of peripheral embolism and stroke

Major signs

- Pulse: often sinus rhythm, but may be atrial fibrillation
- Auscultation: pansystolic murmur at cardiac apex, radiating to axilla. Often associated with third heart sound

Diagnosis

- ECG: atrial fibrillation, but may be normal
- Chest X-ray: cardiac enlargement with variable signs of left atrial enlargement, though these are usually less marked than in mitral stenosis. Pulmonary congestion in severe cases
- Echocardiogram: prolapsing (floppy) mitral valve may be seen; in subvalvular disease the valve often appears normal. Left ventricular and left atrial dilatation. Doppler studies confirm regurgitant jet

Additional investigations

- Transoesophageal echo is sometimes necessary to clarify the severity and mechanism of regurgitation
- Cardiac catheterization is necessary to evaluate coronary arteries in patients aged >50 years being considered for mitral valve replacement surgery

Comments

- In patients with atrial fibrillation, anticoagulation with warfarin is mandatory to protect against stroke

of regional wall motion in response to adrenergic stress. Decreasing systolic wall motion or wall thickening indicates ischaemia and the need for further investigation. Stress echocardiography is also used to identify myocardial 'viability' in the patient with heart failure, and improvement in regional hypokinesis in response to dobutamine infusion, indicating 'hibernating' (and hence potentially salvageable) myocardium likely to respond favourably to revascularization by angioplasty or bypass surgery.

Doppler echocardiography

Doppler echocardiography permits evaluation of the direction and velocity of blood flow within the heart and great vessels. It is widely used for measuring the severity of valvular stenosis and identifying valvular regurgitation and intracardiac shunts through septal defects.

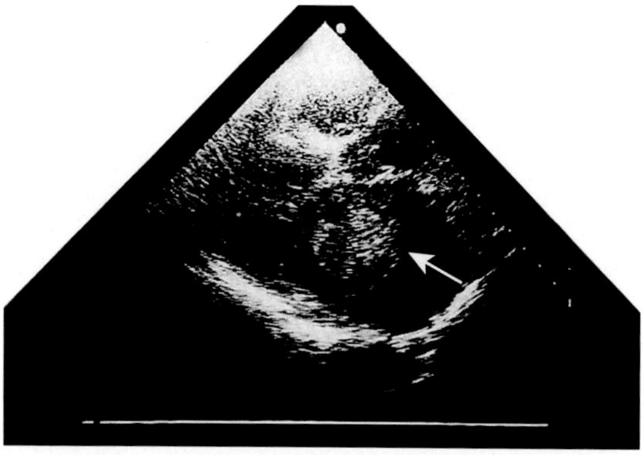

Figure 13.44 Mitral stenosis: 2D echocardiogram (long-axis view). The left atrium is severely dilated and a large thrombus (arrow) is visible, emphasizing the importance of anticoagulation in patients with mitral valve disease and atrial fibrillation.

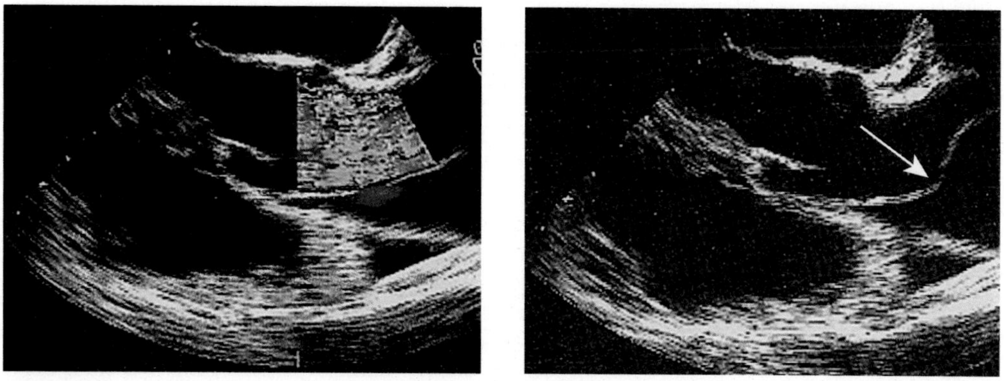

Figure 13.45 Aortic dissection: transoesophageal echocardiogram. Right panel: this long-axis transoesophageal echocardiogram reveals the dilated aortic root and an S-shaped flap (arrow) traversing the lumen. Left panel: same patient with colour Doppler superimposed to show flow in the true lumen.

Principles

Physics

According to the Doppler principle, when an ultrasound beam is directed towards the bloodstream, the frequency of the sound waves reflected from the blood cells is altered. The frequency shift or Doppler effect is related to the direction and velocity of flow. If continuous-wave Doppler is used, blood flow at any point along the path of the ultrasound beam is detected, such that a 'clean' Doppler signal from the area of interest may be difficult to obtain. Pulsed Doppler, however, has a range-gating facility that permits frequency sampling from any specific point within the heart, preselected on the echocardiogram. This lends greater precision to the technique. Nevertheless, pulsed Doppler is less able than continuous-wave Doppler to quantify very high-velocity jets, such as those that occur in aortic stenosis.

Colour-flow mapping

Colour-flow mapping has been a major technological advance. Instead of the unidirectional ultrasound beam used in continuous-wave and pulsed Doppler imaging, the beam is rotated through an arc. Frequency sampling throughout the arc permits the construction of a colour-coded map, red indicating flow towards and blue away from the transducer. Colour-flow data can be superimposed on the standard 2D echocardiogram to identify precisely the patterns of flow within the four chambers of the heart. This simplifies the interpretation of Doppler imaging and provides more useful qualitative data, although it is less useful for quantitative assessment of valve gradients, which requires the precision of conventional Doppler technique.

Clinical applications

In paediatric cardiology, the combination of 2D echocardiography and colour-flow Doppler mapping has made possible the 'non-invasive' diagnosis of a large majority of congenital defects, often without the need for cardiac catheterization. These techniques have also revolutionized the diagnosis of valvular disease in all age groups. In valvular regurgitation, the retrograde flow that occurs after valve closure is readily detected by Doppler echocardiography, although only an approximate estimate of its severity is possible (Fig. 13.46). In valvular stenosis, the peak velocity (as opposed to the volume) of flow across the valve is directly related to the degree of stenosis. Thus, measurement of Doppler flow velocity (ideally by continuous wave) permits quantification of the stenosis by the application of the Bernoulli equation:

$$\text{pressure gradient} = 4 \times \text{velocity}^2$$

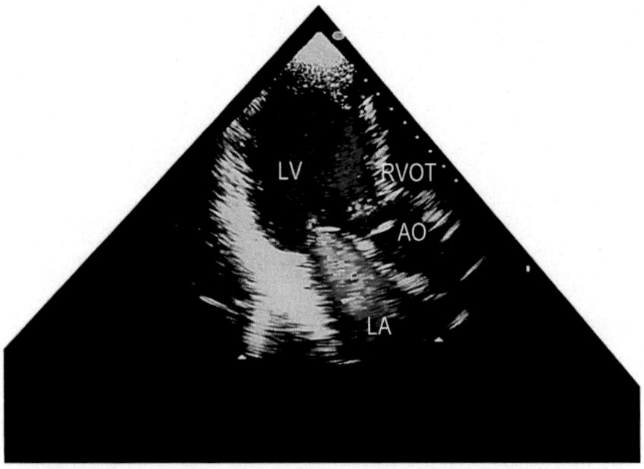

Figure 13.46 Mitral regurgitation: colour-flow Doppler. This is an apical long-axis view of the heart showing a large jet of mitral regurgitation (blue) occupying most of the left atrial cavity (LA).

New developments

In recent years, real time three-dimensional (3D) imaging has emerged as a powerful technique – particularly in the assessment of valvular disease and in guiding percutaneous interventions such as minimally invasive transcatheter aortic valve implantation (TAVI).

Cardiovascular radionuclide imaging

Principles

All radionuclide techniques require the internal administration of a radioisotope; the distribution of radioactivity in the area of interest is then imaged with a gamma camera. Ideally, the isotope should be distributed homogeneously in that part of the cardiovascular system under investigation: thus, isotopes that remain in the intravascular space during imaging are used for radionuclide angiography. In myocardial perfusion scintigraphy, however, isotopes taken up by the myocardium are required. Because of their potential toxicity, isotopes with a short half-life are usually used.

Clinical applications

Radionuclide ventriculography

This method is used for assessment of ventricular function. Red cells labelled with technetium-99m (^{99m}Tc) are allowed to equilibrate in the blood pool and the heart is then imaged under the gamma camera. The waxing and waning of radioactivity within the ventricular chambers during diastole and systole, respectively, permits the construction of a dynamic ventriculogram. Left ventricular contractile function can be evaluated quantitatively by calculating the ejection fraction, or qualitatively by observing wall movement. In clinical practice, this has now been replaced by other techniques for the assessment of left ventricular function such as echocardiography and magnetic resonance imaging.

Myocardial perfusion scintigraphy

This method is used for the diagnosis and assessment of coronary artery disease (Fig. 13.47). In an attempt to provoke myocardial ischaemia the patient is 'stressed' by a standardized exercise test, an intravenous dobutamine infusion or an intravenous adenosine infusion. Isotope is injected intravenously at peak stress and the heart is imaged under a gamma camera. Thallium-201 (^{201}Tl) has now given way to ^{99m}Tc-labelled methoxy-isobutyl-isonitrile (MIBI) which provides better image quality. Isotope is distributed homogeneously in normally perfused myocardium, ischaemic or infarcted areas appearing as scintigraphic defects. If ^{201}Tl is used, repeat imaging after 2-4 hours' rest permits the reassessment of scintigraphic defects; those that disappear (reversible defects) indicate areas of stress-induced ischaemia, while those that persist (fixed defects) indicate infarcted myocardium. If ^{99m}Tc-labelled MIBI is used, resting images for assessment of reversibility require a separate injection of isotope 24 hours after (or before) the stress images.

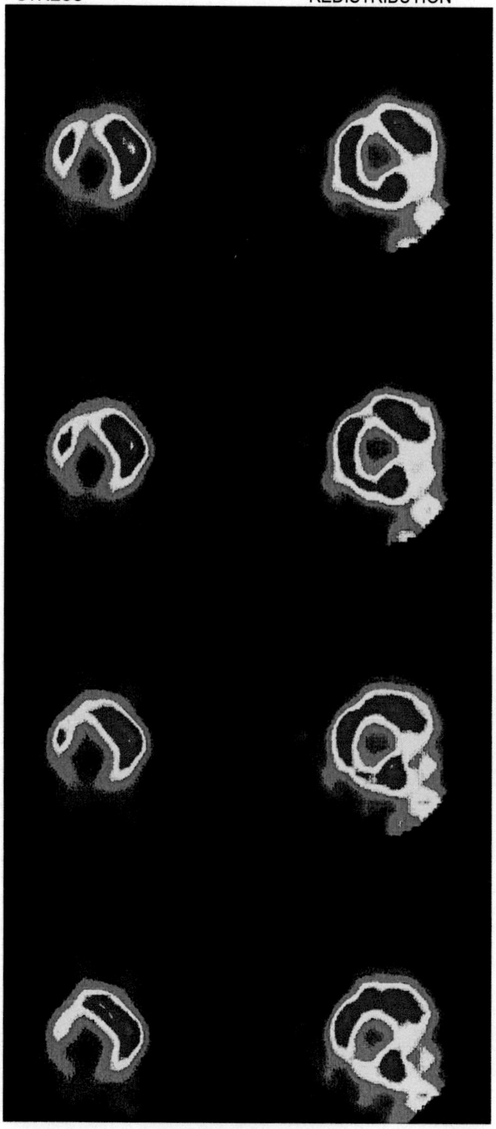

Figure 13.47 Isotope perfusion scan. These are tomographic slices across the short axis of the left ventricle. A posterior wall defect is seen during stress, but it largely disappears during rest as isotope 'redistributes' into the ischaemic area. A smaller fixed defect is seen in the anterior wall, indicating infarction in that territory.

Positron emission tomography

Positron emission tomography (PET) scanning is used to determine myocardial 'viability' in patients with heart failure (see stress echocardiography, above). Simultaneous assessment of myocardial perfusion using ^{13}N ammonia and glucose uptake using a glucose analogue permits the identification of viable but dysfunctional myocardium, in which perfusion is impaired but metabolic activity in terms of glucose uptake remains normal. This perfusion-metabolic 'mismatch' indicates viable muscle likely to respond favourably to revascularization by angioplasty or bypass surgery.

New PET tracers, such as rubidium, can be used to assess myocardial perfusion. A specialist cyclotron is not required for this tracer, reducing the costs involved.

Pulmonary scintigraphy (radioisotope imaging)

Pulmonary scintigraphy is used for the diagnosis of pulmonary embolism (Fig. 13.48). The ^{99m}Tc-labelled microspheres injected intravenously become trapped within the pulmonary capillaries. The normal pulmonary perfusion scintigram shows a homogeneous distribution of radioactivity throughout both lung fields. Pulmonary embolism causes regional impairment of pulmonary flow, which results in a perfusion defect on the scintigram; however, the appearance is non-specific and occurs in many other pulmonary disorders, particularly chronic obstructive pulmonary disease. Specificity is enhanced by simultaneous ventilation scintigraphy (a ventilation/perfusion, or V/Q scan). Inhaled xenon-133 (^{133}Xe) is distributed homogeneously throughout the normal lung, and in pulmonary embolism (unlike other pulmonary disorders), distribution remains homogeneous. Thus, a scintigraphic perfusion defect not 'matched' by a ventilation defect is highly specific for pulmonary embolism. CT pulmonary angiography is now the diagnostic test of choice for pulmonary embolism, but V/Q scanning is still valuable in patients with suspected pulmonary embolism who have severe renal impairment in whom X-ray contrast is contraindicated.

Computed tomography

Principles

CT measures the attenuation of X-rays after they have traversed body tissues. Attenuation is greatest

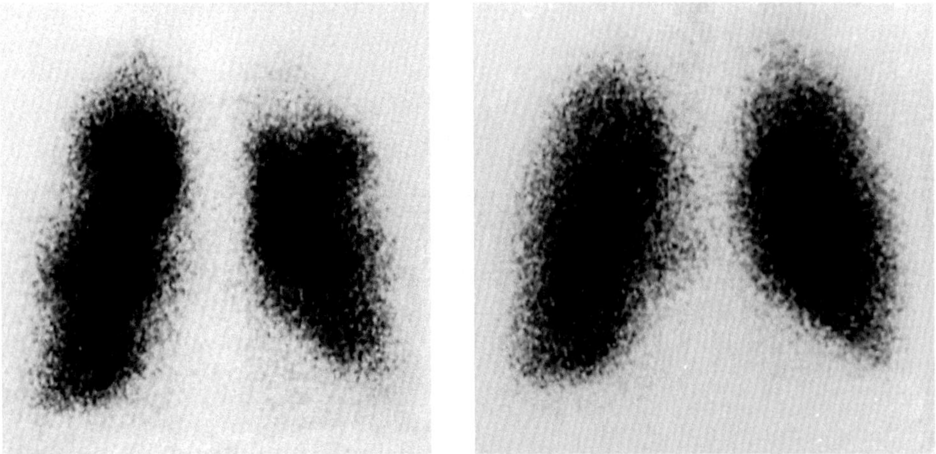

Figure 13.48 Ventilation (right) and perfusion (left) lung scans in pulmonary embolism. Contrast the homogeneous distribution of isotope in the ventilation scan with the regional defects in the perfusion scan.

for tissues such as bone, which are relatively radio-opaque, and least for tissues such as lung or fat, which are relatively radiolucent. From X-ray attenuation measurements, taken as a sensor rotates around the chest, cross-sectional images are constructed. Image resolution is excellent, and contrast injection into a peripheral vein opacifies the blood pool, allowing assessment of the coronary arteries and intracardiac structures. In the past, the clinical application of cardiac CT was limited by image acquisition times of up to 5 seconds, during which the constant motion of the heart degraded the image, and by high radiation doses. The current generation of ultrafast CT scanners with image acquisition times of less than 1 second provide high-resolution cardiac images in both static and video mode while radiation doses have reduced substantially.

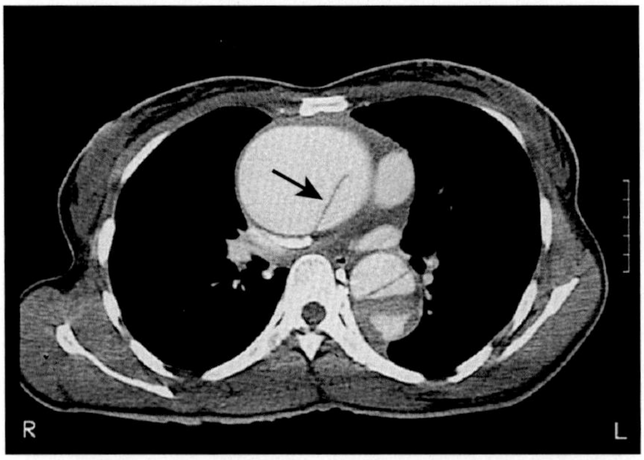

Figure 13.49 Aortic dissection: CT scan (Marfan syndrome). The ascending aorta is dilated and the intimal flap (arrow) clearly visible. This flap extends around the arch (not seen here) into the descending aorta, where again it is clearly visible.

Clinical applications

CT (with contrast enhancement) diagnoses pulmonary embolism and aortic dissection (Fig. 13.49) with a sensitivity of about 95%. It is also used for accurate assessment of pericardial thickness in constrictive disease (Fig. 13.50) and in the diagnosis of cardiac tumours. Recently, multislice CT has emerged as a useful investigation for the diagnosis of coronary artery disease. The quantification of coronary calcification has found application as a marker of coronary risk in asymptomatic or low-risk individuals; a zero calcium score has a high accuracy rate for the exclusion of coronary artery disease. CT coronary angiography is able to diagnose normal coronary arteries or mild plaque disease extremely accurately (Fig. 13.51) but it cannot distinguish reliably between moderate and severe stenoses or determine the degree of stenosis in heavily calcified coronary segments. CT coronary angiography is therefore best used in the assessment of low- to medium-risk patients to 'rule out' significant obstructive coronary artery disease. Additional applications of CT include the evaluation of graft patency

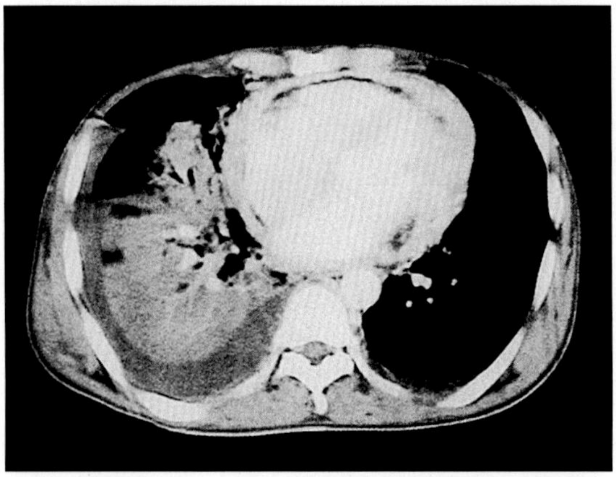

Figure 13.50 Non-calcific pericardial constriction: CT scan. There is consolidation in the right lung and severe pericardial thickening. The patient had pulmonary tuberculosis with pericardial involvement and presented with fever and signs of constriction. Antituberculous therapy caused regression of all symptoms and signs, although the patient is at major risk of developing constriction later as the pericardium becomes fibrotic and calcified.

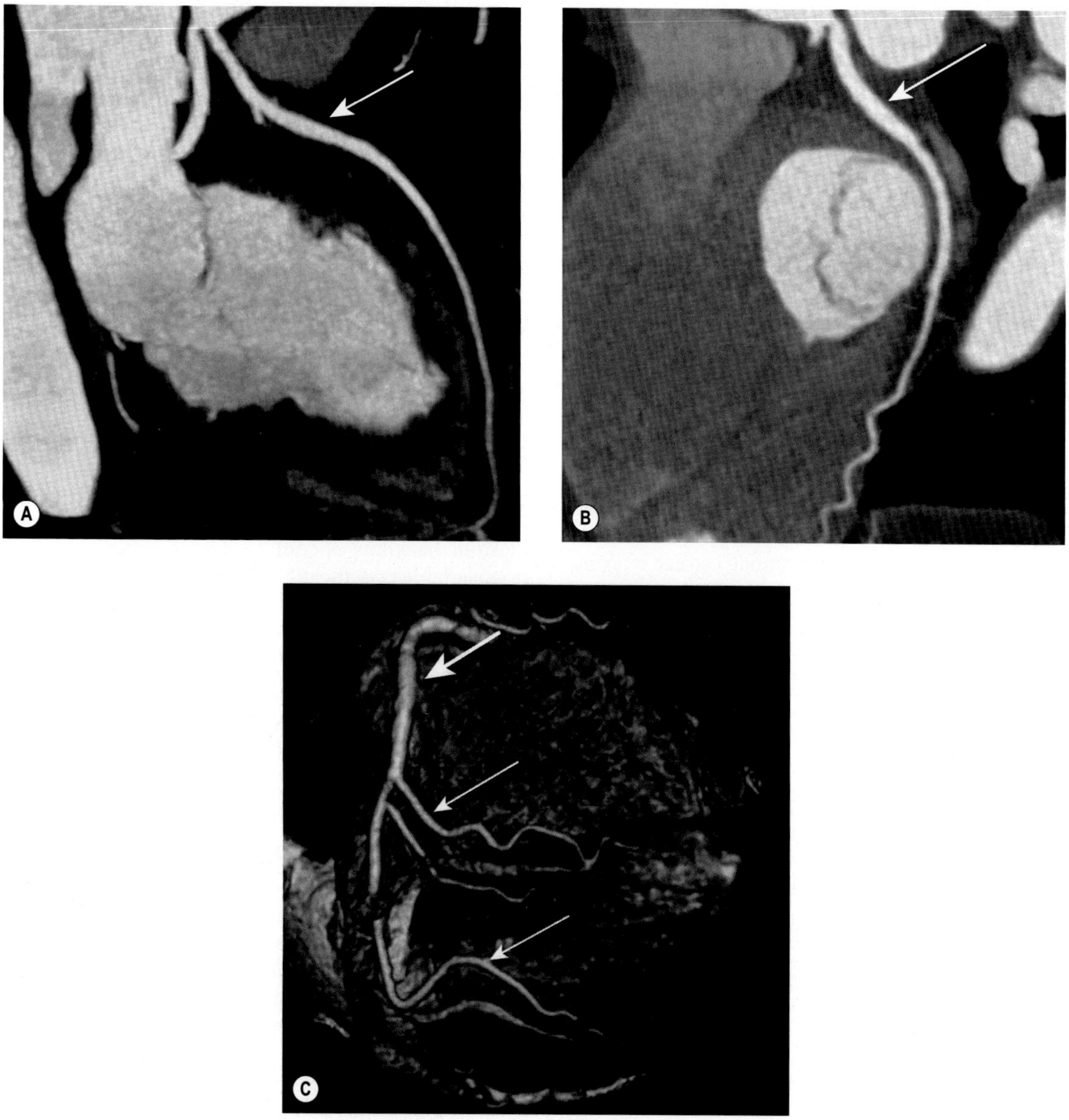

Figure 13.51 CT coronary angiogram: normal study in a 42-year-old man with atypical chest pain and a family history of premature coronary artery disease. **(A)** Multiplanar reformatted image of the left anterior descending artery (arrow). **(B)** Multiplanar reformatted image of the circumflex artery (arrow). **(C)** 3D volume-rendered image of the right coronary artery (large arrow), its posterior descending branch (upper small arrow) and posterior left ventricular branch (lower small arrow).

following coronary bypass surgery and analysis of ventricular wall motion.

Magnetic resonance imaging

Principles

Magnetic resonance imaging (MRI) utilizes the fact that certain nuclei with an intrinsic spin generate magnetic fields and behave like tiny bar magnets. Placed in a magnetic field, these nuclei align and adopt a resonant frequency that is unique to that nucleus and the strength of the magnetic field. If the nuclei are exposed to pulsed radiowaves of that frequency, they resonate and release energy, which allows their location to be determined.

For imaging purposes, the patient lies in a strong magnetic field which is artificially graded. The hydrogen protons of fat and water are imaged and, on exposure to pulsed radiowaves, they resonate at different frequencies in different parts of the imaging zone. Analysis of the emitted frequencies permits the construction of tomographic and 3D images of the heart. If data acquisition is gated to a specific part of the cardiac cycle, motion artefact is eliminated and excellent image resolution can be obtained. Different scanning parameters and patterns of gadolinium enhancement after its intravenous administration allow precise myocardial tissue characterization and detection of myocardial ischaemia.

Clinical applications

Cardiac MRI is now widely used for the assessment of cardiac structure and ventricular function. It can differentiate between myocardial infarction (Fig. 13.52), oedema, fibrosis and fat. MRI is well validated for the assessment of myocardial viability and ischaemia. It is therefore used in the diagnosis of coronary artery disease, myocarditis (Fig. 13.53) and cardiomyopathies. It is also used to guide therapy in patients with documented coronary artery disease; particularly in those with chronic coronary occlusions or multivessel disease, the presence of viability or ischaemia, respectively, provides justification for revascularization. Cardiac MRI does not involve the use of ionizing radiation so it can be used safely for repeated follow-up assessments and it is unique among cardiac imaging modalities in being able to assess myocardial function, viability and ischaemia in a single study. MRI provides an accurate assessment of valve regurgitant fraction and it is also highly sensitive for the diagnosis of aortic dissection (Fig. 13.54), intracardiac tumours and thrombi.

Cardiac catheterization

Catheters introduced into an artery or vein may be directed into the left or right sides of the heart, respectively. Arterial access is gained percutaneously from the femoral or radial artery or by surgical cutdown to the brachial artery. Venous access is usually from the femoral vein. Originally developed for diagnostic purposes, catheter techniques have now found widespread application in the interventional management of cardiovascular disease.

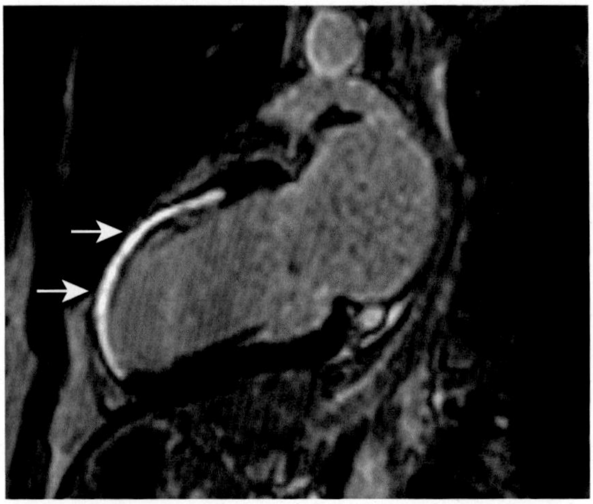

Figure 13.52 Anteroapical myocardial infarction: MRI scan. Delayed gadolinium enhancement (white area, arrows) of the full thickness of the anteroapical left ventricular wall indicating infarcted, non-viable tissue.

Cardiac angiography

Coronary angiography uses relatively small volumes of contrast (5-8 ml) injected manually, but other angiographic procedures require larger amounts (up to 40 ml) introduced by power injection. Digital subtraction techniques permit a reduction in contrast volume but at present have only a limited role in cardiovascular angiographic diagnosis (see below). The current generation of angiographic laboratories uses digital technology to provide high-quality dynamic images of ventricular wall movement, blood flow and intravascular anatomy.

Aortic root angiography

Injection of contrast into the aortic root demonstrates the vascular anatomy in suspected aneurysm or dissection, and also permits evaluation of aortic valve function (Fig. 13.55). The normal aortic valve prevents diastolic backflow of contrast, but in aortic regurgitation, variable opacification of the left ventricle occurs, depending on the severity of the valve lesion.

Left ventricular angiography

Contrast injection into the left ventricle defines ventricular anatomy and wall motion and also permits evaluation of mitral valve function. Dilatation of the ventricle and contractile dysfunction occurs in left ventricular failure. An akinetic segment denotes previous myocardial infarction. Exaggerated contractile function with systolic obliteration of the cavity occurs in hypertrophic cardiomyopathy. Filling defects within the ventricular lumen may indicate thrombus or neoplasm. The normal mitral valve prevents systolic backflow of contrast into the left atrium, but in mitral regurgitation variable atrial opacification occurs, depending on the severity of the valve lesion (Fig. 13.56).

Coronary angiography

Coronary angiography is the most reliable technique for diagnostic imaging of the coronary arteries and assessment of lesion severity. Indications are summarized in Box 13.22. The technique requires selective injection of contrast into the left and right coronary arteries to opacify the lumen (Fig. 13.57), and multiple

Box 13.22 Indications for coronary angiography

- ST elevation myocardial infarction
- High-risk non-ST elevation acute coronary syndromes
- Severe angina unresponsive to medical treatment
- Angina or a positive exercise test following myocardial infarction
- Cardiac arrhythmias when there is clinical suspicion of underlying coronary artery disease
- Preoperatively in patients requiring valve surgery when advanced age (>50 years) or angina suggest a high probability of coronary artery disease

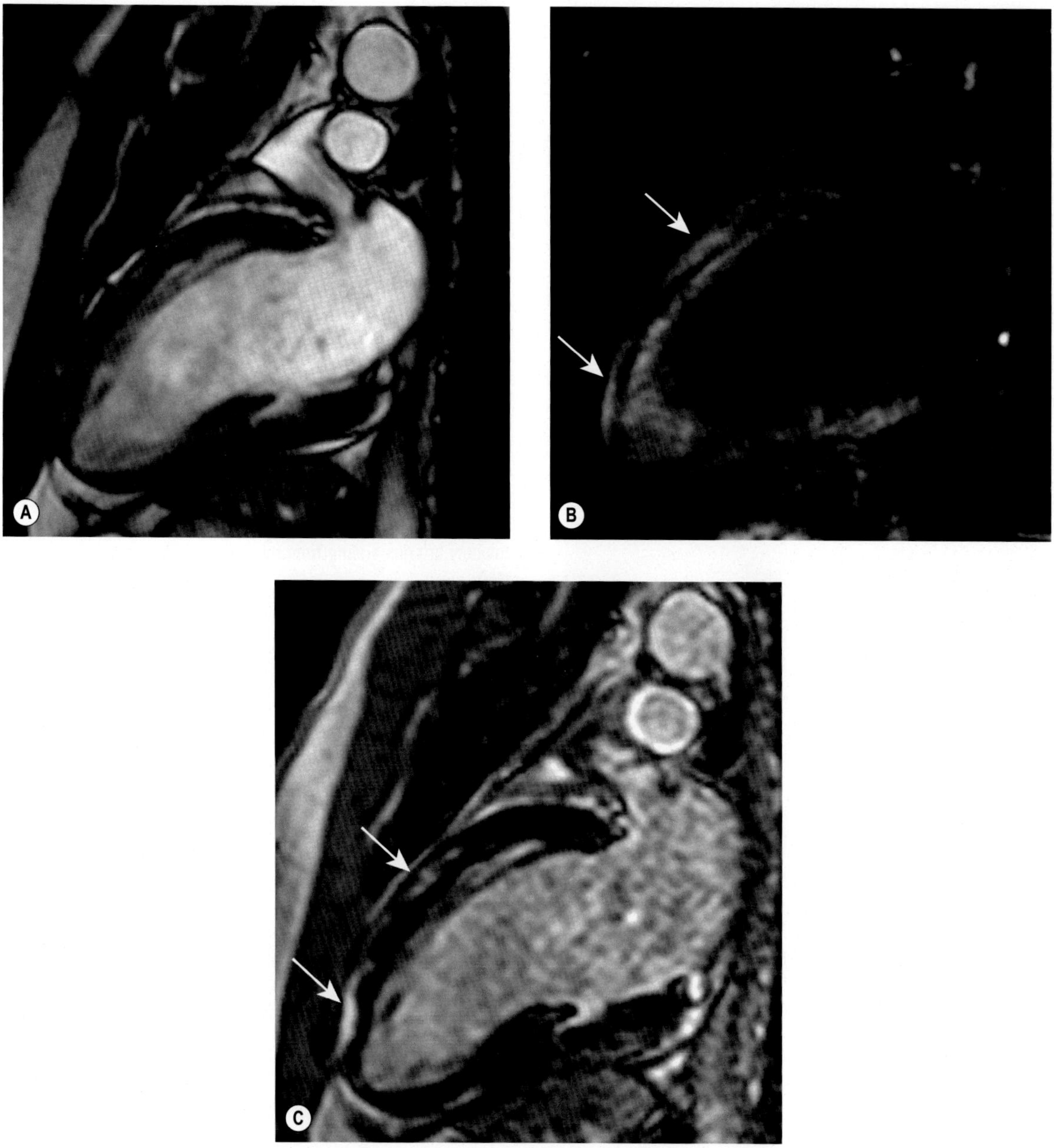

Figure 13.53 Myocarditis: MRI scan. **(A)** Still image from a cine loop of a two-chamber view of the left ventricle. Measurements of systolic function, chamber size and myocardial mass can be made from the cine loops. **(B)** Two-chamber view from the same patient with imaging for water content (T2 weighted) showing regions of myocardial oedema (arrows). **(C)** Late enhancement imaging following gadolinium infusion allows detection of areas of increased interstitial expansion from scar or oedema (arrows). The subepicardial pattern indicates myocarditis.

views in different projections are necessary for a complete study. Intraluminal filling defects or occlusions indicate coronary artery disease, which is nearly always caused by atherosclerosis. In stable patients, coronary angiography often reveals a stenosis or stenoses of intermediate severity. Additional information regarding the functional significance and anatomical severity of the disease is required before treatment decisions can be made. This can be obtained either from non-invasive myocardial perfusion imaging that looks for ischaemia in the territory of the affected artery (see MRI perfusion imaging) or from catheter laboratory-based techniques.

Pressure wire

Pressure wire is a relatively new catheter laboratory-based technology that is increasingly used to assess functional significance and guide management of coronary stenoses. The wire has a pressure sensor 3 cm from its distal tip. The pressure sensor is calibrated and then equalized to the pressure at the

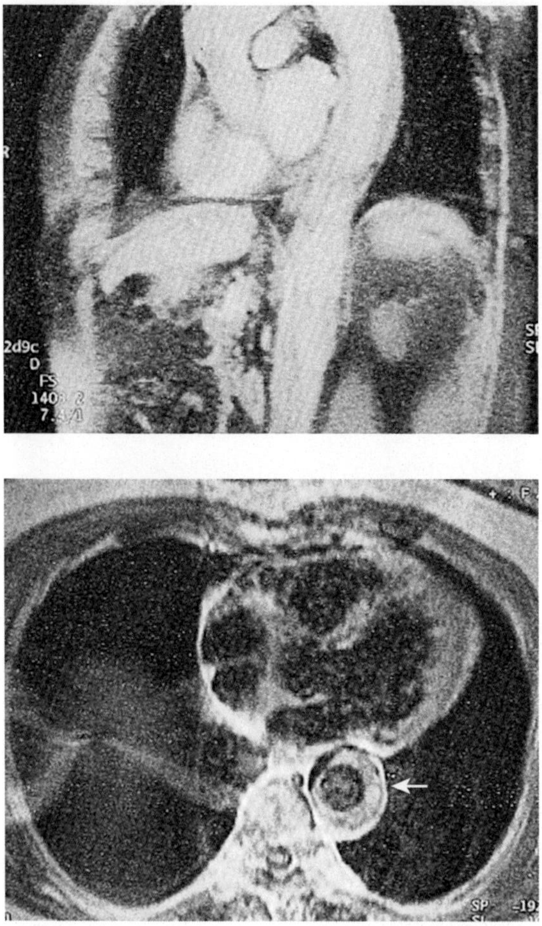

Figure 13.54 Aortic dissection: MRI scan. The upper panel (coronal section) reveals an extensive aortic dissection extending from the aortic root through the arch and into the descending aorta. The lower panel reveals a transverse view through the heart and descending aorta. Note the thrombus in the false lumen surrounding the true lumen in the descending aorta (arrow).

guide catheter tip in the left main stem, before being passed down the artery so that the pressure sensor is distal to the stenosis to be interrogated. Adenosine is administered by intravenous infusion to induce maximal hyperaemia in the myocardial capillary bed and simulate the physiological state during exercise. The fractional flow reserve (FFR) is calculated automatically by computer software from the pressure measured distal to the stenosis referenced against the pressure measured proximal to the stenosis at the guide catheter tip. An FFR <0.75 signifies a stenosis that is likely to cause myocardial ischaemia and the stenosis is deemed functionally significant. Clinical studies have shown that pressure wire-guided management is superior to angiographic-driven decision making, predominantly through avoiding procedure-related myocardial infarction in patients who undergo revascularization.

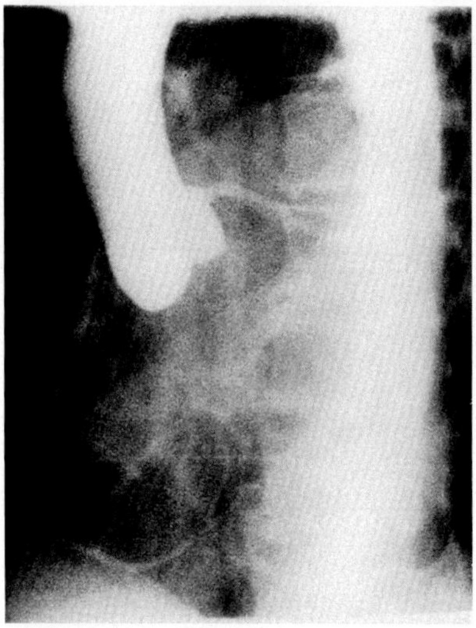

Figure 13.55 Aortic root angiogram: normal study. Contrast injection provides an X-ray image of the ascending aorta. The coronary arteries arising from the sinuses of Valsalva are clearly seen.

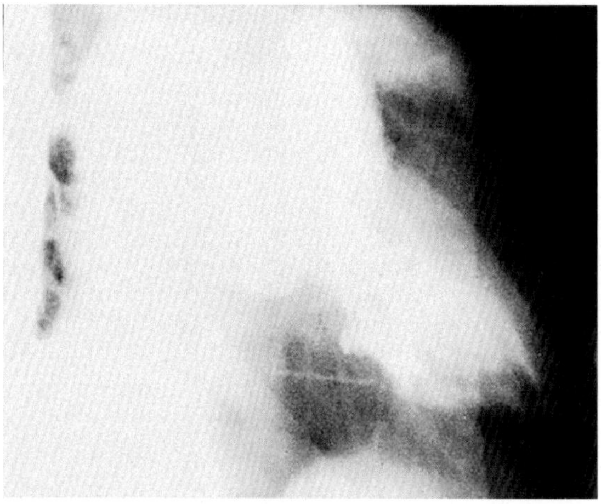

Figure 13.56 Left ventricular angiogram showing mitral regurgitation. Contrast injection into the left ventricle has resulted in prompt opacification of the left atrium owing to backflow across the diseased mitral valve.

Intravascular ultrasound

An ultrasound transducer mounted at the tip of a coronary catheter provides cross-sectional images of the artery. The technique permits accurate measurement of the luminal area and provides information about plaque composition and structure that cannot be obtained from angiographic images (Fig. 13.58). Intravascular ultrasound has a clinical role in quantifying the severity of intermediate stenoses identified on coronary angiography, optimizing stent deployment, assessing instent restenosis and stent thrombosis, and in clarifying the cause of equivocal angiographic appearances due to possible thrombus, dissection, calcium or plaque.

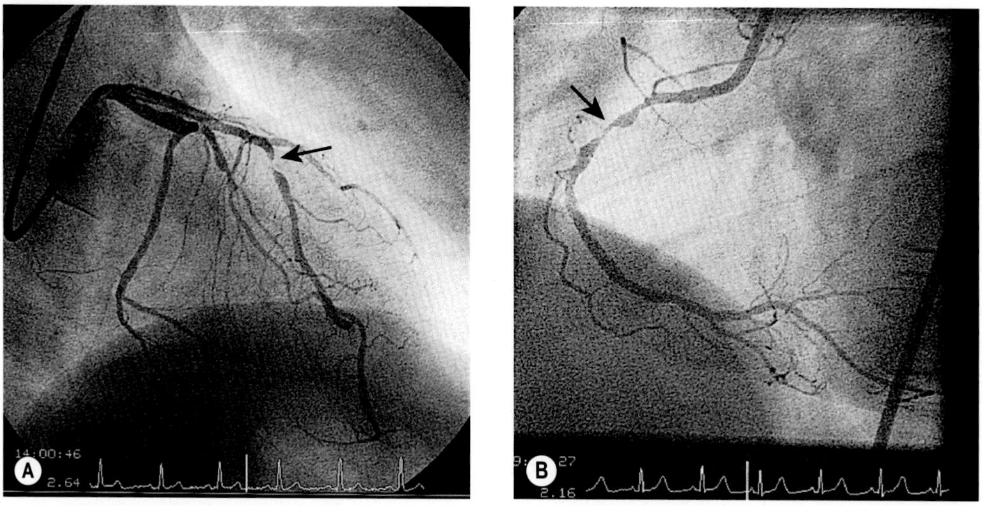

Figure 13.57 Coronary angiograms. **(A)** Left anterior descending disease (arrow). This tight stenosis threatens the coronary supply to the anterior wall of the left ventricle. **(B)** Right coronary artery disease (arrow). Serial stenoses in this dominant right coronary artery threaten the supply to the inferior wall of the heart.

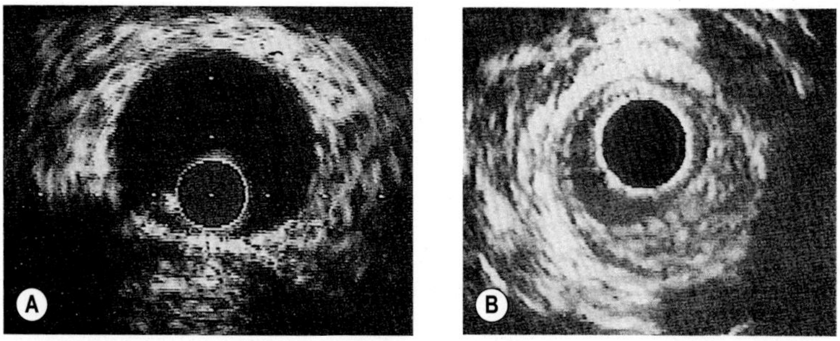

Figure 13.58 Intravascular ultrasound. **(A)** Non-obstructive, calcified plaque between the 5 and 7 o'clock position in a distal segment of the right coronary artery. The ultrasound's transducer is clearly visible at the intersection of the horizontal and vertical centimetre scales. **(B)** Coronary artery disease. A large semilunar, non-calcified coronary plaque that produced an intermediate severity stenosis on coronary angiography is shown extending from the 1 o'clock to the 7 o'clock position, severely reducing the vessel lumen.

Pulmonary angiography

Injection of contrast medium into the main pulmonary artery opacifies the arterial branches throughout both lung fields. The normal flow distribution is homogeneous. Vascular occlusions with regional perfusion defects usually indicate pulmonary thromboembolism (particularly when intraluminal filling defects are present) but may also occur in advanced emphysema. The high diagnostic accuracy of CT pulmonary angiography means that invasive pulmonary angiography is now rarely performed.

Intracardiac pressure measurement

Cardiac catheterization for measurement of blood flow and pressure within the heart and great vessels is widely used both for diagnostic purposes and to guide treatment. The fluid-filled catheter is attached to a pressure transducer, which converts the pressure waves into electrical signals. For measurement of right-sided pressures, the catheter is directed by the venous route into the right atrium and then advanced through the right ventricle into the pulmonary artery. For measurement of left-sided pressures, the catheter is directed by the arterial route into the ascending aorta and advanced retrogradely through the aortic valve into the left ventricle. Because access to the left atrium is technically difficult, left atrial pressure is usually measured indirectly using the pulmonary artery wedge pressure.

The pulmonary artery wedge pressure is obtained during right-heart catheterization by advancing the catheter distally into the pulmonary arterial tree until the tip wedges in a small branch. Alternatively, a catheter with a preterminal balloon (Swan-Ganz catheter) may be used. Inflation of the balloon in the pulmonary artery causes the catheter tip to be carried with blood flow into a more distal branch, which becomes occluded by the balloon. Regardless of which method is used, the wedge pressure recorded at the catheter tip is a more or less accurate measure of the left atrial pressure transmitted retrogradely through the pulmonary veins and capillaries.

Haemodynamic evaluation of valvular stenosis

In the normal heart, there is no pressure gradient across an open valve. Such a gradient usually indicates valvular stenosis (Fig. 13.59) and, as stenosis worsens, the pressure gradient increases. This therefore provides a useful index of the severity of stenosis. However, it must be recognized that the pressure gradient is influenced by the flow through the valve. For example, if cardiac output is very low, the gradient may be

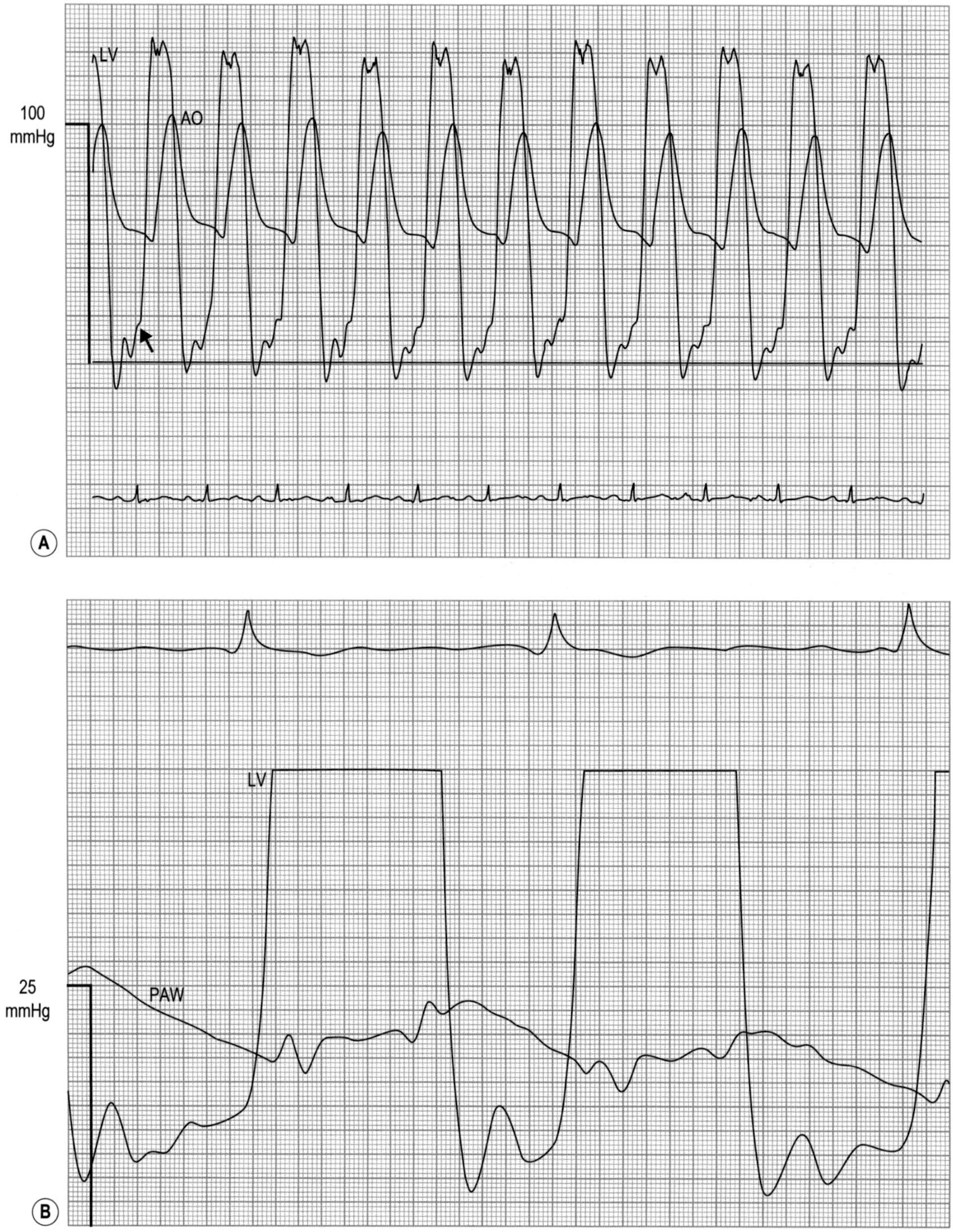

Figure 13.59 Valvular stenosis: pressure signals. **(A)** Aortic stenosis. Simultaneous left ventricular (LV) and aortic (AO) pressure signals. In the normal heart, the pressure signals should be essentially similar throughout systole. Here there is a peak systolic gradient of about 35 mmHg across the aortic valve. Note the prominent 'a' wave (arrow), reflecting the major contribution that atrial systole makes to filling of the hypertrophied, non-compliant ventricle. Note also the pulsus alternans indicating left ventricular failure. **(B)** Mitral stenosis: simultaneous recordings of the pulmonary artery wedge (PAW) and left ventricular (LV) pressure signals. In the normal heart, the pressure signals should be superimposed throughout diastole. Here there is a pressure gradient >10 mmHg, indicating severe mitral stenosis. Note that the patient is in atrial fibrillation and the pressure gradient varies inversely with the RR interval, tending to increase as the RR interval shortens.

small despite the presence of severe stenosis. This applies particularly to the aortic valve because flow velocity is normally high. In patients with poor left ventricular function, the 2D appearances of the valve on echocardiography and estimates of valve area should be considered before concluding that significant aortic stenosis is not present.

Haemodynamic evaluation of intracardiac shunts

Left-to-right intracardiac shunts through atrial or ventricular septal defects introduce 'arterialized' blood into the right side of the heart. This results in an abrupt increase or step-up in the oxygen saturation of venous blood at the level of the shunt, which can be detected by right heart catheterization. Thus, by drawing serial blood samples for oxygen saturation from the pulmonary artery, right ventricle, right atrium and vena cava, the shunt may be localized to the site at which the step-up in oxygen saturation occurs. The magnitude of the step-up is related to the size of the shunt, but precise quantification of the shunt requires measurement of pulmonary and systemic blood flow. The extent to which the pulmonary-systemic flow ratio exceeds 1 is a measure of the size of the shunt.

Haemodynamic evaluation of constriction and tamponade

In constrictive pericarditis and tamponade (Boxes 13.23 and 13.24), diastolic relaxation of the ventricles is impeded, preventing adequate filling. Compensatory increments in atrial pressures occur to help maintain ventricular filling, and because these disorders usually affect both ventricles equally, the filling pressures also equilibrate. Thus, simultaneous left- and right-sided recordings in constrictive pericarditis and tamponade show characteristic elevation and equalization of the filling pressures (atrial or ventricular end-diastolic), with loss of the normal differential (Fig. 13.60). Similar physiology characterizes restrictive cardiomyopathy, in which infiltrative disease (usually amyloid in the UK) impedes relaxation of the ventricles.

Measurement of cardiac output

Measurement of cardiac output is usually calculated by thermodilution using a Swan-Ganz catheter with a right atrial portal and a terminal thermistor positioned in the pulmonary artery. A known volume of cold saline (usually 10 ml) is injected into the right atrium and the temperature reduction in the pulmonary artery is recorded at the thermistor. The contour of the cooling curve is dependent on cardiac output, which is calculated by measuring the area under the curve using a bedside computer.

Cardiac output can also be measured by a variety of non-invasive methods including oesophageal Doppler probe, pulse waveform analysis, bioimpedance

Box 13.23 Constriction

Typical patient

- Middle-aged or elderly patient with a long history of progressive debilitation

Major symptoms

- Dyspnoea and weight loss with abdominal discomfort

Major signs

- Fluid retention with raised JVP (prominent 'x' and 'y' descents), hepatomegaly and peripheral oedema; diastolic filling sound ('pericardial knock'); paradoxical rise in JVP with inspiration (Kussmaul's sign)

Diagnosis

- High level of clinical suspicion
- CT or MRI scan: increased pericardial thickness (±calcification)
- Cardiac catheterization: equalization of diastolic pressures in the four cardiac chambers

Additional investigations

- Chest X-ray: often normal but occasionally shows pericardial calcification on lateral film

Comments

- Tuberculosis no longer commonest cause in developed countries, where most cases are idiopathic

Box 13.24 Tamponade

Typical patient

- Either middle-aged or elderly patient with malignant disease (usually breast or lung) or patients of any age with tuberculosis

Major symptoms

- Dyspnoea and variable circulatory collapse

Major signs

- Low-output state (hypotension, oliguria, cold periphery), tachycardia, paradoxical pulse, raised JVP with rapid 'x' descent, paradoxical rise in JVP on inspiration (Kussmaul's sign)

Diagnosis

- This is a clinical diagnosis, confirmed by echocardiographic demonstration of pericardial effusion

Additional investigations

- ECG: low-voltage QRS complexes with alternating electrical axis
- Tests for aetiological diagnosis: these might include serological tests for rheumatoid and systemic lupus erythematosus and tests for malignant or tuberculous disease

Comments

- Any cause of pericardial effusion may produce tamponade, malignant disease being the commonest cause in developed countries. Pericardiocentesis relieves the tamponade. Pericardial fluid should always be sent for cytological and bacteriological analysis

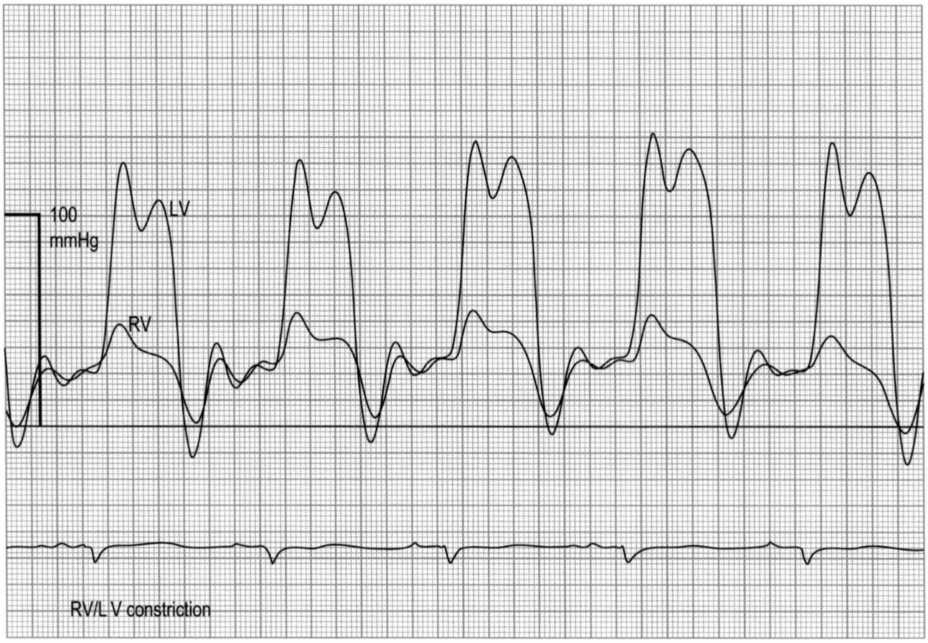

Figure 13.60 Pericardial constriction: left (LV) and right (RV) ventricular pressure signals. Like tamponade and restrictive cardiomyopathy, constriction usually affects both ventricles equally and the diastolic pressures must rise and equilibrate to maintain ventricular filling. Thus, in diastole, the pressure signals are superimposed with a typical 'dip and plateau' configuration ('square root' sign).

and echocardiography. Stroke volume can be calculated using 2D echocardiography from the estimated difference in left ventricular volumes at the end of systole and diastole. Alternatively, Doppler echocardiography can be used to measure stroke volume.

Cardiac output measurement is performed most commonly in intensive care units to characterize cardiovascular status and monitor responses to treatment. It is particularly valuable in the patient in shock whose intravascular volume status cannot be determined by clinical assessment.

Pathology laboratory support

Haematology laboratory

Anaemia exacerbates angina by adversely affecting the myocardial oxygen supply-demand relationship and also exacerbates heart failure by increasing the cardiac work necessary to meet the oxygen demands of metabolizing tissues. Rarely, anaemia is a consequence of, rather than a contributor to, heart disease. In infective endocarditis, a normochromic normocytic anaemia is almost invariable, reflecting the adverse effects of chronic illness on erythropoiesis. Chronic haemolysis occasionally occurs in patients with mechanical prosthetic heart valves and is caused by traumatic erythrocyte damage. Anaemia is usually low grade but if severe may require removal of the prosthesis and substitution with a xenograft.

Biochemistry laboratory

Cardiac enzymes and other markers of myocardial injury

Following myocardial infarction, enzymes and structural proteins released into the circulation by the necrosing myocytes provide biochemical markers of injury. In the UK, until recently, creatine kinase (CK) was the most widely used marker, the MB isoenzyme being the most specific for myocardial injury. However, newer serum markers of myocardial injury, particularly the highly specific troponins T and I, have replaced enzymatic markers. Indeed, these form the basis of the updated definition of myocardial infarction, which is diagnosed in any patient with raised circulating troponins who presents with cardiac chest pain or who develops regional ST elevation on the 12-lead ECG. Implicit in this definition is the fact that myocardial infarction may be diagnosed in patients without ST elevation. In non-ST elevation myocardial infarction (non-STEMI), the increase in circulating troponin concentration is a useful measure of risk, troponin concentration correlating directly with rates of recurrent myocardial infarction and death, and it is widely used to guide decisions about cardiac catheterization and coronary revascularization.

Increased ventricular wall stress (which occurs in heart failure, left ventricular hypertrophy etc.) causes release of natriuretic peptides from the heart (brain natriuretic peptide, BNP and its precursor, N-terminal pro BNP), causing dilatation and natriuresis. High levels are associated with worsening symptoms and prognosis. They can be used to determine whether breathless patients need further cardiological investigations or need to be assessed for lung disease. Patients with low levels of BNP are unlikely to have heart failure.

Renal function

Renal function should always be measured in the cardiac patient. Renal dysfunction is a major cause (and consequence) of hypertension whereas in heart failure, progressive deterioration of renal function is almost inevitable as perfusion of the kidneys becomes threatened. Renal function may also deteriorate in response to treatment with diuretics and angiotensin-converting enzyme (ACE) inhibitors, and careful monitoring is essential as these drugs are introduced. Cardiac drugs that are excreted through the kidneys (e.g. digoxin) should be used cautiously if renal function is impaired. In the patient with established renal failure, accelerated coronary artery disease and heart failure commonly occur, reflecting the combined effects of dyslipidaemia, hypertension, arterial endothelial dysfunction, anaemia and volume loading on the cardiovascular system. Cardiovascular disease is the major cause of death in patients with renal failure.

Electrolytes

Patients with hypokalaemia are at risk of lethal cardiac arrhythmias, while hyperkalaemia may cause bradyarrhythmias and heart block. Patients presenting with acute coronary syndromes commonly have hypokalaemia, due to the effects of sympathoadrenal activation on membrane-bound sodium–potassium ATPase, and this may require correction. For patients taking thiazide or loop diuretics, potassium supplements (or potassium-sparing diuretics) are usually necessary to protect against hypokalaemia unless ACE inhibitors are also given. The combination of an ACE inhibitor and an aldosterone antagonist is used in patients with severe heart failure and can be complicated by hyperkalaemia. Serum potassium should always be measured in patients with hypertension, not only to provide a baseline before the introduction of diuretic therapy but also as a simple screening test for primary aldosteronism. Hyponatraemia is common with chronic diuretic use.

Glucose and lipids

Blood glucose and lipid profiles (triglycerides, total cholesterol and high-density lipoprotein (HDL) and low-density lipoprotein (LDL) cholesterol) should be measured in all patients with suspected vascular disease. In high-risk individuals, particularly those with diabetes, and in all patients with established coronary artery disease, statin therapy is essential regardless of the baseline lipid profile and reduces the cardiovascular event rate by about 25%. Statins lower LDL ('bad') cholesterol, but if HDL ('good') cholesterol is low, treatment with nicotinic acid or fibrates should be added. Treatment of diabetes protects against microvascular complications, and in hyperglycaemic patients with acute myocardial infarction, infusion of insulin and glucose is usually recommended.

Bacteriology laboratory

Blood culture

In suspected infective endocarditis (Box 13.25), treatment must not be delayed beyond the time necessary to obtain three to four blood samples for culture (Table 13.3). Aerobic, anaerobic and fungal cultures should be performed. Occasionally, bone marrow cultures are helpful for detection of *Candida* and *Brucella* endocarditis. *Coxiella* and *Chlamydia* can never be cultured from the blood and must be diagnosed by serological tests. Failure to detect bacteraemia may be due to pretreatment with antibiotics, inadequate sampling (up to six blood samples

Box 13.25 Infective endocarditis

Typical patient

- Elderly man or woman with mitral or aortic valve disease (often not previously recognized)
- Younger patients with congenital heart defects (usually ventricular septal defect or patent ductus arteriosus)
- Patient of any age with prosthetic heart valve or history of intravenous drug abuse

Major symptoms

- Non-specific feverish ('flu-like') illness

Major signs

- Fever and heart murmur (usually aortic or mitral regurgitation)
- Splinter haemorrhages and vasculitic rash may occur
- Clubbing, Osler's nodes and Roth's spots are rare

Diagnosis

- Blood culture: usually provides bacteriological diagnosis
- Echocardiogram: usually reveals valvular regurgitation ± vegetation

Additional investigations

- Haematology: leukocytosis; normochromic, normocytic anaemia
- Inflammatory markers: raised erythrocyte sedimentation rate and C-reactive protein
- Urinalysis: haematuria

Comments

- Formerly a disease of young adults, now seen more commonly in the elderly
- Diagnosis should always be considered in patients with fever and a heart murmur

Table 13.3 Organisms implicated in endocarditis

Organism	Typical source of infection	First choice of antibiotics (pending sensitivity studies)
Streptococcus viridans	Upper respiratory tract	Benzylpenicillin, gentamicin
Streptococcus faecalis	Bowel and urogenital tract	Ampicillin, gentamicin
Anaerobic streptococcus	Bowel	Ampicillin, gentamicin
Staphylococcus epidermidis	Skin	Flucloxacillin, gentamicin
Fungi: *Candida*, histoplasmosis	Skin and mucous membranes	Amphotericin B*, 5-fluorocytosine*
Coxiella burnetii	Complication of Q fever	Chloramphenicol*, tetracycline*
Chlamydia psittaci	Contact with infected birds	Tetracycline*, erythromycin
Acute disease		
Staphylococcus aureus	Skin	Flucloxacillin, gentamicin
Streptococcus pneumoniae	Complication of pneumonia	Benzylpenicillin, gentamicin
Neisseria gonorrhoeae	Venereal	Benzylpenicillin, gentamicin

*These drugs are not bactericidal, and valve replacement is nearly always necessary to eradicate infection.

should be taken over 24 hours) or infection with unusual microorganisms.

Serology

If a recent streptococcal throat infection can be confirmed by demonstrating an elevated serum antistreptolysin O titre, Jones's criteria may be used for the diagnosis of rheumatic fever (Box 13.26). The presence of two major criteria, or one major and two minor criteria, indicates a high probability of rheumatic fever. In suspected viral pericarditis or myocarditis, the aetiological diagnosis depends on the demonstration of elevated viral antibody titres in acute serum samples, which decline during convalescence. Virus may sometimes be cultured from throat swabs and stools.

Acknowledgement

The author would like to acknowledge the significant contribution of Adam D. Timmis and Andrew Archbold, the authors of the equivalent chapter in the previous edition of this textbook, on which this chapter is based.

Box 13.26 Jones's criteria for the diagnosis of rheumatic fever

Major criteria

- Carditis
- Polyarthritis
- Erythema marginatum
- Chorea
- Subcutaneous nodules

Minor criteria

- Fever
- Arthralgia
- Previous rheumatic fever
- Elevated erythrocyte sedimentation rate
- Prolonged PR interval

Gastrointestinal system 14

Andrew Rochford and Michael Glynn

Introduction

The human gastrointestinal (GI) tract is a complex system of serially connected organs approximately 8 m in length, extending from the mouth to the anus, which together with its connected secretory glands, controls the passage, processing, absorption and elimination of food. Symptoms of GI disorders are often non-specific, and signs of abnormality few unless the disease is advanced. The liver, biliary system and pancreas are embryologically part of the GI tract. Symptoms of disease in these organs can also be non-specific but each can give specific clinical features. Finally, from the standpoint of systematic history taking and examination, the kidneys, groin and genitalia are also considered in this chapter.

Symptoms of gastrointestinal disease

In normal health there is some awareness of the functioning of the gut, and this can be partly related to the body's needs. For example, thirst and hunger are common symptoms; the latter may be associated with epigastric discomfort and a dry mouth may suggest the need to drink. Swallowing is normally perceived, and there is temperature sensation in the upper and mid-oesophagus, as well as in the mouth. Vigorous peristaltic contractions in the gut, the movement of gas and fluid in the gut, called borborygmi, and the experience of a sensation of fullness in the colon and rectum prior to defaecation or during constipation and the call to stool are all aspects of the normal sensation of gut activity.

It is always sensible to remember that, although it is often convenient for doctors to classify symptoms according to their anatomical site of origin, patients present with single or groups of symptoms that characterize functional or disease processes. Therefore, history taking that follows these likely processes is more likely to lead to a meaningful diagnosis, particularly in the GI tract and abdomen for which many symptoms are not easily referable to a clear anatomical site.

The common symptoms of GI and abdominal disease are listed in Box 14.1 and are discussed individually below.

Dysphagia (and odynophagia)

Dysphagia is the awareness of something sticking in the throat or retrosternally during swallowing; odynophagia is the term that describes painful swallowing in the oropharynx or oesophagus and may occur with or without dysphagia. Dysphagia often has a significant cause which can be malignant and almost always needs investigation. An oesophageal or upper gastric carcinoma usually presents with dysphagia for solids progressing fairly quickly to liquids and with accompanying weight loss. A benign stricture (or rarely an oesophageal pouch) may follow the same pattern but much less rapidly. Neurogenic dysphagia may present with greater difficulty in swallowing liquids than solids, sometimes associated with aspiration or coughing. Odynophagia may indicate infection of the oesophageal mucosa, classically candida oesophagitis associated with HIV infection and other immuno-compromised states.

Heartburn

Heartburn is due to acid reflux from the stomach into the oesophagus. It causes pain in the epigastrium, retrosternally and in the neck. It is occasionally difficult to distinguish from angina pectoris and may cause atypical chest pain in various sites. It occurs particularly at night when the patient lies flat in bed or after bending or stooping when abdominal pressure is increased. Heartburn may be exacerbated by dietary intake (such as alcohol or very spicy foods) and certain medications (such as bisphosphonates).

Reflux

Reflux is a symptom which occurs without heartburn, when non-acidic fluid or bile regurgitates into the mouth, causing a bitter taste and a disagreeable sensation retrosternally.

Indigestion (dyspepsia)

Dyspepsia is the medical term for indigestion, a symptom which may include epigastric pain,

Box 14.1 Common symptoms of gastrointestinal and abdominal disease

- Dysphagia and odynophagia
- Heartburn and reflux
- Indigestion
- Flatulence
- Vomiting
- Anorexia
- Constipation
- Diarrhoea
- Alteration of bowel pattern
- Abdominal pain
- Abdominal distension
- Weight loss
- Haematemesis
- Rectal bleeding
- Melaena
- Jaundice
- Itching
- Urinary symptoms

heartburn, distension, nausea or 'an acid feeling' occurring after eating or drinking. The symptom is subjective and frequent. In many patients there is no demonstrable cause but it may be associated with *Helicobacter* infection, peptic ulceration, and acid reflux. Upper GI malignancy should be excluded in older patients who present with new onset dyspepsia.

Flatulence

Flatulence describes excessive wind. It is associated with belching, abdominal distension and the passage of flatus per rectum. It is only infrequently associated with organic disease of the GI tract but usually represents a functional disturbance, some of which is due to excessively swallowed air. In some patients it is clearly associated with certain foods such as vegetables.

Vomiting

Vomiting is a neurogenic response triggered by chemoreceptors in the brainstem or reflexly through irritation of the stomach. Vomiting consists of a phase of nausea, followed by hypersalivation, pallor, sweating and hyperventilation. Retching, an involuntary effort to vomit, then occurs followed by expulsion of gastric contents through the mouth and sometimes through the nose. Most nausea and vomiting of GI origin are associated with local discomfort in the abdomen. Non-GI disease, such as raised intracranial pressure or metabolic disturbance, should be suspected if there is painless vomiting not associated with eating.

Anorexia

Anorexia refers to loss of appetite, although some patients with GI disease have an appetite for food but feel full after just a few mouthfuls (a symptom described as early satiety). It often indicates important pathology particularly in the upper GI tract. It is important to recognize the symptom of anorexia as distinct from the psychiatric illness anorexia nervosa.

Constipation

The frequency of bowel action varies greatly from person to person. In developed countries, the statistical norm is between three bowel actions per day and three per week. Constipation is a subjective complaint. Patients may say they feel constipated when they sense that they have not adequately emptied the bowel by defaecation. The term is sometimes used to describe the passage of hard stools, irrespective of stool frequency. In clinical practice, the passage of formed stool less frequently than three times per week is usually taken to indicate an abnormality of bowel frequency, and if unresponsive to simple treatment or if there are associated features, then investigation may be needed.

Diarrhoea

Diarrhoea is also subjective, but the regular passage of more than three stools per day or the passage of a large amount of stool (more than 300 g/day) can certainly be called diarrhoea. It commonly results from dietary indiscretion or from viral or bacterial infection. Causes of chronic diarrhoea include inflammatory bowel disease, in which there may be associated passage of blood or mucus per rectum, or malabsorptive states. Steatorrhoea refers to the passage of pale, bulky stools containing excess fats that commonly float in water and are difficult to flush away.

Abdominal pain

Abdominal pain is a common symptom that often accompanies serious diagnoses but frequently has no definable cause. As with any pain, it is important to characterize its site, intensity, character, areas of radiation, duration and frequency, together with aggravating and relieving factors and associated features. The particular clinical problem of acute abdominal pain is discussed on page 138. The particular characteristics of pain from certain frequent and important causes are given in Box 14.2. Pain that comes in waves is described as colicky and may vary over time. Abdominal pain may also be due to causes that are not specifically in the abdomen such as metabolic disorders (porphyria or lead poisoning) or depression.

Abdominal distension

Abdominal distension has many causes, which include flatus, fluid (e.g. ascites) and pregnancy. Obesity may be perceived as abnormal abdominal distension by the patient but marked enlargement of the major organs or the presence of a large mass lesion should be excluded. Consideration should be given to whether the distension is symmetrical (as seen with ascites) or asymmetrical (as may be the case with marked organomegaly).

Box 14.2 Particular characteristics of pain from frequent and important causes (the regions of the abdomen are shown in Fig. 14.5 – the loin is lateral and posterior to the lumbar area)

- Peptic ulcer: epigastric, burning or gnawing, radiates through to back, meal related, wakes the patient, relieved by antacid
- Gastric cancer: epigastric, severe, partly meal related, not relieved by antacid
- Pancreatic: high epigastric, severe, felt front-to-back, immediately after eating, relieved by sitting forward
- Midgut: periumbilical, colicky, some relation to meals
- Lower gut: periumbilical or suprapubic, colicky, some relief from bowel action
- Biliary: right upper quadrant, severe, colicky (but over a long time period), radiates to right shoulder, accompanied by nausea
- Renal colic: loin-to-groin, colicky, very severe, accompanied by nausea
- Functional: anywhere in the abdomen, colicky, accompanied by bloating, relieved by bowel action

Weight loss

Weight loss may be due to lack of food intake (anorexia, dysphagia or vomiting), malabsorption of nutrients or a systemic effect of important diseases. There are diseases that directly cause malabsorption such as coeliac disease, inflammatory bowel disease or pancreatic exocrine insufficiency. Weight loss is also commonly associated with conditions such as cancer (within or outside the GI tract) or chronic infections such as tuberculosis (within or outside the GI tract).

Haematemesis

Haematemesis is the vomiting of blood and results from bleeding in the upper GI tract (above the duodenojejunal flexure). Blood that lies in gastric juice for a while turns black and may be vomited looking like ground coffee. Observed reports of vomiting blood by the patient or bystander may be unreliable and can be confused with haemoptysis (coughing up blood) or blood coming from the oral cavity.

Rectal bleeding

Bleeding from the sigmoid colon, rectum or anal canal typically causes bright red blood loss that is separate from the stool or just noticeable on the toilet paper; haemorrhoids are the commonest cause. If darker red and mixed with the stool, this usually indicates a source above the rectum, of which carcinoma is the most important cause. Large-volume rectal bleeding (haematochezia) in an ill patient may be from an upper GI source.

Melaena

Melaena describes altered blood that has passed through a significant length of the small bowel and looks jet-black, tarry and has a characteristic smell. It usually indicates bleeding proximal to the ileo-caecal valve but occasionally may originate from a source in the right colon.

Jaundice

Jaundice (or icterus) is a yellowish pigmentation of the skin and conjunctival membranes due to high levels of bilirubin in the blood. Its presence implies disease of the liver or the biliary tract although it may also be the result of excessive haemolysis. In addition to the characteristic colour of the skin and conjunctiva, there may be other associated cutaneous and systemic features of liver disease, often with dark urine (see below).

Urinary symptoms

These are discussed in Chapter 17.

Nutritional assessment

The simplest nutritional assessment is to ask about weight loss and what the patient's weight was before the illness. Patients at risk of weight loss and malnutrition may have GI disease preventing eating, reducing appetite or preventing absorption of nutrients or non-GI disease causing reduced appetite (especially malignancy). Increased energy consumption is also important in some cancer patients and those with severe sepsis, thyrotoxicosis or burns.

A full dietary history is best undertaken by a dietitian, but a full medical clerking in a patient who has lost weight needs to include a simple assessment of the quantity and variety of foods eaten, as well as any restrictions on eating (e.g. poor dentition, social and financial circumstance) or special diets followed for medical reasons (e.g. a gluten-free diet in coeliac disease).

A full examination will include most signs of general and nutrient-specific malnutrition. Some detail of the latter is given in Table 14.1. Body weight and patient height are key parts of the general examination. The two values are used to calculate the body mass index (BMI or Quetelet index). This is defined by body weight (in kilograms), divided by height (in metres) squared. The World Health Organization (WHO) classification of this index is given in Table 14.2. In the UK, the range 20-25 is often regarded as desirable, but the lower level of 18.5 is more applicable internationally. Patients with a BMI >30 should undergo weight loss. In malnourished children, retardation of height lags behind that of weight and the relation between weight and height should always be compared with age using appropriate charts. If height cannot be measured, there are nomograms which relate the length of the forearm (ulna) or knee height (knee to heel) to the true height. In addition, the state of nourishment can be assessed by the more specialized measurements of mid-upper arm

Table 14.1 Principal symptoms and signs due to vitamin and mineral deficiencies

Nutrients	Deficiency syndrome	Principal symptoms/signs
Vitamin A, retinol (carotenoids)	Protein-energy malnutrition	Night blindness, Bitot spots, keratomalacia
Vitamin B_1, thiamine	Wernicke/Korsakoff, beri-beri	Nystagmus, sixth cranial nerve palsy, ataxia (Wernicke's encephalopathy) Symmetrical peripheral neuropathy (dry beri-beri), fulminant cardiac failure, lactic acidosis (Shoshin beri-beri), high output cardiac failure (wet beri-beri)
Vitamin B_2, riboflavin	Ariboflavinosis	Angular stomatitis, glossitis, magenta tongue
Vitamin B3, niacin, nicotinic acid	Pellagra	Dermatitis of sun-exposed areas (including 'Casal's Necklace'), dementia, poor appetite, difficulty sleeping, diarrhoea
Vitamin B_6, pyridoxine	Deficiency associated with isoniazid use	Poor appetite, lassitude, oxaluria, seborrhea, neuropathy
Pantothenic acid		Nausea, abdominal pain, paraesthesiae, burning feet
Biotin		Dermatitis, depression, lassitude, muscle pains, electrocardiogram abnormalities, blepharitis
Folic acid	Deficiency associated with methotrexate use	Macrocytic anaemia, thrombocytopenia and megaloblastic bone marrow
Vitamin B_{12}	Pernicious anaemia	Subacute combined degeneration of the spine, macrocytic anaemia
Vitamin C, ascorbic acid	Scurvy	Poor wound healing, fatigue, limb pain, shortness of breath, difficulty sleeping, gingivitis, perifollicular purpura, hyperkeratosis
Vitamin D, ergo-/cholecalciferol	Rickets/osteomalacia	Bone pain, proximal myopathy, waddling gait, growth retardation
Vitamin E, tocopherol		Haemolysis, posterior column signs, ataxia, muscle wasting, retinitis pigmentosa-like changes, night blindness
Vitamin K, phylloquinone and other menaquinones	Chronic liver disease	Bruising, purpura, coagulopathy
Trace elements		
Iron		Koilonychia, smooth tongue, anaemia, oesophageal web, impaired cognitive development
Zinc	Acrodermatitis enteropathica	Peristomal/perinasal/perineal erythema, thin hair, diarrhoea, apathy, anorexia, growth failure, hypoglycaemia
Copper		Microcytic hypochromic anaemia, neutropenia, scurvy-like bone lesions, osteoporosis
Chromium		Peripheral neuropathy, hyperglycaemia
Selenium		Cardiomyopathy
Iodine		Goitre

Table 14.2 World Health Organization classification of body weight

Category	BMI/Quetelet index
Underweight	<18.5
Healthy weight	18.5-24.9
Overweight	25-29.9
Moderately obese	30-34.9
Severely obese	35-39.9
Morbidly obese	>40

circumference (MUAC), skin-fold thickness, waist circumference and waist/hip ratio.

All UK hospital inpatients are now assessed for their risk of malnutrition. The most common assessment method used by healthcare staff is the Malnutrition Universal Screening Tool (MUST). This involves calculating the patient's BMI and then adding on a score for the percentage of unexpected weight loss and a score for the degree of acute illness. The final score is used to trigger a full dietary assessment and initiation of treatment in those who need it. Patients should be screened weekly whilst in hospital and at every outpatient attendance.

Physical examination of the GI tract and abdomen

General signs

Systemic features of GI disease may be evident on general examination. Peripheral signs of chronic liver disease are listed in Box 14.3. Of these, the most common and useful are spider naevi (Fig. 14.1) (the presence of up to five can be normal) and palmar erythema (Fig. 14.2) (the blotchy appearance often being more important than the overall redness). Inflammatory bowel disease may give rise to clubbing of the hands, arthritis, uveitis and skin changes including erythema nodosum (tender raised red lumps on the extensor surface of the limbs) and the much rarer pyoderma gangrenosum. Anaemia accompanies many GI diseases, as does oedema, and lymphadenopathy can be secondary to GI malignancy.

It is helpful when examining the patient, recording in notes or communicating information to colleagues to remember the surface anatomy of the structures related to the GI tract and abdomen (Figs 14.3 and 14.4) and to think of the abdomen as divided into regions (Fig. 14.5). The two lateral vertical planes pass from the femoral artery below to cross the costal margin close to the tip of the ninth costal cartilage. The two horizontal planes, the subcostal and interiliac, pass across the abdomen to connect the lowest points on the costal margin and the tubercles of the iliac crests, respectively.

Remember that the area of each region will depend on the width of the subcostal angle and the proximity of costal margin to iliac crest, in addition to other features of bodily habitus which vary greatly from one patient to the next.

Box 14.3 Peripheral stigmata (signs) of chronic liver disease

Skin, nails and hands

- Spider naevi – small telangiectatic superficial blood vessels with a central feeding vessel
- Clubbing of the hands
- Leuconychia – expansion of the paler half-moon at the base of the nail
- Palmar erythema – seen on the thenar and hypothenar eminence – often with blotchy appearance
- Bruising
- Dupuytren's contracture – can occur in the absence of liver disease
- Scratch marks – particularly in cholestatic liver disease

Endocrine – due to excess oestrogens

- Gynaecomastia
- Testicular atrophy
- Loss of axillary and pubic hair

Other

- Parotid swelling – particularly in alcohol-related liver disease
- Hepatic foetor – characteristic sweet-smelling breath
- Hepatic flap – a sign of encephalopathy and advanced disease

Inspection

The patient should be lying supine with arms loosely at the sides, the head and neck supported by up to two pillows, sufficient for comfort (Fig. 14.6). A sagging mattress makes examination difficult, particularly palpation. Make sure there is a good light, that the room is warm and that the hands are warm. A shivering patient cannot relax and vital signs, especially on palpation, may be missed.

Stand on the patient's right side, introduce yourself to the patient and with his consent expose the abdomen by turning down all the bed clothes except the upper sheet. The clothing should then be drawn up to just above the xiphisternum and the sheet

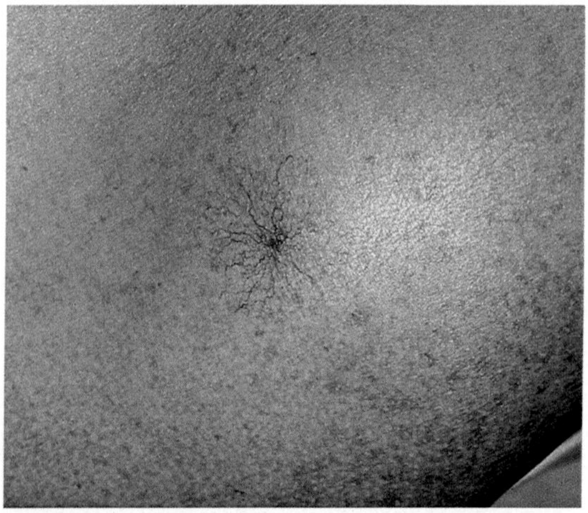

Figure 14.1 A typical spider naevus, with a central arteriole and fine radiating vessels.

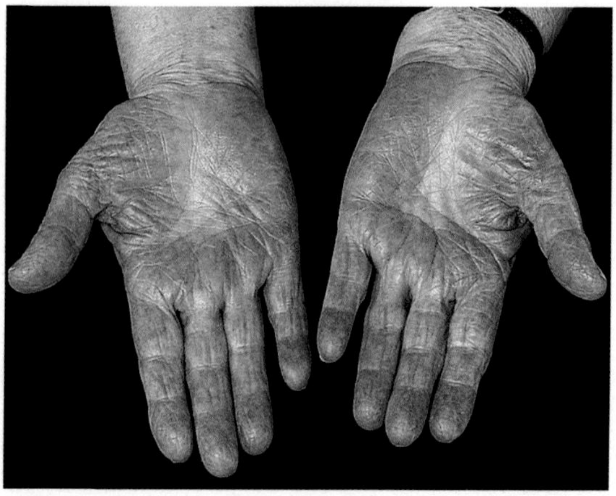

Figure 14.2 Palmar erythema in chronic liver disease (sparing the centre of the palms).

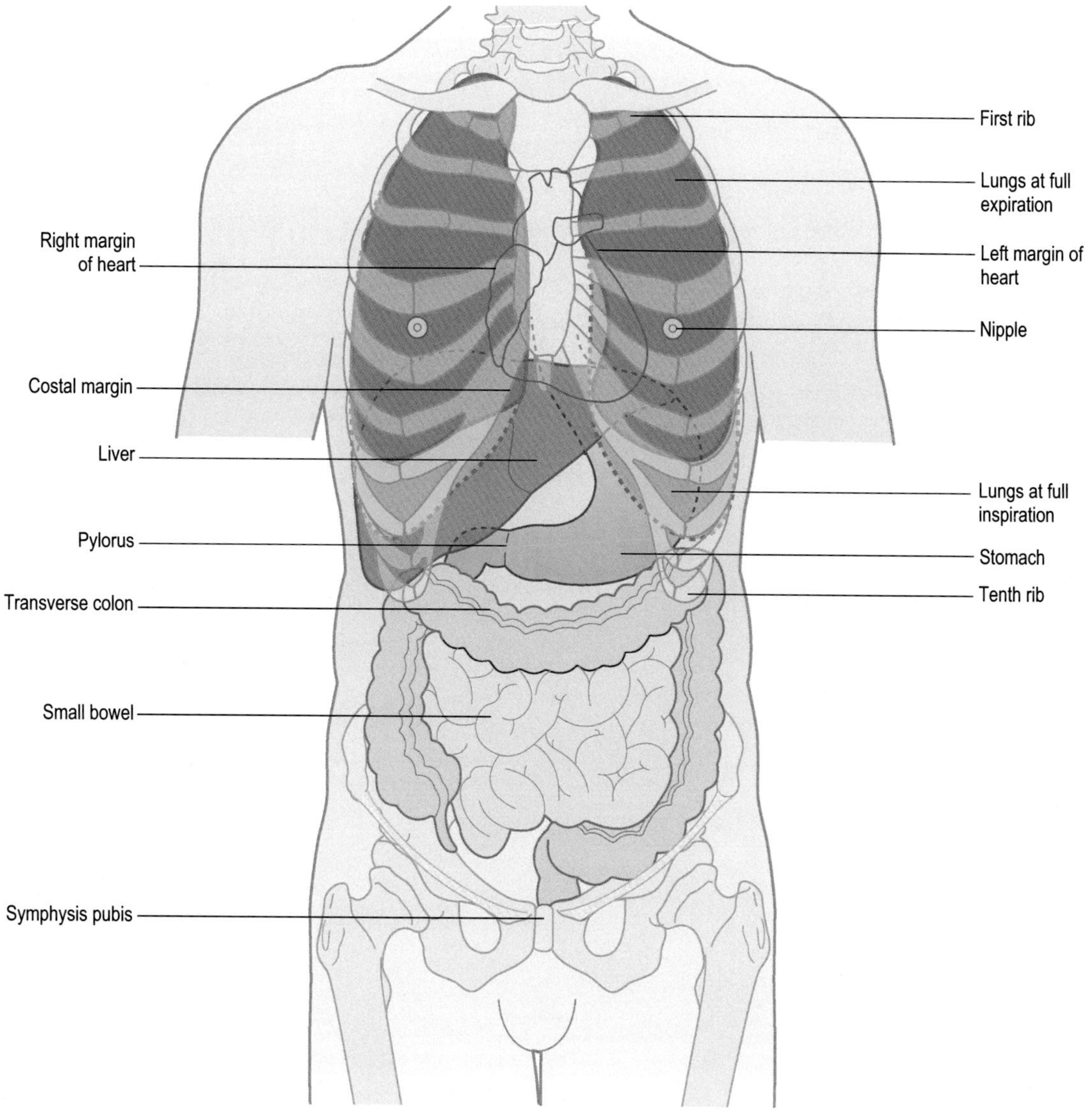

Figure 14.3 Anterior view of the external relationships of the abdominal and thoracic organs.

folded down to the level of the symphysis pubis. Traditional teaching was to expose the patient 'from nipples to knees', but in the modern era when patient dignity is of paramount importance, this approach is not acceptable. However, inspection of the groins and genitalia must not be neglected and needs to be carried out with discretion, with full explanation as to the reasons, and leaving these areas exposed for the minimum time. It is not unusual for a patient to present with intestinal obstruction due to a strangulated femoral or inguinal hernia where the diagnosis has been missed initially due to lack of proper inspection of the groins in an effort to save embarrassment. Inspection is an important and neglected part of abdominal examination. Initially, it is well worthwhile spending 30 seconds observing the abdomen from different positions to note the following features:

Shape

Is the abdomen of normal contour and fullness, or distended? Is it scaphoid (sunken)?

- Generalized fullness or distension may be due to fat, fluid, flatus, faeces or fetus.
- Localized distension may be symmetrical and centred around the umbilicus as in the case of small bowel obstruction, or asymmetrical as in gross enlargement of the spleen, liver or ovary.
- Make a mental note of the site of any such swelling or distension; think of the anatomical structures in that region and note if there is any movement of the swelling, either with, or independent of, respiration.
- Remember that chronic urinary retention may cause palpable enlargement in the lower abdomen.

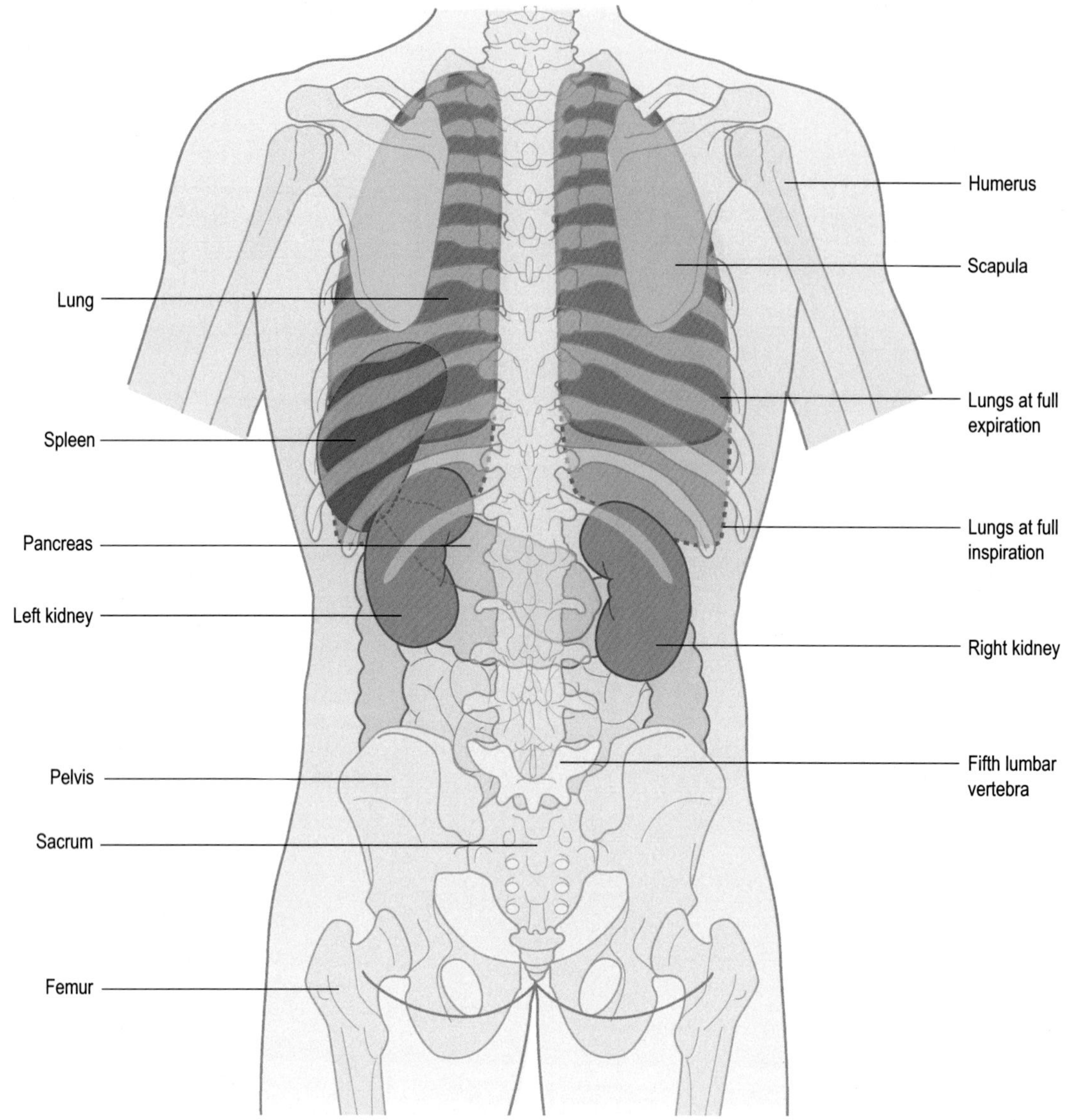

Figure 14.4 Posterior view of the external relationships of the abdominal and thoracic organs. The liver is not shown.

A scaphoid abdomen is seen in advanced stages of starvation and malignant disease.

The umbilicus

Normally the umbilicus is slightly retracted and inverted. If it is everted, then an umbilical hernia may be present and this can be confirmed by feeling an expansile impulse on palpation of the swelling when the patient coughs. The hernial sac may contain omentum, bowel or fluid. A common finding in the umbilicus of elderly obese people is a concentration of inspissated desquamated epithelium and other debris (omphalolith).

Movements of the abdominal wall

Normally there is a gentle rise in the abdominal wall during inspiration and a fall during expiration; the movement should be free and equal on both sides. In generalized peritonitis, this movement is absent or markedly diminished (the 'still, silent abdomen'). To aid the recognition of intra-abdominal movements, shine a light across the patient's abdomen. Even small movements of the intestine may then be detected by alterations in the pattern of shadows cast over the abdomen.

Visible pulsation of the abdominal aorta may be noticed in the epigastrium and is a frequent finding in nervous, thin patients. It must be distinguished from an aneurysm of the abdominal aorta, where pulsation is more obvious and a widened aorta is felt on palpation.

Visible peristalsis of the stomach or small intestine may be observed in three situations:

1 Obstruction at the pylorus. Visible peristalsis may occur where there is obstruction at the pylorus produced either by fibrosis following

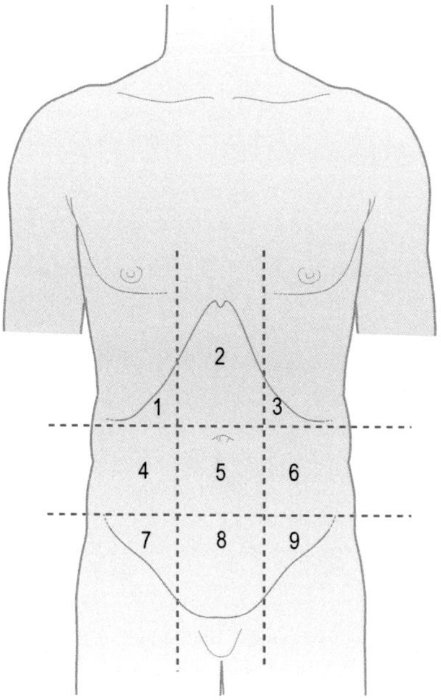

Figure 14.5 Regions of the abdomen. 1 and 3, right and left hypochondrium; 2, epigastrium; 4 and 6, right and left lumbar; 5, umbilical; 7 and 9, right and left iliac; 8, hypogastrium or suprapubic.

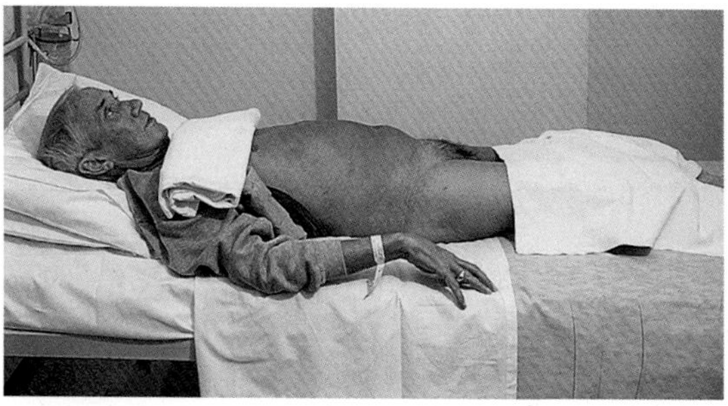

Figure 14.6 Position of the patient and exposure for abdominal examination. Note that the genitalia should be exposed only when necessary.

chronic duodenal ulceration or, less commonly, by carcinoma of the stomach in the pyloric antrum. In pyloric obstruction, a diffuse swelling may be seen in the left upper abdomen but, where obstruction is longstanding with severe gastric distension, this swelling may occupy the left mid and lower quadrants. Such a stomach may contain a large amount of fluid and, on shaking the abdomen, a splashing noise is usually heard ('succussion splash'). This splash is frequently heard in healthy patients for up to 3 hours after a meal, so enquire when the patient last ate or drank. In congenital pyloric stenosis of infancy, not only may visible peristalsis be apparent but also the grossly hypertrophied circular muscle of the antrum and pylorus may be felt as a 'tumour' to the right of the midline in the epigastrium. Both these signs may be

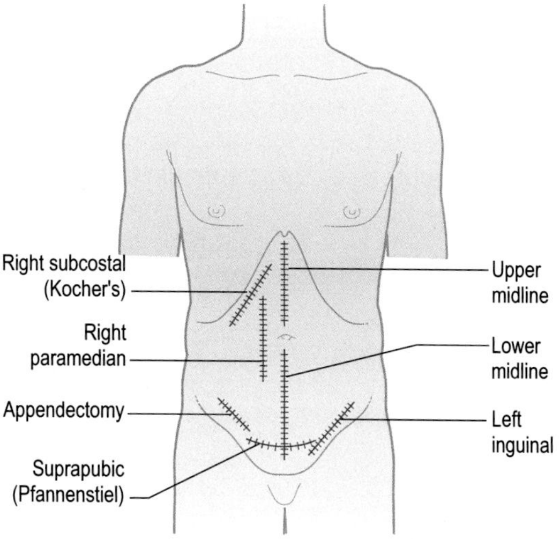

Figure 14.7 Some commonly used abdominal incisions. The midline and oblique incisions avoid damage to the innervation of the abdominal musculature and the later development of incisional hernia.

elicited more easily after the infant has been given a feed. Standing behind the child's mother with the child held on her lap may allow the child's abdominal musculature to relax sufficiently to feel the walnut-sized swelling.

2 Obstruction in the distal small bowel. Peristalsis may be seen where there is intestinal obstruction in the distal small bowel or coexisting large and small bowel hold-up produced by distal colonic obstruction, with an incompetent ileo-caecal valve allowing reflux of gas and liquid faeces into the ileum. Not only is the abdomen distended and tympanitic (hyper-resonant) but the distended coils of small bowel may be visible in a thin patient and tend to stand out in the centre of the abdomen in a 'ladder pattern'.

3 As a normal finding in very thin, elderly patients with lax abdominal muscles or large, wide-necked incisional herniae seen through an abdominal scar.

Skin and surface of the abdomen

In marked abdominal distension, the skin is smooth and shiny. Striae atrophica or gravidarum are white or pink wrinkled linear marks on the abdominal skin. They are produced by gross stretching of the skin with rupture of the elastic fibres and indicate a recent change in size of the abdomen, such as is found in pregnancy, ascites, wasting diseases and severe dieting. Wide purple striae are characteristic of Cushing's syndrome and excessive steroid treatment.

Note any scars present, their site, whether they are old (white) or recent (red or pink), linear or stretched (and therefore likely to be weak and contain an incisional hernia). Common examples are given in Fig. 14.7.

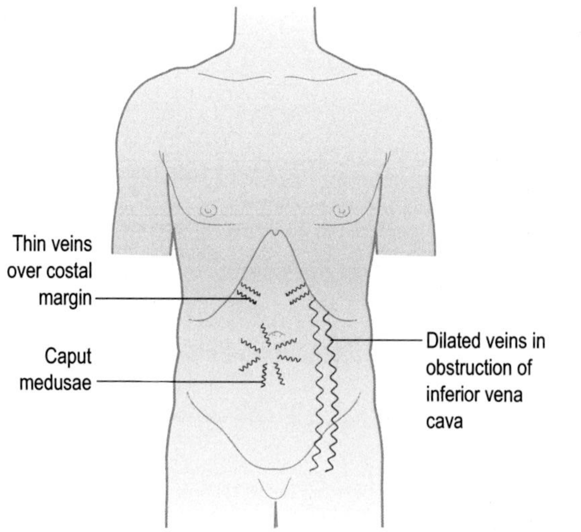

Figure 14.8 Prominent veins of the abdominal wall.

Look for prominent superficial veins, which may be apparent in three situations (Fig. 14.8): thin veins over the costal margin, usually of no significance; occlusion of the inferior vena cava; and venous anastomoses in portal hypertension. Inferior vena caval obstruction not only causes oedema of the limbs, buttocks and groins but, in time, distended veins on the abdominal wall and chest wall appear. These represent dilated anastomotic channels between the superficial epigastric and circumflex iliac veins below and the lateral thoracic veins above, conveying the diverted blood from the long saphenous vein to the axillary vein; the direction of flow is therefore upwards. If the veins are prominent enough, try to detect the direction in which the blood is flowing by occluding a vein, emptying it by massage and then looking for the direction of refill. Distended veins around the umbilicus (caput medusae) are uncommon but signify portal hypertension, other signs of which may include splenomegaly, ascites and other cutaneous manifestations of chronic liver disease. These distended veins represent the opening up of anastomoses between portal and systemic veins and occur in other sites, such as oesophageal and rectal varices.

Pigmentation of the abdominal wall may be seen in the midline below the umbilicus, where it forms the *linea nigra* and is a sign of pregnancy. Erythema *ab igne* is a brown mottled pigmentation produced by constant application of heat, usually a hot water bottle or heat pad, on the skin of the abdominal wall. It is a sign that the patient is experiencing severe persistent pain such as from chronic pancreatitis.

Finally, uncover and inspect both groins and the external genitalia. In male patients inspect and examine the penis and scrotum for any swellings and to ensure that both testes are in their normal position. Then bring the sheet back up to the level of the symphysis pubis.

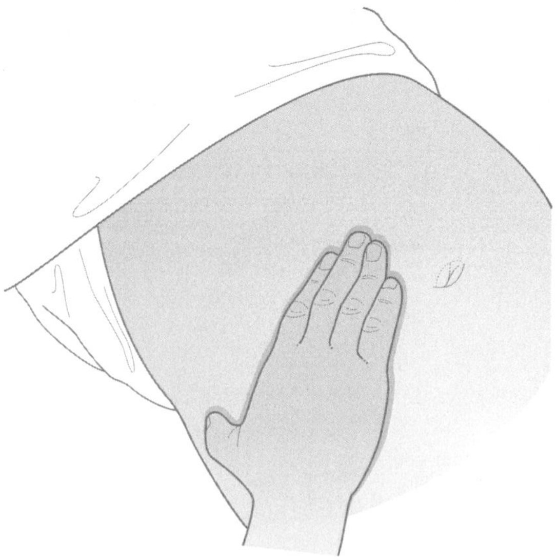

Figure 14.9 Correct method of palpation. The hand is held flat and relaxed and 'moulded' to the abdominal wall.

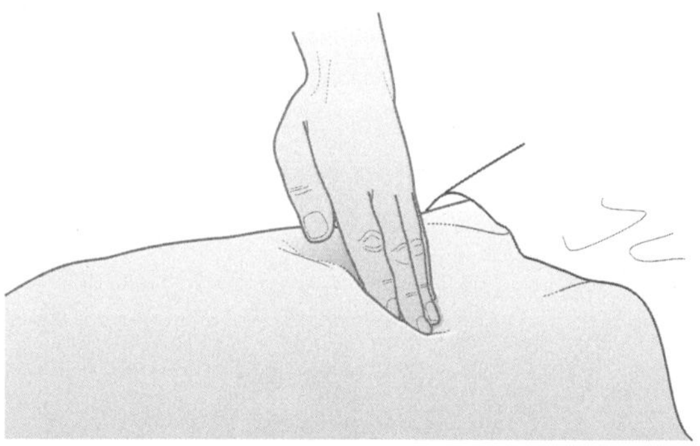

Figure 14.10 Incorrect method of palpation. The hand is held rigid and mostly not in contact with the abdominal wall.

Palpation

Palpation forms the most important part of the abdominal examination. Ask the patient to relax as much as possible, to breathe quietly, and assure him that you will be as gentle as possible. Enquire about the site of any pain and examine this region last. These points, together with unhurried palpation with a warm hand, will give the patient confidence and allow the maximum amount of information to be obtained.

When palpating, the wrist and forearm should be in the same horizontal plane where possible, even if this means bending down or kneeling by the patient's side. The best palpation technique involves moulding the relaxed right hand to the abdominal wall, not to hold it rigid (Fig. 14.9). The best movement is gentle but with firm pressure, with the fingers held almost straight but with slight flexion at the metacarpophalangeal joints and avoiding sudden poking with the fingertips (Fig. 14.10).

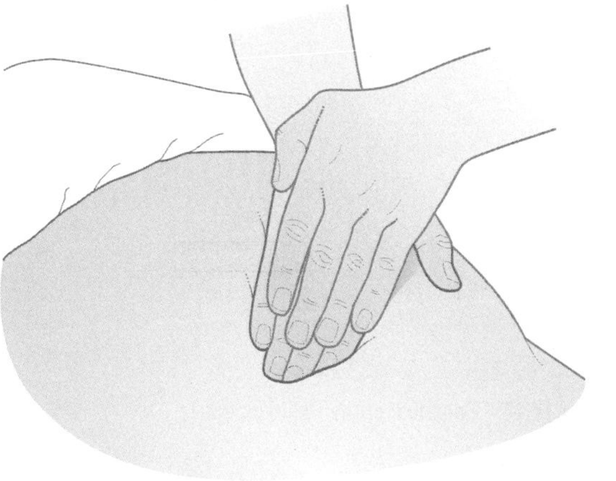

Figure 14.11 Method of deep palpation in an obese, muscular or poorly relaxed patient.

Palpation of intra-abdominal structures is an imperfect process in which the great sensitivity of the sense of touch and pressure is heavily masked by the abdominal wall tissue. It is unusual for structures to be very easily palpable and so it is necessary to concentrate fully on the task and to try to visualize the normal anatomical structures and what might be palpable beneath the examining hand. It may be necessary to repeat the palpation more slowly and deeply. Putting the left hand on top of the right allows increased pressure to be exerted (Fig. 14.11), such as with an obese or very muscular patient.

A small proportion of patients find it impossible to relax their abdominal muscles when being examined. In such cases, it may help to ask them to breathe deeply, to bend their knees up or to distract their attention in other ways. No matter how experienced the examiner, little will be gained from palpation of a poorly relaxed abdomen.

It is helpful to have a logical sequence to follow and, if this is done as a matter of routine, then no important point will be omitted. Always consider the underlying anatomy when examining the abdomen. The following scheme is suggested, which may need to be varied according to the site of any pain:

- Start in the left lower quadrant of the abdomen, palpating lightly, and repeat for each quadrant.
- Repeat using slightly deeper palpation examining each of the nine areas of the abdomen.
- Feel for the left kidney.
- Feel for the spleen.
- Feel for the right kidney.
- Feel for the liver.
- Feel for the aorta and para-aortic glands and common femoral vessels.
- Feel for the urinary bladder.
- Palpate both groins.
- Examine the external genitalia.
- If a swelling is palpable, spend time eliciting its features.

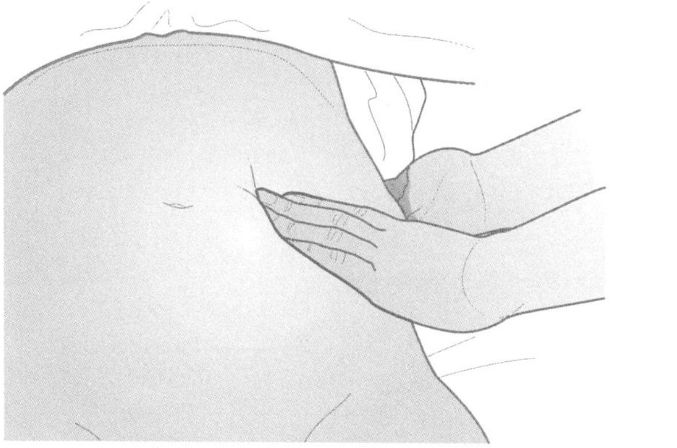

Figure 14.12 Palpation of the left kidney.

All the organs in the upper abdomen (liver, spleen, kidneys, stomach, pancreas, gallbladder) move downward with inspiration (with the spleen moving more downwards and medially). Thus, asking the patient to take a deep breath while examining makes detection of these organs easier. When the patient breathes in, the examining hand should be still so that the organ in question 'comes on to the examining hand' or 'slips by underneath it'.

Left kidney

The right hand is placed anteriorly in the left lumbar region while the left hand is placed posteriorly in the left loin (Fig. 14.12). Ask the patient to take a deep breath in, press the left hand forward and lift the right hand upward and inward. The left kidney is not usually palpable unless either low in position or enlarged. Its lower pole, when palpable, is felt as a rounded firm swelling between both right and left hands (i.e. bimanually palpable) and it can be pushed from one hand to the other, in an action which is called 'ballotting'.

Spleen

Like the left kidney, the spleen is not normally palpable. It has to be enlarged to two or three times its usual size before it becomes palpable and then is felt beneath the left subcostal margin. Enlargement takes place in a superior and posterior direction before it becomes palpable subcostally. Once the spleen has become palpable, the direction of further enlargement is downwards and towards the right iliac fossa (Fig. 14.13). Place the flat of the left hand over the lowermost rib cage posterolaterally, thus restricting the expansion of the left lower ribs on inspiration and concentrating more of the inspiratory movement into moving the spleen downwards. The right hand is placed beneath the costal margin well out to the left. Press in deeply with the fingers of the right hand beneath the costal margin, at the same time exerting considerable pressure medially and downwards with the left hand (Fig. 14.14), and then ask the patient to breathe in deeply. Repeat this manoeuvre with

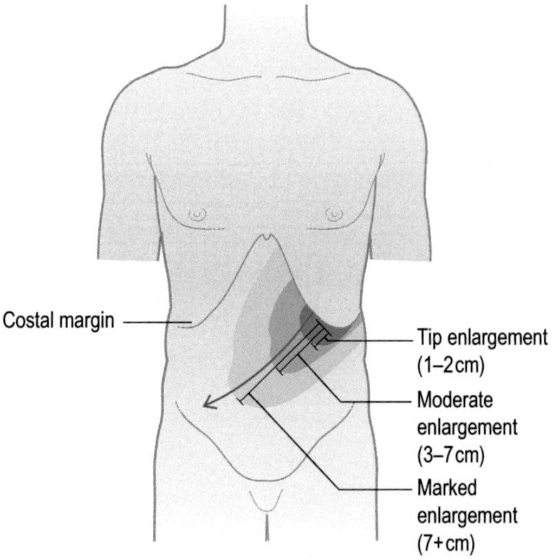

Figure 14.13 The direction of enlargement of the spleen. The spleen has a characteristic notched shape and the organ moves downwards during full inspiration.

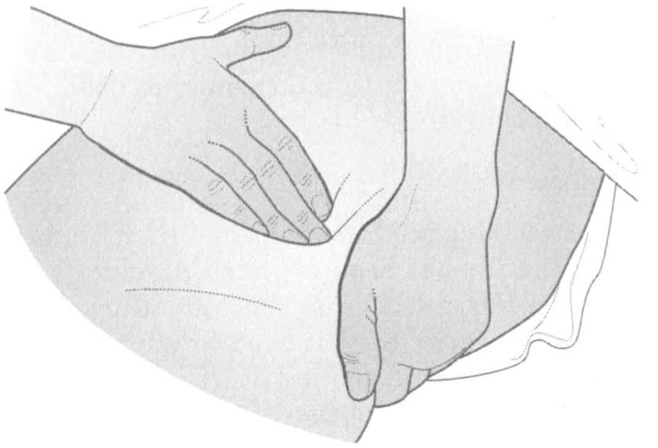

Figure 14.14 Palpation of the spleen. Start well out to the left.

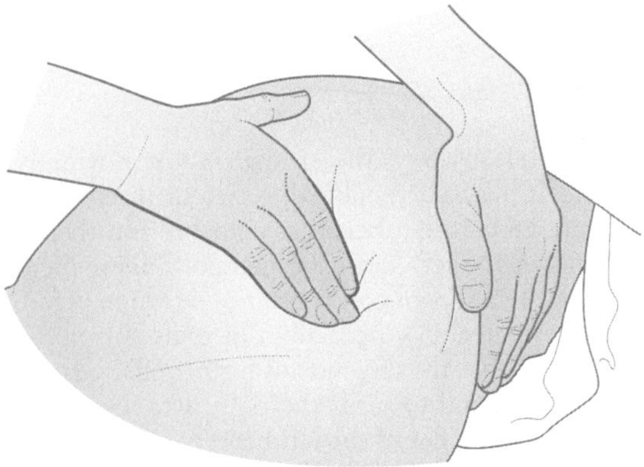

Figure 14.15 Palpation of the spleen more medially than in Fig. 14.14.

the right hand being moved more medially beneath the costal margin on each occasion (Fig. 14.15). If enlargement of the spleen is suspected from the history and it is still not palpable, turn the patient half on to the right side, ask him to relax back on to your left hand, which is now supporting the lower

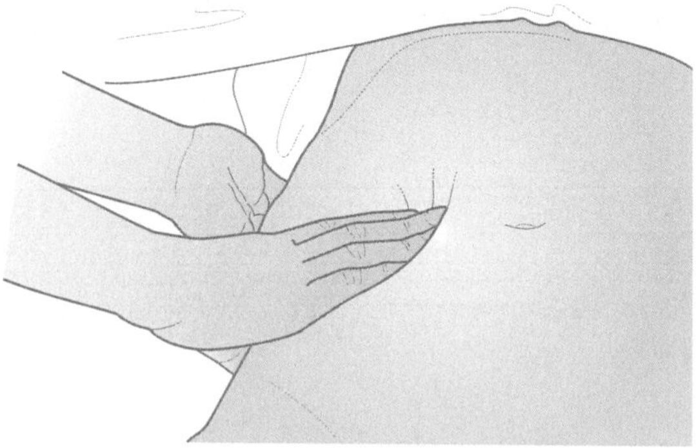

Figure 14.16 Palpation of the right kidney.

ribs, and repeat the examination as above. Alternatively the spleen may be very large and the lower edge may be much lower than at first suspected. It may help to ask the patient to place the left hand on your right shoulder while palpating for the spleen.

In minor degrees of enlargement, the spleen will be felt as a firm swelling with smooth, rounded borders. Where considerable splenomegaly is present, its typical characteristics include a firm swelling appearing beneath the left subcostal margin in the left upper quadrant of the abdomen, which is dull to percussion, moves downwards on inspiration, is not bimanually palpable, whose upper border cannot be felt (i.e. one cannot 'get above it') and in which a notch can often, though not invariably, be felt in the lower medial border. The last three features distinguish the enlarged spleen from an enlarged kidney; in addition, there is usually a band of colonic resonance anterior to an enlarged kidney.

Right kidney

Feel for the right kidney in much the same way as for the left. Place the right hand horizontally in the right lumbar region anteriorly with the left hand placed posteriorly in the right loin. Push forwards with the left hand, lift the right hand inward and upward (Fig. 14.16) and ask the patient to take a deep breath in. The lower pole of the right kidney, unlike the left, is commonly palpable in thin patients and is felt as a smooth, rounded swelling which descends on inspiration and is bimanually palpable and may be 'ballotted' (bounced back and forth between the two examining hands).

Liver

Place both hands side by side flat on the abdomen in the right subcostal region lateral to the rectus with the fingers pointing towards the ribs. If resistance is encountered, move the hands further down until this resistance disappears. Exert gentle pressure and ask the patient to breathe in deeply. Concentrate on whether the edge of the liver can be felt moving downwards and under the examining hand (Fig. 14.17).

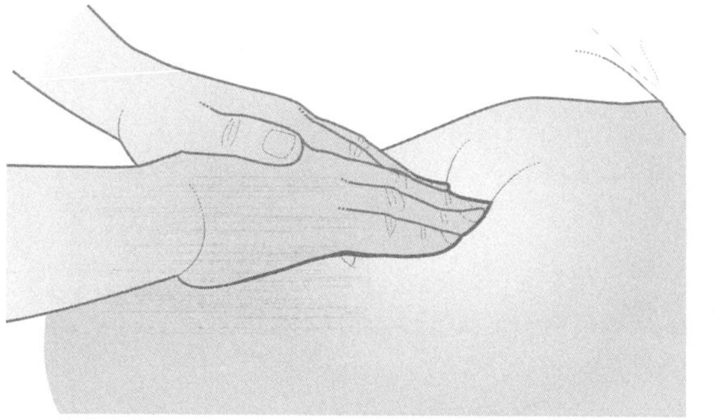

Figure 14.17 Palpation of the liver: preferred method.

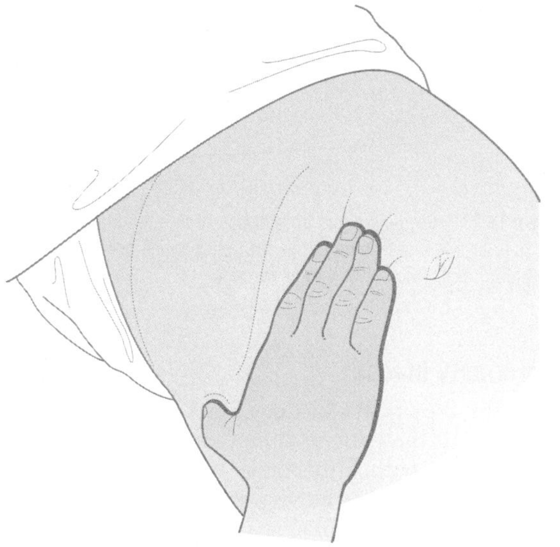

Figure 14.18 Palpation of the liver: alternative method.

Repeat this manoeuvre working from lateral to medial regions to trace the liver edge as it passes upwards to cross from right hypochondrium to epigastrium. Another commonly employed method of feeling for an enlarged liver is to place the right hand below and parallel to the right subcostal margin. The liver edge will then be felt against the radial border of the index finger (Fig. 14.18). The liver is often palpable in normal patients without being enlarged. The lower edge of the liver can be clarified by percussion (see below), as can the upper border in order to determine overall size: a palpable liver edge can be due to enlargement or displacement downwards by lung pathology. Hepatomegaly conventionally is measured in centimetres palpable below the right costal margin, which should be determined with a ruler if possible. Alternatively, displacement measured in fingerbreadths is an acceptable way of describing hepatomegaly.

Try to discern the character of the liver surface (i.e. whether it is soft, smooth and tender as in heart failure, very firm and regular as in obstructive jaundice and cirrhosis, or hard, irregular, painless and sometimes nodular as in advanced secondary carcinoma). In

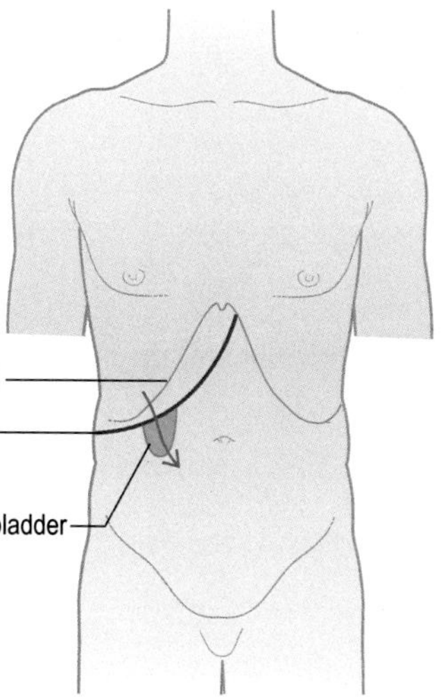

Figure 14.19 Palpation of an enlarged gallbladder, showing how it merges with the inferior border of the liver so that only the fundus of the gallbladder and part of its body can be palpated.

tricuspid regurgitation, the liver may be felt to pulsate. Occasionally a congenital variant of the right lobe projects down lateral to the gallbladder as a tongue-shaped process called Riedel's lobe. Though uncommon, it is important to be aware of this because it may be mistaken either for the gallbladder itself or for the right kidney.

Gallbladder

The gallbladder is palpated in the same way as the liver. The normal gallbladder cannot be felt. When it is distended, however, it forms an important sign and may be palpated as a firm, smooth, or globular swelling with distinct borders, just lateral to the edge of the rectus abdominis near the tip of the ninth costal cartilage. It moves with respiration. Its upper border merges with the lower border of the right lobe of the liver or disappears beneath the costal margin and therefore can never be felt (Fig. 14.19). When the liver is enlarged or the gallbladder grossly distended, the latter may be felt not in the hypochondrium but in the right lumbar or even as low down as the right iliac region.

The ease of definition of the rounded borders of the gallbladder, its comparative mobility on respiration, the fact that it is not normally bimanually palpable and that it seems to lie just beneath the abdominal wall helps to identify such a swelling as the gallbladder rather than a palpable right kidney. A painless gallbladder can usually be palpated in the following clinical situations:

- In a jaundiced patient with carcinoma of the head of the pancreas or other malignant causes of obstruction of the common bile duct (below the entry of the cystic duct), the ducts above the obstruction become dilated, as does the gallbladder (see Courvoisier's law, below).

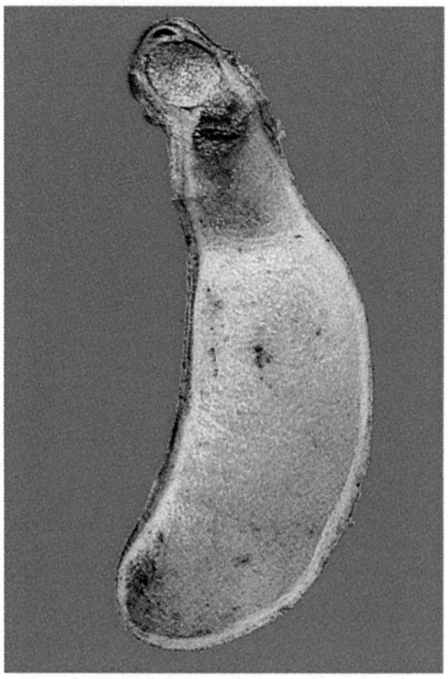

Figure 14.20 A mucocele of the gallbladder that is distended, pale and thin walled.

- In mucocele of the gallbladder, a gallstone becomes impacted in the neck of a collapsed, empty, uninfected gallbladder and mucus continues to be secreted into its lumen (Fig. 14.20). Eventually, the uninfected gallbladder is so distended that it becomes palpable. In this case, the bile ducts are normal and the patient is not jaundiced.
- In carcinoma of the gallbladder, the gallbladder may be felt as a stony, hard, irregular swelling, unlike the firm, regular swelling in the two above-mentioned conditions.

Murphy's sign

In acute inflammation of the gallbladder (acute cholecystitis), severe pain is present. Often an exquisitely tender but indefinite mass can be palpated; this represents the underlying acutely inflamed gallbladder walled off by greater omentum. Ask the patient to breathe in deeply and palpate for the gallbladder in the normal way; at the height of inspiration, the breathing stops with a gasp as the mass is felt. This represents Murphy's sign. The sign is not found in chronic cholecystitis or uncomplicated cases of gallstones.

Courvoisier's law

Courvoisier's law states that in the presence of jaundice, a palpable gallbladder makes gallstone obstruction of the common bile duct an unlikely cause (because it is likely that the patient will have had gallbladder stones for some time and these will have rendered the wall of the gallbladder relatively fibrotic and therefore non-distensible). However, the converse is not true, because the gallbladder is not palpable in many patients who do turn out to have malignant bile duct obstruction.

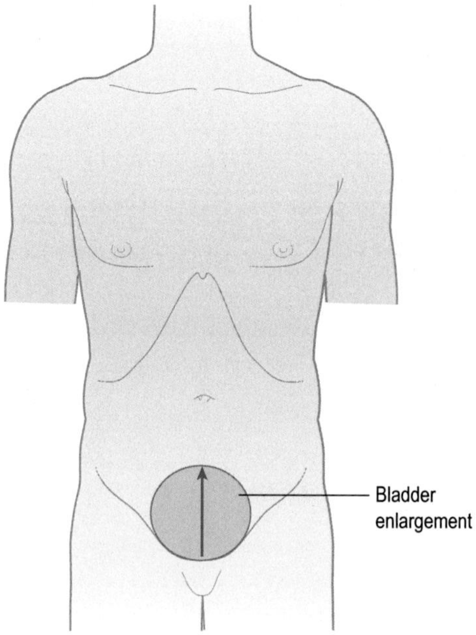

Figure 14.21 Physical signs in retention of urine: a smooth, firm and regular swelling arising out of the pelvis which one cannot 'get below' and which is dull to percussion.

The urinary bladder

Normally the urinary bladder is not palpable. When it is full and the patient cannot empty it (retention of urine), a smooth, firm, regular oval-shaped swelling will be palpated in the suprapubic region and its dome (upper border) may reach as far as the umbilicus. The lateral and upper borders can be readily identified, but it is not possible to feel its lower border (i.e. the swelling is 'arising out of the pelvis'). The fact that this swelling is symmetrically placed in the suprapubic region beneath the umbilicus, that it is dull to percussion and that pressure on it gives the patient a desire to micturate, together with the signs above, confirm such a swelling as the bladder (Fig. 14.21).

In women, however, a mass that is thought to be a palpable bladder has to be differentiated from a gravid uterus (firmer, mobile side to side), a fibroid uterus (may be bosselated and firmer) and an ovarian cyst (usually eccentrically placed to left or right side).

The aorta and common femoral vessels

In most adults, the aorta is not readily felt, but with practice it can usually be detected by deep palpation a little above and to the left of the umbilicus. In thin patients, particularly women with a marked lumbar lordosis, the aorta is more easily palpable. Palpation of the aorta is one of the few occasions in the abdomen when the fingertips are used as a means of palpation. Press the extended fingers of both hands, held side by side, deeply into the abdominal wall in the position shown in Fig. 14.22; identify the left wall of the aorta and note its pulsation. Remove both hands and repeat

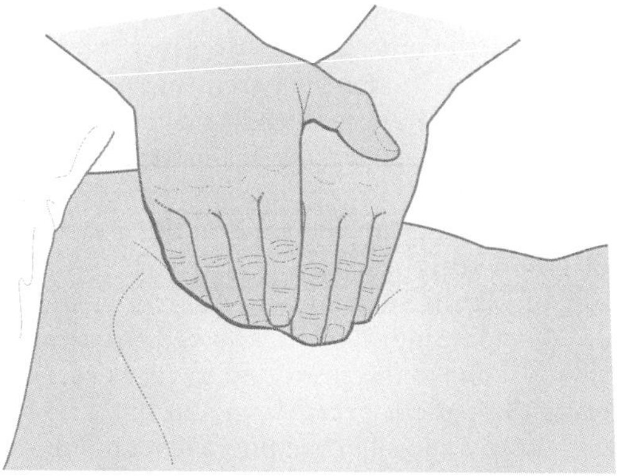

Figure 14.22 Palpation of the abdominal aorta.

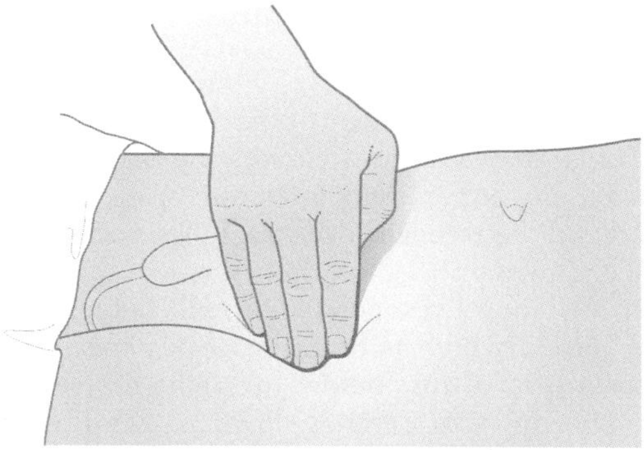

Figure 14.23 Palpation of the femoral vessels.

the manoeuvre a few centimetres to the right. In this way the pulsation and width of the aorta can be estimated. It is difficult to detect small aortic aneurysms; where a large one is present, its presence and width may be assessed by placing the extended fingertips on either side of it with the palms flat on the abdominal wall and the fingers pointing towards each other. When the fingertips are either side of an aneurysm, it should be clear that they are being separated by each pulsation and not just moved up and down (this latter manoeuvre can involve very deep palpation and the patient should be warned).

The common femoral vessels are found just below the inguinal ligament at the mid-point between the anterior superior iliac spine and symphysis pubis. Place the pads of the right index, middle and ring fingers over this site in the right groin and palpate the wall of the vessel. Note the strength and character of its pulsation and then compare it with the opposite femoral pulse (Fig. 14.23).

Lymph nodes lying along the aorta (para-aortic nodes) are palpable only when considerably enlarged. They are felt as rounded, firm, often confluent fixed masses in the umbilical region and epigastrium along the left border of the aorta. Pulsations of the aorta are transmitted through the nodes which separates them from the expansile pulsations palpated in aneurysmal dilatation.

Causes of diagnostic difficulty on palpation

In many patients, especially those with a thin or lax abdominal wall, faeces in the colon may simulate an abdominal mass. The sigmoid colon is frequently palpable, particularly when loaded with hard faeces. It is felt as a firm, tubular structure about 12 cm in length, situated low down in the left iliac fossa, parallel to the inguinal ligament. The caecum is often palpable in the right iliac fossa as a soft, rounded swelling with indistinct borders. The transverse colon is sometimes palpable in the epigastrium. It feels somewhat like the pelvic colon but rather larger and softer, with distinct upper and lower borders and a convex anterior surface. A faecal 'mass' will usually have disappeared or moved on repeat examination and may retain an indentation with pressure (not the case with a colonic malignancy).

In the epigastrium, the muscular bellies of rectus abdominis lying between its tendinous intersections can mimic an underlying mass and give rise to confusion. This can usually be resolved by asking the patient to tense the abdominal wall (by lifting the head off the pillow), when the 'mass' may be felt to contract.

What to do when an abdominal mass is palpable

When a mass in the abdomen is palpable, first make sure that it is not a normal structure, as described above. Consider whether it could be due to enlargement of the liver, spleen, right or left kidney, gallbladder, urinary bladder, aorta or para-aortic nodes. The aim of examination of a mass is to decide the organ of origin and the pathological nature. In doing this, it is helpful to bear in the mind the following points:

Site

Feeling the swelling while the patient lifts his head and shoulders off the pillow to tense the anterior abdominal wall will differentiate between a mass in the abdominal wall and within the abdominal cavity.

Note the region occupied by the swelling. Think of the organs that normally lie in or near this region and consider whether the swelling could arise from one of these organs. For instance, a swelling in the right upper quadrant most probably arises from the liver, right kidney, hepatic flexure of colon or gallbladder.

If the swelling is in the upper abdomen, try to determine if it is possible to 'get above it'; that is, to feel the upper border of the swelling as it disappears above the costal margin, and similarly, if it is in the lower abdomen, whether one can 'get below it'. If one cannot 'get above' an upper abdominal swelling, a hepatic, splenic, renal or gastric origin should be suspected. If one cannot 'get below' a lower abdominal mass, the swelling probably arises in the bladder, uterus, ovary or, occasionally, upper rectum.

Size and shape

As a general rule, gross enlargement of the liver, spleen, uterus, bladder or ovary presents no undue difficulty in diagnosis. On the other hand, swellings arising from the stomach, small or large bowel, retroperitoneal structures such as the pancreas, or the peritoneum (see section on mobility, below) may be difficult to diagnose. The larger a swelling arising from one of these structures, the more it tends to distort the outline of the organ of origin (e.g. a large renal mass can feel as if it is arising from intraperitoneal organs).

Surface, edge and consistency

The pathological nature of a mass is suggested by a number of features. A swelling that is hard, irregular in outline and nodular is likely to be malignant, while a regular, round, smooth, tense swelling is likely to be cystic. A solid, ill-defined and tender mass suggests an inflammatory lesion such as may be seen in ileocaecal Crohn's disease.

Mobility and attachments

Swellings arising in the liver, spleen, kidneys, gallbladder and distal stomach all show downward movement during inspiration, due to the normal downward diaphragmatic movement, and such structures cannot be moved with the examining hand. Tumours of the small bowel and transverse colon, cysts in the mesentery and large secondary deposits in the greater omentum are not usually influenced by respiratory movements, but may easily move on palpation.

When the swelling is completely fixed, it usually signifies one of three things:

1 A mass of retroperitoneal origin (e.g. pancreas).
2 Part of an advanced tumour with extensive spread to the anterior or posterior abdominal walls or abdominal organs.
3 A swelling resulting from severe chronic inflammation involving other organs (e.g. diverticulitis of the sigmoid colon or a tuberculous ileocaecal mass).

In the lower abdomen, the side-to-side mobility of a fibroid or pregnant uterus rapidly establishes such a swelling as uterine in origin and as not arising from the urinary bladder.

Is it bimanually palpable or pulsatile?

Bimanually palpable swellings in the lumbar region are usually renal in origin. Occasionally, however, a posteriorly situated gallbladder or a mass in the postero-inferior part of the right lobe of the liver may give the impression of being bimanually palpable. Carefully note whether a swelling is pulsatile and decide if any pulsation comes from the mass or is transmitted through it.

Percussion

Details of how to percuss correctly are given in Chapter 12. The normal percussion note over most of the abdomen is resonant (tympanic) except over the liver, where the note is dull. A normal spleen is not large enough to render the percussion note dull. A resonant percussion note over suspected enlargement of liver or spleen weighs against there being true enlargement.

In obese patients, tympanic areas of the abdomen may not give a truly resonant percussion note and palpation of organs such as a large liver is more difficult. If hepatomegaly is suspected, rhythmic percussion just above the suspected lower border of the liver, as the patient breathes in and out deeply, can elicit a note cyclically changing between dull to hollow, and eliciting this change may be more certain than the character of the fixed and unchanging note.

Defining the boundaries of abdominal organs and masses

Liver

The upper and lower borders of the right lobe of the liver can be mapped out accurately by percussion. Start anteriorly, at the fourth intercostal space, where the note will be resonant over the lungs, and work vertically downwards.

Over a normal liver, percussion will detect the upper border, which is found at about the fifth intercostal space (just below the right nipple in men). The dullness extends down to the lower border at or just below the right subcostal margin, giving a normal liver vertical height of 12-15 cm. The normal dullness over the upper part of the liver is reduced in severe emphysema, in the presence of a large right pneumothorax and after laparotomy or laparoscopy.

Spleen

Percussion over a substantially enlarged spleen provides rapid confirmation of the findings detected on palpation (see Fig. 14.14). Dullness extends from the left lower ribs into the left hypochondrium and left lumbar region.

Urinary bladder

The findings in a patient with retention of urine are usually unmistakable on palpation (see Fig. 14.21). The dullness on percussion and clear difference from the adjacent bowel provides reassurance that the swelling is cystic or solid and not gaseous.

Other masses

The boundaries of any localized swelling in the abdominal cavity or in the walls of the abdomen can sometimes be defined more accurately by percussion than palpation, as for the urinary bladder.

Detection of ascites and its differentiation from ovarian cyst and intestinal obstruction

There are three common causes of diffuse enlargement of the abdomen:

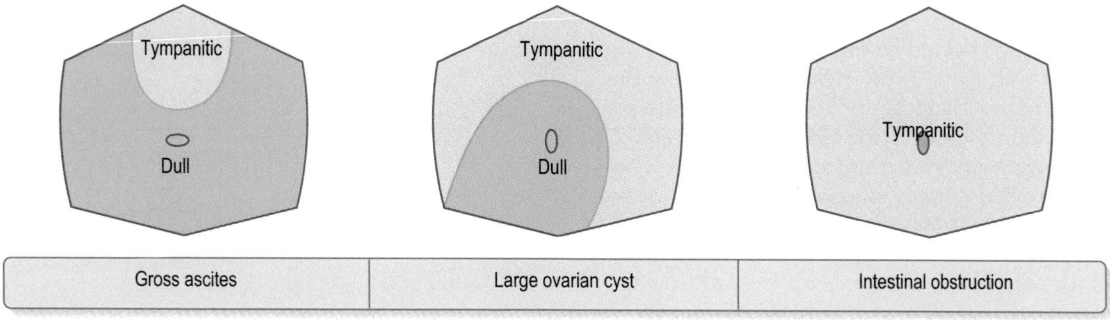

Figure 14.24 Three types of diffuse enlargement of the abdomen.

Box 14.4 Clinical features of marked abdominal swelling

Gross ascites
- Dull in flanks
- Umbilicus everted and/or hernia present
- Shifting dullness positive
- Fluid thrill positive

Large ovarian cyst
- Resonant in flank
- Umbilicus vertical and drawn up
- Large swelling felt arising out of pelvis which one cannot 'get below'

Intestinal obstruction
- Resonant throughout
- Colicky pain
- Vomiting
- Recent cessation of passage of stool and flatus
- Increased and/or 'tinkling' bowel sounds

1 The presence of free fluid in the peritoneum (ascites).
2 A massive ovarian cyst.
3 Obstruction of the large bowel, distal small bowel or both.

Percussion rapidly distinguishes between these three causes, as can be seen in Fig. 14.24. Other helpful symptoms or signs which are usually present are listed in Box 14.4.

The use of ultrasound to assess ascites has shown that probably more than 2 litres of ascites needs to be present to be detected clinically. It is unreliable to diagnose ascites unless there is sufficient free fluid present to give generalized enlargement of the abdomen. The cardinal sign created by ascites is shifting dullness. A fluid thrill may also be present but it would be unwise to diagnose ascites based on this sign without the presence of shifting dullness.

To demonstrate shifting dullness, have the lie patient supine. Place your fingers in the longitudinal axis on the midline near the umbilicus and begin percussion, moving your fingers laterally towards the right flank. When dullness is first detected (in normal individuals, dullness is only over the lateral abdominal musculature), keep your fingers in that position and ask the patient to roll on to his left side. Wait a few seconds for any peritoneal fluid to redistribute and, if ascites is present, the percussion note will become resonant. This shift in the area of dullness can be confirmed by finding the left border of dullness with the patient still on his left side and seeing if it shifts when the patient returns to the supine position or by repeating the original manoeuvre but towards the other side of the abdomen.

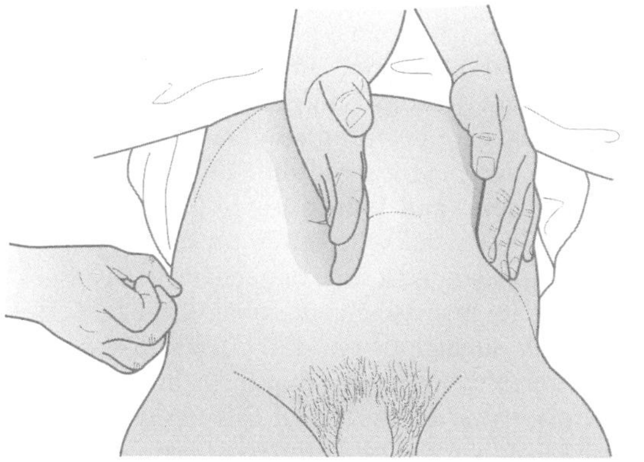

Figure 14.25 Eliciting a fluid thrill. (The hand in the middle of the abdomen is that of an assistant.)

To elicit a fluid thrill, the patient is again laid supine. Place one hand flat over the lumbar region of one side, and get an assistant to put the side of his hand longitudinally and firmly in the midline of the abdomen. Then flick or tap the opposite lumbar region (Fig. 14.25). A fluid thrill or wave is felt as a definite and unmistakable impulse by the detecting hand held flat in the lumbar region. (The purpose of the assistant's hand is to dampen any impulse that may be transmitted through the fat of the abdominal wall.) As a rule, a fluid thrill is felt only when there is a large amount of ascites present which is under tension, and it is not a very reliable sign.

Auscultation

Auscultation of the abdomen is for detecting bowel sounds and vascular bruits.

Bowel sounds

The stethoscope should be placed on one site on the abdominal wall (just to the right of and below the umbilicus is best) and kept there until sounds are heard. It should not be moved from site to site. Normal bowel sounds are heard as intermittent low- or medium-pitched gurgles interspersed with an occasional high-pitched noise or tinkle.

In simple acute mechanical obstruction of the small bowel, the bowel sounds are excessive and exaggerated. Frequent, loud, low-pitched gurgles (borborygmi) are heard, often rising to a crescendo of high-pitched tinkles and occurring in a rhythmic pattern with peristaltic activity. The presence of such sounds occurring at the same time as the patient experiences bouts of colicky abdominal pain is highly suggestive of small bowel obstruction. In between the bouts of peristaltic activity and colicky pain, the bowel is quiet and no sounds are heard on auscultation.

If obstruction progresses leading to bowel necrosis, peristalsis ceases and sounds lessen in volume and frequency. In generalized peritonitis, bowel activity rapidly disappears and a state of paralytic ileus ensues, with gradually increasing abdominal distension. The abdomen is 'silent' but one must listen for several minutes before being certain that there are no sounds. Frequently, towards the end of this period, a short run of faint, very high-pitched tinkling sounds is heard. This represents fluid spilling over from one distended loop to another and is characteristic of ileus.

A succussion splash may be heard without a stethoscope and also on auscultation when there is pyloric stenosis, in advanced intestinal obstruction with grossly distended loops of bowel and in paralytic ileus. Have the patient lie supine and place the stethoscope over the epigastrium. Shake the abdomen briskly from side to side and, if the stomach is distended with fluid, a splashing sound will be heard.

Vascular bruits

Listen for bruits by light application of the stethoscope above and to the left of the umbilicus (aorta), the iliac fossae (iliac arteries), epigastrium (coeliac or superior mesenteric arteries), laterally in the mid-abdomen (renal arteries) or over the liver (increased blood flow in liver tumours – classically primary liver cancer). If an arterial bruit is heard, it is a significant finding which indicates turbulent flow in the underlying vessel, due to stenosis, aneurysm or a malignant circulation.

The groins

Once the groins have been inspected, ask the patient to turn his head away from you and cough. Look at both inguinal canals for any expansile impulse. If none is apparent, place the left hand in the left groin so that the fingers lie over and in line with the inguinal canal; place the right hand similarly in the right groin (Fig. 14.26). Now ask the patient to give a loud cough and feel for any expansile impulse with each hand. When a patient coughs, the muscles of the abdominal wall contract violently and this imparts a definite, though not expansile, impulse to the palpating hands which is a source of confusion to the inexperienced. Trying to differentiate this normal contraction from a small, fully reducible inguinal hernia is difficult, and the matter can usually be resolved only when the patient is standing up.

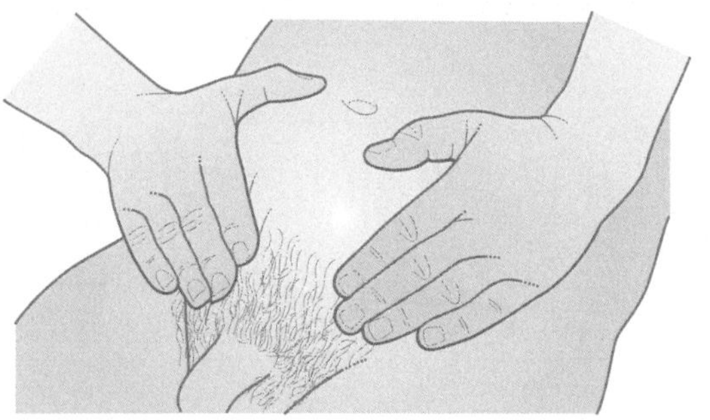

Figure 14.26 Palpating the groins to detect an expansile impulse on coughing.

The femoral vessels have already been felt (see Fig. 14.23) and auscultated. Now palpate along the femoral artery for enlarged inguinal nodes, feeling with the fingers of the right hand, and carry this palpation medially beneath the inguinal ligament towards the perineum. Then repeat this on the left side.

What to do if a patient complains of a lump in the groin

A patient who complains of a lump in the groin should be examined both lying down and standing up. A lump in the groin or scrotum is a common clinical problem in all age groups. Most lumps in the groin are due either to herniae or to enlarged inguinal nodes; inguinal herniae are considerably more common than femoral, with an incidence ratio of 4:1. In the scrotum, hydrocele of the tunica vaginalis or a cyst of the epididymis are common causes of painless swelling; acute epididymo-orchitis is the most frequent cause of a painful swelling. Generalized diseases such as lymphoma may present as a lump in the groin. Usually the diagnosis of a lump in the groin or scrotum can be made simply and accurately.

Ask the patient to stand in front of you, get him to point to the side and site of the swelling and note whether it extends into the scrotum. Ask him to turn his head away from you and give a loud cough; look for an expansile impulse and try to decide whether it is above or below the crease of the inguinal ligament. If an expansile impulse is present on inspection, it is likely to be a hernia, so move to whichever side of the patient the lump in the groin is on. Stand beside and slightly behind the patient. If the right groin is being examined, place the left hand over the right

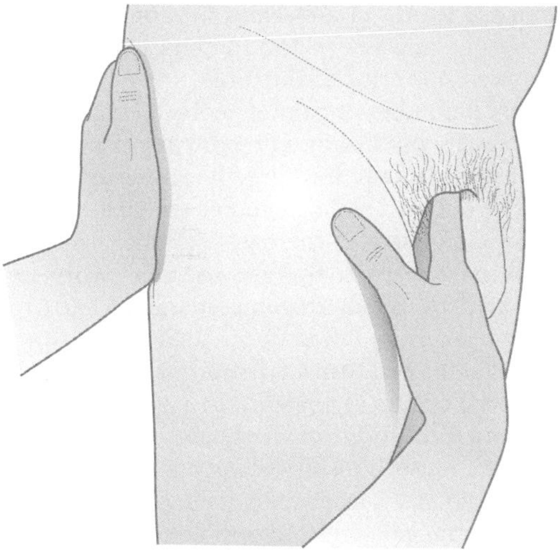

Figure 14.27 Locating the pubic tubercle. Note the position of the examiner, at the side of the patient, with one hand supporting the buttock.

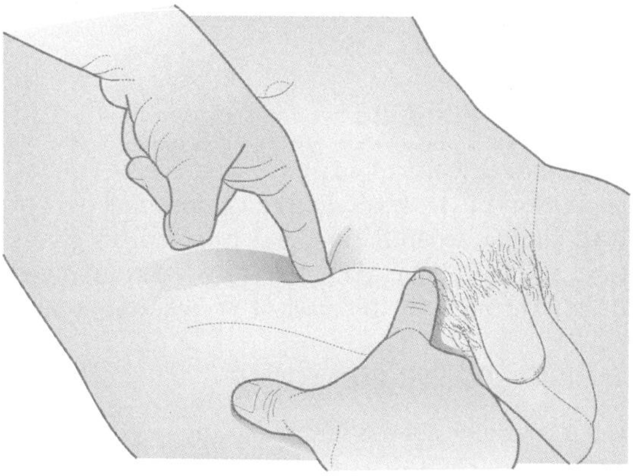

Figure 14.28 Left hand: index finger occluding the deep inguinal ring. Right hand: index finger on the pubic tubercle.

buttock to support the patient, the fingers of the right hand being placed obliquely over the inguinal canal. Now ask the patient to cough again. If an expansile impulse is felt, then the lump must be a hernia.

Next decide whether the hernia is inguinal or femoral. The best way to do this is to determine the relationship of the sac to the pubic tubercle. To locate this structure, push gently upwards from beneath the neck of the scrotum with the index finger (Fig. 14.27) but do not invaginate the neck of the scrotum as this is painful. The tubercle will be felt as a small bony prominence 2 cm from the midline on the pubic crest. In thin patients, the tubercle is easily felt but this is not so in the obese. If difficulty is found, follow up the tendon of adductor longus, which arises just below the tubercle.

If the hernial sac passes medial to and above the index finger placed on the pubic tubercle, then the hernia must be inguinal in site; if it is lateral to and below, then the hernia must be femoral in site.

If it has been decided that the hernia is inguinal, then one needs to know these further points:

- What are the contents of the sac? Bowel tends to gurgle and is soft and compressible, while omentum feels firmer and is of a doughy consistency.
- Is the hernia fully reducible or not? It is best to have the patient lie down to decide this. Ask the patient if he is 'able to push the hernia back in' and, if so, ask him to do so and confirm yourself. (It is more painful if the examiner reduces it.)
- Is the hernia direct or indirect? Again, it is best to have the patient lie down to decide this. Inspection of the direction of the impulse is often diagnostic, especially in thin patients. A direct hernia tends to bulge straight out through the posterior wall of the inguinal canal, while in an indirect hernia the impulse can often be seen to travel obliquely down the inguinal canal. Another helpful point is to place one finger just above the mid-inguinal point over the deep inguinal ring (Fig. 14.28). If a hernia is fully controlled by this finger, it must be an indirect inguinal hernia.

Apart from a femoral hernia, the differential diagnosis of an inguinal hernia includes a large hydrocele of the tunica vaginalis, a large cyst of the epididymis (one should be able to 'get above' and feel the upper border of both of these in the scrotum), an undescended or ectopic testis (there will be an empty scrotum on the affected side), a lipoma of the cord and a hydrocele of the cord.

In considering the differential diagnosis of a femoral hernia, one must think not only of an inguinal hernia but of a lipoma in the femoral triangle, an aneurysm of the femoral artery (expansile pulsation will be present), a saphenovarix (the swelling disappears on lying down, has a bluish tinge to it, there are often varicose veins present and there may be a venous hum), a psoas abscess (the mass is fluctuant and may be compressible beneath the inguinal ligament to appear above it in the iliac fossa) and an enlarged inguinal lymph node. Whenever the latter is found, the feet, legs, thighs, scrotum, perineum and the pudendal and perianal areas must be carefully scrutinized for a source of infection or primary tumour.

The examination is completed by examining the opposite groin in a similar manner.

The male genitalia

The examination of the genitalia is important in men presenting with abnormalities in the groin and in many acute or subacute abdominal syndromes. Thus, disease of the genitalia may lead to abdominal symptoms, such as pain or swelling. It is vital to give a careful and ongoing explanation of what is involved and why throughout this part of the examination. A detailed description of the examination of the male genitalia is given in Chapter 17.

The female genitalia

These are described in Chapters 5 and 17. As in men, examination of the genitalia is an important part of overall clinical examination, and it is vital to give a careful and ongoing explanation of what is involved and why throughout this part of the examination.

The anus and rectum

The left lateral position is best for routine examination of the rectum (Fig. 14.29). Make sure that the buttocks project over the side of the couch with the knees drawn well up and that a good light is available. Put on disposable gloves and stand behind the patient's back, facing the patient's feet. Explain to the patient what you are about to do, that you will be as gentle as possible and that you will stop the examination, if requested, at any time.

Inspection

Separate the buttocks carefully and inspect the perianal area and anus. Note the presence of any abnormality of the perianal skin, such as inflammation or excoriation, which may vary in appearance from mild erythema to a raw, red, moist, weeping dermatitis or, in chronic cases, thickened white skin with exaggeration of the anal skin folds. The latter form anal skin tags, which may follow not only severe pruritus but also occur when prolapsing haemorrhoids have been present over a period of time. Tags should not be confused with anal warts (condylomata acuminata), which are sessile or pedunculated papillomata with a red base and a white surface. Anal warts may be so numerous as to surround the anal verge and even extend into the anal canal. Note any 'hole' or dimple near the anus with a telltale bead of pus or granulation tissue surrounding it, which represents the external opening of a fistula-in-ano. It is usually easy to distinguish a fistula-in-ano from a pilonidal sinus, where the opening lies in the midline of the natal cleft but well posterior to the anus.

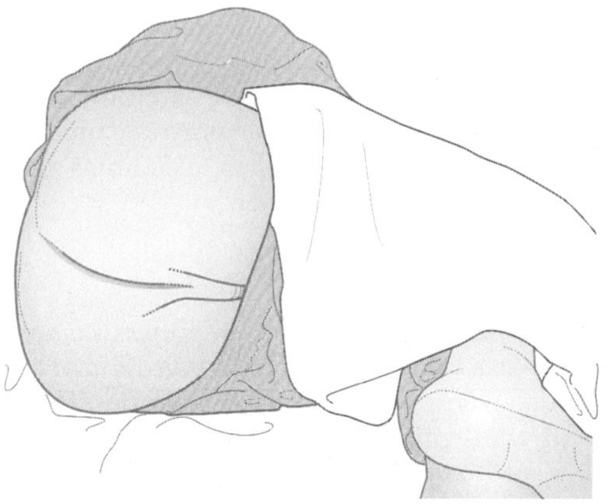

Figure 14.29 Left lateral position for rectal examination.

There are a number of painful anorectal conditions that can usually be diagnosed readily on inspection. An anal fissure usually lies directly posterior in the midline. The outward pathognomonic sign of a chronic fissure is a tag of skin at the base (sentinel haemorrhoid). If pain allows, the fissure can easily be demonstrated by gently drawing apart the anus to reveal the tear in the lining of the anal canal.

A perianal haematoma (thrombosed external haemorrhoid) occurs as a result of rupture of a vein of the external haemorrhoidal plexus. It is seen as a small (1 cm), tense, bluish swelling on one aspect of the anal margin and is exquisitely tender to the touch. In prolapsed strangulated haemorrhoids, there is gross swelling of the anal and perianal skin, which looks like oedematous lips, with a deep red or purple strangulated haemorrhoid appearing in between, and sometimes partly concealed by, the oedema of the swollen anus. In a perianal abscess, an acutely tender, red, fluctuant swelling is visible which deforms the outline of the anus. It is usually easy to distinguish this from an ischiorectal abscess where the anal verge is not deformed, the signs of acute inflammation are often lacking and the point of maximum tenderness is located midway between the anus and ischial tuberosity.

Note the presence of any ulceration. Finally, if rectal prolapse is suspected, ask the patient to bear down (as if trying to pass stool) and note whether any pink rectal mucosa or bowel appears through the anus or whether the perineum itself bulges downwards. Downward bulging of the perineum during straining on bending down or in response to a sudden cough indicates weakness of the pelvic floor musculature, usually due to denervation of these muscles. This sign is often found in women after childbirth, in women with faecal or urinary incontinence and in patients with severe chronic constipation.

Digital rectal examination (palpation)

Put a generous amount of lubricant on the gloved index finger of the right hand, place the pad of the finger (not the tip) flat on the anus (Figs 14.30 and 14.31) and press firmly and slowly (flexing the finger) in a slightly backwards direction. After initial resistance, the anal sphincter relaxes and the finger can be passed into the anal canal. If severe pain is elicited when attempting this manoeuvre, then further examination should be abandoned as it is likely the patient has a fissure and the rest of the examination will be very painful and unhelpful.

Feel for any thickening or irregularity of the wall of the canal, making sure that the finger is carefully turned through a full circle (180° each way). Assess the tone of the anal musculature; it should normally grip the finger firmly. If there is any doubt, ask the patient to contract the anus on the examining finger.

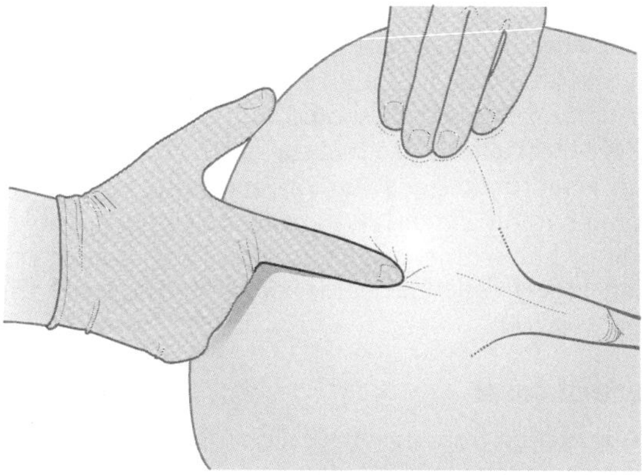

Figure 14.30 Correct method for insertion of the index finger in rectal examination. The pad of the finger is placed flat against the anus.

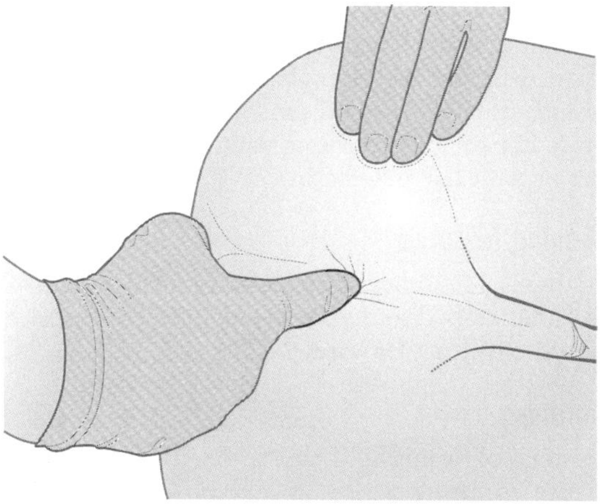

Figure 14.31 Incorrect method of introduction of the finger into the anal canal.

A cough will induce a brisk contraction of the external anal sphincter which should be readily appreciated. In the old and infirm with anal incontinence or prolapse, almost no appreciable contraction will be felt. With experience it is usually possible to feel a shallow groove just inside the anal canal which marks the dividing line between the external and internal sphincter. The anorectal ring may be felt as a stout band of muscle surrounding the junction between the anal canal and rectum.

Now pass the finger into the rectum. The examiner's left hand should be placed on the patient's right hip and later it can be placed in the suprapubic position to exert downward pressure on the sigmoid colon. Try to visualize the anatomy of the rectum, particularly in relation to its anterior wall. The rectal wall should be assessed with sweeping movements of the finger through 360°, 2, 5 and 8 cm inwards or until the finger cannot be pushed any higher into the rectum. Repeat these movements as the finger is being withdrawn. In this way it is possible to detect malignant ulcers, proliferative and stenosing carcinomas, polyps and villous adenomas. The hollow of the sacrum and coccyx can be felt posteriorly. Laterally, on either side, it is usually possible to reach the side walls of the pelvis. In men, one should feel anteriorly for the rectovesical pouch, seminal vesicles (normally not palpable) and the prostate. In a patient with a pelvic abscess, however, pus gravitates to this pouch, which is then palpable as a boggy, tender swelling lying above the prostate. Malignant deposits will feel hard and, in infection of the seminal vesicles, these structures become palpable as firm, almost tubular swellings deviating slightly from the midline just above the level of the prostate.

Assessment of the prostate gland is important. It forms a rubbery, firm swelling about the size of a large walnut. Run the finger over each lateral lobe, which should be smooth and regular. Between the two lobes lies the median sulcus, which is palpable as a faint depression running vertically between each lateral lobe. While it is possible to say on rectal examination that a prostate is enlarged, accurate assessment of its true size only comes with a lot of experience. In carcinoma of the prostate, the gland loses its rubbery consistency and becomes hard, while the lateral lobes tend to be irregular and nodular and there is distortion or loss of the median sulcus.

The cervix is felt as a firm, rounded mass projecting back into the anterior wall of the rectum. This is often a disconcerting finding for the inexperienced. The body of a retroverted uterus, fibroid mass, ovarian cyst, malignant nodule or a pelvic abscess may all be palpated in the pouch of Douglas (rectouterine pouch), which lies above the cervix. This aspect of rectal examination forms an essential part of pelvic assessment in female patients.

On withdrawing the finger after rectal examination, look at it for evidence of mucus, pus and blood, either fresh or altered. If in doubt, wipe the finger on a white swab. Finally, make sure to wipe the patient clean before telling the patient that the examination is completed and also tell him to be careful as he rolls to the supine position as he will be very near the edge of the couch or bed.

The acute abdomen

History

The patient usually presents with acute abdominal pain (which is also discussed in Chapter 9). Any pain, its site, severity, radiation, character, time and circumstances of onset and any aggravating or relieving features are all important.

Site

When the visceral peritoneum is predominantly involved in an acute process, pain is often referred in a developmental distribution, and so when assessing acute abdominal pain it is often helpful to think of the embryological development of the gut. Foregut structures are proximal to the duodenojejunal flexure and pain from here will often be felt in the upper abdomen. The small bowel and the colon around to the mid-transverse originate from the mid-gut and may produce pain in the periumbilical region, such as in the early phases of acute appendicitis. Pain from structures developing from the hind-gut will be felt in the lower abdomen. As any disease process advances and the parietal peritoneum is irritated, pain is felt at the site of the affected organ, such as in the right iliac fossa in the later stages of acute appendicitis.

Ask the patient to point to the site of maximal pain with one finger. If pain is experienced mostly in the upper abdomen, think of perforation of a gastric or duodenal ulcer, cholecystitis or pancreatitis. If pain is located in the mid-abdomen, disease of the small bowel is likely. Pain in the right iliac fossa is commonly due to appendicitis and pain in the left iliac fossa to diverticulitis. In women, the menstrual history is important as low abdominal pain of acute onset is often due to salpingitis, but rupture of an ectopic pregnancy should also be considered. The coexistence of severe back and abdominal pain may indicate a ruptured or dissecting abdominal aneurysm; alternatively, acute severe pancreatitis should be considered. The former is associated with cardiovascular collapse whilst the latter is associated with systemic inflammatory response syndrome (SIRS).

Severity

Try to assess the severity of the pain. Ask whether it keeps the patient awake. In women who have had children, compare the severity with labour pains. Sometimes comparison to the pain of a fractured bone is useful. Asking a patient to score the pain on a scale of 0-10 is useful for ongoing assessment and monitoring of effectiveness of treatment.

Radiation

If pain radiates from the right subcostal region to the shoulder or to the interscapular region, inflammation of the gallbladder (cholecystitis) is a likely diagnosis. If pain begins in the loin but then is felt in the lumbar region, a renal stone or renal infection should be considered. Pain beginning in the loin and radiating to the groin is likely to be due to a ureteric calculus, and umbilical pain radiating to the right iliac fossa is usually due to appendicitis. Central upper abdominal pain, later radiating through to the back, is common in pancreatitis.

Character and constancy

Constant severe pain felt over many hours is likely to be due to infection. For example, diverticulitis or pyelonephritis can present in this manner. Colicky pain, on the other hand (i.e. pain lasting a few seconds or minutes and then passing off, leaving the patient free of pain for a further few minutes), is typical of small bowel obstruction. If such pain is suddenly relieved after a period of several hours of severe pain, perforation of a viscus should be considered. Large bowel obstruction produces a more constant pain than small bowel obstruction, but colic is usually prominent. Biliary and renal colic are also of variable severity but with a longer period of variation than small bowel colic and come on more quickly than they wear off.

Mode of onset

In obstruction from mechanical disorders such as that due to biliary or ureteric stone or obstruction of the bowel from adhesions or volvulus, the onset of colicky pain is usually sudden. It is often related to activity or movement in the previous few hours. In infective and inflammatory disorders, the pain usually has a slower onset, sometimes over several days, and there is no relation to activity. Alcohol excess or recent ingestion of a rich, heavy meal sometimes precedes pancreatitis. The ingestion of aspirin or non-steroidal anti-inflammatory drugs is sometimes a precipitating feature in patients presenting with perforated peptic ulcer or with haematemesis.

Relieving features

Abdominal pain relieved by rest suggests an infective or inflammatory disorder. Pancreatic pain is classically relieved by sitting forward.

Vomiting

A history of vomiting is not in itself very helpful because vomiting occurs as a response to pain of any type. However, effortless projectile vomiting often denotes pyloric stenosis or high small bowel obstruction. In peritonitis, the vomitus is usually small in amount but vomiting is persistent. There may be a faeculent smell to the vomitus when there is low small bowel obstruction. In bowel obstruction, vomiting may be an early or late sign depending on the level of obstruction. Persistent vomiting with associated diarrhoea strongly suggests gastroenteritis. It is unusual for patients with a perforated ulcer to vomit.

Micturition

Increased frequency of micturition occurs both in urinary tract infections and in other pelvic inflammatory disorders as well as in patients with renal infections or ureteric stones. In the latter, haematuria commonly occurs. The presence of air or faeculent discolouration of urine is highly suspicious of an entero-vesical fistula.

Appetite and weight

In patients with a chronic underlying disorder, such as abdominal cancer, there may be a history of anorexia and weight loss, although weight loss also occurs in a variety of other disorders. A dietary history is important for progressive weight loss but a sudden loss of appetite clearly indicates a disorder of sudden onset.

Other features

It is important to note whether there have been previous episodes of abdominal pain and whether or not they have been severe. The patient may have noticed swellings at the site of a hernial orifice, indicating the likelihood of an obstructed hernia, or there may be a history of blunt or penetrating abdominal trauma. Sometimes the patient may be aware of increasing abdominal distension, a phenomenon indicating intestinal obstruction or paralytic ileus probably associated with an inflammatory or infective underlying bowel disorder. Food poisoning may be suggested by a history of ingestion of unusual or under-prepared foods or a meal in unfamiliar surroundings. The menstrual history should never be forgotten, particularly in relation to the possibility of an ectopic pregnancy. Enquiry should always be made as to a purulent vaginal discharge, indicating salpingitis, or of discharge of mucus, pus or blood from the rectum, suggesting inflammatory bowel disease.

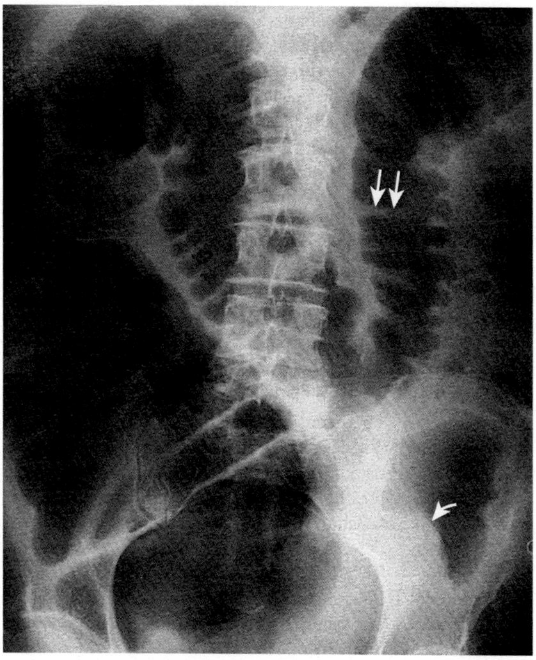

Figure 14.32 Plain X-ray of the abdomen. Obstruction of the large bowel due to carcinoma of the sigmoid colon. Most of the colon is dilated with gas, indicating obstruction, but there appears to be no gas below the sigmoid region.

Examination

There are certain features that are important in all patients presenting with an acute abdominal crisis. An assessment of the vital signs and of the patient in general is essential. The physical signs found on inspection and on auscultation of the abdomen have already been discussed above in the relevant sections.

Guarding

Guarding is an involuntary reflex contraction of the muscles of the abdominal wall overlying an inflamed viscus and peritoneum, producing localized rigidity. It indicates localized peritonitis. What is felt on examination is spasm of the muscle, which prevents palpation of the underlying viscus. Guarding is seen classically in uncomplicated acute appendicitis. It is very important to distinguish this sign from voluntary contraction of muscle.

Rigidity

Generalized or 'board-like' rigidity is an indication of diffuse peritonitis. It can be looked upon as an extension of guarding, with involuntary reflex rigidity of the muscles of the anterior abdominal wall. It is quite unmistakable on palpation, as the whole abdominal wall feels hard and 'board like', precluding palpation of any underlying viscus. The least downward pressure with a palpating hand in a patient with generalized rigidity produces severe pain. It may be differentiated from voluntary spasm by getting the patient to breathe: if there is voluntary spasm, the abdominal wall will be felt to relax during expiration.

Rebound tenderness

Rebound tenderness is present if when palpating slowly and deeply over a viscus and then suddenly releasing the palpating hand, the patient experiences sudden pain. Rebound tenderness is not always a reliable sign and should be interpreted with caution, particularly in those patients with a low pain threshold, but is often a useful adjunct to detecting peritoneal inflammation.

Percussion

The absence of dullness over the liver can indicate free intraperitoneal gas and hence a perforated viscus.

Radiology

A plain X-ray of the abdomen is an important immediate investigation in the diagnosis of the acute abdomen, especially in suspected perforation or obstruction (Fig. 14.32). An erect chest X-ray may also demonstrate free air under the diaphragm although this is not always completely reliable.

Examination of abdominal fluids

Examination of vomit

The character of the vomit varies with the nature of the food ingested and the absence or presence of bile, blood or intestinal obstruction. In pyloric stenosis, the vomit is usually copious and sour-smelling, containing recognizable food eaten many hours before and exhibiting froth on the surface after standing. The presence of much mucus gives vomit a viscid consistency. Brisk haematemesis such as from a large vessel in an ulcer will cause the patient to vomit essentially pure blood. Bright red blood that is 'vomited' nearly always originates from the naso- or oropharynx and not from the stomach. Slower upper-GI bleeding leads to the blood mixing with gastric juice and becoming darker with an appearance likened to ground coffee.

Vomit which contains dark green bile may resemble vomit which contains blood but usually red and green parts can be distinguished. Faeculent vomit, characteristic of advanced intestinal obstruction, is brown in colour, rather like vomited tea, and has faecal odour. Vomit containing formed faeces is rare but indicates a communication between the stomach and transverse colon, usually from a colonic carcinoma.

Examination of faeces

Examination of the faeces is all too easily omitted. No patient with bowel disturbance has been properly examined until the stools have been inspected.

Faecal amount

Note whether the stools are copious or scanty, and whether they are hard, formed, semi-formed or liquid. Faecal character is usually defined using the Bristol Stool Chart; this standardized descriptor is of particular use in monitoring progress in infective or inflammatory diarrhea.

Faecal colour

Black stools may be produced by altered blood or the ingestion of iron or bismuth. In haemorrhage occurring high up in the intestine, the altered blood makes the stools dark, tarry-looking and with the characteristic and offensive smell of melaena. Pallor of the stools may be due to lack of entrance of bile into the intestine, as in obstructive jaundice; to dilution and rapid passage of the stool through the intestine as in diarrhoea; or to an abnormally high fat content as in malabsorption.

Faecal odour

The stools in jaundice are often very offensive. Cholera stools, on the other hand, contain very little organic matter and are almost free from odour. The stools of acute bacillary dysentery are almost odourless, while those of amoebic dysentery have a characteristic odour, something like that of semen. Melaena stools have a characteristic smell.

Abnormal stools

Watery stools are found in all cases of profuse diarrhoea and after the administration of purgatives. In cholera, the stools – known as rice-water stools – are colourless, almost devoid of odour, alkaline in reaction and contain a number of small flocculi consisting of shreds of epithelium and particles of mucus. Purulent or pus-containing stools are found in severe dysentery or ulcerative colitis. Slimy stools are due to the presence of an excess of mucus and point to a disorder of the large bowel. The mucus may envelop the faecal masses or may be intimately mixed with them.

Bloody stools vary in appearance according to the site of the haemorrhage. If the bleeding takes place high up, the stools look like tar. In an intussusception, they may look like red-currant jelly. Large bowel bleeding above the rectum may produce darker red visible blood whereas bleeding from the rectum or anus may streak the faeces bright red, and haemorrhoidal bleeding may just be found on the toilet paper. A brisk upper-GI bleed can lead to bright red rectal bleeding (haematochezia).

The stools of bacillary dysentery initially consist of faecal material mixed with blood and pus, later of blood and pus without faecal material. Those of amoebic dysentery characteristically consist of fluid faecal material, mucus and small amounts of blood. The stools of steatorrhoea are very large, pale and putty- or porridge-like, sometimes frothy with a visible oily film, and often float. They are apt to stick to the sides of the toilet and are difficult to flush away.

Tests for faecal occult blood

Several methods are available. For reasons of ease of use and safety, the guaiac test (Haemoccult) is the most widely used. A filter paper impregnated with guaiac turns blue in the presence of haemoglobin when hydrogen peroxide is added. The test depends on the oxidation of guaiac in the presence of haemoglobin. Other substances with peroxidase activity, including dietary substances such as bananas, pineapple, broccoli and radishes, can produce a false-positive reaction, and ascorbic acid may cause false-negative results. Therefore, dietary preparation is necessary for accurate screening, for example, when screening a population in the early detection of colonic cancer. In ordinary clinical use, the test is sensitive to faecal blood losses of about 20 ml per day. This test can be used on patients on a normal diet but it may not detect small amounts of GI bleeding. The test may be negative in the presence of lesions which bleed intermittently or slightly, particularly those situated in the upper GI tract. Spectroscopic methods and isotopic methods using radiolabelled red cells that can localize the source of bleeding in the gut are also available.

Tests for faecal fat

Fat is present in food as neutral fat or triglyceride. It is split to greater or lesser degrees by lipases, mainly from the pancreas, into glycerol and fatty acids. Some of the fatty acids, if unabsorbed, combine with bases to form soaps. Fat may therefore be found in the faeces as neutral fat, fatty acids and soaps.

The estimation of the proportion of split and unsplit fats present has been found unreliable as a method of distinguishing pancreatic from non-pancreatic steatorrhoea because of the effects of bacterial activity on neutral fats.

For the estimation of the fat in the stools, the patient may be placed on a diet containing 50 g of fat per day. The fat present in the stools collected over at least 3 days is then estimated and should not exceed 6 g/day (11-18 mmol/day). It has been found that equally reliable results are obtained if the patient eats a normal diet, provided a 3-5 day collection is made.

Faecal fat testing has largely been replaced by the measurement of faecal elastase which, if reduced below a reference value, usually indicates pancreatic exocrine insufficiency.

Stool microbiology

Reliable microbiological examination of the stool is vital for accurate diagnosis of acute and chronic diarrhoea. All stool samples for microbiological examination should get to the laboratory as fresh as possible, and if amoebic or similar infection is suspected, then microscopy should be performed with the stool still as close to body temperature as possible (a 'hot' stool).

Any microbiological finding must be correlated with the history, as many patients are healthy carriers of organisms that can be pathogenic in other situations. If *Clostridium difficile* infection is suspected in a patient with diarrhoea following the use of antibiotics, the laboratory must be asked to look for the *Clostridium* toxin in preference to the organism.

Aspiration of peritoneal fluid

Aspiration of peritoneal fluid (paracentesis abdominis) is undertaken for diagnostic and therapeutic purposes. Most patients with significant ascites should have an initial diagnostic aspiration to help differentiate the causes. Cirrhotic patients with ascites whose condition deteriorates need the complication of spontaneous bacterial peritonitis excluded because it has no specific signs, has a significant mortality and substantially affects prognosis. Therapeutic paracentesis may be needed in cirrhotic patients for whom diuretics are contraindicated or have not worked, and in patients with ascites due to malignancy.

The patient should be lying flat or propped up at a slight angle. The aspiration is usually performed in the flanks, a little outside the mid-point of a line drawn from the umbilicus to the anterior superior iliac spine. With suitable sterile precautions, the skin at the point chosen should be infiltrated with local anaesthetic and the anaesthetic then injected down to the parietal peritoneum. For a simple diagnostic puncture, a 20-ml syringe and an 18-gauge needle can be used; clotting and platelet abnormalities do not require correcting. If a significant quantity of fluid is intended to be drained, efforts should be made to normalize haematological abnormalities (liaison with a haematologist may be required) to minimize risk of haemorrhage. A trochar and flanged cannula or catheter (which can be fixed to the skin with adhesive dressing) should be employed (a peritoneal dialysis or suprapubic catheter is often suitable). A diagnostic tap should be performed before inserting the trochar and cannula to ensure that fluid can be obtained at the chosen site. A tiny incision should be made in the anaesthetized area of the skin before the trochar and cannula are inserted. The cannula is attached to a drainage bag and the drainage rate should be limited to 1 litre/hour. Because of the risk of infection, the drainage catheter should not be left *in situ* for more than 6 hours. Human albumin solution is usually used to replace volume (8 g/l ascites removed). In general, diuretics are preferable to therapeutic drainage for the management of chronic ascites, but the latter can have a place in therapy.

The fluid withdrawn is sent for bacteriological and cytological examination and chemical analysis. Transudates, such as occur in heart failure, cirrhosis and nephrotic syndrome, normally have a protein content under 25 g/l (i.e. less than two-thirds the concentration of albumin in the plasma). Exudates occurring in tuberculous peritonitis or in the presence of secondary malignancy usually contain more than 25 g/l of protein. This method of distinction, however, is somewhat unreliable. It is now routine to calculate the serum-albumin ascites gradient (SAAG); a value of ≥11 g/l suggests that the ascites is secondary to portal hypertension.

Lymphocytes in the fluid are characteristic features of tuberculous peritonitis but acid-fast bacilli are often not seen on staining. Blood-stained fluid strongly suggests a malignant cause, and malignant cells may also be demonstrated (Fig. 14.33). If pancreatic pathology is suspected, the amylase content of the fluid should be measured.

In ascites due to cirrhosis, 10 ml of the sample should be inoculated into blood culture bottles. However, in spontaneous bacterial peritonitis, the cultures are often negative and the diagnosis is primarily based on the finding of >250 or more neutrophils per mm^3 fluid and an unexpectedly high protein content, results which should lead to the use of appropriate broad-spectrum antibiotics.

Special techniques in the examination of the GI tract

There are a number of common and important methods of examining the oesophagus, stomach and duodenum, the small and large intestine, the liver, gallbladder, biliary tree and pancreas.

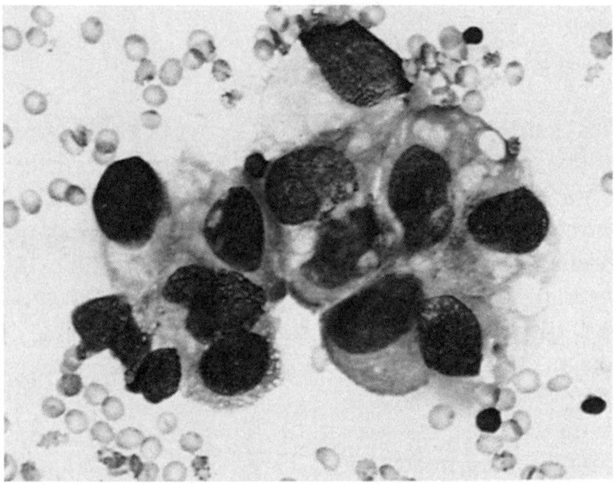

Figure 14.33 Ascites cytology. A group of tumour cells showing random orientation and large abnormal nucleoli indicating malignancy. Ascitic fluid from patient with ovarian carcinoma. May-Grünwald-Giemsa stain ×160.

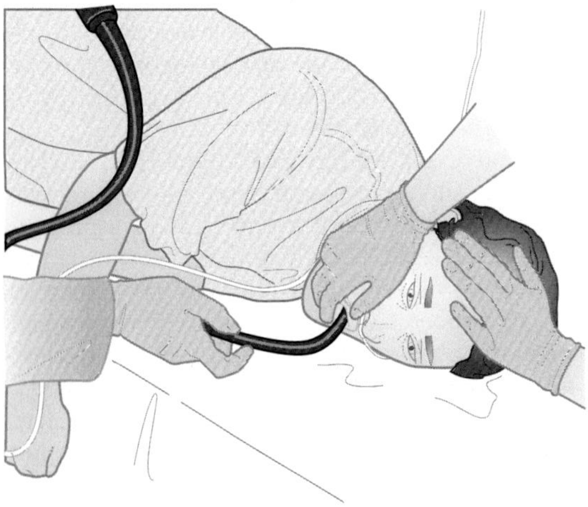

Figure 14.34 A patient undergoing endoscopy of the upper GI tract. The plastic guard between the teeth prevents the instrument from being bitten. The patient may have received pharyngeal local anaesthetic spray or light sedation with midazolam.

Upper gastrointestinal endoscopy

In the last 40 years or so, the developments of the fibreoptic endoscope, and more recently of video-endoscopy, have revolutionized the assessment of the upper GI tract (Fig. 14.34). With these instruments it is possible to inspect directly as far as the proximal small bowel, with or without conscious sedation and local pharyngeal anaesthesia. Because of the ability to photograph and biopsy any suspicious lesions, this technique is the investigation of choice for demonstrating structural abnormalities in the upper gut. Therapeutic endoscopy is now the treatment of choice for bleeding varices, oesophageal obstruction and in most cases of bleeding peptic ulcer (Fig. 14.35). In inoperable cancer of the oesophagus, palliative prostheses (stents) can be inserted endoscopically. Enteral nutrition may be delivered via percutaneous endoscopic gastrostomy tubes.

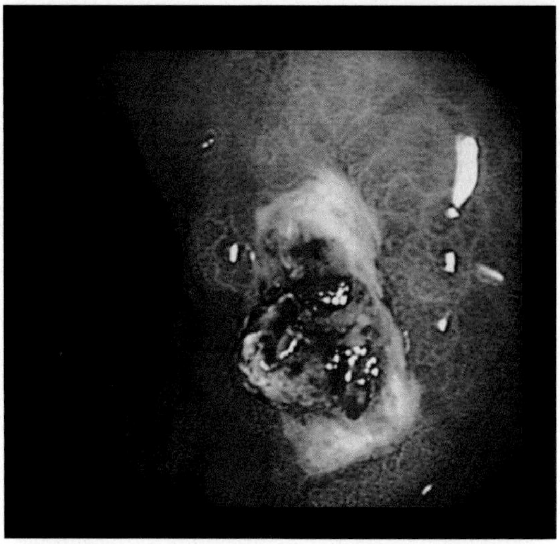

Figure 14.35 Endoscopic view of a duodenal ulcer that has recently bled with a visible blood vessel on its surface.

Oesophageal function studies

The oesophageal phase of swallowing can be assessed by barium swallow and may show slowing or arrest of transit of the food bolus in the oesophagus. In special clinical applications, manometric studies of pressure changes during swallowing are used to localize functional abnormalities in the coordination of oesophageal peristalsis, for example achalasia and oesophageal spasm. In patients with epigastric and retrosternal discomfort (heartburn) related to eating or to lying supine, reflux of acid from the stomach into the lower oesophagus should be suspected. Acid reflux can best be detected by monitoring the pH in the lower oesophagus during a 24-hour period. The pH measuring probe, passed via the nose, is placed in the lower oesophagus, 5 cm above the oesophago-gastric junction, for 24 hours and the pH recorded continuously. The patient indicates when pain is experienced by pressing an electronic marker on the recorder to see if there is a correlation with the degree of acidity. This investigation has found a major clinical application in the differential diagnosis of acid reflux pain from atypical cardiac pain. A combined pH and impedance recording can also detect non-acid reflux.

Gastric secretory studies and serum gastrin levels

Measurement of acid secretion by the stomach was formerly frequently used for the assessment of patients with peptic ulcer disease, and for the diagnosis of hyperacidity caused by the rare gastrin-secreting tumours (Zollinger-Ellison syndrome), but serum gastrin estimation is now the investigation of choice.

In normal subjects, the basal acid output is no more than a few millilitres per hour, containing up to 10 mmol/l of hydrogen ions. The maximal acid output, measured during 1 hour after the administration of pentagastrin (6.0 mg/kg body weight), a synthetic analogue of the naturally occurring human hormone gastrin, may reach 27 mmol/l/h in males, and 25 mmol/l/h in females. In most patients with Zollinger-Ellison syndrome, the ratio of basal to maximum acid secretion is raised as much as sixfold.

Measurement of serum gastrin is made fasting, after quite a long period without acid-suppression therapy, and collected into special preservative. In Zollinger-Ellison patients, the level of gastrin in the serum is increased above 100 ng/l. Serum gastrin levels are also increased in renal failure, pernicious anaemia, after vagotomy and during acid-suppression therapy.

Tests for *Helicobacter pylori*

The role of infection by *Helicobacter pylori* in the pathogenesis of gastric and duodenal ulceration is well documented, although an exact causative link is less well understood. *H. pylori* is a Gram-negative spiral bacillus. The organism is found in the gastric antrum in about 60% of patients with gastritis or gastric ulceration and in almost all patients with duodenal ulceration. There are many asymptomatic carriers in the general population. Patients carrying *H. pylori* in the stomach will have IgG antibodies in the serum and these will remain present for a long period after successful treatment; serological testing is therefore no longer recommended. *H. pylori* can be detected by microscopy or culture of gastric mucosal biopsies obtained during endoscopy and by stool antigen testing.

H. pylori is rich in urease. In a simple clinical test, a gastric biopsy is placed in contact with a pellet or solution containing urea and a coloured pH indicator. The colour of the substrate changes when the pH is greater than 6, indicating the conversion of urea to ammonia by urease in *H. pylori*. A variant of this method utilises ^{13}C-labelled urea given to the patient by mouth. The patient's breath is monitored for labelled carbon dioxide, indicating breakdown of the ingested urea by urease-containing organisms in the upper-GI tract. In the community and before endoscopy is indicated or performed, detection of the stool antigen for *H. pylori* is now the most widely used method. ^{13}C-labelled urea breath testing should be used to confirm successful eradication.

H. pylori can be rendered undetectable but not eradicated by acid-suppression therapy, which should be stopped 2 weeks before any testing for reliable results (other than stool antigen testing or histology of gastric biopsies).

Radiology of the upper gastrointestinal tract

Plain radiographs

Plain radiographs of the chest and abdomen with the patient supine and in the erect position are of great value in cases of suspected peritonitis due to a perforated viscus, when gas may be seen under the diaphragm, usually on the right side (Fig. 14.36). A plain abdominal X-ray is useful in suspected intestinal obstruction or ileus when dilated bowel loops may be seen with fluid levels appearing on the erect X-ray. It is important to use a plain abdominal X-ray to exclude toxic megacolon in fulminant colitis.

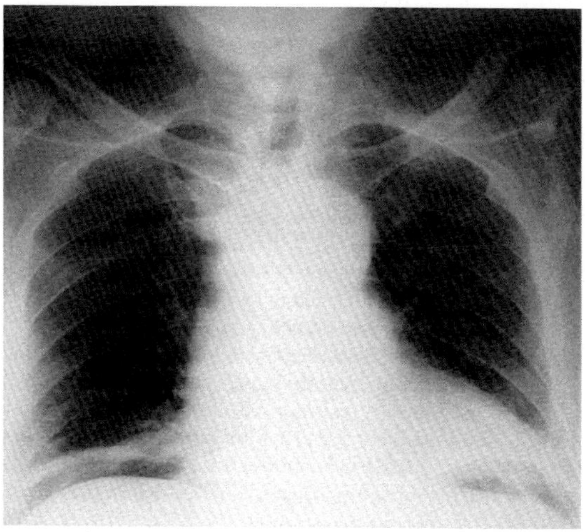

Figure 14.36 Plain X-ray of the chest showing gas under the right and left diaphragms after perforation of the duodenal ulcer. The patient was admitted in shock with abdominal pain and abdominal rigidity.

Barium swallow

The direct observation of the passage of a radiopaque barium solution through the pharynx and oesophagus into the stomach remains an important investigation of dysphagia. In addition to structural abnormalities such as neoplasia or stricture, disorders of motor function can be detected which might otherwise escape diagnosis. Lack of progress of barium through an apparently normal lower oesophageal sphincter on swallowing in a patient with dysphagia usually indicates the presence of achalasia, a disorder of neuromuscular coordination of the oesophageal body and failure of the lower sphincter to relax.

A careful radiological assessment of the stomach and duodenum, which has been coated with swallowed barium and then inflated with a gas-forming tablet, has the ability to demonstrate benign ulcers and tumours as well as assessing gastric outflow. However, the ability to take endoscopic biopsies has meant that barium radiology is now a secondary investigation to upper GI endoscopy.

Small intestine

Barium follow-through studies

The small intestine may be studied by taking sequential X-rays of the abdomen after swallowing barium contrast. Abnormalities in the transit time to the colon and in small bowel pattern (e.g. dilation, narrowing, increase in transverse barring or flocculation) may be demonstrated in malabsorptive states. Areas of narrowing with proximal dilatation, fistulae and mucosal abnormalities may be produced by Crohn's disease. Small bowel diverticula or neoplasms may also be demonstrated. The amount and type of barium used for examination of the stomach/duodenum and of the small bowel is different, and so a barium follow-through should be requested as a specific examination and not as an add-on to a barium meal.

Small-bowel enema

Small-bowel enema is an alternative to the barium follow-through examination and involves intubating the duodenum and passing small quantities of a non-flocculating barium suspension down the tube. This method is useful for detecting isolated focal lesions and strictures but in most centres has been replaced by MR enterography and/or double balloon enteroscopy.

Radioisotope studies

In inflammatory bowel disease, the location of the disease and a measure of its activity can be obtained by radioisotope studies using the patient's own white blood cells that have been radiolabelled.

Selective angiography of gastrointestinal arteries

Angiography is occasionally used in the investigation of haematemesis or melaena when gastroscopy and colonoscopy fail to identify the bleeding source. It is most useful if performed when the patient is actively bleeding but may be of value if an aneurysm or abnormal tumour vasculature is present, and it can occasionally detect angiomas. It is an invasive technique that demands a great deal of skill on the part of the radiologist. It is sometimes possible to use therapeutic embolization to treat haemorrhage.

Small intestine endoscopy and biopsy

Samples of small intestine mucosa are valuable for histological diagnosis in various types of malabsorption. Direct biopsy of the lower duodenum at conventional upper GI endoscopy is usually sufficient for diagnosis of coeliac disease but jejunal tissue can also be obtained using push-type flexible enteroscopes. Endoscopic techniques for biopsying have now largely replaced remote biopsy by the Crosby capsule. If necessary, full-thickness jejunal biopsies, useful for diagnosing neuromuscular gut disorders, can be obtained by laparoscopy. Excellent endoscopic images of the whole of the small bowel can now be obtained by wireless capsule endoscopy but, as yet, biopsies are not possible by this method.

If coeliac disease is suspected, serum antibodies to gliadin, reticulin, endomysial and tissue transglutaminidase antigens are a useful screening test (provided there is no IgA deficiency), but a biopsy is essential to fully complete or fully exclude the diagnosis. The low-power view of the villi is as important as the detailed histology. Other malabsorption problems such as Whipple's disease and chronic giardiasis may also be seen on duodenal biopsy.

Magnetic resonance scanning

Magnetic resonance scanning is now replacing barium radiology for assessing areas of stricturing and inflammation in the small bowel.

Colon, rectum and anus

Proctoscopy

The anal canal and lower rectum can be readily visualized with a rigid proctoscope. Place the patient in the position described for rectal examination and gently pass the lubricated instrument to its full depth. Remove the obturator and inspect the mucosa as the instrument is slowly withdrawn and air gently insufflated. Haemorrhoids are seen as reddish/blue swellings which bulge into the lumen of the instrument. Asking the patient to strain down as the proctoscope is withdrawn exaggerates any haemorrhoids. The internal opening of an anal fistula, an anal or low rectal polyp and a chronic anal fissure are other abnormalities that may be seen.

Rigid sigmoidoscopy and other tests in chronic diarrhoea

Proctitis, polyps and carcinomas may be seen and biopsies taken. Sigmoidoscopy is particularly useful in the differential diagnosis of diarrhoea of colonic origin. Granularity, loss of vascular pattern and ulceration with bleeding may indicate the presence of ulcerative colitis, aphthous ulceration may suggest Crohn's disease, and multiple rounded white macules may be diagnostic of pseudomembranous colitis due to *Clostridium difficile* toxin, usually following antibiotic treatment. In suspected amoebic dysentery, the mucous membrane should be inspected and portions of mucus and scrapings from the ulcerated mucosa may be removed and examined microscopically for amoebic cysts.

Urine tests for purgative abuse are useful in the investigation of persistent unexplained diarrhoea but not widely available.

Barium enema

Prior to barium enema, the patient must have his bowel prepared with a vigorous laxative, as residual stool or fluid can be mistaken for polyps and other lesions. Impending obstruction is a contraindication to this laxative preparation. A plain X-ray of the abdomen should always be taken in patients with suspected perforation or obstruction before considering a contrast study (see Fig. 14.32).

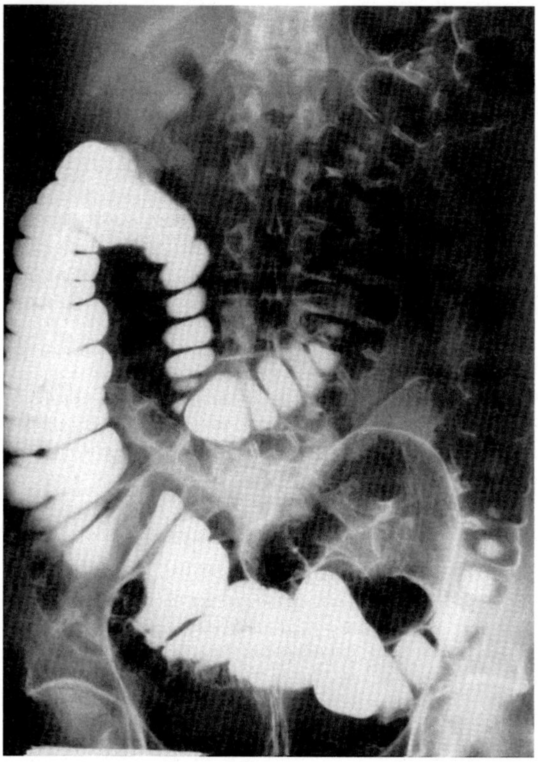

Figure 14.37 Barium enema with air contrast. The right colon is outlined by barium sulfate and the rectum, left colon and part of the transverse colon are outlined by air with a thin mucosal layer of barium sulfate. Note the normal haustral pattern in the colon and the smooth appearance of the rectum. The anal canal can also be seen.

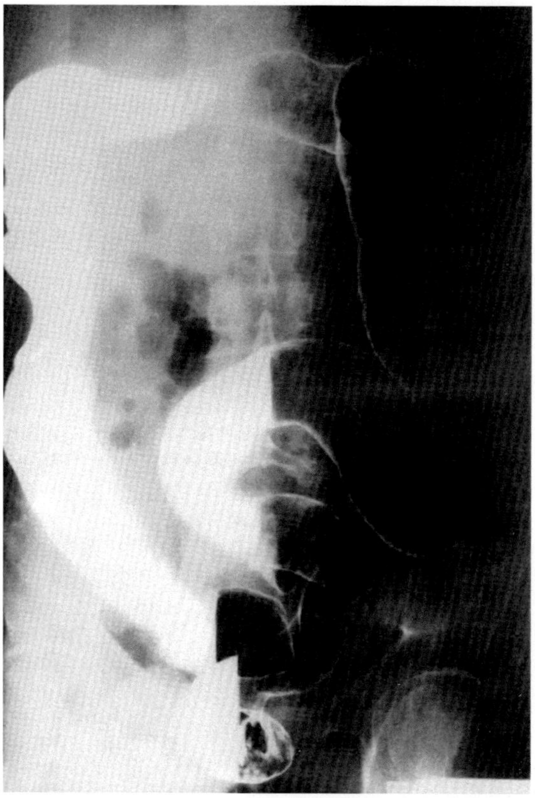

Figure 14.38 Barium enema with air contrast. In this patient with ulcerative colitis, the normal mucosal pattern and the haustra themselves have been obliterated. The patient is lying on his right side so that there are clear fluid levels in the barium sulphate suspension in the bowel.

Barium suspension is introduced via a tube into the rectum as an enema and the patient is repositioned to move the contrast around the rest of the colon. Radiological screening is performed with the barium *in situ* and after it has been evacuated. By this means, obstruction to the colon, tumours, diverticular disease, fistulae and other abnormalities can be recognized.

Following evacuation, air is introduced into the colon. This improves visualization of the mucosa and is especially valuable for detecting small lesions such as polyps and early tumours (Figs 14.37 and 14.38).

Patients often find the preparation and procedure uncomfortable and there is a very small risk of perforating the colon. The inability to take diagnostic samples and the advent of CT colonography means that barium enemas are now rarely used for diagnostic purposes.

Colonoscopy and flexible sigmoidoscopy

As in the upper gut, the use of flexible fibreoptic and video instruments has revolutionized the investigation of the colon. Both sigmoidoscopes and colonoscopes are available. The former instrument may be employed in an outpatient setting after a simple enema preparation; the latter requires more extensive colon preparation (similar to barium enema X-ray) but is also an outpatient procedure. Conscious sedation may be used. These techniques are invaluable for obtaining tissue for diagnosis of inflammatory and neoplastic disease and for removal of neoplastic polyps (Figs 14.39 and 14.40). Dilation of strictures, stenting or other thermal treatments of obstructing tumours can also be applied during endoscopy.

A skilled colonoscopist should reach the caecum in >90% of examinations attempted and the terminal ileum in 50%. There is a small risk (1:1000) of colonic perforation associated with the colonoscopy.

The liver

Biochemical tests in liver disorders

Biochemical tests are used in the differential diagnosis of jaundice, to detect liver cell damage in other disorders and to monitor the results of medical and surgical treatments of the liver, pancreas and biliary systems. Tests include plasma bilirubin, alkaline phosphatase, serum aminotransferases, plasma proteins and prothrombin time. Serum gamma glutamyl transferase levels are especially sensitive to

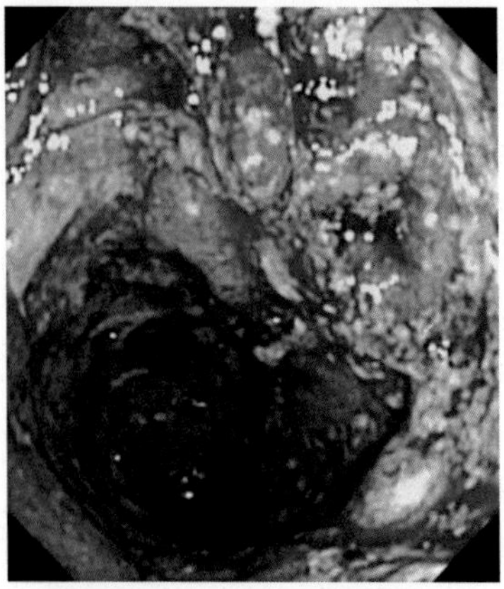

Figure 14.39 View of colonic epithelium at colonoscopy, showing severe ulcerative colitis with extensive ulceration and bleeding.

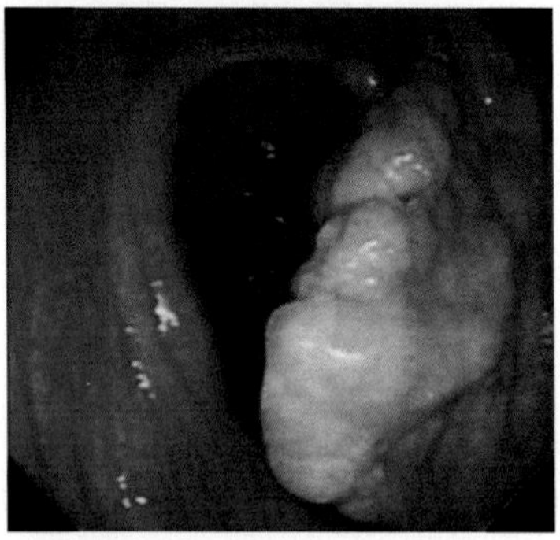

Figure 14.40 Colonoscopic view of a tubulovillous adenoma.

liver dysfunction as, for example, in alcohol-related liver disease.

Smooth muscle antibodies are commonly present in the blood in chronic active hepatitis, and other autoantibody studies are used in the investigation of chronic inflammatory liver disease. Anti-mitochondrial antibodies are found in the blood in primary biliary cirrhosis in over 90% of cases.

Liver disease due to excess iron or copper accumulation can be detected by measurements of these metals and their carrier proteins in blood (or urine for copper). In primary haemochromatosis, genetic studies are very useful in diagnosis. Serum alpha-foetoprotein is often raised in primary liver cell cancer, which can complicate any cause of cirrhosis, or the carriage of hepatitis B or C.

Viral hepatitis

The presence of ongoing carriage of viral hepatitis is initially detected by antigen testing (for hepatitis B) and by antibody testing for hepatitis C, D and E. Active infection is detected by finding IgM antibody (for hepatitis A, B, D and E), and by polymerase chain reaction (PCR) testing for the viral RNA (hepatitis C). At least two antigens and antibodies of hepatitis B can be detected (surface and E) which give information about activity and ongoing disease and, in the latter, detection of the viral DNA is helpful.

Needle biopsy of liver

Percutaneous needle biopsy is the standard technique for obtaining liver tissue for histological examination. While needle biopsy can be conducted under local anaesthesia (sometimes with mild sedation), it should be carried out only in hospital by fully experienced staff. Generally, the method is safe and reliable but there is a tiny but definite mortality from the procedure due to leakage of bile and/or blood into the peritoneal cavity from the puncture site. The procedure should therefore always be regarded as a potentially dangerous investigation for which there should be a clear beneficial indication for the patient and should be performed by an appropriately trained operator. Liver biopsy under ultrasound guidance is preferable and can allow targeting of specific abnormalities and give confidence of a safer procedure. Contraindications to biopsy include patients with abnormal clotting times or thrombocytopaenia, obstructive jaundice or ascites.

Ultrasound scanning

In ultrasound scanning a probe emitting ultrasonic pulses is passed across the abdomen. Echoes detected from within the patient are received with a transducer, amplified and suitably displayed. This technique is the most commonly used non-invasive imaging modality for the liver. It can identify cirrhosis and small metastases and is helpful in the diagnosis of fluid-filled lesions such as cysts and abscesses. Fine needle aspiration of suspicious lesions can be undertaken under direct ultrasound guidance for cytology and for drainage of fluid, bile or pus.

The gallbladder is most easily investigated by ultrasound. It appears as an echo-free structure. If stones are present, they are usually easily seen as mobile and echo-dense with a characteristic 'acoustic shadow' behind them. Ultrasound detects 95% of gallbladder stones but only about 50% of stones in the bile ducts themselves. Ultrasound is particularly valuable in detecting dilation of the bile duct which may be due to partial or complete obstruction by gallstones or tumour. Ultrasound has replaced oral cholecystography for imaging the gallbladder.

Ultrasound is the usual initial technique for investigating the pancreas, is particularly useful in the diagnosis of true and pseudopancreatic cysts and is an essential tool for percutaneous needle biopsy. However, images may be obscured by overlying bowel gas and the tail of the pancreas is poorly visualized. Ultrasound is used extensively for examining other intra-abdominal, pelvic and retroperitoneal organs and increasingly for imaging the bowel in inflammatory conditions such as in Crohn's disease. Blood flow patterns (such as in the portal vein) can be assessed by ultrasound using the Doppler principle.

Isotope scanning

Technetium-labelled red blood cells can be used to detect the location of sources of bleeding in the GI tract. Isotopes taken up in the bile (hepatobiliary iminodiacetic acid, HIDA) can give images of the gallbladder and biliary tree, and give some information as to the functioning of these organs. Technetium-labelled white cells can be used to localize inflamed bowel segments in inflammatory bowel disease, and both the small and large bowel can be imaged with the same test. (Isotope liver scans have largely been superseded by the use of ultrasound.)

Computed tomography scanning

Computed tomography (CT) can be used to produce cross-sectional images of the liver and other intra-abdominal and retroperitoneal organs. It is particularly helpful in assessing patients with cancer of the oesophagus, stomach, pancreas and colon (Fig. 14.41). Because it can be combined with injection of vascular contrast, it can be helpful in assessing intra-abdominal vascular abnormalities. It can facilitate guided biopsy of abnormalities, and drainage of fluid and other collections. It is also increasingly being used to image the bowel, particularly if there is suspected obstruction, and is widely used in assessing patients with an acute abdomen. Clinicians should be aware of the radiation exposure associated with CT scanning and caution should be exercised for younger patients in particular.

Positron emission tomography scanning

Radiolabelled isotopes that are taken up by cell metabolism are injected intravenously and the radiation that is detected is reconstructed into a cross-sectional image by the same techniques as for CT. It is a particularly sensitive technique for staging cancers, particular if the CT images are acquired at the same time.

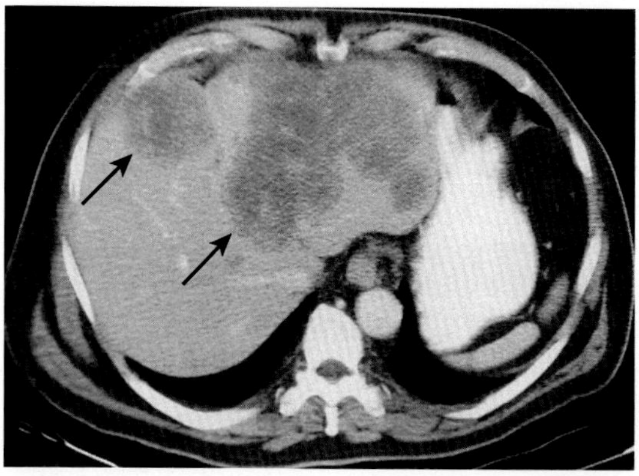

Figure 14.41 CT demonstrating liver metastases from colonic carcinoma. Large, lobulated, non homogeneous masses (arrows) replace most of the left lobe of the liver.

Endoscopic ultrasound

Endoscopic ultrasound is more sensitive in staging the mucosal depth of penetration of cancers in the oesophagus and stomach than CT scanning and is frequently better at lymph node detection but is less effective at detecting distant metastases. It is also valuable in assessing biliary and pancreatic abnormalities. Endoscopic ultrasound has the advantage of guiding fine needle aspiration cytology as well as other endoscopic interventions.

Magnetic resonance imaging

Magnetic resonance cholangiopancreatography (MRCP) can give high-quality images of the bile duct and pancreatic duct. The safety of this non-invasive technique has reduced the need for more invasive and hazardous examinations such as endoscopic retrograde cholangiopancreatography (ERCP), which is reserved for patients requiring therapeutic intervention. Magnetic resonance is increasingly used to image the small bowel in Crohn's disease and also to characterize liver lesions.

Endoscopic retrograde cholangiopancreatography (ERCP)

Using a special side-viewing duodenoscope, the duodenal papilla is identified and a cannula passed through it into the common bile duct. Radiopaque contrast is then injected into the cannula and the whole of the biliary system is visualized. The technique is useful in the rapid diagnosis and localization of the different causes of jaundice due to obstruction of the main bile ducts. Needle or forceps biopsy and brush cytology may give a specific diagnosis of strictures of the biliary tree. ERCP has an important therapeutic role in the treatment of jaundice because it allows the removal of bile duct stones or the placement of stents which are tubes that facilitate the passage of bile into the duodenum past obstructing lesions such as tumours of the pancreas or bile duct. More novel techniques allow direct visualization of the biliary system. Such therapies often involve performing a sphincterotomy during ERCP using a cutting diathermy wire passed into the bile duct via the ampulla. The sphincterotomy opens the ampulla and may allow the delivery of stones in the bile duct.

The entire pancreatic duct system can be visualized at ERCP. The technique is therefore valuable in the diagnosis of chronic pancreatitis. In patients with pancreatic carcinoma, a needle biopsy can be performed at ERCP, and brush cytology of the pancreatic duct may also provide histological confirmation of the diagnosis. ERCP carries a small mortality and may be complicated by pancreatitis, bleeding, perforation or infection. Prophylactic antibiotics should be used if there is biliary obstruction. The advent of magnetic resonance imaging of the bile and pancreatic ducts now means that essentially all ERCPs are therapeutic.

Percutaneous transhepatic cholangiography

Percutaneous transhepatic cholangiography complements the use of ERCP in patients with jaundice due to obstruction of the main bile ducts, although is usually only possible if the intrahepatic bile ducts are seen to be dilated on ultrasound. The site of the obstruction due to tumours of the head of the pancreas or benign and malignant bile duct strictures can be accurately localized and differentiated. This technique is usually only used if ERCP fails. It also has a therapeutic function. Transhepatic drains can be placed to treat cholangitis and sepsis, stents can be placed to relieve obstruction, gallstones can be removed and wires can be passed into the duodenum to facilitate stenting at ERCP.

Pancreatic function tests

Pancreatic function tests are now rarely used. In suspected pancreatic malabsorption, a therapeutic trial of pancreatic supplementation may be the easiest confirmatory test. If a definitive test is required, the pancreolauryl test can be used, a test which relies on the urine collection of a substance which can be absorbed only after GI breakdown by pancreatic enzymes. In chronic pancreatitis, faecal elastase may be reduced. Measurement of the blood amylase or lipase concentration is still valuable in the diagnosis of acute pancreatitis.

Locomotor system

15

Stephen Kelly

Introduction

Musculoskeletal symptoms are a major cause of pain and disability, accounting for a quarter of all GP consultations in the UK, and have significant economic consequences. Common musculoskeletal conditions such as back pain and osteoarthritis are the dominant causes of chronic pain, disability and work loss in the UK and many other countries, consuming considerable health and social service resources. In addition, inflammatory arthritis and connective tissue disorders may present with musculoskeletal symptoms. As such, it is critical that clinicians are able to appropriately assess patients with such symptoms and initiate appropriate management or referral to a specialist centre. Early diagnosis and treatment of inflammatory arthritis, such as rheumatoid arthritis, has been consistently shown to improve patients' long-term outcome with the early initiation of disease modifying therapy. The autoimmune rheumatic disorders, although much less common, cause significant morbidity with the potential for end-organ damage which may be fatal if not recognized and treated early.

The objectives of performing a musculoskeletal assessment are:

- to make an accurate diagnosis
- to assess the severity and consequences of the condition
- to construct a clear management plan.

Taking an effective structured history and making a simple, focused examination is likely to be more important than imaging and serology, which on their own may be falsely reassuring. Although modern musculoskeletal medicine uses complex imaging and immunological investigations, in most patients with locomotor disorders, diagnosis can be achieved at the bedside without complex investigations.

General assessment: the 'GALS' locomotor screen

This brief screening examination, which should take 1-2 minutes, has been devised for use in routine clinical assessment. This brief global assessment of the gait, arms, legs and spine (GALS) is typically used by both non-specialist and specialist alike (Box 15.1). The routine requires some practise to become proficient, but once achieved, it has been shown to be highly sensitive in detecting significant abnormalities of the musculoskeletal system. It involves inspecting carefully for joint swelling and abnormal posture, as well as assessing the joints for normal movement. Typically, the clinician will then focus on particular areas of interest with more dedicated and targeted examinations.

Screening history

If answers to the following four questions are negative, a musculoskeletal disorder is unlikely:

1. Do you have any pain or stiffness in your muscles, joints or back?
2. Have you ever had gout or arthritis?
3. Can you dress yourself completely without difficulty?
4. Can you walk up and down stairs without difficulty?

Positive answers imply the need for a more detailed assessment, as described in this chapter.

Screening examination

Gait

Watch the patient walking and turning back towards you. Normal: symmetry, smooth movement, arm swing, no pelvic tilt, normal stride length, ability to turn quickly.

With the patient standing in the anatomical position, observe from behind, from the side, and from in front. Muscle symmetry should be noted along with limb alignment. Spine and limb alignment can be observed as well as abnormalities in the feet such as pes plans or pes cavus.

Common gait abnormalities are listed in Table 15.1.

Spine

Inspect the standing patient. Normal on inspection: no scoliosis, symmetrical paraspinals, normal shoulder and gluteal muscle bulk and symmetry, level iliac crests, normal cervical and lumbar lordosis. Movement: finger to floor distance less than 15 cm, lumbar expansion greater than 6 cm, ear touches acromion.

Table 15.1 Gait abnormalities

Type	Description	Causes
Antalgic	Avoiding weight bearing on affected side	Pain related to arthritis or tendonitis
Spastic	Leg swings outwardly from hip with extended knee	Hemiplegia related to CVA
Shuffling	Small shuffling steps, speeding up (festination), reduced arm swing and difficulty turning	Parkinson's disease
Ataxic	Wide based gait, swaying torso	Cerebellar disease. Peripheral sensory ataxia (typically worsens with loss of visual input)
Waddling (Trendelenburg)	Exaggerated lateral movement of trunk and circumduction of hip to compensate for weak abductors	Bilateral gluteus medius tendinopathy
High stepping (foot drop)	Excessive hip and knee flexion to accommodate failure of ankle dorsiflexion	Peroneal neuropathy (multiple causes)

Box 15.1 GALS checklist

Gait
- Observe gait
- Observe patient in anatomical position

Arms
- Observe movement – hands behind head
- Observe backs of hands and wrists
- Observe palms
- Assess power grip and strength
- Assess fine precision pinch
- Squeeze MCPJs

Legs
- Assess full flexion and extension
- Assess internal rotation of hips
- Perform patellar tap
- Inspect feet
- Squeeze MTPJs

Spine
- Inspect spine
- Assess lateral flexion of neck
- Assess lumbar spine movement

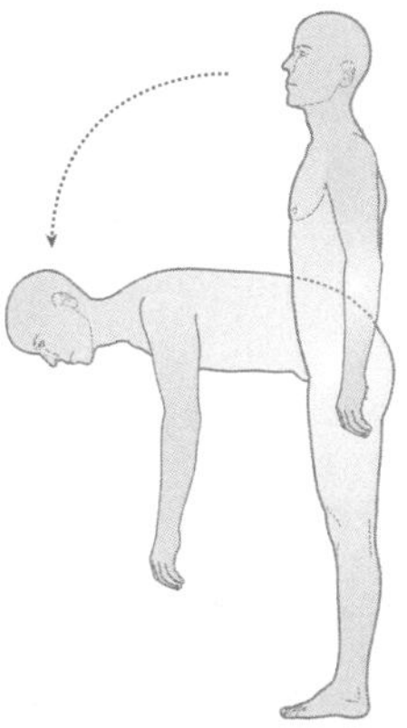

Figure 15.1 Inspect patient from behind and side, observing for normal spinal curves, then ask the patient to 'bend forwards to try to touch your toes'.

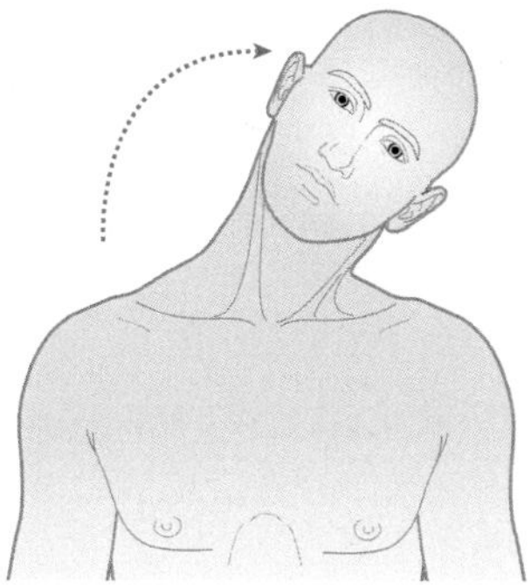

Figure 15.2 From the front, ask the patient to 'place your ear on your right then your left shoulder'.

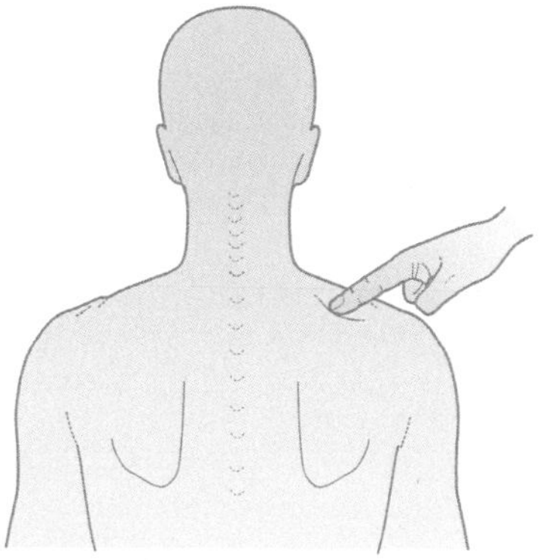

Figure 15.3 Gently press the mid-point of each supraspinatus to elicit the hyperalgesia of fibromyalgia.

- From behind – look for abnormal spinal and paraspinal anatomy and look at the legs.
- From the side – look for abnormal spinal posture, then ask the patient to bend down and touch his toes (Fig. 15.1).
- From the front – ask the patient to 'put your ear on your left then right shoulder' and watch the neck movements (Fig. 15.2).
- Gently press the mid-point of each supraspinatus muscle to elicit tenderness (Fig. 15.3).

Arms

Ask the patient to follow instructions as in Table 15.2 (see Figs 15.4-15.9).

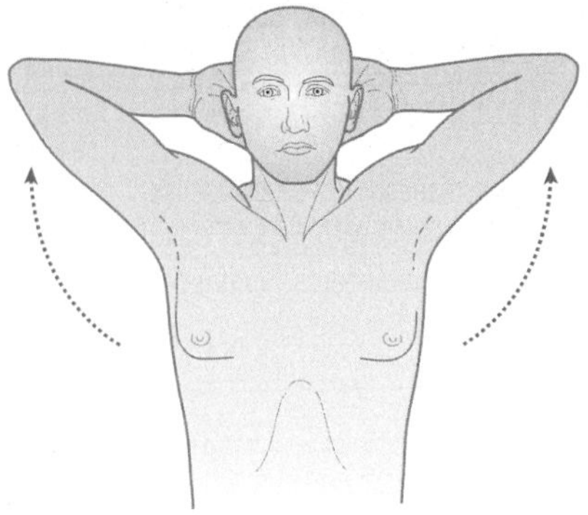

Figure 15.4 'Put your hands behind your head, elbows back.' Observe for pain or restricted movement.

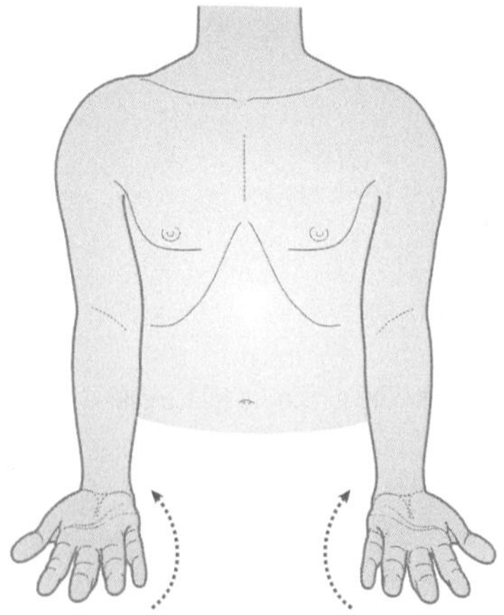

Figure 15.5 'Put your hands out, palms down, and then turn your hands over.'

Table 15.2 Instructions for examining arms

Instruction	Normal outcome
'Raise arms out sideways and up above your head'	180° elevation through abduction without wincing
'Touch the middle of your back'	Touches above T10 with both hands
'Straighten your elbows right out'	Elbows extend to 180° or slightly beyond (females) symmetrically
'Place hands together as if to pray, with elbows right out'	90° wrist extension and straight fingers
'The same with hands back to back'	90° wrist flexion
'Place both hands out in front, palms down, fingers out straight'	No wrist/finger swelling/ deformity, 90° pronation
Metacarpophalangeal (MCP) cross-compression	No tenderness
'Turn hands over'	90° supination No palmar swellings, wasting or erythema
'Make a fist and hide your nails'	Can hide fingernails
'Pinch index, middle finger and thumb together'	Can do
Also look for swelling between the heads of the metacarpals and gently squeeze across the MCP joints to elicit tenderness	Tenderness may be elicited

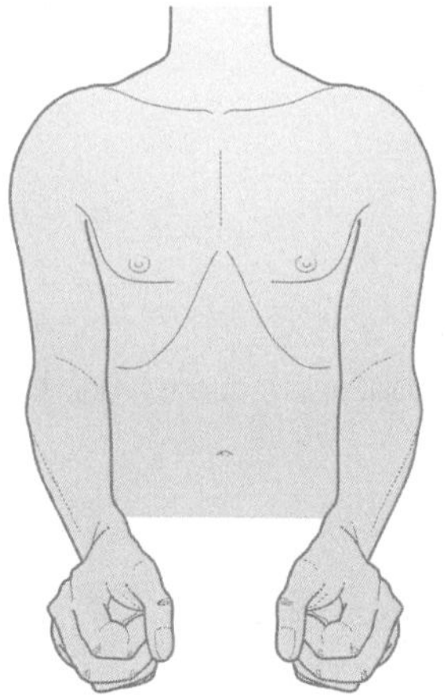

Figure 15.6 'Make a fist with both hands.'

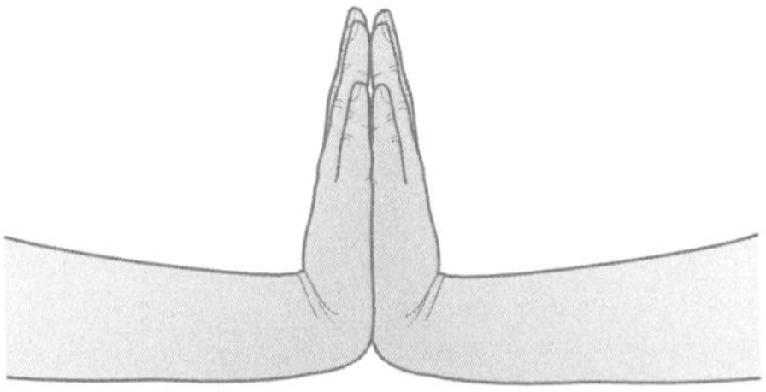

Figure 15.7 'Place your hands together as if to pray, with elbows right out.'

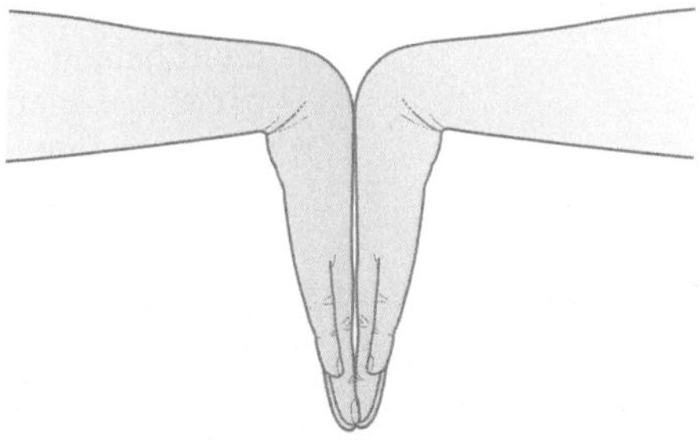

Figure 15.8 'Do the same with your hands back to back.'

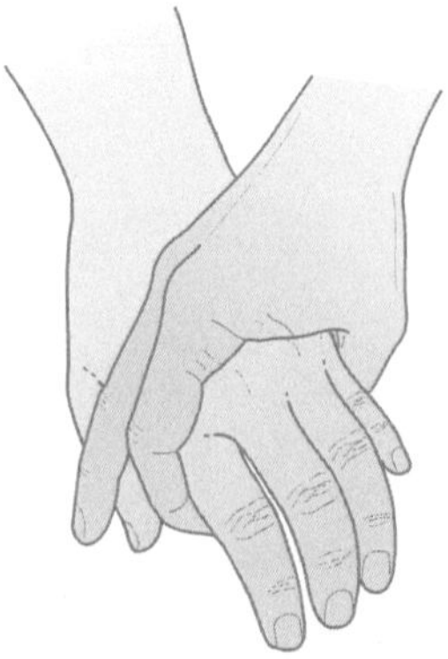

Figure 15.9 Look for swelling between the heads of the metacarpals and gently squeeze across the metacarpophalangeal joints to elicit tenderness.

Legs

With the patient still standing:

- Examine the lower limbs for swelling, deformities or limb shortening. Normal: no knee deformity, anterior or popliteal swelling, no muscle wasting, no hindfoot swelling or deformity.
- Then, with the patient lying on a couch, continue the examination following the instructions in Table 15.3 (see Figs 15.10-15.14).

This examination can be conducted in approximately 2 minutes, especially if the clinician performs the movements and asks the patient to follow them. The precise order of the examination is not important and clinicians usually develop their own pattern of examination.

Table 15.3 Instructions for examining legs

Instruction	Normal outcome
Flex hip and knee, holding knee	No bony crepitus, 140° knee flexion
Passively rotate hips	90° total pain-free rotation
Bulge test/patellar tap	No detectable fluid
Palpate popliteal fossa	No swelling
Inspect feet	No deformity, callosities or forefoot widening (daylight sign)
Test subtalar and ankle movement	Pain-free calcaneal mobility at subtalar joint, dorsiflexion beyond plantigrade and 30° plantarflexion

Children

Children should have their height and weight measured and plotted on centile charts to assess growth. When examining children, the assessment

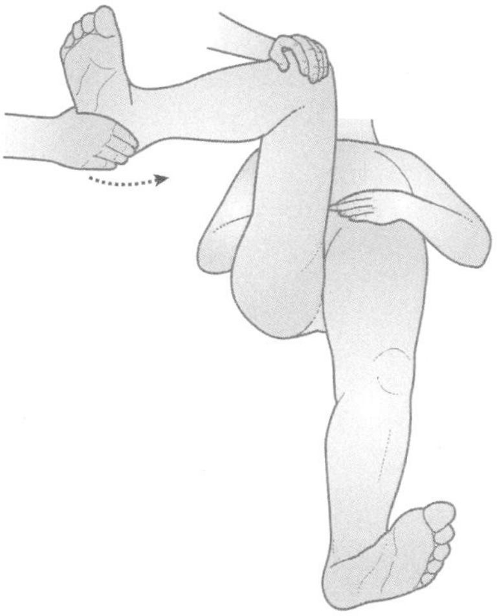

Figure 15.10 Gently flex the hips and knees, feeling for crepitus at the knee during movement, and look for pain and restriction of movement. Look for knee effusion.

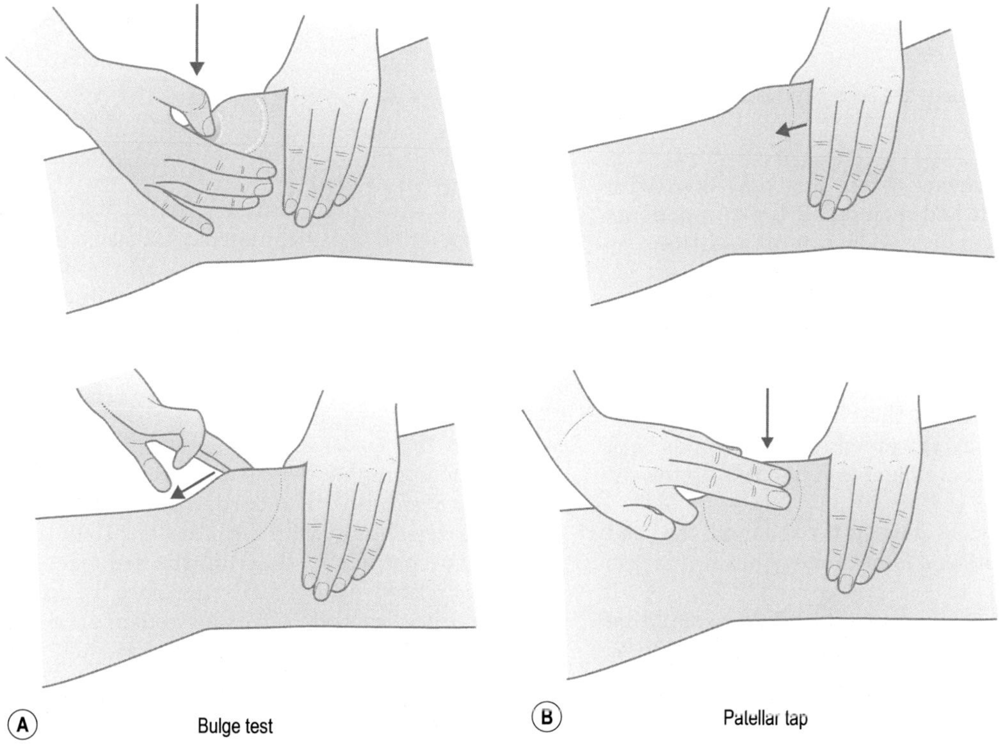

Figure 15.11 **(A)** Bulge test and **(B)** patellar tap.

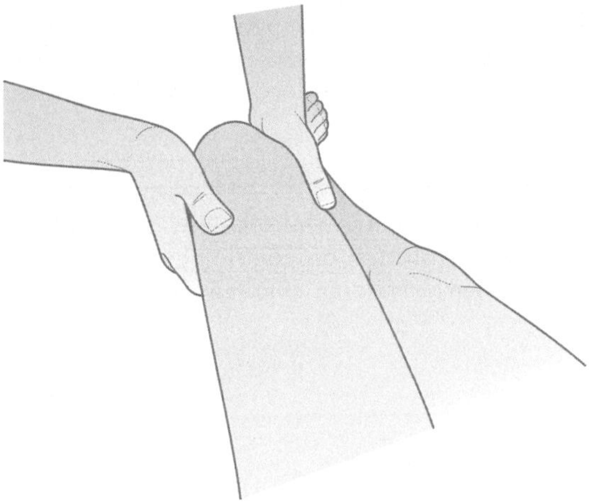

Figure 15.12 Palpate popliteal fossa.

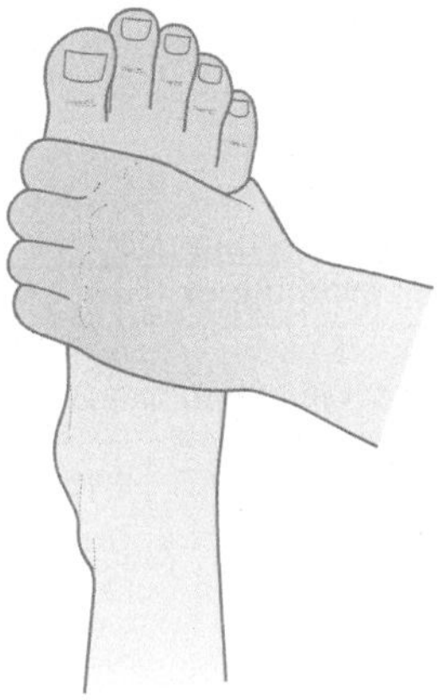

Figure 15.14 Squeeze across metacarpophalangeal (MTP) joints and inspect the soles of the feet.

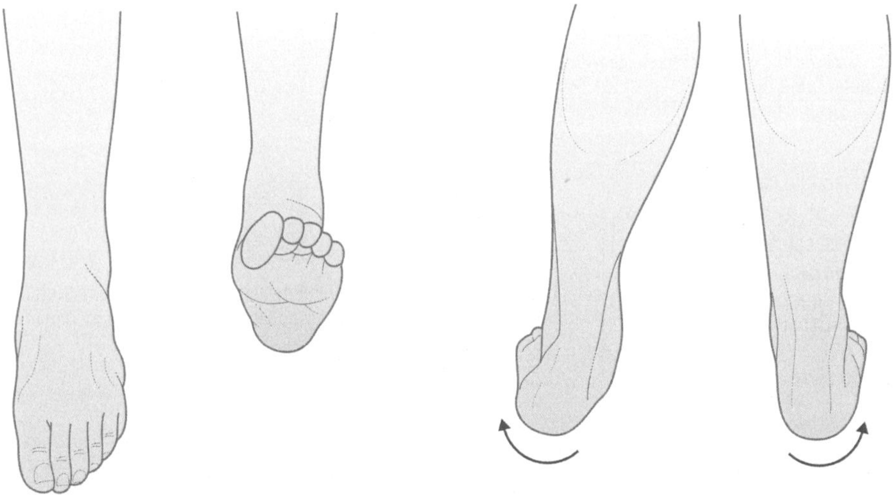

Figure 15.13 Test subtalar and ankle movement.

of the musculoskeletal system should be done with a parent present and include all the components of the adult version with minor additions as follows:

Gait

Ask the child to walk on his tiptoes and then on the heels.

From the front, ask the child to put his hands together (as if praying) and also put his hands back to back and then have him reach his arms up toward the sky.

Additionally, when assessing the spine, ask the child to open his mouth and insert three of his own fingers into it.

Symmetry is key and any asymmetry should be assessed for pathology. It is normal for toddlers to be 'bow-legged', 'knock-kneed' and 'flat-footed'. Various foot and toe appearances are also normal, including in-toeing, out-toeing and 'curly' toes. These appearances usually resolve as the child grows.

Recording the results

The incorporation of a brief musculoskeletal examination into the routine examination should lead to a more detailed assessment if any abnormalities are found (Table 15.4).

Specific locomotor history

General demographic details such as age, sex and occupation should be recorded. Start the full musculoskeletal history with the presenting complaint and ask the patient to describe the sequence of symptoms, related features and events since the onset. Characteristic diagnostic points may emerge. Pain is a common presenting complaint and as such the clinician is expected to explore this fully. Using the WILDA (Words, Intensity, Location, Duration, Aggravating/alleviating factors) pain assessment approach may be helpful in drawing out key aspects

Table 15.4 How to record the locomotor screen routinely in the medical record

Screening questions:	pain	0
	gout or arthritis	0
	dressing	✓
	walking	✓
with positive answers being elaborated.		
Examination:		
A (Appearance)	M (Movement)	
G ✓		
A ✓	✓	
L ✓	✓	
S ✓	✓	
with abnormal findings indicated, e.g. in rheumatoid arthritis:		
A (Appearance)	M (Movement)	
G ✗		
A ✗	✗	
L ✗	✗	
S ✓	✓	
Slow painful gait.		
Synovitis of MCP, MTP, wrists and knee joints.		

of the patient's history and clarify the nature of the complaint. (See also Chapter 11.)

Words

'I have pain' is not descriptive enough to inform a clinician about the character of the pain symptoms. Patients may have more than one type of pain and should be encouraged to describe their pain as much as possible. Neuropathic pain can be described as burning, shooting, tingling, radiating, lancinating or numbness. Somatic pain may be described as dull or throbbing and can usually be well localized. Somatic pain is most commonly described in the context of musculoskeletal pain afflicting joints and the spine.

Pain described as squeezing, pressure, cramping, distention, dull, deep, and stretching is visceral in origin.

Intensity

It may be useful to use a simple visual analogue scale or ask the patient to rate his pain on a 0 to 10 scale. This may allow for monitoring and assessing progression of the underlying disorder.

Location

An accurate location of pain is often very helpful although it must be remembered that joint pain may radiate. Patients should be asked, 'Where is your pain?' or 'Do you have pain in more than one area?'

Pain may be referred or radiate from an affected joint (Box 15.2).

Box 15.2 Common patterns of joint pain radiation

Pain may be referred or radiate from an affected joint, e.g.:

- Neck pain may radiate through the occiput to the vertex or to the shoulder and down the arm, with paraesthesiae if there is nerve-root impingement.
- Shoulder joint pain may radiate to the elbow and below.
- Thoracic spine nerve root pain may radiate around the chest and mimic cardiac pain.
- Lumbar spinal root pain may radiate through the buttock and leg to the knee and below, with paraesthesiae in the foot with a large disc prolapse – this is called 'sciatica'.
- Hip-joint pain may radiate to the knee and below.
- Knee pain may radiate above and below the joint.

Duration

The temporal description of pain is important in understanding the route cause. Pain may be constant, episodic or a combination of both. Is the patient ever pain free? Can he clearly identify the time of onset and is there a pattern periodicity? For example, an osteoporotic vertebral fracture may be acute and self-limiting which contrasts with the severe, constant and gnawing pain of a spinal metastatic deposit that prevents sleep.

Aggravating/alleviating factors

Aggravating and alleviating factors are often very helpful when trying to make a diagnosis. Back pain or stiffness which improves with exercise may point to an inflammatory cause whereas pain which worsens after use is often describe in the setting of degenerative arthritis.

Back pain is the most common musculoskeletal complaint and as such deserves further consideration. When taking a history of a patient's back symptoms it is important to identify potential 'red flags' which mandate further imaging or investigations to exclude a potentially sinister underlying diagnosis. If red flag signs are present, then referral to a specialist for further evaluation is advised and a patient should be advised to rest and to avoid physical activity until then. Importantly, nerve root pain (unilateral sciatica) is not itself a cause for alarm, and conservative treatment should be effective. A list of red flag symptoms associated with back pain can be found in Table 15.5, with potential associated causes.

Pain may be referred or radiate from an affected joint (Box 15.2). With these pain patterns in mind, the joints above and below the apparently affected area should be examined.

Chronic pain syndromes

Chronic pain syndromes need to be distinguished from other rheumatic disorders and a careful history

Table 15.5 Red flag symptoms associated with back pain with potential associated causes

Red flag	Potential cause
Elderly (>65) or young (<40) patient	Elderly patient – osteoporosis Young patient – inflammatory arthritis
Immunocompromised	Infection
Trauma	Fracture or displacement
History of cancer	Malignancy/metastasis
Nocturnal pain	Malignancy
Systemically unwell (temperature/weight loss/night sweats)	Infection
Thoracic pain	Inflammatory – ankylosing spondylitis Infection/malignancy Aortic dissection/pancreatitis
Saddle anaesthesia/ bilateral sciatica/ progressive neurological deficit	Cauda equina or cord compression
Bladder, bowel or sexual dysfunction	Cauda equina or cord compression

is essential. A number of pain descriptors used by patients can indicate the influence of non-organic amplifying factors. For example, at least in the English language, words like 'searing', 'torturing' and 'terrifying' can be used by patients with chronic widespread pain and fibromyalgia. Fibromyalgia falls under the umbrella term central sensitization syndromes (CSS) and so may present with overlapping symptoms with other conditions such as irritable bowel syndrome, chronic fatigue and TMJ disorders. These debilitating disorders are often accompanied by poor sleep patterns, severe fatigue and depressed mood. The difficulty of cultural, religious and linguistic influences in interpreting pain should not be underestimated.

Joint disease

A combination of pain and stiffness, leading to loss of function, is a classic feature of joint disease. Usually one component predominates, as with stiffness in inflammation and pain in mechanical joint problems. Therefore, specific questions will establish whether symptoms are non-inflammatory (e.g. osteoarthritis) or inflammatory (e.g. rheumatoid arthritis). As with any condition, the good clinician will also draw out the consequences of the disorder in terms of the impact on the patient's day-to-day function and quality of life. The effect on relationships, work and social activities will help the clinician to gauge the severity of the problem and possibly elicit issues of stress and psychosocial pressure.

Non-inflammatory joint disease

Pain of a non-inflammatory origin is more directly related to function and use and usually improves with rest. This is in contrast to inflammatory joint pain which is often present at rest as well as on use and tends to vary from day to day and from week to week. Stiffness, particularly in the morning or after a period of inactivity, is often reported in a patient's history and typically lasts no more than 30 minutes. However, in severe cases the duration may be much longer. Subjective joint swelling may be described and indeed patients with knee osteoarthritis may present with a significant effusion. Joint swelling in this context tends to be more intermittent than the persistent joint swelling and warmth seen in inflammatory conditions.

Locking of a joint may occur. In the knee, this means that the knee becomes locked in such a way that it will not extend fully, although it may flex. In other joints, locking is less well defined and simply means that at some point through its range of motion the joint becomes stuck, usually associated with pain and often followed by swelling. Locking is due to material within the joint interfering with movement at the articular surfaces. In the knee, this is usually part of one of the menisci or a cartilaginous loose body.

Inflammatory joint disease

Early morning stiffness

Early morning joint stiffness that persists for more than 30 minutes is an important symptom of active inflammatory joint disease. Ask about redness (rubor), warmth (calor), tenderness/pain (dolor) and swelling (tumour), the classic features of inflammation.

Distribution of joint disease

The pattern of joint involvement is important. Common patterns are monoarticular (single joint), pauciarticular (up to four joints), polyarticular (many joints) and axial (spinal involvement). The pattern of joint involvement often aids in making a list of likely differential diagnoses. For example, rheumatoid arthritis is typically a symmetrical inflammatory arthritis of the small and large joints often presenting with metacarpal-phalangeal, wrist and metatarsal-phalangeal joint involvement. There are only a few causes of an exactly symmetrical arthropathy (Box 15.3). An asymmetrical inflammatory arthritis presentation is often seen in spondyloarthropathies such as reactive arthritis. An inflammatory monoarthritis presentation must elicit a suspicion of infection alongside other potential conditions such as gout or psoriatic arthritis. A history of fever or sweating may be helpful and if possible, synovial fluid should be aspirated from the joint to look for infection. Other conditions have such a classic history that it is diagnostic. For example, acute inflammation in the first metatarsophalangeal joint (hallux) suggests a diagnosis of gout (Box 15.4).

Box 15.3 Importance of distribution of joint involvement in differential diagnosis of pauciarthritis or polyarthritis

Typically symmetrical

- Upper and lower limbs: rheumatoid arthritis, systemic lupus erythematosus
- Especially upper limbs: haemochromatosis (hand: index, middle metacarpophalangeal joints)

Typically asymmetrical

- Psoriatic arthritis

Typically lower limb and asymmetrical

- Spondyloarthritis (e.g. ankylosing spondylitis, reactive arthritis)
- Document any associated features

Box 15.4 Acute gout

A 48-year-old publican presented with sudden severe pain and swelling of his left big toe. He was unable to bear weight or wear a shoe and said that he could not even bear the weight of his bedclothes on the toe at night. His past history included hypertension, for which he was taking a thiazide diuretic, and his alcohol intake was excessive. On examination, he had tophi on the ears (Fig. 15.15) and the left first metatarsophalangeal joint was red, hot, swollen and exquisitely painful to touch. Aspiration of the joint revealed urate crystals.

Box 15.5 Polymyalgia rheumatica

A 74-year-old woman presented with a 2-month history of pain around her hips and shoulders. The key points in the history were that these regions were extremely stiff for 4 hours each morning and inability to turn over in bed, and that there was no joint swelling. Clinically there was pain and some limitation of movement at the shoulders and hips but no synovitis. Her erythrocyte sedimentation rate was 96 mm/1st hour, and she had a dramatic response within 2 days to a moderate dose of prednisolone.

Box 15.6 Historical pointers to the differential diagnosis of monoarticular inflammatory joint disease

First attack

- Exclude infection by aspiration for culture and crystals
- If negative culture but high-risk group, biopsy, e.g. tuberculosis in Asian immigrants or immunosuppressed patients

Recurrent attacks

- Flitting (gonococcal arthritis, rheumatic fever)
- Episodic (crystal arthritis, palindromic rheumatism)

Persistent synovitis with none of the above features

- Look for systemic features and check serology (e.g. rheumatoid factor or antinuclear antibody)

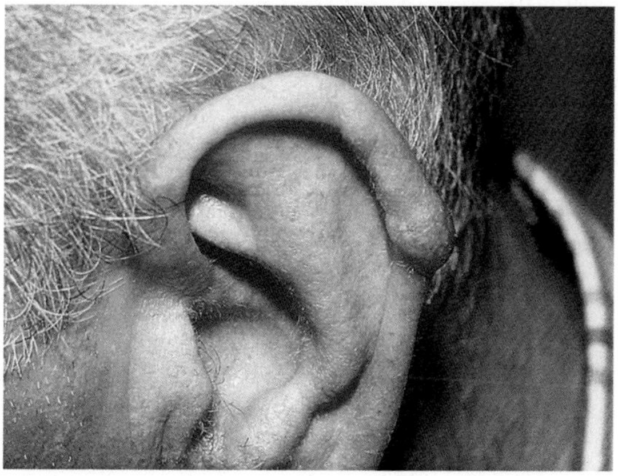

Figure 15.15 Gouty tophus on the ear. Other sites include the elbows, fingers and toes.

The pain and stiffness of the shoulder and hip girdles in polymyalgia rheumatica is also typical (Box 15.5). The pattern of the spondyloarthropathies can also be diagnostic with inflammatory sacroiliac and spinal pain and stiffness, lower limb arthritis, Achilles tendinitis and plantar fasciitis.

Recurrent attacks of joint pain

Ask if the same joint is always involved. If not, define the patterns of involvement, the severity and duration of the episodes and any associated clinical symptoms.

Episodic joint pain

Ask if attacks of joint pain are acute and associated with redness around the joint, with the attacks lasting about 48 hours (occasionally up to 1 week) and migrating to other joints. This is typical of palindromic rheumatism, which may progress to rheumatoid arthritis. Recurrent painful swelling of the same joint may be indicative of a crystal arthropathy such as gout or calcium pyrophosphate disease.

Flitting or migratory joint pains

The term 'flitting' or migratory joint pains is used to describe inflammation beginning in one joint and then involving others, usually one at a time for about 3 days each. Gonococcal arthritis should be considered; this is characterized by typical fleeting skin lesions and urethritis, in addition to joint pain. In rheumatic fever, there is associated cardiac involvement, and erythema marginatum and subcutaneous nodules may occur.

The other features in the history that should be brought out are best considered under the differential diagnosis of polyarthritis (Box 15.6). Many arthropathies may have a monoarticular presentation.

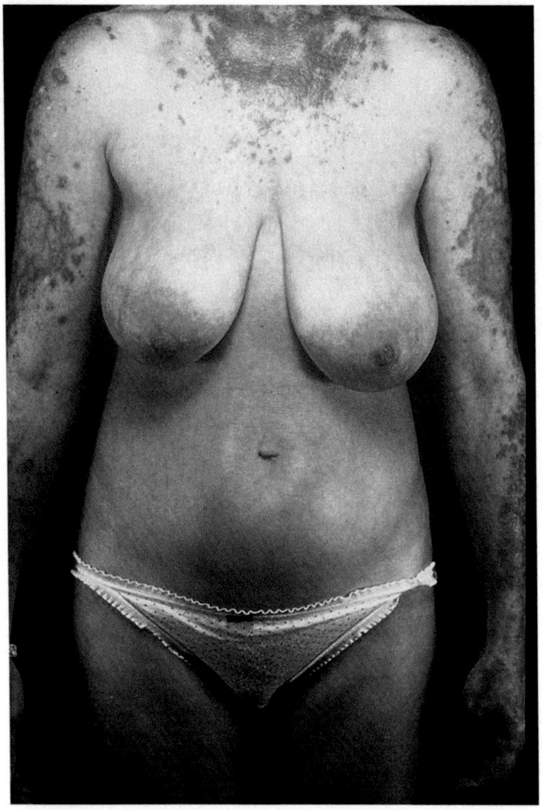

Figure 15.16 Extensive rash in sun-exposed areas in a woman with systemic lupus erythematosus and anti-Ro antibodies.

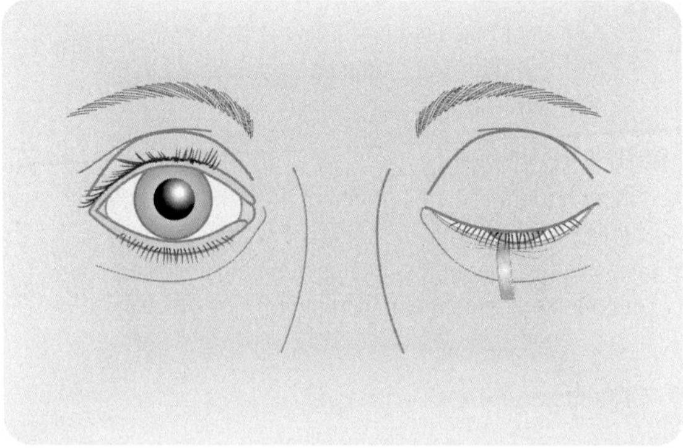

Figure 15.17 Schirmer's test – a sterile strip of filter paper is hooked over the lower eyelid. Less than 5 mm of wetness after 5 minutes is abnormal and is associated with autoimmune rheumatic disease.

Inflammatory connective tissue diseases

The autoimmune rheumatic disorders, such as systemic lupus erythematosus (SLE), Sjögren's syndrome, inflammatory myopathies, systemic sclerosis and the vasculitides, are multisystem disorders. It is critical that a full systems enquiry and physical examination are performed when inflammatory connective tissue is suspected. Associated features of these conditions include systemic symptoms such as weight loss, malaise or fevers, and rash, especially if the latter is photosensitive or vasculitic (Fig. 15.16). Alopecia, oral and genital ulceration, Raynaud's phenomenon and symptoms of neurological, cardiac, pulmonary and gastrointestinal involvement may occur. Dry eyes and dry mouth (sicca symptoms) are common and can be documented with Schirmer's test (Fig. 15.17). Renal disease is a serious complication of the autoimmune rheumatic disorders, especially in SLE and the systemic vasculitides. Clinical assessment should always include measuring blood pressure and dip-testing the urine for blood and protein and microscopy of the urine sediment for casts or dysmorphic red cells if this is positive. Ear, nose and throat involvement with sinusitis, facial pain and deafness is common in Wegener's granulomatosis and Churg–Strauss syndrome. A history of arterial and venous thromboses or miscarriages, especially in the context of livedo reticularis, should raise the suspicion of the antiphospholipid syndrome.

Soft tissue symptoms

Soft tissue problems are common and usually consist of pain, a dull ache, tenderness or swelling. In the elderly these symptoms often appear spontaneously, but in younger people there is usually a history of injury or overuse, through either occupation (e.g. tenosynovitis of the long flexor tendons of the hand) or sport (e.g. Achilles tendinitis in runners, shoulder rotator cuff tendinopathy in swimmers or throwers). It is important to define the exact site of the symptoms and the factors that either make them worse or induce relief. The mechanism of injury is also important and can help guide a focused examination. The localization of symptoms to specific soft tissue structures can be confirmed by careful examination (Box 15.7). The possible structures involved are joint, tendon, ligament, bursa and muscle. Local palpation may be enough to accurately locate bursitis or enthesitis (inflammation at the attachment of a ligament or tendon to bone). Movement of the joint region often elicits pain or discomfort in a particular direction which can direct the clinician to the affected structure. Subacromial bursitis typically produces pain when the shoulder is abducted to 80° and resolves at 130-140°, described as a painful arc, whereas anterior and posterior movements are maintained.

The bones

Bone pain is characteristically deep seated and localized, but referred pain may confuse the clinical picture. In the case of fractures, unless pathological, there will almost always be a history of injury. In athletes, however, a fracture may be due to chronic overuse, as in stress fractures of the tibia or metatarsals in runners. The spontaneous onset of pain may suggest Paget's disease (with bony enlargement, e.g. skull or

Box 15.7 Localization of the site of articular and extra-articular features

Joint

- Diffuse pain and tenderness
- Generalized joint swelling
- Restriction of movement, usually in all directions of movement (specific to each joint)

Tendon

- Localized pain/tenderness at attachment (enthesis) or in the tendon substance
- Swelling, tendon sheath or paratendon
- Pain on resisted movement
- Sometimes pain on stretch (e.g. Achilles)

Ligament

- Localized pain/tenderness at attachment or in ligament substance
- Pain on stretch
- Instability, if major tear

Bursa

- Localized tenderness
- Pain on stretching adjacent structures

Muscle

- Localized or diffuse pain and tenderness
- Pain on resisted action
- Pain on stretch (e.g. hamstring)

Box 15.8 Examination of the musculoskeletal system

General observations

- Gait
- Posture
- Mobility
- Deformity
- Independence: use of wheelchair or walking aids
- Muscle wasting
- Long bones

Fractures

- Joints
- Tendons
- Skin

tibia) or metastatic deposits. Infection must also be considered, particularly in younger patients or in immunodeficiency states. Consider also congenital or familial disorders as predisposing factors, for example multiple osteochondromata or brittle bone disease (osteogenesis imperfecta).

Examination: general principles

Observe the patient entering the room (Box 15.8). Abnormalities of gait and posture may provide clues

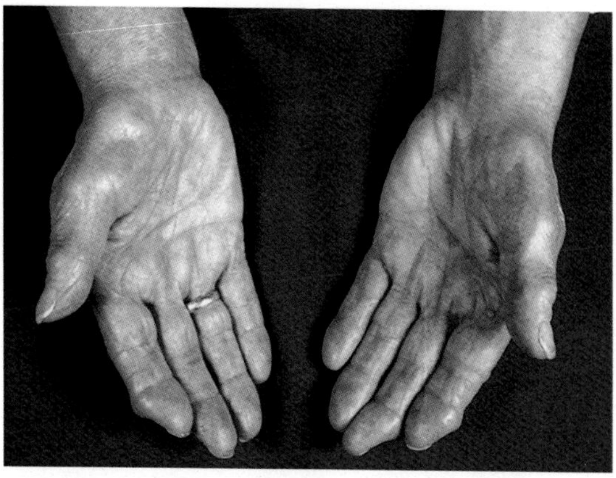

Figure 15.18 Thenar wasting due to carpal tunnel syndrome. This is often associated with osteoarthritis. Note nodal change on the terminal interphalangeal joints of the index fingers.

that can be pursued in history taking. Observation of any difficulty in undressing and getting onto the examination couch will further help in assessment. The patient must always be asked to stand and walk, even when it is obvious that this may be difficult. Note how much help the patient requires from others or from sticks, crutches, etc. The musculoskeletal system includes the muscles, bones, joints and soft-tissue structures such as tendons and ligaments. Remember that although muscle-wasting may be due to primary muscle disease (e.g. polymyositis), it is more commonly secondary to disuse, perhaps because of a painful joint, or to neuropathy due to nerve root compression or peripheral neuropathy (Fig. 15.18). Examination of the muscles is discussed further in Chapter 16.

The bones

The examination of the bones should always be directed by information obtained from the history.

Inspection

Look for any alterations in shape or outline and measure any shortening. In Paget's disease (osteitis deformans), bowing of the long bones, particularly the tibia (Fig. 15.19) and femur, is associated with bony enlargement and, usually, increased local temperature. The skull is also commonly involved, but this may not be apparent until the disease is advanced. Early involvement of the skull bones can be detected on X-rays (Fig. 15.20). Alterations in the shape of bones also occur in rickets as a result of epiphyseal enlargement. Deformity of the chest in rickets is due to osteochondral enlargement (rickety rosary).

Localized swellings of long bones may be caused by infections, cysts or tumours. Spontaneous fractures may occasionally be the presenting symptom in the diagnosis of secondary carcinoma, multiple myeloma, generalized osteitis fibrosa cystica (hyperparathyroidism) or osteogenesis imperfecta.

Palpation

On palpation, bone tenderness occurs in local lesions when there is destruction, elevation or irritation of the periosteum, as in generalized osteitis fibrosa cystica, myelomatosis, bone infections, occasionally in carcinomatosis of bones and, rarely, in leukaemia. Injury is the commonest cause.

Fractures

Fractures are common and may involve any bone. They are painful, distressing for the patient and expensive for the community (Box 15.9). Fractures in healthy bones commonly involve the long bones and are usually due to trauma. Fractures of the wrists, hips and vertebrae are more frequently complications

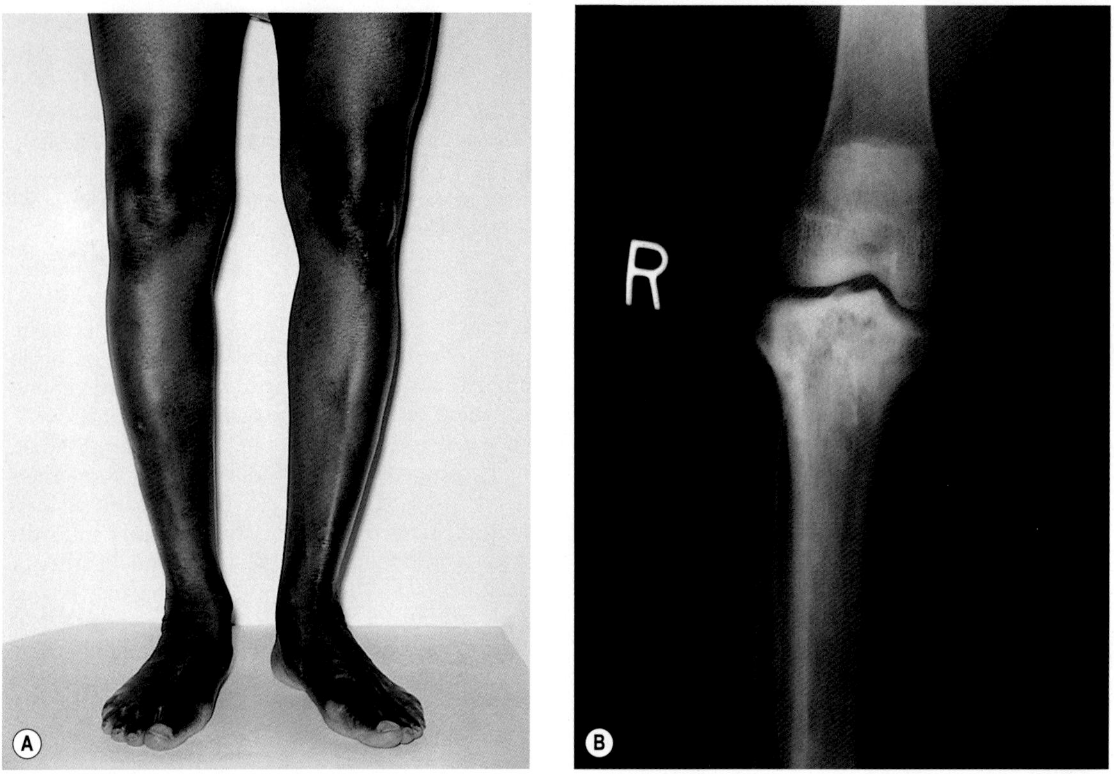

Figure 15.19 Paget's disease of the right tibia. Note tibial bowing and bony enlargement **(A)** and bony enlargement sclerosis with some patchy porosis in the X-ray of the upper tibia **(B)**.

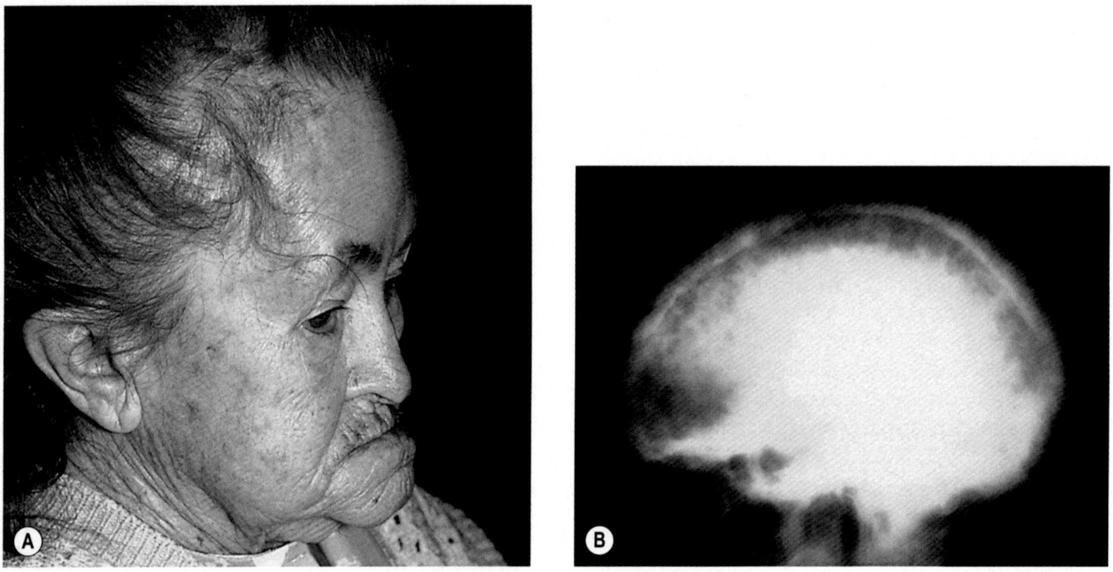

Figure 15.20 Paget's disease, causing deformity of the skull **(A)**. Note the thickened skull vault with remodelled bone **(B)**.

Box 15.9 Fractures: clinical features

Type
- Closed
- Compound (open)

Complications
- Accompanying soft-tissue injury (indirect)

Features
- Haemorrhage
- Deformity
- Pain
- Crepitus
- Restricted movement

Cause
- Traumatic
- Spontaneous (osteoporosis or metabolic)
- Pathological

of bone disease, such as osteoporosis. Multiple rib fractures, caused by falls, may be found in heavy alcohol users but may only be seen as healed lesions on chest X-ray. Fractures occur without apparent trauma when a bone is weakened by disease, especially with metastatic malignant deposits in bone (pathological fractures). Traumatic fractures invariably present with local pain, swelling and loss of function, but pathological fractures may be relatively silent. The history will reveal the circumstances of the trauma, whether accidental or due to physical abuse, and should be carefully documented, if necessary, with diagrams or digital photographs of the clinical findings. If clinical photographs are taken, prior written consent is needed.

Examination of suspected fracture

Fractures may be open (compound) or closed. In closed fractures, the surrounding soft tissues are intact. In open fractures, the bone communicates with the surface of the skin, either because the primary injury has broken the overlying skin or because deformation at the fracture site has caused the bone ends to penetrate the skin. There is a major risk of infection when the fracture site communicates with the open air.

Deformity is an obvious feature in the majority of fractures although in some patients this may be difficult to appreciate due to a large body habitus. Comparison with the contralateral limb is often helpful. Deformity may be clinically characteristic, as in Colles' fracture, in which there is a fracture of the distal end of the radius characterized by dorsal displacement and angulation, shortening of the wrist and rotation of the fragment, well summarized in the description 'dinner-fork deformity'. Certain fractures may show little deformity; for example, a fracture of the femoral shaft may be accompanied by only slight deformity, as there is often little separation of the bones at the fracture site and other features are disguised by the thick overlying muscle. A fractured neck of the femur causes deformity through external rotation of the foot and shortening of the leg.

Most fractures are characterized by local tenderness and swelling, unless the overlying muscle mass is large such as at the hip. Bony crepitus, due to abnormal motion at the fracture site, is a feature of fractures, but this should not be elicited unless absolutely necessary for diagnosis because it is very painful. However, if it is perceived or has been recognized by the patient, it is diagnostic.

A fracture of the bone may damage the neighbouring soft tissues directly or, alternatively, a fracture may be a marker of severe injury in which direct damage to the soft tissues such as the nerves and vessels may have taken place. A neuromuscular assessment distal to the fracture site is imperative. The presence or absence of pulses and cutaneous sensation and the colour and perfusion of the limb must always be recorded and any changes over time reported. Limb ischaemia distal to a fracture is a surgical emergency. Voluntary movement at joints distal to a fractured long bone, such as ankle movement in a fractured femur, should be noted. If this is absent, nerve injury must be suspected.

The joints

Examination of the joints can be summarized simply as 'look, feel and move' (i.e. inspection, palpation and range of movement). With practice, the clinician can develop a systematic review of the joints – for example the jaw, cervical spine, shoulder girdle and upper limb, thoracic and lumbar spine, pelvis and lower limb – so that inconspicuous but important joints, such as the temporomandibular, sternoclavicular and sacroiliac joints, will not be overlooked. Compare the corresponding joints on the two sides of the body and always take care to avoid causing undue discomfort.

Inspection

The detection of joint inflammation is a crucial clinical skill. Inflammation is often associated with redness of the joint and with tenderness and warmth. Look also for swelling or deformity of the joint. The overall pattern of joint involvement should be recorded. Examine the contralateral joint where possible and note whether the distribution is symmetrical, as is usual in rheumatoid arthritis (Fig. 15.21), or asymmetrical, as in psoriatic arthropathy or gout (Fig. 15.22). The seronegative spondyloarthropathies (Fig. 15.23) tend to involve predominantly the joints of the lower limb.

Palpation

On palpation of a joint, check first for tenderness. Then determine whether the swelling is due to bony

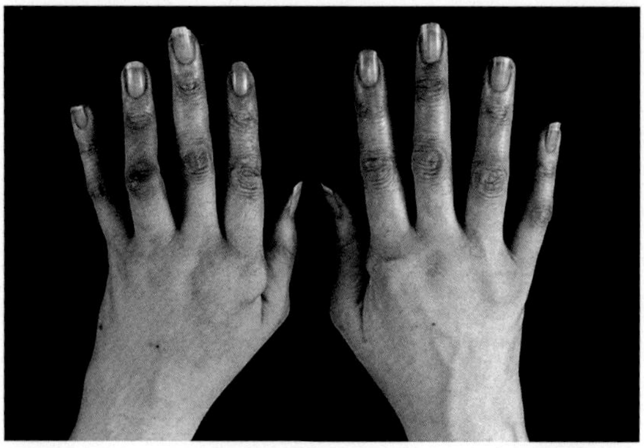

Figure 15.21 Symmetrical joint involvement due to rheumatoid arthritis.

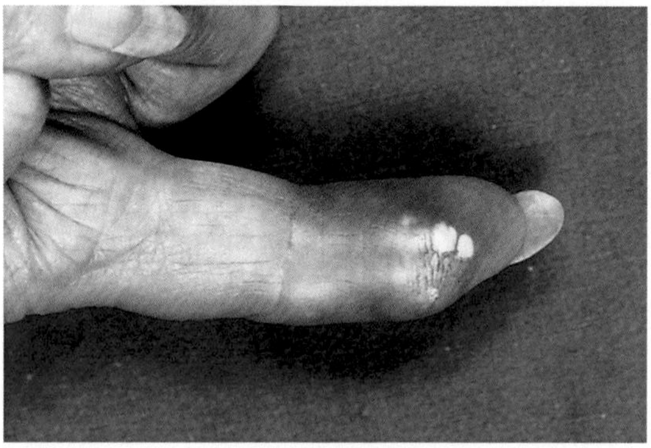

Figure 15.22 Gouty tophus of the index finger.

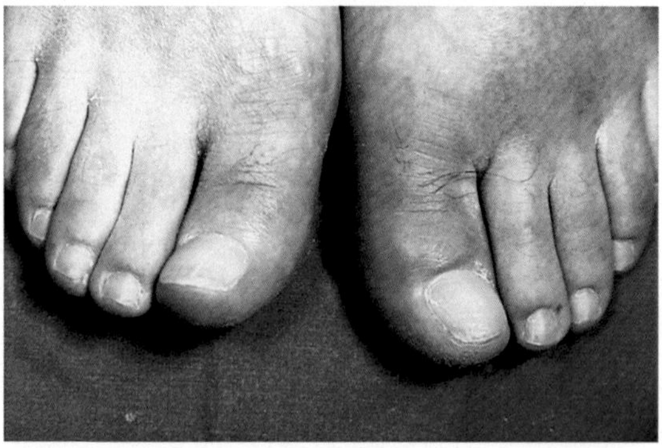

Figure 15.23 Acute synovitis of the interphalangeal joint in reactive arthritis of the left hallux. Differential diagnosis includes gout.

enlargement or osteophytes (e.g. Heberden's nodes, Fig. 15.24), thickening of synovial tissues, such as occurs in inflammatory arthritis, or effusion into the joint space. Joint effusions usually have a characteristically smooth outline and fluctuation is usually easily demonstrable. Palpation of the whole joint is important as this may reveal localized enthesitis (lateral epicondylitis at the elbow) or reveal localized effusions (Baker's cyst in the posterior aspect of the knee joint).

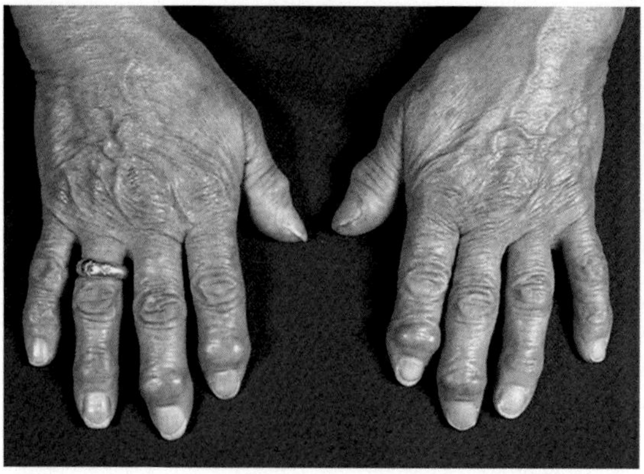

Figure 15.24 Nodal osteoarthritis (Heberden's nodes).

Box 15.10 Assessment of joint tenderness

- Grade 1: The patient says the joint is tender
- Grade 2: The patient winces
- Grade 3: The patient winces and withdraws the affected part
- Grade 4: The patient will not allow the joint to be touched

Tenderness and enlargement of the ends of long bones, particularly the radius, ulna and tibia, can occur in hypertrophic pulmonary osteoarthropathy: a chest X-ray is essential. Gross disorganization of a joint – nearly always the foot and ankle joints – associated with an absence of deep pain and position sense occurs in neuropathic (Charcot) joints. Charcot joints probably arise from recurrent painless injury and overstretching and are a feature of severe chronic sensorimotor neuropathy.

Joint tenderness may be graded depending on the patient's reaction to firm pressure of the joint between finger and thumb (Box 15.10). Grade 4 tenderness occurs only in septic arthritis, crystal arthritis and rheumatic fever.

If tenderness is present, localize it as accurately as possible and determine whether it arises in the joint or in neighbouring structures, for example in the supraspinatus or bicipital tendon rather than the shoulder joint. Other rheumatic conditions produce different types of pain. For example, in conditions such as complex regional pain syndrome (CRPS) type I (previously known as reflex sympathetic dystrophy), hyperalgesia (abnormal and excessive pain to mildly painful stimuli) and allodynia (a sensation of pain to stimuli not normally painful, e.g. light touch) may often be seen, together with altered sweating and discoloration. In fibromyalgia, there is widespread diffuse muscle and joint tenderness but no inflammation. A number of characteristic trigger points may be tender around the neck, trunk, and upper and lower limbs.

Tendon sheath crepitus

Tendon sheath crepitus is a grating or creaking sensation defined by palpating the tendon while the patient is asked to contract the muscle tendon complex involved. It is particularly common in the hand and is seen in rheumatoid arthritis and systemic sclerosis. In tenosynovitis of the long flexor tendons in the palm, tendon sheath crepitus may be associated with the trigger phenomenon, in which the finger becomes caught in flexion and has to be pulled back into extension. Tendon sheath effusions can be distinguished from joint swelling by their anatomical location in association with tendons but where there is doubt an ultrasonographic assessment will provide clarity.

Joint crepitus

Joint crepitus can be detected by feeling the joint with one hand while moving it passively with the other. This may indicate osteoarthritis or loose bodies (cartilaginous fragments) in the joint space but should be differentiated from non-specific clicking of joints.

Range of movement

When examining joints for range of movement, it is usually sufficient to estimate the degree of limitation based on comparison with the normal side or on the examiner's previous experience. For accurate description, the actual range of movement should be measured with a protractor (goniometer). Both active and passive movement should be assessed. Active movement, however, may give a poor estimation of true range of movement because of muscle spasm due to pain. If pain is very severe on attempting active movement and other findings suggest a fracture, take an X-ray before attempting any further examination. In testing the range of passive movement, always be gentle, particularly when the joints are painful. The direction of joint movement, particularly in ball and socket joints, may provide additional information as to the underlying lesion.

Limitation of movement in a joint may be due to pain, muscle spasm, contracture, inflammation, increased thickness of the capsular or periarticular structures, effusion into the joint space, bony overgrowths, bony ankylosis, mechanical factors such as a torn meniscus or to painful conditions quite unconnected with the joint.

Extra-articular features of joint disease

Some of the extra-articular features of joint disease are listed in Box 15.11.

Subcutaneous nodules

Subcutaneous nodules are associated with several conditions (Box 15.12). If gout is suspected, inspect the helix of the ear for tophi caused by the subcutaneous deposition of urate, which may also be found overlying joints or in the finger pads (see Figs 15.15 and 15.22). Subcutaneous nodules in rheumatoid arthritis are firm and non-tender; they may be detected by running the examining thumb from the point of the elbow down the proximal portion of the ulna (Fig. 15.25). They can also be found at other pressure and frictional sites, such as bony prominences, including the sacrum and in the hands. If an olecranon bursa swelling is found, feel also in its wall, as rheumatoid nodules, tophi or occasionally xanthomata may be found within the swelling. Subcutaneous nodules are not specific to rheumatoid arthritis and may occur in patients with SLE, systemic sclerosis

Box 15.11 Extra-articular features of joint disease

- Cutaneous nodules
- Cutaneous vasculitic lesions
- Lymphadenopathy
- Oedema
- Tendon sheath effusions
- Enlarged bursae
- Ocular inflammation
- Diarrhoea
- Urethritis
- Orogenital ulceration
- Alopecia

Box 15.12 Types of subcutaneous nodules

- Gouty tophi caused by urate deposition
- Rheumatoid nodules
- Vasculitic nodules in SLE and systemic vasculitis
- Xanthomatous deposits (hypercholesterolaemia)

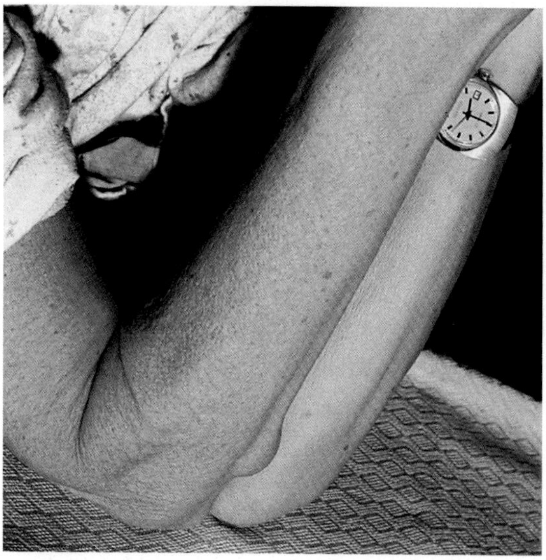

Figure 15.25 Rheumatoid nodule overlying the olecranon of the right arm.

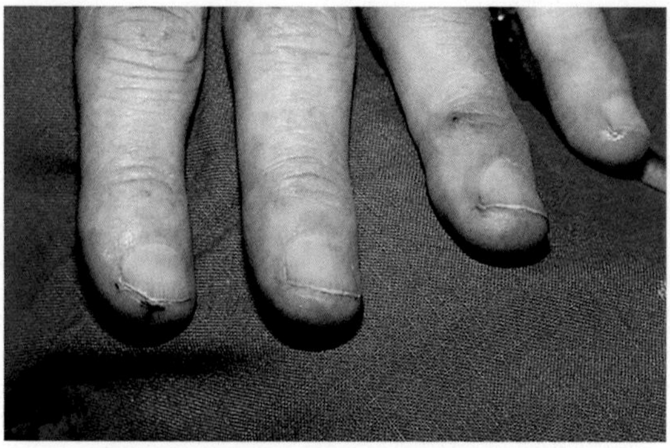

Figure 15.26 Nail-fold vasculitis in rheumatoid arthritis. This also occurs in SLE and other systemic vasculitides.

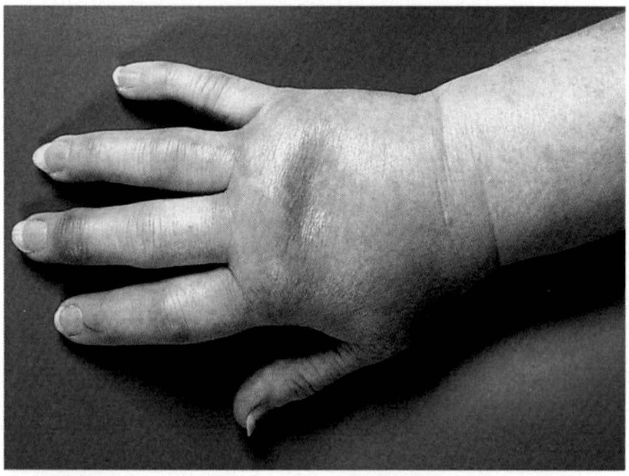

Figure 15.27 Pitting oedema, right hand.

and rheumatic fever. Ultrasonographic appearance may be helpful in distinguishing subcutaneous nodules and may facilitate a guide aspiration if necessary.

Cutaneous vasculitic lesions

Cutaneous vasculitic lesions may be seen in rheumatoid arthritis, SLE, Sjögren's syndrome and the systemic vasculitides. They may be small, punched-out necrotic lesions, palpable purpura or vasculitic ulcers, especially on the lower limbs. Small vessel involvement is typically seen at the nail fold (cutaneous infarct; Fig. 15.26) but also occurs at pressure sites. Splinter haemorrhages, the classic feature of bacterial endocarditis, may also be a feature of vasculitis and the antiphospholipid syndrome.

Lymphadenopathy

Lymphadenopathy may be found proximal to an inflamed joint, not only in septic arthritis but also in rheumatoid arthritis. Generalized lymphadenopathy, sometimes with splenomegaly, is common in active SLE.

Local oedema

Local oedema is sometimes seen over inflamed joints (Fig. 15.27), but other causes of oedema must be excluded. Pitting leg oedema may indicate cardiac failure, pericardial effusion or nephrotic syndrome, which can complicate rheumatoid arthritis and SLE.

Other soft-tissue swellings

Tendon sheath effusions are distinguished from joint swellings by their location in association with tendons. Enlarged subcutaneous bursae may be found over pressure areas, particularly at the olecranon surface of the elbow, owing to inflammatory joint disease or secondary to friction. Deeper bursae may be defined only by finding local tenderness or by stressing adjacent tissues (e.g. greater trochanter bursitis).

Examination of individual joints

The range of movement of joints is described in the following pages. All motion should be measured in degrees from a neutral or zero position, which must be defined whenever possible and compared with the opposite side. Some special features seen at individual joints are set out in each section.

The spine

General examination of the vertebral column

Inspection

Examine the patient both in standing and in sitting in the erect posture. The normal thoracolumbar spine has an S-shaped curve. If there is an abnormality, note which vertebrae are involved and at what level any vertebral projection is most prominent. Note the presence of any local projections or angular deformity of the spine. Torticollis, if present, is usually obvious, resulting form muscle spasm of the sternocleidomastoid, trapezius and other neck muscles. This places the neck in a tilted, rotated, partially flexed position.

Palpation

The major landmarks are the spinous processes of C7 (the vertebra prominens) and the last rib, which articulates with the 12th thoracic vertebra. In many patients, however, the last rib cannot be felt distinctly, and this is therefore rather untrustworthy as a guide to this level.

The neutral position of the spine is an upright stance with head erect and chin drawn in. Note any curvature of the spinal column, whether as a whole or of part of it. Abnormal curvature may be in an anterior, posterior or lateral direction (Fig. 15.28). Anterior curvature (convex forward) is termed lordosis. There are natural lordotic curves in the cervical and lumbar regions. Posterior curvature (convex backward) is termed kyphosis. The thoracic spine usually exhibits a slight smooth kyphosis, which increases in the elderly and especially in osteoporosis. It must be distinguished from a localized angular deformity

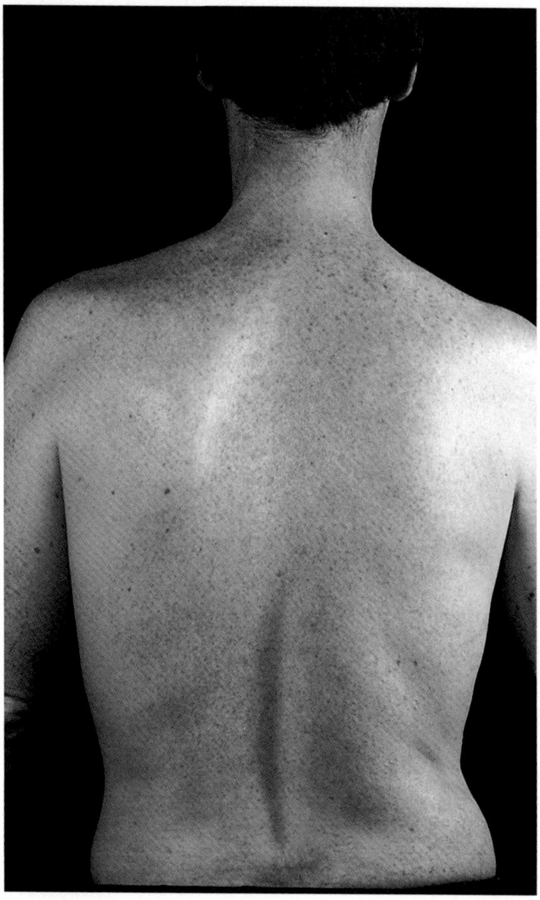

Figure 15.28 Scoliosis of the lumbar spine due to prolapsed intervertebral disc.

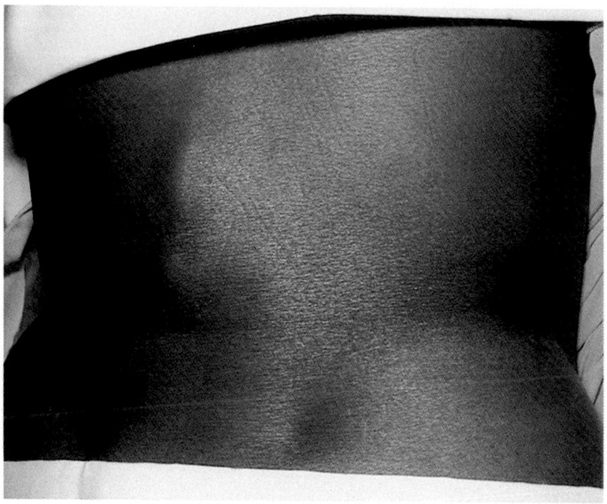

Figure 15.29 Gibbus of the lumbar spine due to tuberculosis.

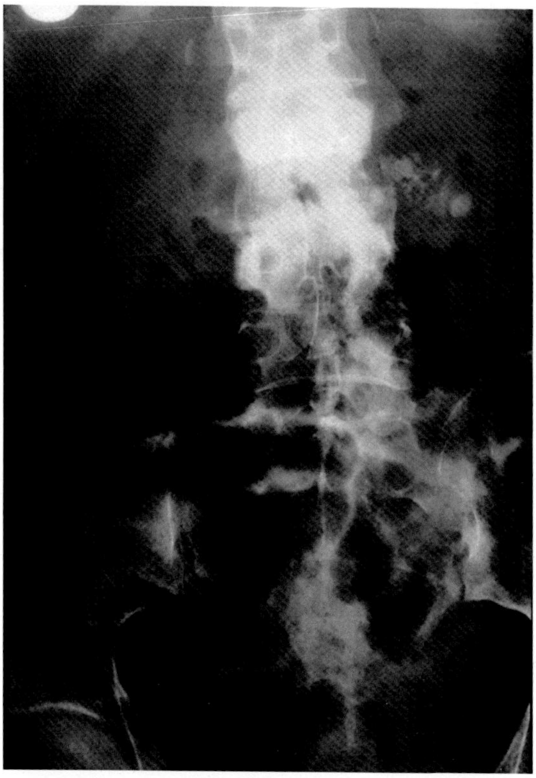

Figure 15.30 X-ray of tuberculous discitis. This shows the underlying deformity shown in Fig. 15.29. There is tuberculous infection of the intervertebral disc, causing the spinal deformity.

(gibbus, Fig. 15.29) caused by a fracture, by Pott's disease (spinal tuberculosis, Fig. 15.30) or by a metastatic malignant deposit.

Lateral curvature is termed scoliosis (see Fig. 15.28) and may be towards either side. It is always accompanied by rotation of the bodies of the vertebrae in such a way that the posterior spinous processes come to point towards the concavity of the curve. The curvature is always greater than appears from inspection of the posterior spinous processes. In scoliosis due to muscle spasm (e.g. with lumbosacral disc protrusion syndromes), the spinal curvature and rotational deformity decrease in flexion. When scoliosis is caused by inequality of leg length, it disappears on sitting, because the buttocks then become level. Scoliosis secondary to skeletal anomalies shows in spinal flexion as a 'rib hump' due to the rotation. Kyphosis and scoliosis are often combined, particularly when the cause is an idiopathic spinal curvature, beginning in adolescence.

The cervical spine

The following movements should be tested (Fig. 15.31):

- Rotation (ask the patient to look over one then the other shoulder).
- Flexion (ask the patient to touch chin to chest).
- Extension (ask the patient to look up to the ceiling).
- Lateral bending (ask the patient to bend the neck sideways and to try to touch the shoulder with the ear without raising the shoulder).

Note any pain or paraesthesiae in the arm reproduced by neck movement, especially on gentle

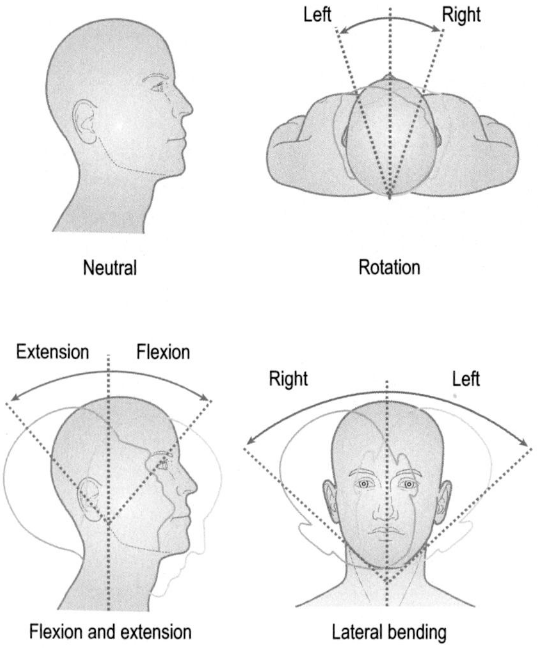

Figure 15.31 Movements of the neck.

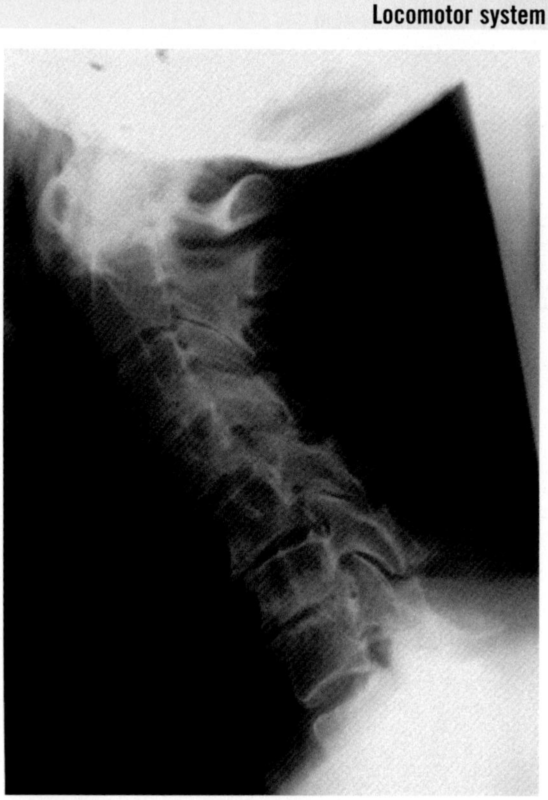

Figure 15.32 Lateral X-ray of cervical spine showing degenerative spondylosis with narrowing of the disc spaces and reversed cervical lordosis between C4 and C6.

sustained extension or lateral flexion, suggesting nerve-root involvement. If indicated, check for any associated neurological deficit, particularly of radicular or spinal cord type.

In rheumatoid arthritis, particular care is necessary when examining the neck, as atlantoaxial instability may lead to damage to the spinal cord when the neck is flexed. If there is any doubt about neck stability in a patient with rheumatoid arthritis, arrange for lateral X-rays of the cervical spine in flexion and extension, together with a view of the odontoid peg through the mouth, and defer clinical examination.

In patients with cervical injury, never try to elicit range of motion of the neck. Instead, splint the neck, take a history, look for abnormality of posture (usually in rotation) and check neurological function in the limbs, including both arms and both legs. Imaging the neck in the lateral (Fig. 15.32) and anteroposterior planes, *without* moving the neck, is essential and may be done with plain radiography or, in trauma patients, with computed tomography or magnetic resonance imaging (MRI) to assess injury to the cord. Only if imaging is normal should neck movements be examined.

The thoracic and lumbar spine

The main movement at the thoracic spine is rotation, whereas the lumbar spine can flex, extend and bend laterally. The following movements should be tested (Fig. 15.33):

- Flexion (ask the patient to try to touch his toes, without bending at the knees).
- Extension (ask the patient to bend backwards).

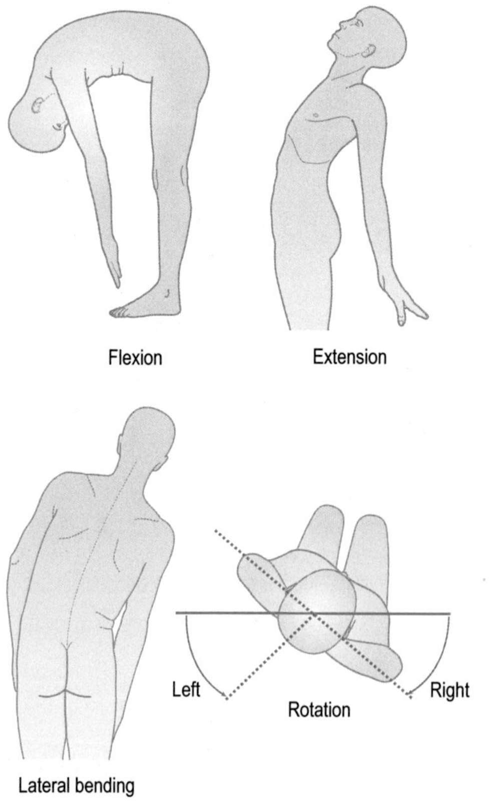

Figure 15.33 Movements of the lumbar and dorsal spine.

- Lateral bending (ask the patient to run the hand down the side of the thigh as far as possible.
- Thoracic rotation (ask the seated patient, with arms crossed, to twist round to the left and right as far as possible).

In flexion, the normal lumbar lordosis should be abolished. It is important to distinguish between flexion at the lumbar spine and compensated flexion at the hips which may deceive the examiner if only a cursory examination is carried out. A more objective assessment of lumbar spine flexion can be performed by marking a vertical 10-cm line on the skin overlying the lumbar spinous processes and the sacral dimples and measuring the increase in the line length on flexion (modified Schober's test); this should normally be 5 cm or more. Painful restriction of spinal movement is an important sign of cervical and lumbar spondylosis but may also be found in vertebral disc disease or other mechanical disorders of the back or neck in association with muscle spasm. A useful clinical aphorism is that a rigid lumbar spine should always be investigated for serious pathology, such as infection (e.g. staphylococcal or tuberculous discitis), malignancy or inflammation (e.g. ankylosing spondylitis). Spinal movements may be virtually absent in ankylosing spondylitis (Fig. 15.34), but in the early stages of this condition lateral flexion of the lumbar spine is typically affected first. In mechanical or osteoarthritic back problems, flexion and extension are reduced more than lateral movements. In prolapsed intervertebral disc lesions, sustained gentle lumbar extension may reproduce the low back pain and sciatic radiation.

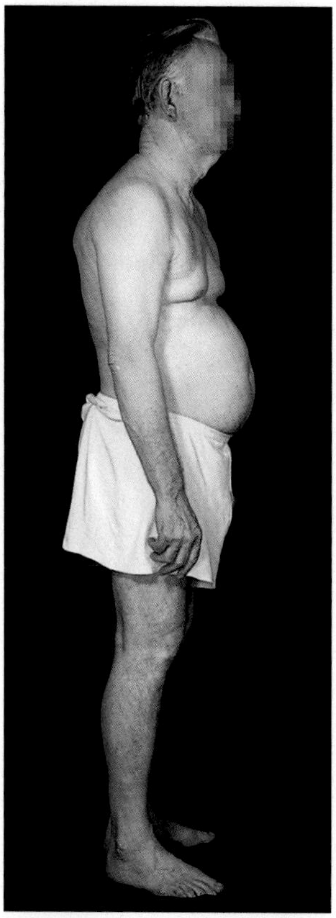

Figure 15.34 Ankylosing spondylitis. Note dorsal kyphosis and protuberant abdomen due to poor chest expansion with abdominal breathing.

Chest expansion is a measure of costovertebral movement and should be recorded using a tape measure with the patient's hands behind his head to reduce the possibility of muscular action in the shoulder girdle giving a false reading. The examiner stands behind the patient and the tape measure is placed around the chest at the level of the xiphisternal joint. The patient is asked to exhale and the tape is tightened before a maximum inhalation. An increase of 5 cm is expected in adults. Reduced chest expansion is a characteristic early feature in ankylosing spondylitis. Obviously, this may also be a feature of primary pulmonary disease, such as emphysema.

Examination of the back is completed by assessing straight leg raising (SLR) and strength, sensation and reflex activity in the legs. Pain and limitation on SLR is a feature of a prolapsed intervertebral disc when there is irritation or compression of one of the roots of the sciatic nerve. Tight hamstring muscles may cause a similar picture, but if there is severe pain, it is more considerate to lower the leg to just below the limit of SLR and then to see whether gentle passive dorsiflexion of the foot brings back the same pain. If in doubt, dorsiflex the foot once the limit of SLR has been reached. This further stretches the sciatic nerve (the pain increases) but does not affect the hamstrings (Lasègue's sign). The femoral stretch test is a useful confirmatory test and is performed with the patient lying prone: if there is a prolapsed disc at that level, flexion at the knee will produce pain in the lower lumbar spine. Sacral sensory loss must always be carefully assessed because, if there is a large central lumbosacral disc protrusion, bilateral limitation of SLR may be associated with bladder or bowel dysfunction and sacral anaesthesia. This combination is an emergency and requires immediate investigation and treatment.

The sacroiliac joints

The surface markings of these joints are two dimples low in the lumbar region. Test for irritability in the following ways:

- Direct pressure over each sacroiliac joint.
- Firm pressure with the side of the hand over the sacrum.
- Inward pressure over both iliac bones with the patient lying on one side, in an attempt to distort the pelvis.
- Flex the hip to 90° and exert firm pressure at the knee through the femoral shaft (this should only be done if the hip and knee are not painful).

In the last three, a positive test is only indicated by the patient localizing discomfort to the sacroiliac joint.

The shoulder

Shoulder examination involves the assessment of a number of other joints in addition to the glenohumeral articulation. Abduction of the shoulder in particular involves movement at the sternoclavicular, acromioclavicular, glenohumeral and scapulothoracic joints. Pain is also referred and the shoulder examination should be accompanied by an examination of the cervical spine as radicular pain may be localized by the patient at the shoulder and vice versa.

Inspection of the shoulder should be from the posterior, lateral and anterior positions. Where possible the contralateral shoulder should be exposed and comparisons made in muscle bulk.

Palpation of the shoulder should include the long head of biceps tendon in the bicipital groove, acromio-clavicular joint, clavicle, sternoclavicular joint and the acromion.

The neutral position is with the arm to the side, elbow flexed to 90° and forearm pointing forwards. Because the scapula is mobile, true shoulder (glenohumeral) movement can be assessed only when the examiner anchors the inferior angle of the scapula between finger and thumb on the posterior chest wall. The following movements should be tested (Fig. 15.35):

- Flexion
- Extension
- Abduction
- Rotation in abduction
- Rotation in neutral position
- Elevation (also involving scapular movement)

In practice, internal rotation can best be compared by recording the height reached by each thumb up the back, representing combined glenohumeral and scapular movement. Similarly, external rotation can be assessed by the ability to get the hand to the back of the neck. Limitation of external rotation is a good sign of true glenohumeral disease, which may occur in adhesive capsulitis (frozen shoulder) or erosive damage from inflammatory arthritis.

Note any pain during the range of movement. In supraspinatus tendinitis, a full passive range of movement is found but there is a painful arc on abduction, with pain exacerbated on resisted abduction (see Fig. 15.35). Other tendon involvement should also be defined by pain on resisted action.

Subacromial impingement due to a bursitis or rotator cuff abnormality may produce severe pain at

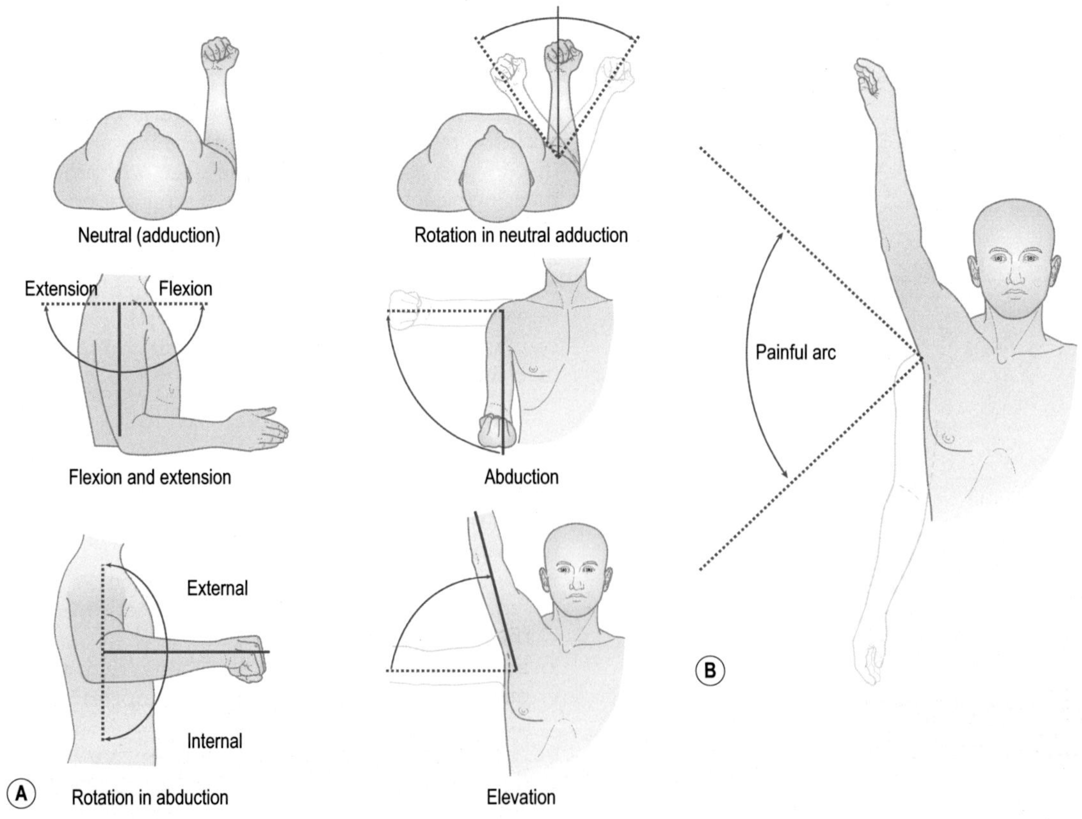

Figure 15.35 **(A)** Movements of the shoulder. **(B)** Painful arc of supraspinatus tendinitis.

the end of abduction, blocking full elevation. Acute bursitis, however, may be so painful that no abduction is allowed (grade 4 discomfort). Acromioclavicular joint pain is always very localized and is typically felt in the last 10° of elevation (170-180° arc).

Special tests in shoulder examination

Supraspinatus

The supraspinatus muscle can be tested using the 'empty can' test which involves forward flexion of the arm to 90° and abduction to 30° with the thumb pointing upwards. The shoulder is then internally rotated so that the thumb is now facing downwards. The examiner places his hand on the arm and exerts downward pressure while the patient resists. Weakness or significant pain may indicate a muscle tear and further imaging is recommended (US or MRI). It is recommended that both arms be used in this test for comparison purposes.

Subscapularis

The patient is asked to place his hand behind the back with the dorsum of the hand resting in the region of the mid-lumbar spine (mainly internal rotation at the glenohumeral joint). The ability to actively lift the dorsum of the hand off the back constitutes a normal test with no dysfunction or rupture of subscapularis.

Infraspinatus and teres minor

Hornblower's sign is an inability to externally rotate the elevated arm. This movement indicates severe infraspinatus and teres minor weakness.

Long head of biceps

Hueter sign may indicate a ruptured tendon. The patient is seated with the elbow extended and forearm supinated. The elbow is then flexed by the patient against resistance. If the tendon is ruptured, a biceps 'ball' develops.

Yergason's test indicates if there is bicipital tendinitis. The patient's elbow is flexed and the forearm pronated. The examiner holds the arm at the wrist while the patient actively supinates against resistance. If this resisted movement produces pain located to the bicipital groove area, then pathology within the long head of biceps tendon sheath is likely.

The elbow

The neutral position is with the forearm in extension. The following movements should be tested (Fig. 15.36):

- Flexion.
- Hyperextension.

Medial (golfer's elbow) and lateral (tennis elbow) epicondylitis are the most common causes of elbow pain. They are characterized by pain on active use but if severe may be associated with night pain.

Examination must define localized epicondylar tenderness with pain on resisted movement. Wrist extension exacerbates lateral epicondylar tenderness and wrist flexion exacerbates medial epicondylar tenderness. An elbow effusion may be palpated in the posterior triangle formed by the epicondyles and the olecranon.

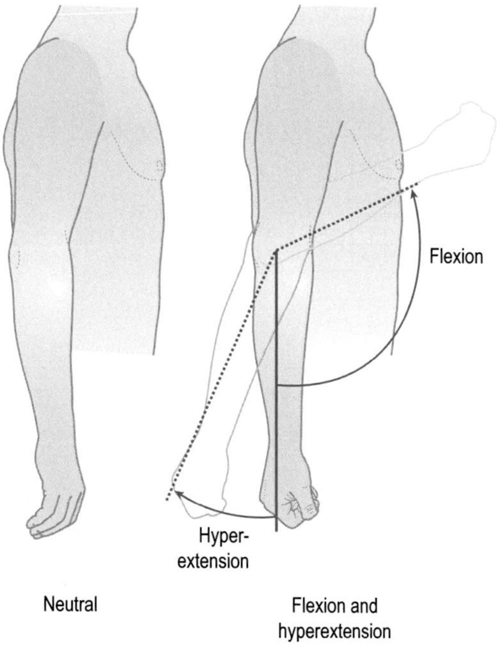

Figure 15.36 Movements of the elbow.

Placing the thumb and second and third fingers on the lateral, medial epicondyles and olecranon, respectively, with the joint in an extended position produces a straight alignment. In a flexed position these three points form a triangular shape. Disturbance of this geometric shift may indicate a supracondylar fracture.

The forearm

The neutral position is with the arm by the side, elbow flexed to 90° and thumb uppermost. The following movements should be tested (Fig. 15.37):

- Supination.
- Pronation.

The wrist

Inspection of the wrist may reveal clear evidence of joint swelling or localized tenosynovitis. The distal ulna is usually visible as a smooth, rounded protrusion. Loss of the normal anatomical landmarks may suggest joint or tendon inflammation.

Palpation of the wrist for warmth and swelling should be performed as well as specific palpation for tendon and bone discomfort. Palpation over the anatomical snuff box resulting in pain may indicate a scaphoid fracture if there is a history of trauma. Tenderness along the ulnar aspect of the wrist may

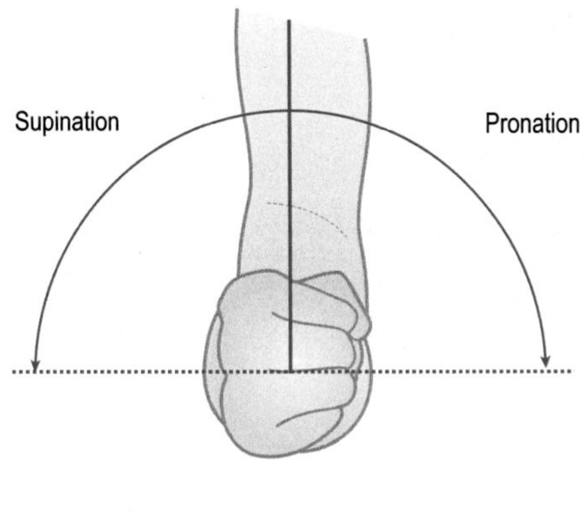

Figure 15.37 Movements of the forearm.

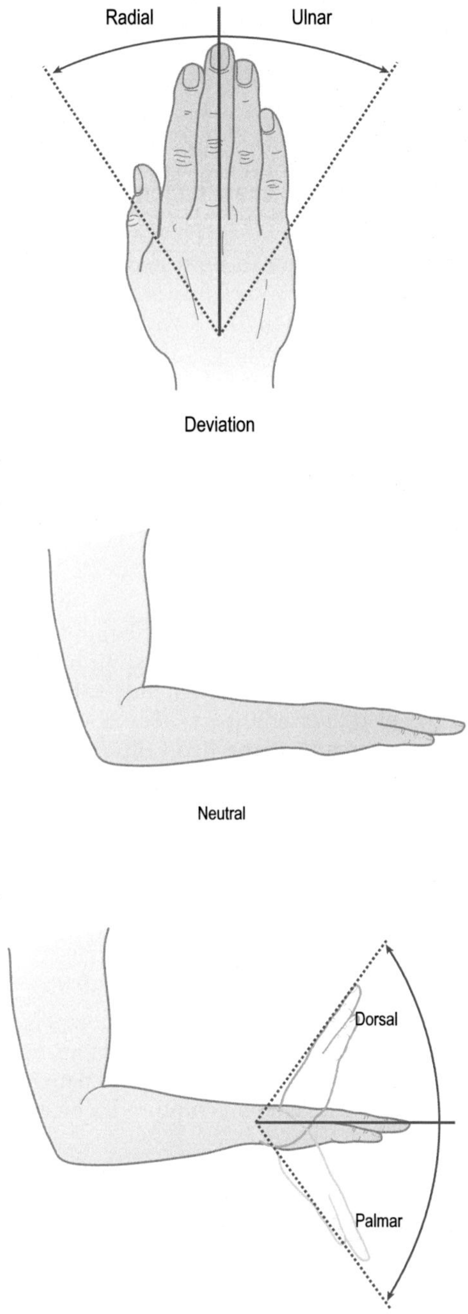

Figure 15.38 Movements of the wrist.

suggest inflammation of the extensor carpi ulnas tendon, commonly involved in early rheumatoid arthritis. At the distal end of the anatomical snuff box the base of the thumb (1st carpal-metacarpal joint) can be palpated, which is a commonly affected joint in generalized osteoarthritis in middle-aged and older patients.

The neutral position is with the hand in line with the forearm, and palm down. The following movements should be tested (Fig. 15.38):

- Dorsiflexion (extension).
- Palmar flexion.
- Ulnar deviation.
- Radial deviation.

Even minor limitation of wrist flexion or extension can be detected by comparing movement in both wrists (Fig. 15.39). Limitation of the wrist joints is usually due to inflammatory arthritis. Primary osteoarthritis of the wrist is rare, but secondary degenerative change is common.

The fingers

When identifying fingers, use the names thumb, index, middle, ring and little. Numbering tends to lead to confusion. The neutral position is with the fingers in extension. Test flexion at the metacarpophalangeal (MCP), proximal interphalangeal (PIP) and distal interphalangeal (DIP) joints (Fig. 15.40).

In fractures of the fingers, the commonest deformity is rotational. If the finger will flex, make sure it points to the scaphoid tubercle (all the fingers will point individually in this direction). If it will not flex, look end-on at the nail and make sure it is parallel with its fellows.

The thumb (carpometacarpal joint)

The neutral position is with the thumb alongside the forefinger, and extended. The following movements should be tested (Fig. 15.41):

- Extension.
- Flexion (measured as for the fingers).
- Opposition.
- Abduction (not illustrated; movement at right angles to plane of palm).

The hand

Deformities in joint disease

Examination of the individual joints of the hand may be less informative than inspection of the hand as a

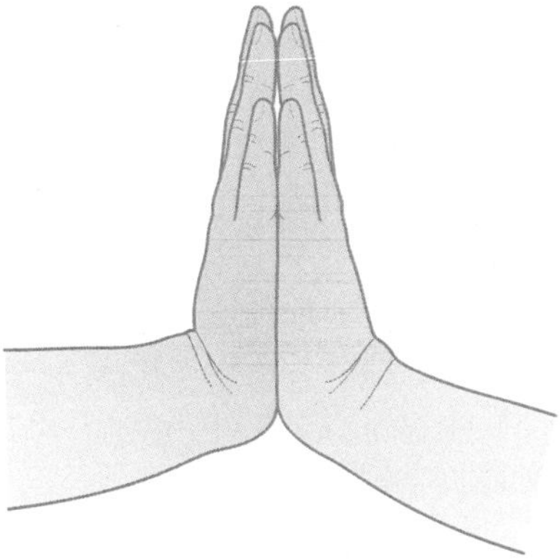

Figure 15.39 Minor limitation of left wrist extension compared with the right. Note the slightly different angulation of the left forearm.

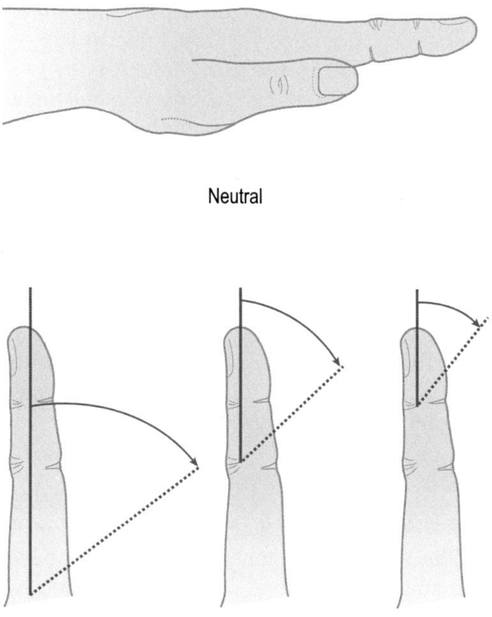

Figure 15.40 Movements of the fingers.

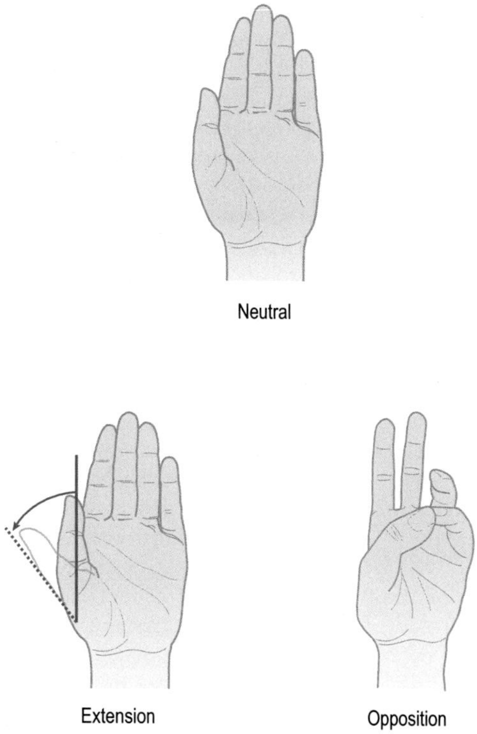

Figure 15.41 Movements of the thumb.

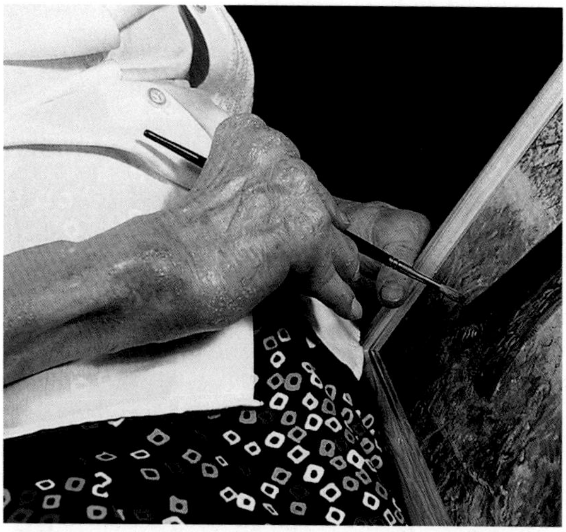

Figure 15.42 Functional ability. Severe joint deformity due to psoriatic arthropathy but retention of function and artistic ability.

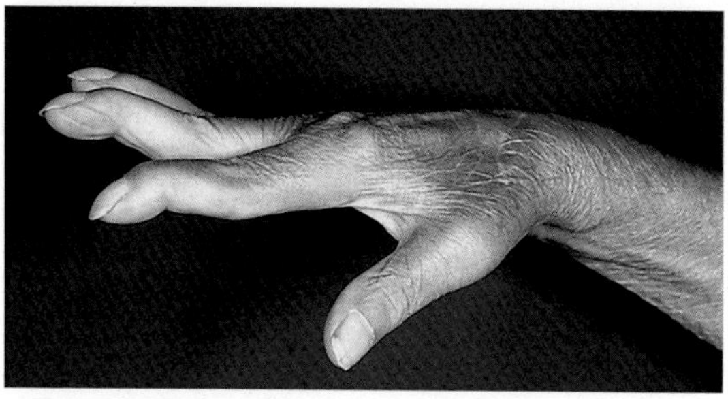

Figure 15.43 Swan-neck deformity of the right hand. Note also wasting of the small muscles of the hand owing to disuse in this patient with rheumatoid arthritis.

whole (Fig. 15.42). The combination of Heberden's nodes and thumb carpometacarpal arthritis occurs in osteoarthritis (see Fig. 15.24). Pain and subluxation of the carpometacarpal joint is a typical feature of primary nodal osteoarthritis, leading to a 'square hand' appearance on making a fist.

A variety of patterns of deformity are characteristic of long-standing rheumatoid arthritis. For example, metacarpophalangeal joint subluxation, ulnar deviation of the fingers at the metacarpophalangeal joints, 'swan neck' (Fig. 15.43) and 'boutonnière' deformities (flexed proximal and hyperextended distal interphalangeal joints) of the fingers are typical in advanced disease. This is due to the head of the phalanx sliding dorsally between the lateral slips of the extensor tendon, the middle slip having been damaged. In psoriatic arthritis, terminal interphalangeal joint swelling may occur, with psoriatic pitting and ridging of the nail (onychopathy) on that digit. Jaccoud's arthropathy produces a similar appearance to swan neck and boutonniere deformity alongside thumb subluxation and ulnar deviation. However, these deformities are reducible when the patient is asked to make a fist as a result of no underlying structural joint damage. This arthropathy may be seen in SLE and Sjögren's syndrome.

Deformities due to neuropathy

The hand may adopt a posture typical of a nerve lesion (see Ch. 16). Slight hyperextension of the medial metacarpophalangeal joints with slight flexion of the interphalangeal joints is the 'ulnar claw hand' of an ulnar nerve lesion. There is wasting of the small muscles of the hypothenar eminence, with loss of sensation of the palmar and dorsal aspects of the little finger and of the ulnar half of the ring finger. In a median nerve lesion, the thenar eminence (abductor pollicis brevis) will be flattened (see Fig. 15.18) and sensory impairment will be found on the palmar surfaces of the thumb, index, middle and radial half of the ring fingers. Remember that carpal tunnel syndrome may be a presenting feature of wrist inflammation.

Assessment of hand function

Assessment of hand function (see Fig. 15.42) should include testing hand grip and pinch grip (between index and thumb). The latter may be decreased in lesions in the line of action of the thumb metacarpal, particularly scaphoid fractures.

The hip

The neutral position is with the hip in extension and the patella pointing forwards. Ensure the pelvis does not tilt by placing one hand over it while examining the hip with the other. Look for scars and wasting of the gluteal and thigh muscles. The hip joint is too deeply placed to be accessible to palpation. Hip movements to be tested are listed in Box 15.13 (Fig. 15.44).

Additional examination of the hip joint

- Test for flexion deformity. With one hand flat between the lumbar spine and the couch, flex the normal hip fully to the point of abolishing the lumbar lordosis. The spine will come down onto the hand, pressing it onto the couch. If there is a flexion deformity on the opposite side, the leg on that side will move into a flexed position (Thomas' test).
- Trendelenburg test. Observe the patient from behind and ask him to stand on one leg. In health, the pelvis tilts upwards on the side with the leg raised. When the weight-bearing hip is abnormal, owing to pain or subluxation, the pelvis sags downwards due to weakness of the hip abductors on the affected side.
- Measurement of 'true' and 'apparent' shortening. The length of the legs is measured from the anterior superior iliac spine to the medial malleolus on the same side. Any difference is termed 'true' shortening and may result from disease of either the hip joint or the neck of the femur on the shorter side. 'Apparent' shortening is due to tilting of the pelvis and can be measured by comparing the lengths of the two legs, measured from the umbilicus, provided there is no true shortening of one leg. Apparent shortening is usually due to an abduction deformity of the hip. Femoral or tibial shortening may be demonstrated with the patient lying on a couch and looking across both knees held equally flexed.

Box 15.13 Hip movements to be tested

- Flexion: measured with knee bent. Opposite thigh must remain in neutral position. Flex the knee as the hip flexes.
- Abduction: measured from a line that forms an angle of 90° with a line joining the anterior superior iliac spines.
- Adduction (measured in the same manner).
- Rotation in flexion.
- Rotation in extension.
- Extension: attempt to extend the hip with the patient lying in the lateral or prone position.

The knee

MRI scans of the normal knee are illustrated in Fig. 15.45. The neutral position is complete extension. Observe any valgus (lateral angulation of the tibia) or varus (medial angulation) deformity on the couch and on standing. Look for muscle wasting. The quadriceps, especially the medial part near the knee, wastes rapidly in knee joint disease. Swelling may be obvious, particularly if it distends the suprapatellar pouch. Check the apparent height of the patella and watch to see if it deviates to one side in flexion or extension of the knee. Feel for tenderness at the joint margins, not forgetting the patellofemoral joint. Palpate the ligaments, remembering that the medial collateral ligament is attached 8 cm below the joint line. Measure the girth of the thigh muscles 10 cm above the upper pole of the patella.

Joint swelling

The presence of swelling in the knee joint may be confirmed by the patellar tap test or, for small effusions, by the bulge test, in which the medial parapatellar fossa is emptied by pressure of the flat of the hand sweeping proximally. The bulge is seen to

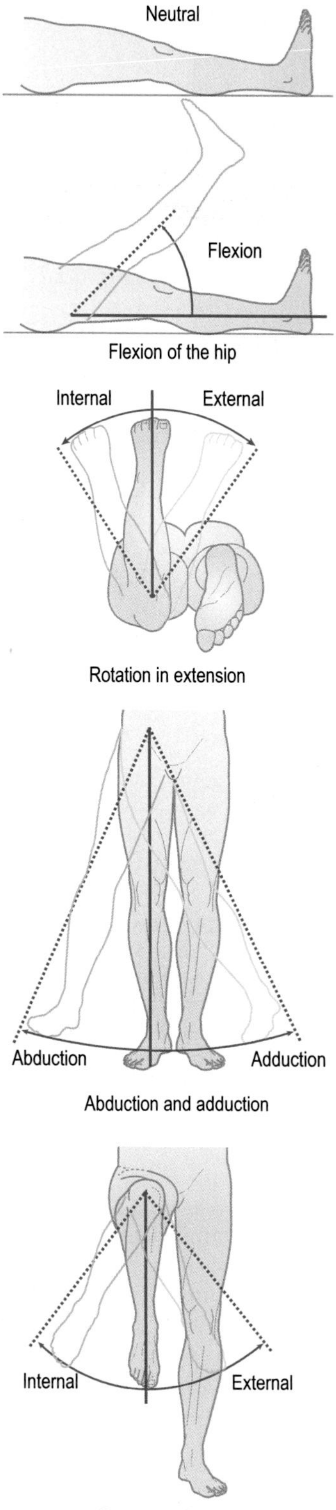

Figure 15.44 Movements of the hip.

refill as the suprapatellar area is emptied by pressure from the flat hand. Posterior knee joint (Baker's) cysts, particularly in rheumatoid arthritis, may be palpable in the popliteal fossa. They sometimes rupture, producing calf pain, and may then mimic a deep vein thrombosis. When intact, large posterior knee cysts can sometimes cause venous obstruction.

The movements of the knee are flexion and extension (Fig. 15.46). Loss of flexion can be documented by loss of the angle of flexion or loss of heel-to-buttock distance, either in the crouching position or on the couch. Loss of extension is detected by inability to get the back of the knee onto the flat examining couch. Hyperextension must be sought by lifting the foot with the knee extended and comparing with the normal side. Lack of full extension by comparison with the normal constitutes fixed flexion deformity. Loose bodies in the joint cause crepitus, interruption of movement (locking) and pain and effusion (Fig. 15.47).

Testing for stability

Cruciate ligaments

Anterior/posterior drawer test. The patient should be situated on the couch with the knee placed in 90° flexion. If there is a posterior sag on inspection, this may provide a false-positive anterior drawer sign. Place both hands around the upper part of the leg with both thumbs placed on the tibial tuberosity and fingers around the posterior aspect of the knee. With your forearm resting on the shin, firmly pull the tibia anterior. If there is significant forward movement of the tibia plateau, this suggests an anterior cruciate tear. Pushing backwards with posterior movement of the tibial plateau may suggest a posterior cruciate pathology.

Collateral ligaments

The collateral ligaments are best assessed with the knee in 30° of flexion. Place your right hand on the lower limb (medial mid-calf) and left hand on the upper lateral thigh. Gradually apply opposing force to detect excessive medial movement of the lower limb. This tests the integrity of the medial collateral ligament. Reverse hand positions (left hand on lateral mid-calf and right hand on medial lower thigh) and repeat the movement to test the lateral collateral ligament. Pain on testing indicates possible enthesitis or tear. Excessive movement can be seen in the context of joint hypermobility which should be considered as part of the overall examination.

The ankle

The ankle is a hinge joint with movement only in the sagittal plane. The neutral position is with the outer border of the foot at an angle of 90° with the leg and midway between inversion and eversion. Observe the patient from behind in the standing position. With any long-standing ankle disorder, there will be a loss of calf muscle bulk.

Look at the position of the foot with the patient standing. The heel may tilt outwards (valgus deformity)

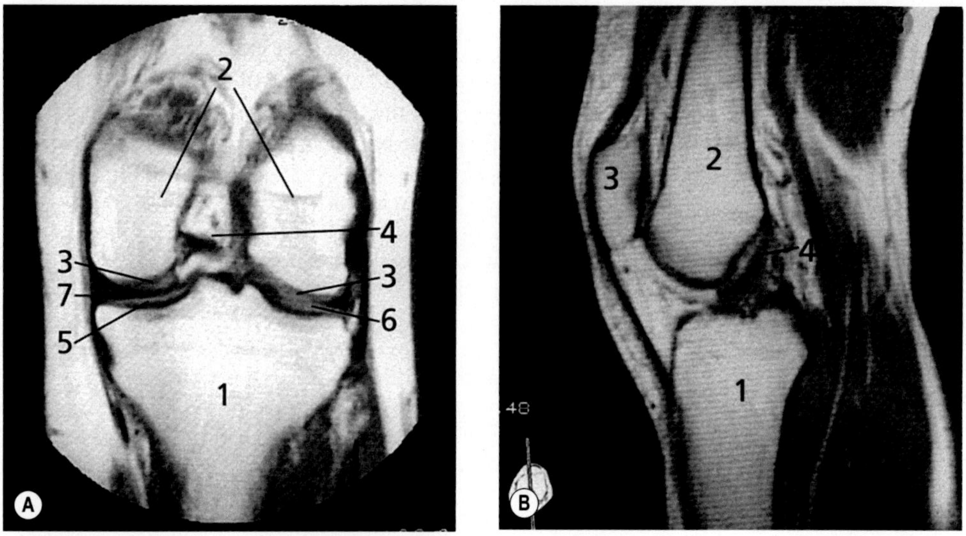

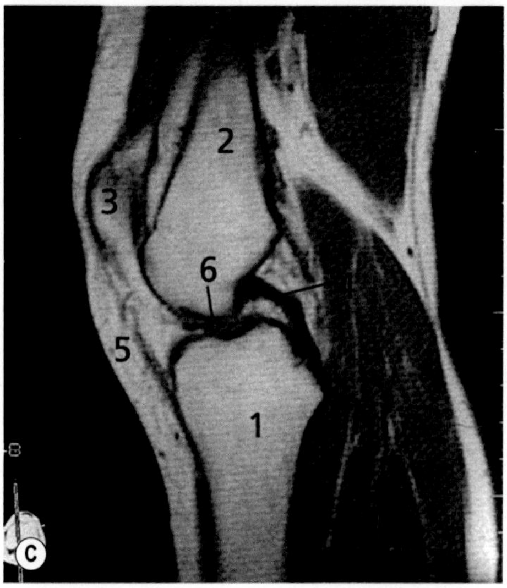

Figure 15.45 MRI scans of the normal knee (MR image, T1-weighted). **(A)** Scan to show the medial (5) and lateral (6) menisci, origin of the anterior cruciate ligament (4) and the articular cartilages (3) and synovial fluid (7). Other structures shown are (1) tibia, (2) articular surfaces of femur. **(B)** The anterior cruciate ligament (4). Other structures shown are (1) tibia, (2) femur, (3) patella. **(C)** The posterior cruciate ligament (4). Other structures shown are (1) tibia, (2) femur, (3) patella, (5) patellar tendon, (6) joint space.

in subtalar joint damage. Inward (varus deformity) is much less common and usually not so painful. Flattening of the longitudinal arch of the foot (pes planus) also produces valgus at the heel, but the foot curves laterally as well because the change is in the mid-tarsal joints in addition to the subtalar joint.

The following movements should be tested (Fig. 15.48):

- Dorsiflexion: test with the knee in flexion and extension to exclude tight calf muscles.
- Plantarflexion: place a finger on the head of the talus to be sure that it is moving. A hypermobile subtalar joint can mimic movement in an arthrodesed ankle.

The foot

Remember that complaints apparently relating to the foot may be features of systemic disease, such as gout, or of referred vertebral problems such as a prolapsed intervertebral disc. Look for abnormalities of posture.

Callosities are areas of hard skin under points of abnormal pressure. The most common site is beneath the metatarsal heads because loss of the normal soft tissue pad allows abnormal loading. There may be abnormal spread of two adjacent toes (daylight sign: Fig. 15.49) on weight-bearing if there is synovitis between the metatarsal heads. Check for lateral deviation of the big toe (hallux valgus), usually associated with abnormal swelling at its base (a bunion). There may be deformities affecting any or all toes, with abnormal curvature (claw toes), fixed flexion of the terminal joint (hammer toes) or overriding.

The foot consists of three regions: hind foot (subtalar joint), mid-foot (tarsal joints) and fore-foot (MTP, PIP, DIP joints). The following movements should be tested (Fig. 15.50):

- Subtalar inversion and eversion: cup the heel in the hands and move it in relation to the tibia

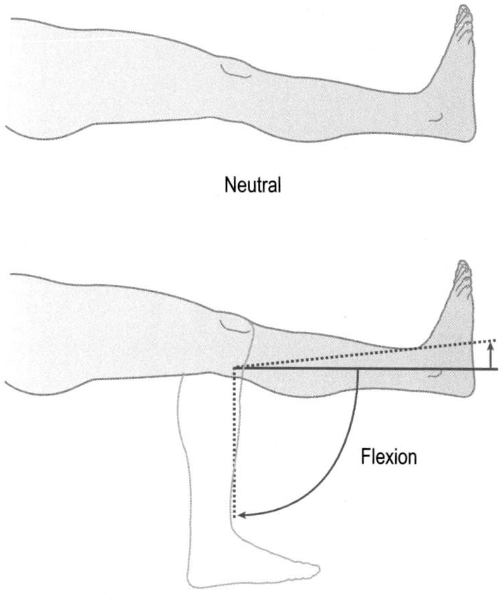

Figure 15.46 Movements of the knee.

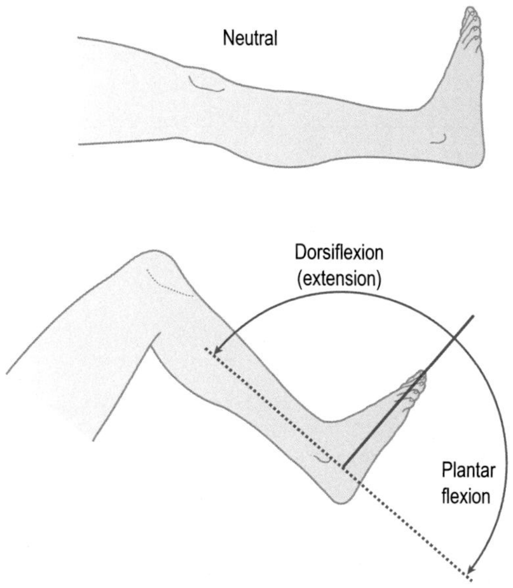

Figure 15.48 Movements of the ankle.

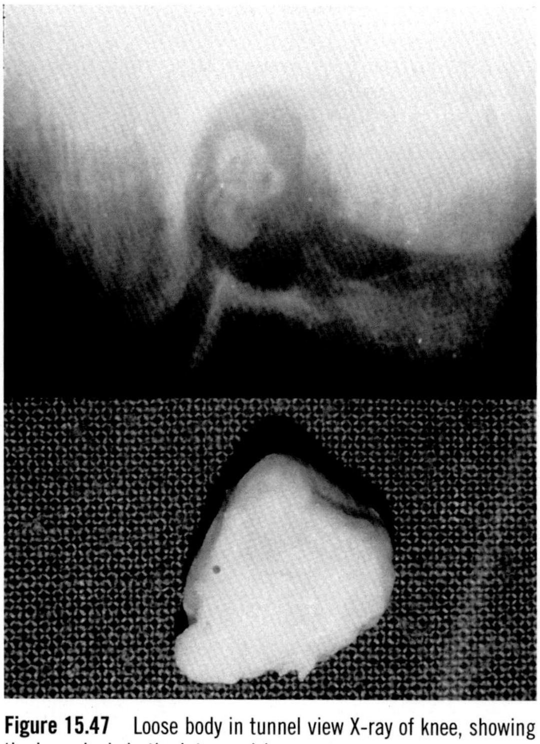

Figure 15.47 Loose body in tunnel view X-ray of knee, showing the loose body in the intercondylar space.

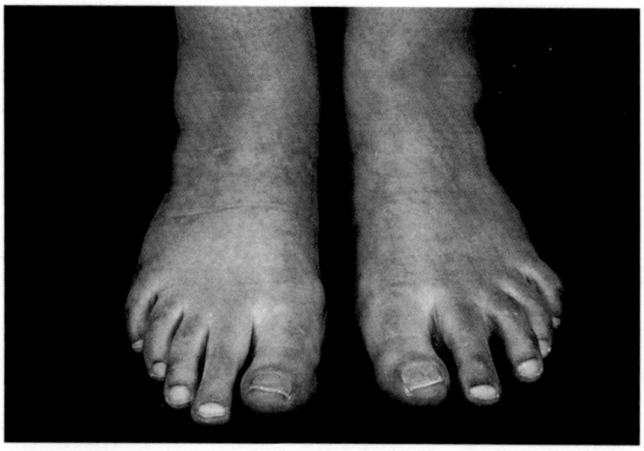

Figure 15.49 Daylight sign due to metatarsophalangeal joint synovitis in rheumatoid arthritis.

without any up and down movement; this eliminates movement at the ankle or mid-tarsal joints.

- Mid-tarsal inversion/eversion and adduction/abduction: hold the os calcis in the neutral position in one hand and grasp and rotate the forefoot in the other.
- Metatarsophalangeal and interphalangeal flexion/extension.

Also look for tenderness or swelling at the Achilles tendon insertion on the back of the calcaneum and for plantar tenderness at the site of the plantar fascial insertion. Inflammation of these attachments (enthesopathy) is common in ankylosing spondylitis and other spondyloarthropathies.

Achilles tendon rupture

Thompson test: This test requires positioning the patient in the prone position with the feet hanging off the table. The clinician then squeezes the patient's calf muscle which should shorten the Achilles tendon causing the ankle to plantar flex. It is important to note that false negative results may occur in older injuries, where organization of a hematoma can cause some reconstitution of the tendon or with an incomplete partial tear. Patients may still be able to walk

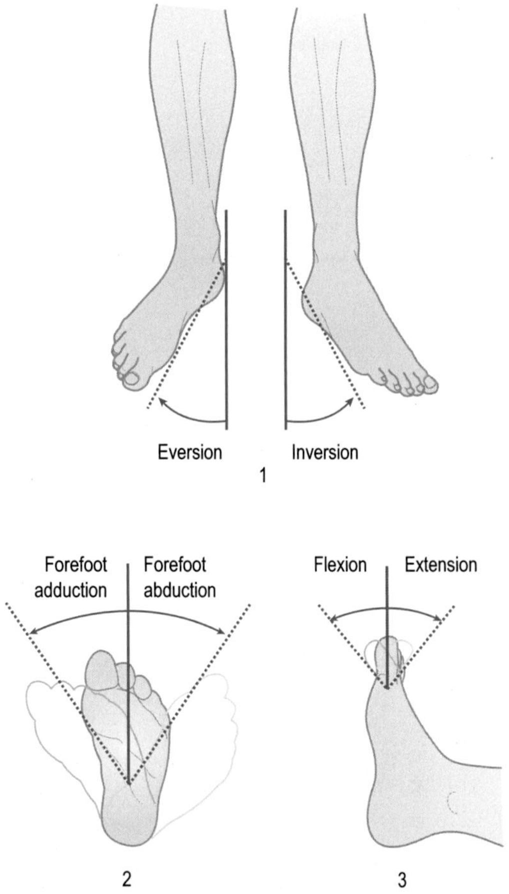

Figure 15.50 Movements of the foot.

and actively plantar flex the ankle despite significant Achilles tendon tear. When an index of suspicion of an Achilles tear or rupture arises, imaging with ultrasound or MRI is recommended.

The gait

It is best to study gait with the patient's legs and feet fully exposed and *without* socks, shoes or slippers. Ask the patient to walk away from you, to turn around at a given point and then to walk towards you.

Abnormalities of gait are usually due either to joint problems in the legs or to neurological disorder, although alcohol intoxication or malingering may occasionally cause difficulty. A full examination of the legs and feet should reveal any local cause, which may range from a painful corn to osteoarthritis of the hip. Abnormalities due to neurological disorders are described in Chapter 16.

Hypermobility

There is a wide variation in the range of normal joint movement, associated with age, sex and race. Excessive laxity or hypermobility of the joints (Fig. 15.51) can be defined in about 10% of healthy subjects and is frequently familial. It is also a feature of two inherited connective tissue disorders, Marfan syndrome and Ehlers-Danlos syndrome. Repeated trauma, haemarthrosis or dislocation may produce permanent joint damage. Hypermobility is often generalized but may occur at a single joint and must be considered if considerable joint lax is demonstrated on examination.

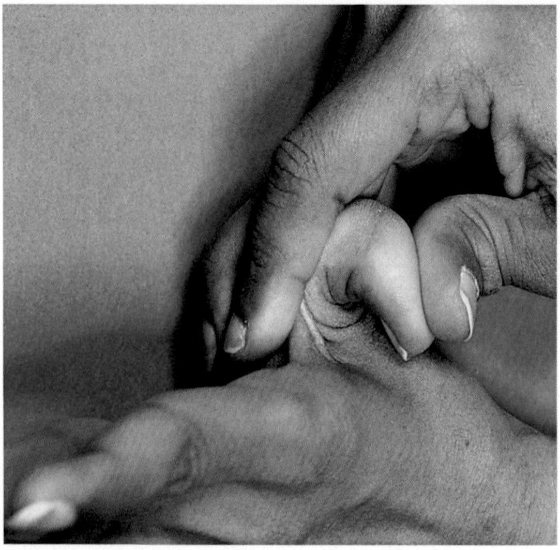

Figure 15.51 Hyperextensibility of the digits in Ehlers-Danlos syndrome.

Work-related musculoskeletal disorders

Musculoskeletal pain arising as a result of a patient's occupation is an increasingly recognized cause of disability and economic loss. For example, spinal pain may be ascribed to poor seating in sedentary occupations. Likewise, an occupational history of repetitive movements may be relevant to upper limb pain. Assessment by an occupational health physician and an occupational therapist may be needed to consider workplace alterations.

Investigations in rheumatic diseases

When a full history and examination have been completed, investigations should be considered to support the working diagnosis or to distinguish between different possible diagnoses. They can broadly be defined as:

- tests in support of inflammatory disease
- diagnostic tests including biopsies and imaging investigations.

Tests in support of inflammatory disease

The acute-phase reactant tests that are used in the assessment of inflammatory disease activity and in the subsequent monitoring of the patient are listed in Box 15.14.

Box 15.14 Common biochemical tests for inflammatory rheumatic conditions

Acute-phase reactant tests that are used in the assessment of inflammatory disease activity and in the subsequent monitoring of the patient:

- Erythrocyte sedimentation rate (ESR). This is a useful screening test although it has poor specificity, being affected by the levels of haemoglobin, globulins and fibrinogen. Higher mean values are seen in healthy elderly individuals.
- C-reactive protein (CRP). This is a more specific indicator of inflammation and is a good marker of the acute-phase response. A high ESR with a normal CRP is a useful pointer towards autoimmune rheumatic diseases, especially SLE.
- Plasma viscosity. This is a more specific measure of the acute-phase response than ESR, but may not be as widely available.
- Anaemia and thrombocytosis. Anaemia of chronic disease and a high platelet count often occur in inflammatory disease but are non-specific. Other abnormalities on blood count, such as neutropenia, thrombocytopenia and lymphopenia, are common in SLE.
- Serum complement. Low levels of serum complement reflect activation due to immune complex deposition; this may be a marker of disease activity in autoimmune diseases such as SLE. Hereditary complement deficiencies are also associated with SLE.
- Muscle enzymes. Elevated creatine kinase levels occur in most patients with inflammatory myopathy.

Diagnostic tests

Diagnostic tests differentiate between specific diseases and are relatively specific investigations.

Tests for rheumatoid factor

Rheumatoid factors are autoantibodies in the form of immunoglobulin (Ig) directed against other immunoglobulin G (IgG) molecules. IgM rheumatoid factor can be detected by its ability to clump particles coated with human IgG (latex test). This test is positive in about 80% of patients with rheumatoid arthritis. Results are reported as a titre, 1:80 or higher being a positive result. The original Rose-Waaler haemagglutination test used sheep erythrocytes coated with rabbit IgG to detect IgM (titres of 1:32 or more are positive); it has now been replaced by other tests. Enzyme-linked immunosorbent serum assay (ELISA) techniques are much more sensitive but produce positive results in many other conditions. Anti-citrullinated protein/peptide antibodies (ACPA) are a specific marker for rheumatoid arthritis and their presence indicates a poor prognosis, with patients at greater risk of joint damage, disability and loss of function.

These rheumatoid factor screening tests are useful where a diagnosis of rheumatoid arthritis is suspected, but they are not specific. Rheumatoid factor is frequently found in patients with other connective tissue diseases, for example SLE and Sjögren's syndrome, or other inflammatory disorders such as subacute bacterial endocarditis and some viral infections.

Approximately 50% of patients with rheumatoid arthritis who present to a rheumatologist are positive for rheumatoid factor or anti-CCP antibodies when they initially present, rising to 70-80% at a later time point. Therefore a negative serology test does not exclude rheumatoid arthritis as a diagnosis.

Antinuclear antibody tests

Antinuclear antibody (ANA), often referred to as antinuclear factor (ANF), is a very useful screening test for SLE as it is positive in up to 95% of patients. It is, however, non-specific, being positive in many other autoimmune rheumatic disorders, including about 20% of patients with rheumatoid arthritis. A positive test in children with arthritis may be associated with chronic iridocyclitis, which is frequently asymptomatic. Slit-lamp examination of the eye is mandatory to confirm the diagnosis.

The ANA test detects antibodies to intracellular nuclear and cytoplasmic antigens and is carried out by incubating the patient's serum with cells such as Hep-2 cells. After washing, a fluorescent antiserum to human IgG is used to detect human antibody adhering to the intracellular and nuclear antigens. A titre of 1:80 or more is significant, and adequate standardization is important.

DNA-binding test

Different immunochemical techniques (Farr assay or ELISA) may be used to detect antibodies to native double-stranded DNA. Another method is indirect immunofluorescence using the protozoon *Crithidia luciliae*, where the kinetoplast at the tail containing DNA fluoresces. The test is usually reserved for patients with a positive ANA test and is specific for SLE but not as sensitive as ANA. Occasionally it is positive in patients in whom the clinical suspicion of SLE is very high but the ANA test is negative.

Antibody tests to extractable nuclear antigens (ENA)

Box 15.15 shows tests that may be indicated by a speckled staining pattern in the ANA test. They can be summarized in terms of their clinical associations. Other diagnostic antibody tests are shown in Box 15.16.

Uric acid

A consistently normal plasma uric acid level (<375 mmol/l in women, <425 mmol/l in men) usually excludes the diagnosis of untreated gout. Raised levels occur in many circumstances and do not in themselves establish the diagnosis of gout (see below). On a low-purine diet, the 24-hour urinary

Box 15.15 Extractable nuclear antigen (ENA) tests

These tests may be indicated by a speckled staining pattern in the ANA test. They can be summarized in terms of their clinical associations:

- Anti-Ro (SSA) and anti-La (SSB), typically in Sjögren's syndrome. Also seen in SLE, where they are associated with photosensitivity, and the neonatal lupus syndrome, which may result in congenital heart block and neonatal rashes.
- Anti-Sm in 5-10% of patients with SLE; a very specific marker if present.
- Anti-RNP (ribonucleoprotein) in some cases of SLE. Also picks out a group of patients who have clinical features of other autoimmune rheumatic disorders and who are therefore often diagnosed as mixed connective-tissue disease (MCTD). The test can be considered a marker for the combination of clinical features, but the major clinical component of the condition will define management.
- Anticentromere antibody is found in limited cutaneous systemic sclerosis or 'CREST syndrome' (calcinosis, Raynaud's phenomenon, oesophageal symptoms, sclerodactyly and telangiectasiae).
- Anti-Scl 70 (DNA topoisomerase I) and anti-RNA polymerase are found in scleroderma and are associated with severe disease.

urate excretion should not exceed 600 mg. Higher levels indicate 'overproduction' of urate and a risk of renal stone formation.

Synovial fluid examination

Synovial fluid may be obtained for examination from any joint in which it is clinically detectable. The knee is the most convenient source: after infiltration with a local anaesthetic, a 21-gauge needle is inserted into the joint between the patella and the femoral condyle. For smaller, more inaccessible joints, such as the wrist or MCP, an ultrasound guided aspiration should be considered. The aspirated fluid should be placed in a plain sterile container; if a cell count is required, some of the fluid should be mixed with ethylenediaminetetra-acetic acid (EDTA) anticoagulant.

An injured joint can also be aspirated (Box 15.17). The joint swollen after injury may reveal clear pink fluid suggesting a meniscal lesion, or show frank blood. The latter is usually indicative of a torn anterior cruciate ligament. If blood is aspirated, look at its surface for fat globules. This is derived from the marrow and confirms an intra-articular fracture. Synovial fluid examination is diagnostic in two conditions – bacterial infections and crystal synovitis – and every effort should be made to obtain fluid when either of these is suspected. Polarized light microscopy can differentiate between the crystals of urate in gout and those of calcium pyrophosphate dihydrate in pseudogout. Outside these conditions, synovial fluid examination is unlikely to be diagnostic. Frank blood may point to trauma, haemophilia or villonodular synovitis, whereas inflammatory (as opposed to degenerative) arthritis is suggested by opaque fluid of low viscosity, with a total white cell count >1000/ml, neutrophils >50%, protein content >35 g/l and the presence of a firm clot. Culture of this fluid may produce a bacterial growth, usually of staphylococci,

Box 15.16 Other helpful immunology tests in rheumatic disease

- Antineutrophil cytoplasmic antibodies are a marker for vasculitic conditions. Two immunofluorescence staining patterns occur:
  1. Cytoplasmic or c-ANCA, with specificity for proteinase 3 (a neutrophil enzyme), is specific for Wegener's granulomatosis (Fig. 15.52)
  2. Perinuclear or p-ANCA, with specificity for myeloperoxidase (and some other neutrophil enzymes), occurs in microscopic polyangiitis and other vasculitic diseases (and inflammatory bowel disease).
- Antiphospholipid antibodies include anticardiolipin antibodies, β2 glycoprotein 1 antibodies and the lupus anticoagulant tests and are associated with the antiphospholipid syndrome, characterized by arterial and venous thromboses and, in women, recurrent pregnancy loss and pregnancy morbidity. A false positive VDRL (see Ch. 17) may also be found in these patients.
- Anti-Jo 1 (histidyl t-RNA synthetase) is a marker for the idiopathic inflammatory myopathies such as dermatomyositis and polymyositis, especially when complicated by interstitial lung disease.
- Cryoglobulins are detected by clotting whole blood at 37°C and cooling the serum to 4°C and looking for a precipitate which is usually an IgM rheumatoid factor. Cryoglobulins are associated with vasculitis, infections such as hepatitis C and myeloproliferative disorders.
- Human leukocyte antigen (HLA) typing: the association of tissue antigen HLA-B27 with ankylosing spondylitis remains the strongest association in medicine. Although about 95% of ankylosing spondylitis patients in the UK possess the B27 antigen, it is also found in 8% of the normal population. Ankylosing spondylitis, therefore, remains a clinical diagnosis, supported by typical radiographic findings. However, in early disease, in children with peripheral arthritis or where the clinical findings are atypical, HLA-B27 typing may provide supportive diagnostic value.
- Antistreptolysin-O (ASO) test: the presence in the serum of this antibody in a titre greater than 1/200, rising on repeat testing after about 2 weeks, indicates a recent haemolytic streptococcal infection.
- Viral titres. Certain viruses, notably parvovirus and Coxsackie virus, may cause transient musculoskeletal symptoms which may be mistaken for systemic diseases. Rising viral titres may be useful in the differential diagnosis.

Box 15.17 Findings in synovial fluid after aspiration of the knee joint

- Cloudy fluid or pus: bacterial infection (see text)
- Urate or pyrophosphate crystals: gout or pseudogout
- Pink fluid: torn meniscus
- Blood: trauma, haemophilia, villonodular synovitis

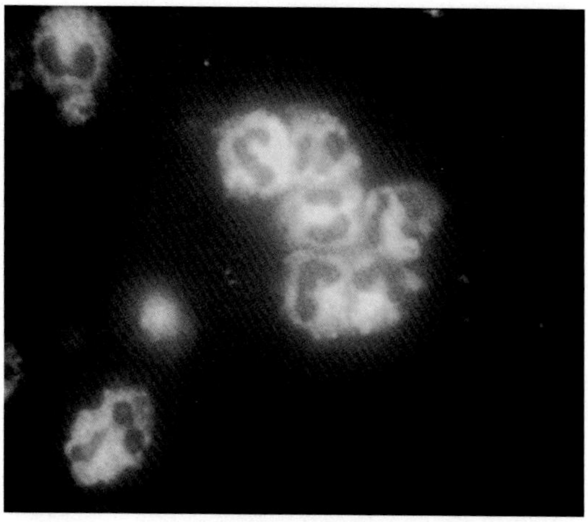

Figure 15.52 Antineutrophil cytoplasmic autoantibodies with cytoplasmic staining (c-ANCA). This pattern has a high predictive value for a diagnosis of Wegener's granulomatosis.

but occasionally *Mycobacterium tuberculosis* or other organisms.

Biopsies useful in differential diagnosis

Box 15.18 shows tests that may be useful in the differential diagnosis of rheumatic diseases.

Radiological examination

Certain general principles are important, particularly as clinicians may be asked to give an opinion on radiographs of limbs after traumatic injury, whether minor or more serious (Box 15.19). Common problems are shown in Figs 15.54-15.57. A systematic approach is essential (Box 15.20).

Bone density (Table 15.6) may be normal, reduced (osteopenia) or increased (osteosclerosis). These changes are easy to detect if focal, but difficult if diffuse. When a focal bone lesion (Box 15.21) is noted, look at its position in the bone and at its margins, and note whether there is any focal matrix calcification, whether the cortex of the bone is intact and whether there is any periosteal reaction around it. Most solitary bone lesions in young people are benign and show no periosteal reaction or swelling around them, and no associated soft-tissue swelling. Aggressive (malignant) bone lesions are more common in the elderly. Certain bone metastases have a

Box 15.18 Biopsy procedures and tissue harvesting that may be useful in the differential diagnosis of rheumatic diseases

- Muscle biopsy should be considered in patients with inflammatory myopathies such as dermatomyositis, polymyositis and inclusion body myositis. Electromyography may show typical features of myopathy and biopsy may be guided by MRI of muscles (Fig. 15.53).
- Rectal biopsy can be useful in the diagnosis of amyloidosis secondary to chronic inflammatory disease, but renal biopsy may still be necessary if the cause of renal impairment is not clear.
- Renal biopsy is essential in the vasculitides or SLE where active glomerulonephritis is suspected. Vasculitis may also be confirmed on renal biopsy but, in general, tissues found to be abnormal on clinical examination or by further investigation (e.g. skin, muscle, sural nerve or liver) should be considered first for diagnostic biopsy in undifferentiated systemic vasculitis.
- Biopsy of a lip minor salivary gland may be useful to confirm Sjögren's syndrome.
- Temporal artery biopsy is often diagnostic in patients with clinical features of temporal (giant cell) arteritis. This is the investigation of choice.
- Synovial biopsy is of little value in the differential diagnosis of inflammatory polyarthritis but should be considered in any unusual monoarthritis to exclude infection, particularly tuberculous, or rare conditions such as sarcoid, amyloid arthropathy or villonodular synovitis. This may be performed by arthroscopy or using a semi-automated guillotine needle under ultrasound guidance.
- Bone biopsy. May be useful in the diagnosis of osteomalacia, malignancy, renal osteodystrophy and Paget's disease. The bone marrow can also be aspirated at the same time if necessary.

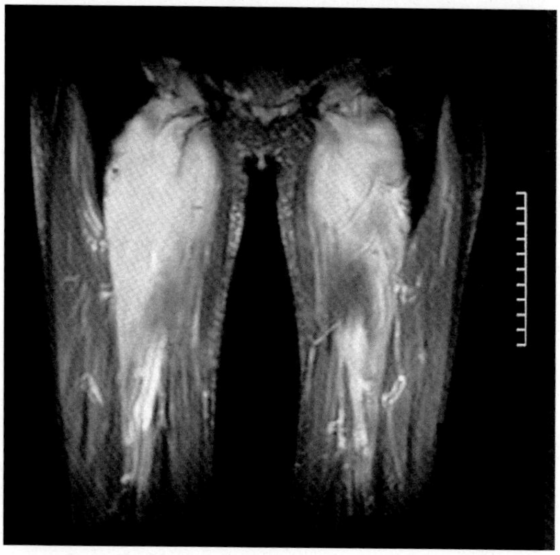

Figure 15.53 MRI scan of thigh muscles showing high signal lesions of inflammatory myositis.

Box 15.19 General principles of musculoskeletal imaging

- Use a systematic approach (see Box 15.13)
- Age, sex and clinical information are essential in interpretation
- Radiographs reveal bones and soft tissues
- Always obtain two views, at right angles, in trauma patients
- Radiographs may be normal even in the presence of disease
- Diffuse abnormalities are difficult to detect
- Bone-based and joint-based disease must be differentiated
- Normal variants can be confused with pathology

Box 15.20 Systematic approach to musculoskeletal imaging

- Bone density
- Soft tissues
- Joints
- Bone
- Periosteum

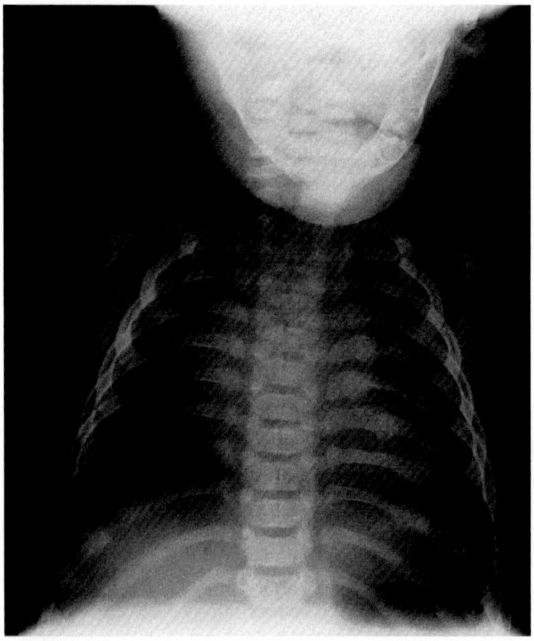

Figure 15.54 Healed fracture of posterior left and right ribs in a 6-month-old infant, classic non-accidental injury (NAI).

characteristic appearance (Box 15.22). Isotope imaging is useful in detecting multiple sites of bony involvement in generalized disease and in metastatic cancer. CT imaging is also sensitive in detecting and analysing bony lesions, as it provides good images of the bony margins of the lesions and of the associated soft tissues. MRI is used to assess the extent of the lesion and any local soft tissue invasion.

Box 15.21 Benign and malignant bone lesions

Benign

- Young person
- Single lesion
- Well-defined margin
- Intact cortex
- No periosteal reaction
- No growth
- Asymptomatic

Malignant

- Older age
- Multiple lesions
- Poorly defined margin
- Destroyed cortex
- Periosteal reaction
- Soft-tissue extension of lesion
- Lesions painful

Box 15.22 Bone metastases

- Expansile – thyroid, kidney, breast, bronchus, melanoma and myeloma
- Sclerotic – prostate and breast
- Lytic – breast, bronchus, kidney, thyroid and melanoma
- Mixed – breast, bladder, or previously treated (irradiated) bone lesions

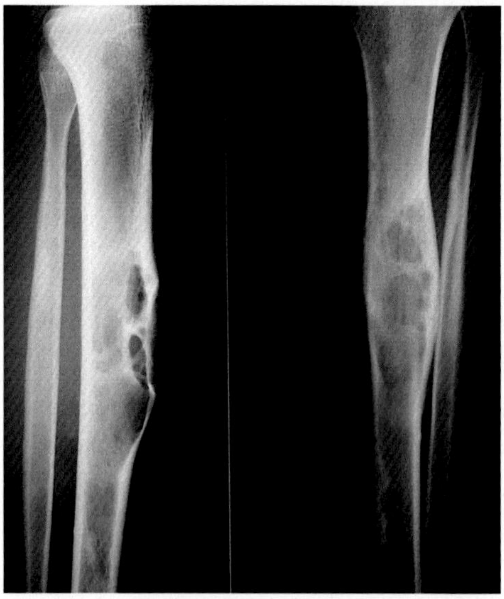

Figure 15.55 Benign bone tumour (adamantinoma). Note the solitary well-defined lucent lesion with a sclerotic margin and the absence of matrix calcification.

The commonest use of plain radiographs is to document joint pathology such as osteoarthritis (joint space narrowing, periarticular sclerosis, subchondral cysts and osteophytes) or inflammatory conditions such as rheumatoid arthritis (joint space narrowing,

Table 15.6 Abnormal bone density

Generalized osteopenia	Generalized osteosclerosis	Benign focal lucent lesions	Benign focal sclerotic lesions
Ageing osteoporosis	Osteopetrosis (marble bone disease)	Simple bone cyst, aneurysmal bone cyst	Bone island
	Metastatic bone disease, e.g. prostate and breast cancer	Fibrous cortical defect	Callus after fracture
Disuse, e.g. trauma and neurogenic paralysis, osteogenesis imperfecta	Dietary causes, e.g. hypervitaminosis A, fluorosis	Non-ossifying fibroma	Paget's disease of bone
Acquired metabolic bone disease, e.g. rickets, osteomalacia, hyperparathyroidism	Acquired metabolic bone disease, e.g. renal osteodystrophy	Enchondroma	Bone infarction Osteoid osteoma
Myeloma	Myelofibrosis, sickle cell disease	Fibrous dysplasia, giant cell tumour of bone	Fibrous dysplasia

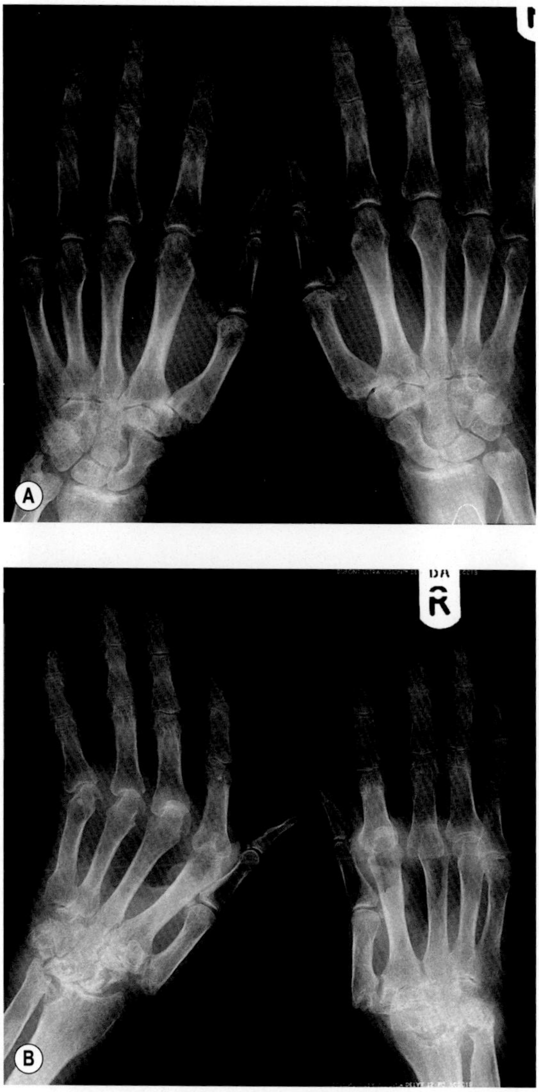

Figure 15.56 **(A)** Early rheumatoid arthritis: local osteopenia, loss of joint spaces, soft-tissue swelling. **(B)** Late rheumatoid arthritis: erosion of periarticular surfaces and ulnar subluxation.

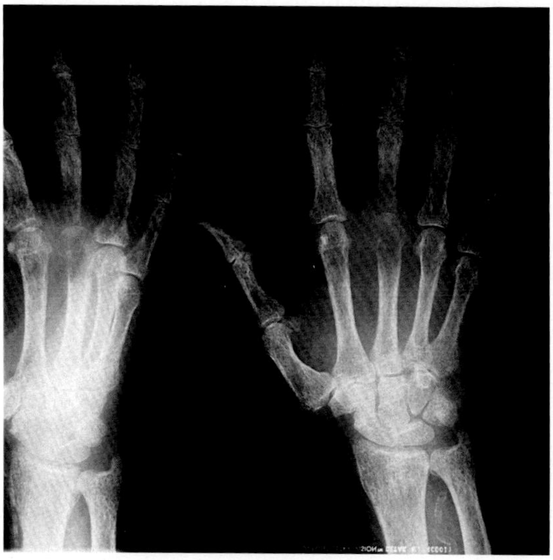

Figure 15.57 Renal osteodystrophy: generalized demineralization, terminal phalangeal and subperiosteal bone resorption and vascular calcification.

peri-articular osteopenia, erosions and subsequent boney ankylosis). Imaging of the hands and feet is most commonly performed when investigating an inflammatory arthritis, as subclinical inflammation and joint description may occur in the absence of frank joint inflammation. Osteoarthritis requires a more focused approach to imaging of symptomatic joints. While imaging changes characteristic of degenerative joint disease can be detected by plain radiographs, they do not correlate well with symptom severity.

Fractures

X-rays are often the first investigation in suspected fractures and in joint disease. In traumatic fractures, X-rays are diagnostic and are used to check alignment of the fracture and healing. X-rays of a fracture are also important in excluding pathological fracture associated with metabolic bone disease, a focal benign bone lesion or neoplastic invasion by metastases. When there is clinical doubt after a non-diagnostic X-ray, an MRI scan often reveals the underlying fracture and is the investigation of choice. Radiographs taken to confirm or exclude a fracture must be taken in two planes. It is essential that either the whole limb is turned or the imaging equipment rotated. The limb must not be twisted at the fracture site. When looking for a fracture, run a pen tip or its equivalent around the cortex of the bone as seen on the film (without leaving marks). Any break in continuity will reveal itself; do not confuse an epiphysis with a fracture. Note soft-tissue swelling and distension of joints. Always seek a radiology opinion if in doubt.

In joint disease, MRI is the imaging method of choice because it can visualize all the soft-tissue components of the joints. Osteopenia is a non-specific feature of disuse but also occurs in relation to affected joints in rheumatoid arthritis and Still's disease of children. Involvement of the distal interphalangeal joint is a feature of psoriatic arthropathy. In rheumatoid disease, the involvement of joints is usually symmetrical, and the wrist is particularly susceptible.

Only radiographs likely to yield specific information should be requested. However, in unilateral joint disease, it is useful to examine both sides for comparison (Fig. 15.58). In patients with inflammatory polyarthritis, three routine films are helpful in the diagnosis and assessment of progression, with both hands and wrists on one plate and both feet on another to compare bone density and to look for periosteal reaction or erosive change, and one of the full pelvis (Fig. 15.59) to show the sacroiliac and hip joints. In the absence of so-called 'red flag' signs, for example, weight loss, night pain, fevers or neurological signs, most spinal radiographs are unnecessary.

Specialized radiology

The following imaging techniques can provide precise information about localized pathology but are dependent on the clinician making a clear diagnostic request with as much clinical information as possible:

- High-resolution ultrasound is of value in defining soft-tissue structures, including muscles and tendons, and provides an excellent means for guiding aspiration of joint effusions and biopsy procedures. Ultrasound has been consistently demonstrated to be more sensitive than clinical examination in the context of joint inflammation and provides considerable additional information in the diagnosis and management of inflammatory arthritis. Grey-scale synovial thickening and power Doppler signal reflect histologically defined synovitis and can be used to differentiate between true joint pathology and fibromyalgia and other pain syndromes. In addition, this imaging modality has the unique capacity to be used in a dynamic fashion allowing tendon,

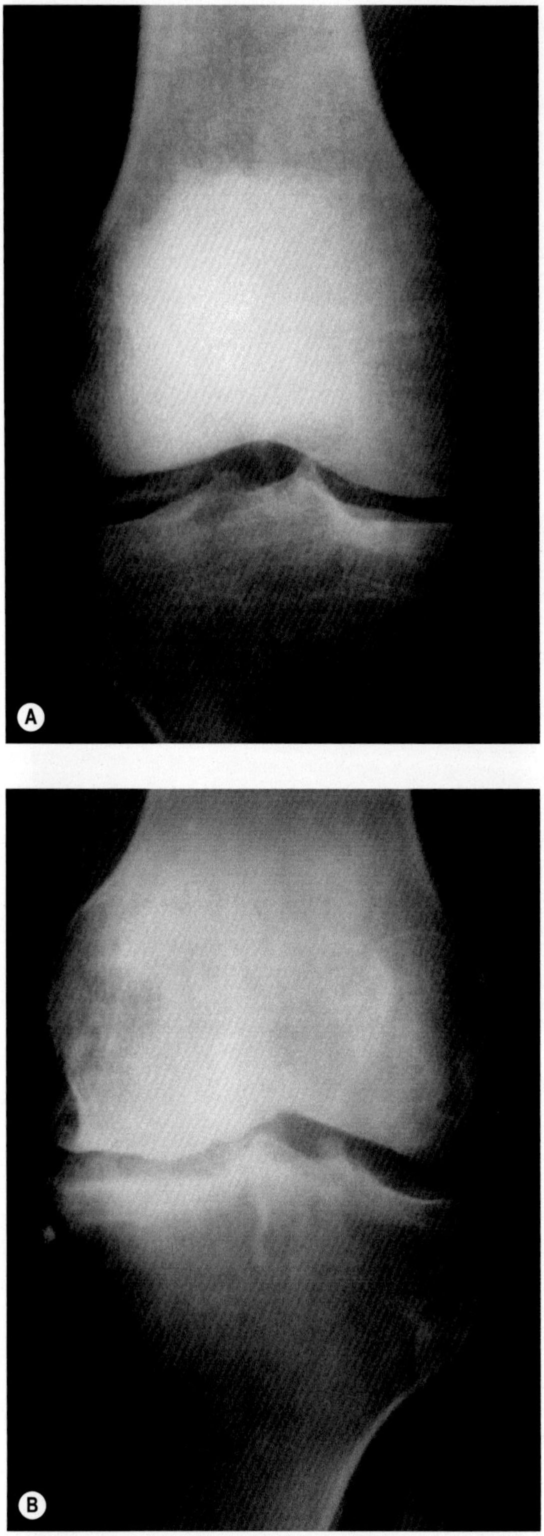

Figure 15.58 Left and right knee joints. The X-rays show normal joint anatomy but with chondrocalcinosis **(A)** and osteoarthritic change **(B)** on the opposite side. Note the increased bone density and narrowing of the joint space.

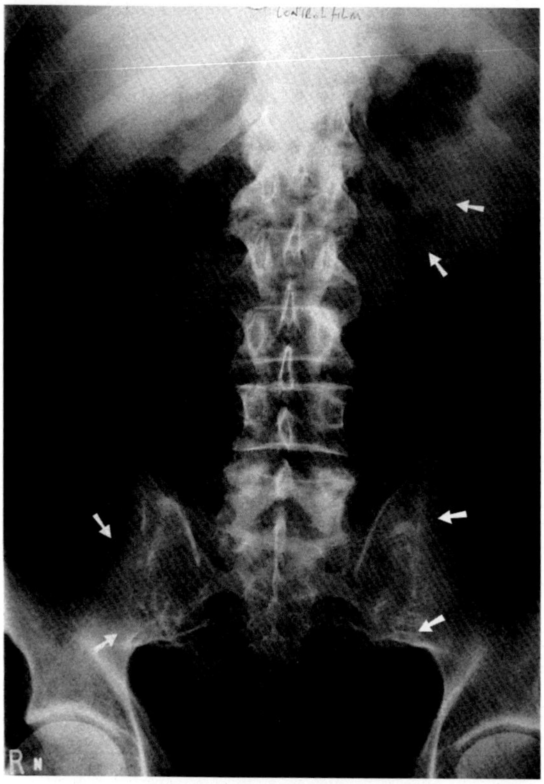

Figure 15.59 X-ray of lumbosacral spine and upper pelvis. There is fusion of several vertebrae, and of the sacroiliac joints (arrows) from ankylosing spondylitis. The renal papillae on the left are calcified, evidence of previous papillary necrosis from prolonged analgesic use.

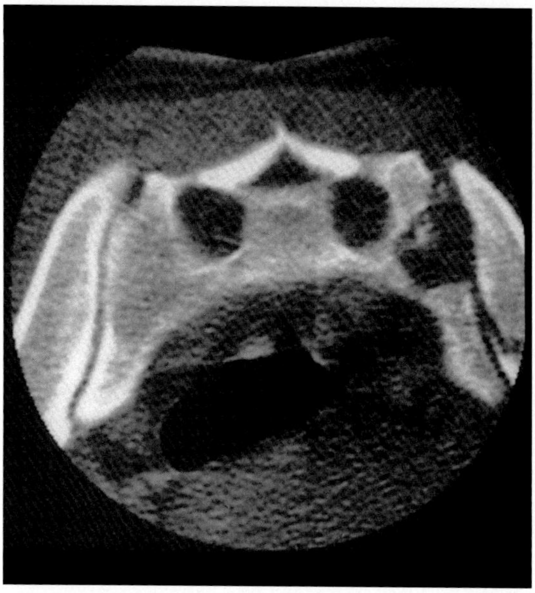

Figure 15.60 CT scan of sacroiliac joints, showing distinctive lesion on the left side with a sequestrum due to tuberculosis.

ligament and joint function to be observed in real time. Rotator cuff pathology at the shoulder is amenable to ultrasound imaging and is often the first imaging investigation of choice when assessing the integrity of the muscle and tendons of these structures. Ultrasound can detect erosions and joint damage at a very early stage of disease before X-ray changes are demonstrated.

- CT. The combination of superior tissue contrast and tomographic technique permits definition of soft-tissue structures obscured by overlapping structures, including intervertebral discs and other joints normally difficult to visualize, such as sacroiliac (Fig. 15.60), sternoclavicular and subtalar. Bone pathology is particularly well characterized on CT imaging, e.g. malignancy, erosive disease or fracture.
- MRI has unique advantages in evaluating the musculoskeletal system, but it is vital that the clinician defines the pathology suspected, as correct positioning and sequence selection (T-weighting) are vital in optimizing image quality. MRI is increasingly used to image the major joints in the limbs, especially the knee (see Fig. 15.45), hip, shoulder and elbow.

In the context of inflammatory arthritis, MRI imaging has much to recommend it as an imaging modality. There is a clear relationship with bone marrow oedema on MRI and the subsequent development of erosive arthritis providing an early indicator of potential poor prognosis. Erosive disease, when present, is detected earlier than with plain radiographs and changes in synovial inflammation can be readily detected after therapeutic intervention. A standardized, validated scoring system has been developed (RAMRIS - Rheumatoid Arthritis MRI Scoring) which encompasses multiple elements of MRI detected synovial inflammation and joint damage.

Enhancement by the use of intravenous paramagnetic contrast (e.g. gadolinium) has further improved definition in spinal imaging.

MRI is invaluable when assessing the degree of spinal involvement in spondyloarthropathies, such as ankylosing spondylitis, particularly in early disease where radiography ankylosis is absent. Both costovertebral and sacroiliac joints are readily imaged with good sensitivity for inflammatory pathology.

It is of particular value in the non-invasive investigation of disc disease (Fig. 15.61), including spinal infection, and is a sensitive technique for the diagnosis of avascular necrosis. MRI scanning of the brain and spine is the single most important investigation in neuroimaging, as the neural tissues themselves, together with supporting tissues, are well visualized. Bone is less well seen with this technique. As a rule of thumb, most abnormalities appear dark on T1-weighted images and white on T2-weighted images. Some common problems are shown in Figs 15.53, 15.61 and 15.62.

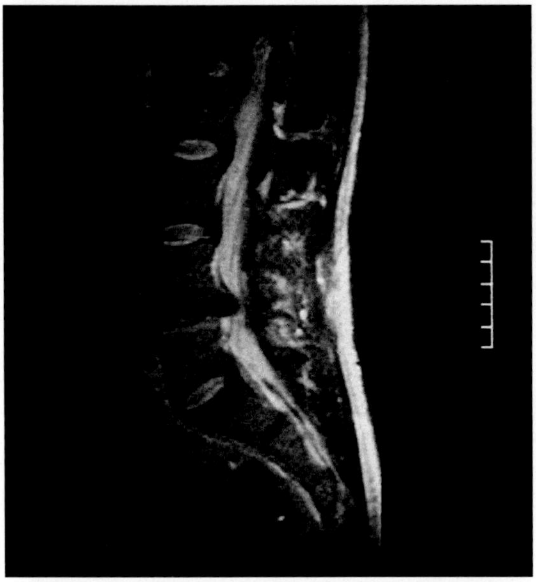

Figure 15.61 A lumbar spine MRI scan. There is a disc protrusion at L4/5 with degeneration of the disc itself, shown by the less bright signal in the intervertebral disc at this level.

- Isotopic scanning (scintigraphy) can be used in the diagnosis of acute (e.g. infection or stress fracture) or multiple (e.g. metastases) bone lesions by use of the first 2-minute (dynamic blood flow) phase, second 10-minute (blood pool) phase and third 3-hour late phase (osteoblastic) (Fig. 15.63) following intravenous injection of diphosphonate compounds. Tomographic scintigraphy can further refine definition of the isotope uptake (e.g. in stress fracture of the pars interarticularis). Radionucleotide bone scans are more sensitive than plain radiographs for the diagnosis of Paget's disease and in polyostotic cases help to quantify the overall burden of disease. Scintigraphy has a high sensitivity to metabolically active lesions; however, it is relatively non-specific and is often used in conjunction with other imaging modalities.
- Dual-energy X-ray absorptiometry (DEXA) is widely used to assess bone mineral density

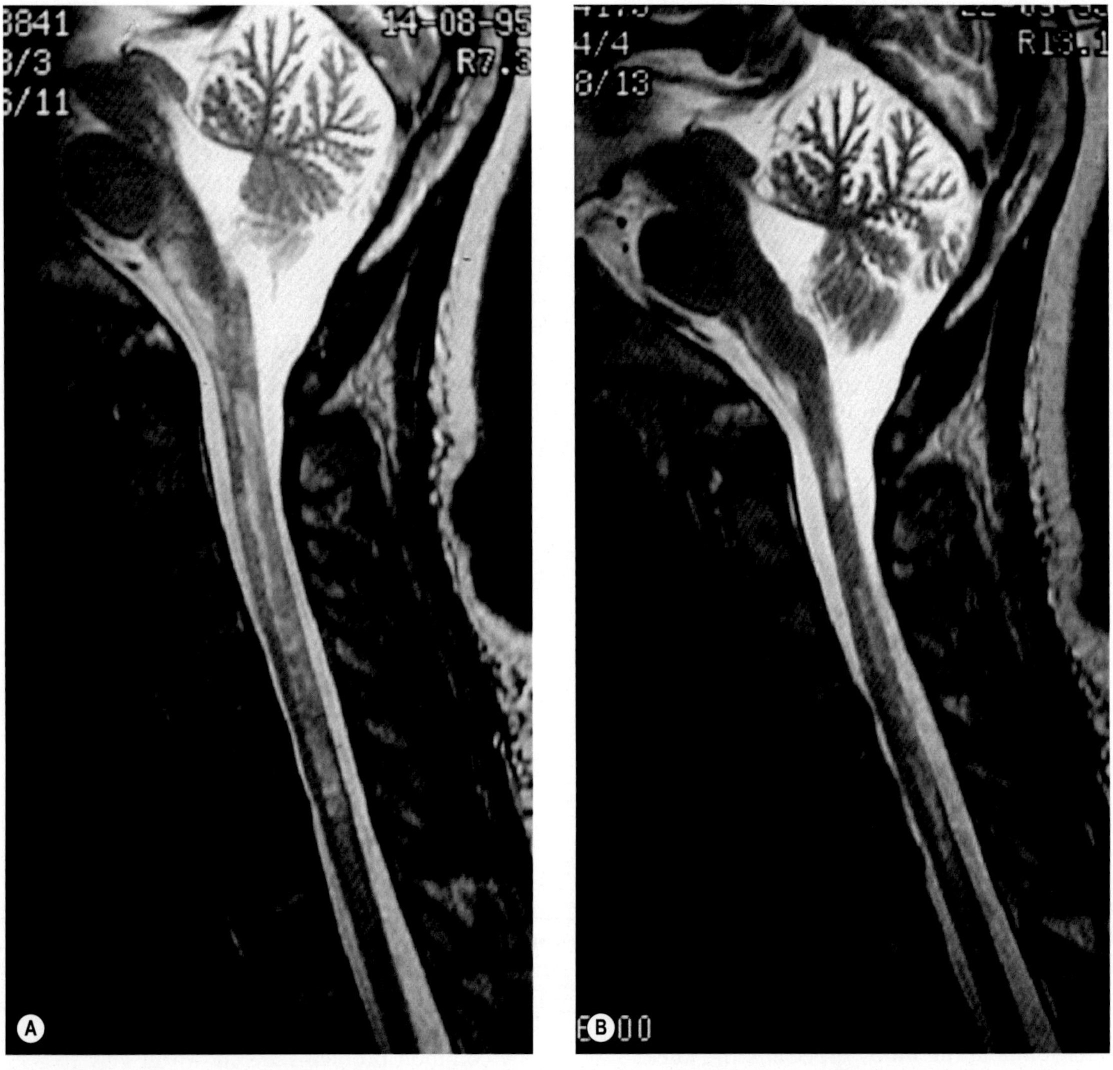

Figure 15.62 MRI of cervical spine in a patient with transverse myelitis due to SLE **(A)** before and **(B)** after immunosuppression.

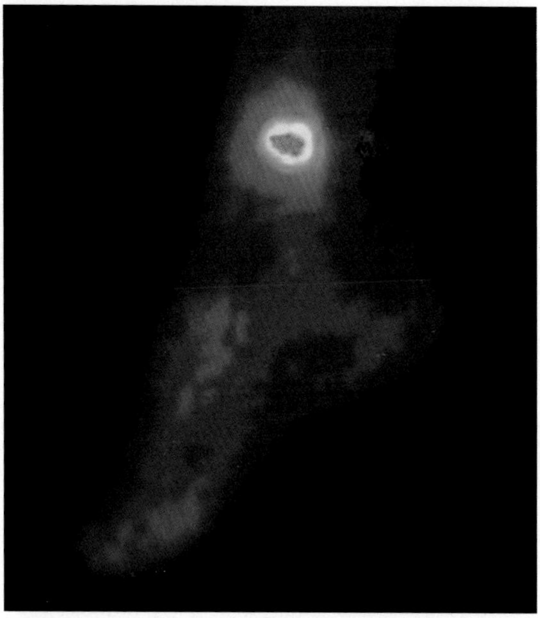

Figure 15.63 Technetium bone scan in a distance runner, showing focally increased uptake in the lower tibia owing to a stress fracture.

in metabolic bone disease and osteoporosis. Scans recorded with long intervals (e.g. every 2-3 years) between them may be used to assess the effects of therapy. Results are expressed in relation to a normal reference range.

- Positron emission tomography (PET) scanning is becoming more widely available but remains expensive. This is a type of scintigraphic molecular imaging based mostly on the uptake of radiolabeled glucose by metabolically active structures. FDG-PET scans are mostly used in rheumatology investigations and have better signal-to-noise ratio than standard isotope bone scanning. The combined technology of CT and PET scanning allows the acquisition of structural information simultaneously with metabolic activity. It is extremely sensitive in detecting malignancy and is also proving useful in documenting large vessel inflammation in disorders such as Takayasu's arteritis and giant cell arteritis. The radiation exposure is considerable and as such this imaging modality should be used cautiously and appropriately.

Nervous system 16

Rodney W.H. Walker

Introduction

In recent years there have been impressive advances throughout the field of neurology – in delineating disease entities and understanding their aetiology and pathogenesis; in diagnostic methods, particularly imaging and genetic testing; and in treatment and management. However, in spite of advances in investigations, careful clinical assessment remains of central importance.

The fundamental importance of the clinical history and examination cannot be overemphasized. In the diagnosis of neurological disease it is the history, rather than the examination, that is paramount, so it is even more important for this to be comprehensive. History taking has not changed significantly, but clinical neurological examination continues to evolve. Significant contributions have come from clinical assessment scales, some of which have been so successful as to have become internationally institutionalized, for example the Glasgow Coma Scale and the Mini-Mental State Examination (although the latter has recently been patented). On the other hand clinical signs of limited sensitivity, specificity, reliability and localizing value can be dispensed with.

A thorough neurological examination does involve doing more than is the case for other systems. Some basic neuroanatomical knowledge is necessary, but most clinical neurology need not be daunting. In new patients presenting for diagnosis, a sensible formulation of the nature of the problem on the basis of the history and examination is critical in order to request appropriate investigations, should they be necessary. Modern imaging undoubtedly has been the biggest revolution in clinical neurology in recent years, but injudicious use of imaging frequently leads to confusion, delay in diagnosis and sometimes harm. Similar considerations apply to the other major investigational modalities.

This chapter will discuss some aspects of neurological history, concentrate on neurological examination and the formulation of the nature of the neurological diagnosis and include some remarks on neurological investigations. Not covered in this chapter are coma, delirium and dementia.

The neurological history

The essentials of history taking have been covered elsewhere, but there are some points particularly salient to neurological conditions. The repertoire of neurological symptoms is actually quite limited, although perhaps larger than that of other specialties. Box 16.1 lists the usual ones, and each should be specifically enquired about in taking a neurological history.

The time course of evolution and sometimes resolution of neurological symptoms very frequently indicates the nature of the problem, and so this needs to be clarified as precisely as possible. Thus, sensory or motor symptoms which start abruptly and are at their most marked at or very soon after their onset strongly suggest a vascular causation (transient ischaemia or ischaemic or haemorrhagic stroke). In contrast, similar symptoms evolving over a few days, reaching a plateau in severity and then slowly receding typify inflammatory central nervous system (CNS) demyelination (a first episode or a relapse of multiple sclerosis). Subacute (developing over weeks to months), progressive symptoms can be caused by many kinds of pathology, but neoplasia is always a prime concern.

These statements are true enough to be clinically useful, although there are exceptions. For example, one of the reasons for requesting cranial imaging in all stroke patients is to exclude a benign or malignant tumour or other pathology which has caused a stroke-like presentation. Neurodegenerative conditions always develop insidiously with gradual progression, but occasionally patients present acutely. For example, motor neuron disease can present acutely with ventilatory failure. Alzheimer's disease commonly becomes evident after an episode of acute delirium caused by an intercurrent illness.

Two common neurological presentations require a history not only from the patient but also, if at all possible, from others: attacks of loss of consciousness and memory impairment.

The three most common causes of attacks of reduced consciousness or awareness that lead to neurological consultations are neurocardiogenic

Table 16.1 Points which help to distinguish syncope from seizures involving loss of consciousness. Minor injury, incontinence and sleepiness after the event do not distinguish well.

Syncope	Seizure
In neurocardiogenic syncope, characteristic prodromal features include: tinnitus, muffled hearing, dimming of vision, loss of vision while still conscious, widespread altered sensation, dizziness (may be described as spinning), lightheadedness, feeling of impending faint, weakness	The symptoms of focal seizure activity which precede a secondarily generalized attack may or may not be remembered after the attack is over
Marked pallor	Usually little or no pallor
Sweating (but not in those with autonomic failure)	Vocalization at onset of generalized convulsion (GC)
Any convulsion is brief (seconds)	Apnoea
Rapid recovery of lucidity and memory (registration and recall)	Cyanosis associated with GC
Patient comes round on the ground where he fell	Stertorous breathing
A second attack immediately on being sat up after the first attack is very suggestive of neurocardiogenic syncope	Tongue biting
Neurocardiogenic syncope is commonly set off by pain, squeamishness, gastrointestinal illness, public places indoors (clubs, restaurants, trains), prolonged standing	Postictal amnesia – paramedical staff present when patient 'comes round', or patient 'comes round' in hospital (although he walked to the ambulance)

Box 16.1 Neurological symptoms

- Cognitive symptoms, especially memory impairment
- Headache
- Loss of awareness
- Loss of consciousness
- Alteration of perception, including déjà vu
- Dizziness, vertigo
- Loss of balance
- Falls
- Loss of sense of smell
- Loss of taste
- Loss of vision
- 'Positive' visual symptoms, including components of migraine auras, unformed and formed hallucinations
- Double vision
- More than double vision (polyopia, palinopsia)
- Oscillopsia (a visual sensation of stationary objects swaying back and forth)
- Deafness
- Tinnitus
- Difficulty with speech
- Difficulty swallowing
- Weakness
- Abnormal movements of muscles (including cramp, fasciculations)
- Abnormal movements of parts of the body (including tremor, dystonia, myoclonus)
- Clumsiness
- Impairment of control of limbs
- Altered sensation
- Loss of sensation
- Pain
- Symptoms of postural hypotension
- Impairment of sexual function
- Impairment of bladder control
- Impairment of bowel control

syncope, epilepsy and psychogenic non-epileptic attacks. It is far more informative to hear a description from a witness than to request potentially misleading and inappropriate investigations. Obtaining the witness's account may require a telephone call; this is time well invested. Table 16.1 summarizes some points which help to distinguish syncope from seizures.

Memory impairment is a common complaint. Distinguishing between the worried, but well, and those with real impairment is greatly facilitated by information provided by close family or other informants. In general, if a patient is brought to a doctor by a relative who complains that the patient has memory impairment, there is most often an organic disorder, usually dementia. In contrast, many but not all patients who come to a doctor by themselves with the same complaint have good cognitive function. Furthermore, it is the relative who can report on changes in personality, behaviour, self-care and capacity which may be crucial to the diagnosis.

The most frequent symptom leading to neurological referral is headache. It is also a common reason for attending an emergency department. The vast majority of headaches are not caused by life-threatening disorders such as aneurysmal subarachnoid haemorrhage, meningitis or brain tumour, but are caused by common primary headache syndromes, particularly migraine. Table 16.2 outlines some of the features which may help to distinguish headaches of different sorts.

Vertigo (a hallucination of movement) is an important symptom and requires careful characterization. It indicates a disorder of one or both labyrinths, vestibular nerves, vestibular nuclei in the brainstem or, rarely, the cerebrum. A clear-cut description of a spinning feeling usually signifies true vertigo. Patients

Table 16.2 Headaches: points to consider in the history

Aspect of history	Feature	Diagnosis
Region/location	Focal, retro-orbital	Cluster headache
		Migraine
		Retro-orbital lesion
	Focal, frontal	Sinus pathology
	Occipital	Chiari malformation/cerebellar tonsillar ectopia Intracranial hypotension Cervical spondylosis Occipital neuralgia Migraine
	Unilateral	Migraine
		Chronic paroxysmal hemicrania (CPH)
		Hemicrania continua
	Generalized	Migraine
		Tension-type headache
Temporal aspects	>50% of days	Chronic daily headache (chronic migraine; tension-type headache)
	Attacks of hours/days	Migraine
	Attacks of up to 1 hour	Cluster headache
	Many attacks, lasting minutes	CPH
	Attacks of seconds	Trigeminal neuralgia
	Worse on waking	Raised intracranial pressure
		Sleep apnoea
	New, acute/subacute onset	Meningitis
		Abscess
		Encephalitis
	Explosive onset, severe	Subarachnoid haemorrhage (SAH)
Character and severity	Tight band around head, bland, featureless, not very severe	Tension-type headache
	Throbbing, moderately severe	Migraine
	Extremely severe, constant	Cluster headache
	Severe, stabbing, lancinating	Trigeminal neuralgia
Provoking/ relieving factors	Provoked by alcohol	Migraine
		Cluster headache
	Occur at night, start in sleep	Migraine
		Cluster headache
		Hypnic headache
	Relieved by sleep	Migraine
	Triggered by touching or moving the face	Trigeminal neuralgia
	Caused by cough	Chiari malformation
		Idiopathic cough headache
	Exertion	Exacerbates migraine
		Benign exertional headache
	Orgasm	Benign coital headache (SAH has to be excluded in a severe single attack)

Continued

Table 16.2 Continued

Aspect of history	Feature	Diagnosis
Associated symptoms	Nausea, vomiting, photophobia, phonophobia	Migraine
	Migraine aura (visual, sensory, etc.)	Migraine
	Neck stiffness, photophobia, vomiting, symptoms of fever	Meningitis
	Tear production ipsilateral to a unilateral headache	Migraine
		Cluster headache
		SUNCT*
	Ipsilateral conjunctival injection	Cluster headache
		SUNCT*
	Visual obscurations	Raised intracranial pressure with papilloedema
	Persistent focal neurological symptoms	Intracranial lesion
General health	Indications of systemic neoplasia	Metastasis
	Polymyalgia and weight loss	Giant cell arteritis

*SUNCT, short-lasting, unilateral, neuralgiform headache attacks with conjunctival injection and tearing (a rare disorder).

are more likely to complain of dizziness or giddiness than vertigo, and both dizziness and giddiness mean different things to different patients, including vertigo, oscillopsia (a visual sensation that stationary objects are swaying back and forth), lightheadedness, loss of balance or even sometimes headache. It is always important to establish whether a patient with vertigo has positional vertigo. Enquiring whether the patient's symptom is provoked by sitting from a lying position or standing from a sitting position will not distinguish vertigo from postural hypotension or ataxia, as all give rise to symptoms on rising. Symptoms brought on by lying down or turning over in bed or looking up at a high shelf or the sky more certainly signify real positional vertigo. It is not uncommon for patients with loss of balance to complain of dizziness; such patients will spontaneously comment that they feel secure sitting in a chair but dizzy as soon as they stand up and move around.

Focal weakness is self-explanatory. Many patients complain of feeling generally weak when they have no loss of muscle strength at all. Some patients become weak without realizing it. Thus, patients with unilateral or bilateral quadriceps weakness may present with falls rather than complain of weakness. Patients with bilateral ankle dorsiflexion weakness may complain of being off balance or of tripping rather than weakness. Exertional weakness or worsening of weakness is characteristic of neuromuscular junction disorders but also occurs in cauda equina compression (spinal canal stenosis), spinal cord compression (cervical spondylotic myelopathy) and in multiple sclerosis and sometimes other disorders, so it is not specific but can be diagnostically helpful and so should be asked about.

Sensory symptoms may be negative (a reduction or absence of normal sensation) or positive (an abnormal sensation which is felt, e.g. buzzing, tingling, 'pins and needles', pain). In ordinary usage, the word numb would seem to be unambiguous, but some patients who are weak without sensory loss refer to numbness (particularly in Bell's palsy) and, conversely, patients with sensory migraine auras may be misdiagnosed as having hemiplegic migraine because of their impression of paralysis even though they can move the affected limbs. Patients who seem imprecise have some justification; the *Shorter Oxford Dictionary* defines numb as 'deprived of feeling, or of the power of movement' so it is important to clarify exactly what the patient is describing.

As a rule, transient ischaemic attacks which involve the parietal cortex give rise to brief negative sensory symptoms. Conversely, focal sensory seizures are characterized by positive sensory symptoms.

Most organic neurological disorders which give rise to sensory symptoms involve structural or functional damage to nerves somewhere, whether it be in peripheral nerves, nerve roots, spinal cord or brain. Hypersensitivity (hyperaesthesia) to all modalities of sensation is therefore improbable or impossible. Patients who appear to have very sensitive skin as a result of a lesion (e.g. herpes zoster radiculitis) have combinations of paraesthesia, hypoaesthesia, dysaesthesia, allodynia, hyperalgesia and hyperpathia. Some of these terms are not without their ambiguities. Table 16.3 provides a definition for each.

Lhermitte's symptom (often called Lhermitte's sign) is a paroxysm of positive sensory symptoms – an electric shock feeling or a shower of paraesthesiae shooting down the spine and/or into the upper or lower limbs triggered by neck flexion. It is indicative of a cervical spinal cord lesion, commonly a multiple sclerosis plaque, although other cord lesions (e.g. spondylotic cord compression) and even cobalamin deficiency may also produce this symptom.

Table 16.3 Nomenclature of cutaneous sensory symptoms

Hypoaesthesia	Reduced cutaneous sensation of any modality
Paraesthesia	Spontaneous abnormal sensation including, tingling, pins and needles and pain
Neuralgia	Pain in the distribution of a nerve or nerve root
Dysaesthesia	An abnormal perception of a sensory stimulus, e.g. touch causes tingling or pain
Allodynia	Pain caused by a stimulus that does not normally cause pain
Hyperalgesia	An abnormally intense perception of a mildly painful stimulus
Hyperpathia	Perseveration, augmentation and, on occasion, spread of pain
	The pain threshold is normal or sometimes high
	The threshold for perceiving pain may be raised and there may be delay in perceiving a painful stimulus, but once perceived, the pain is severe and prolonged and may spread
Hyperaesthesia	An ambiguous term, best avoided

Neurological examination is poor at identifying and characterizing disorders of the autonomic nervous system, making it particularly important that autonomic function (including bladder and bowel control and sexual function) is addressed in the history.

The neurological examination

Aspects of neurological examination can start from the moment the patient is first encountered, before and during the taking of the history, such as noting an abnormality of gait, difficulties with speech, parkinsonism or a hyperkinetic movement disorder. There is no such thing as a comprehensive neurological examination – it would take hours or days. However, too many patients without neurological symptoms have no neurological examination at all, which on occasions proves regrettable. Consider, for instance, the case of a man who develops areflexic weakness some days after a hernia operation. How helpful would it be to know that the reflexes had been normal at the time of preoperative clinical clerking? A suggested minimal neurological examination for non-neurological patients would be assessments of the binocular visual fields, the eye movements, the biceps, triceps, knee and ankle reflexes, the plantar reflexes and funduscopy. Most patients attending for a neurological consultation (with problems such as headache or epilepsy) have no neurological signs. A minimal routine neurological examination for such patients should include assessments of vision, the cranial nerves, motor and sensory examination and examination of gait. Bear in mind that many patients with early cognitive impairment are adept at concealing it, so that without probing, it can be missed.

For most patients, it is best to be systematic with regard to neurological examination, adhering to a routine well rehearsed by the examiner and familiar to those with whom the examiner will communicate. Thus, even if the patient's problem is foot drop, it is entirely valid to start with examination of cranial nerves but sensible to explain to the patient that you are going to start at the top and work down. Certain situations require flexibility; patients with any degree of impairment of consciousness need assessment of their delirium or coma from the outset. In patients presenting with cognitive impairment, it is best to start the examination with cognitive assessment. It is important in all neurological patients to pay attention to and document mobility, and in patients presenting with a gait disorder it is appropriate to examine the gait first. For most other patients, an appropriate order of examination is cranial nerves, speech if necessary, motor system, sensory system and gait, followed by cognitive testing if relevant.

Cranial nerve examination

Examination of the 12 cranial nerves actually involves an assessment of much more than just the nerves and nuclei, particularly with respect to the sensory visual system and eye movements. The naming and numbering of cranial nerves and their nuclei is in some measure idiosyncratic and confusing; for example, there is no olfactory nerve as such and the eighth cranial nerve is actually two nerves, as is the seventh. Within the brainstem, trigeminal sensory nuclei receive fibres not just from the fifth cranial nerve but also from the seventh, ninth and tenth nerves.

The olfactory (I) nerves

Olfactory receptor cells are bipolar sensory neurons situated under the nasal epithelium. Their central axons project in numerous bundles, not as a discrete nerve, up through the cribriform plate of the skull into the olfactory bulb on the inferior surface of the frontal lobe. These project via the olfactory tract to parts of the temporal lobe and frontal lobe.

Examination of the olfactory nerves

For ordinary clinical purposes, olfaction is tested using a small number of bottles containing either a fragrant or pungent smelling substance such as lemon, clove or asafoetida. Each nostril should be tested separately. A necessary precondition is that a rhinological disorder does not preclude the test. Ideally the patient should identify the smell rather than just report that it can be smelt. There is little value in routinely testing olfaction; it is uncommon to detect an abnormality and even less common for an abnormality to contribute to a diagnosis. A subfrontal tumour such as a meningioma may cause unilateral anosmia, but other features of the history and examination will mandate the imaging which should establish that diagnosis. Subfrontal meningiomas can cause bilateral anosmia, so imaging is indicated in a patient presenting just with anosmia unless another cause is clearly evident. Olfactory nerve fibres passing through the cribriform plate are not uncommonly sheared as a result of head injury, frequently leading to permanent bilateral anosmia. Anosmia is commonly neurodegenerative, occurring particularly in Lewy body disease, so its presence in a patient with parkinsonism increases the likelihood that the patient has idiopathic (Lewy body) Parkinson's disease. Endocrinologists test olfaction when Kallman's syndrome is suspected.

The optic (II) nerves (see also Chapter 20)

The optic nerve runs from the back of the globe of the eye to the apex of the orbit and into the skull through the optic canal to the optic chiasm, where it is joined by the optic nerve from the other eye. Directly above the optic chiasm is the hypothalamus. Directly below is the pituitary gland. The pituitary stalk runs from the hypothalamus to the pituitary gland just behind the optic chiasm, between the optic tracts. Sensory afferents from all points of the retina run in the nerve-fibre layer on the inner surface of the retina to enter the optic nerve at the optic disc. Fibres from the temporal retina (nasal visual half-field) are placed laterally while those from the nasal retina (temporal visual half-field) are medial. Fibres from the upper half of the retina run in the upper half of the optic nerve. At the optic chiasm, fibres from the nasal half of the retina (temporal visual half-field) cross (decussate) to the contralateral optic tract, while the fibres from the temporal half of the retina do not cross but proceed posteriorly into the ipsilateral optic tract (Fig. 16.1). Starting within the chiasm and continuing further posteriorly within the optic tract, fibres which convey matching information from each eye (i.e. homonymous fibres, representing equivalent parts in the temporal retina for one eye, nasal retina for the other eye) become aligned with each other. Thus, each optic nerve conveys information from its respective eye, but every part of the sensory visual system behind the optic chiasm on each side deals with vision for the contralateral binocular visual half-field.

The majority of optic tract fibres pass, via the lateral geniculate nucleus, to the occipital cortex. The lower part of the visual radiation transmits visual information from the inferior temporal retina of the ipsilateral eye and inferior nasal retina of the other eye. A few optic tract fibres pass via the superior colliculus to

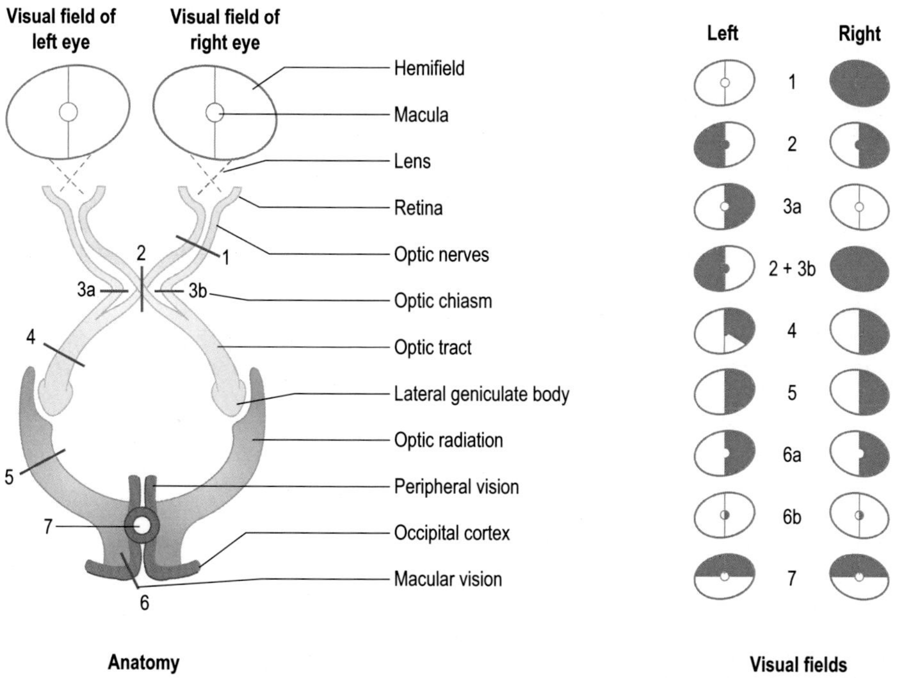

Figure 16.1 A diagram of the sensory visual pathways. Sites of lesions and the visual field defects they produce are shown. 1. Optic nerve lesion. 2. Optic chiasm lesion (bitemporal hemianopia). 3a or 3b. Uniocular nasal hemianopia (rare). 3a plus 3b. Binasal hemianopia (very rare). 4. Optic tract lesion (incongruous homonymous hemianopia). 5. Visual radiation (homonymous quadrantanopia or hemianopia). 6a. Occipital cortex lesion sparing the occipital pole (homonymous hemianopia with macular sparing). 6b. Occipital pole lesion (homonymous paracentral hemiscotoma). 7. A bilateral occipital cortex lesion (homonymous altitudinal hemianopia).

the midbrain to mediate the afferent limb of the pupillary light reflex via connections to the Edinger-Westphal nuclei.

Visual acuity and colour vision

Visual acuity is of neurological as well as ophthalmological importance, since optic nerve disease may lead to any degree of loss of acuity. For ordinary clinical neurological purposes, the acuities measured using the Snellen chart are adequate. Severe loss of acuity (less than 6/60, the top letter on the Snellen chart) is documented as ability to count fingers at 1 metre, ability to perceive hand movements, perception of light only and no perception of light.

Acquired unilateral loss of colour vision is a characteristic feature of optic neuropathy, and loss of colour vision can occur when visual acuity is well preserved. Thus, testing colour vision using Ishihara plates may be a sensitive bedside test for mild optic neuropathy.

Visual fields

Assessment of the visual fields is a key part of the neurological examination and need not take very long to perform. Field defects of importance are commonly missed because they have not been looked for adequately. Increasingly, opticians measure visual fields, but it cannot always be assumed that a recent ophthalmological assessment will have included the visual fields.

Visual field defects in one eye indicate a retinal or optic nerve disorder. They may affect any part of the field of the affected eye or nerve. Lesions at the optic chiasm or lesions behind the chiasm in the optic tracts, visual radiations or occipital cortex give rise to visual field defects affecting both eyes. Unilateral retrochiasmal lesions give rise to field defects affecting the contralateral binocular half-field, and the defects are homonymous (i.e. they affect equivalent parts of the temporal half-field of one eye and the nasal half-field of the other). Congruity refers to the extent to which the defects in the two half-fields match each other exactly. A congruous homonymous hemianopia indicates a lesion in the occipital cortex, while a non-congruous homonymous hemianopia is more likely to occur with an optic tract lesion.

When ophthalmologists do visual field testing, they tend to do Goldman perimetry or to obtain automated Humphrey fields, and the results of these tests are very useful, but in the clinic or on the ward, neurologists and general physicians test visual fields by simple confrontation field testing, comparing the patient's fields with their own, assuming their own to be normal.

Examination of the visual fields

It is best to start by testing the binocular visual fields (i.e. the patient and examiner both have both eyes open). Start by asking the patient to look at your face. Ensure that he avoids the common temptation to look to either side. Hold your hands up one on each side at face level, with your hands about 1 m apart and ask the patient whether he can see both hands. This simple test will detect a dense homonymous hemianopia. Next ask the patient to look into your eyes. Switch from hands held up to index fingers held up and move them up so that they are situated in the right and left superior quadrants of vision. Instruct the patient to point at the finger which wiggles. Getting the patient to point is better than asking him to say whether it is the right or left finger which is moving – very many muddle left and right in this situation. First wiggle one finger, then the other, to check the integrity of the superior quadrants. Failure of the patient to see one of the fingers wiggling suggests a homonymous quadrantanopia. If that happens, carry on wiggling the finger which has not been registered by the patient and move it first across the midline to make sure that it becomes visible at the midline and then go back and do the same, this time moving the finger down into the inferior quadrant, where the finger will be visible if the patient has a quadrantanopia or remain unseen if the patient has a homonymous hemianopia. If the patient sees each finger wiggling consecutively in each of the upper quadrants, then wiggle both fingers simultaneously and ask the patient what is happening. If the patient only sees the wiggling of the finger on one side consistently, then he has visual inattention – an occipitotemporal or occipitoparietal disorder. Having tested the superior quadrants, move down to the inferior quadrants to test them in the same way. With a cooperative patient, all of this takes only a matter of seconds to do. The technique described will not detect a bitemporal hemianopia, optic nerve lesions or retinal disorders; these require testing of the field for each eye separately.

The best way to test the monocular visual fields at the bedside is to use a pin with a bright red pinhead of about 5-8 mm diameter. The patient needs to be positioned such that light is not shining from behind the examiner into the patient's eyes, so as to interfere with his ability to see the colour of the pinhead. The margin of the field is defined by the points at which perception of the colour of the pinhead changes from black to red. Ask the patient to cover one eye with the palm of his hand (or cover the eye with your own hand) and then to look with his open eye straight into your own confronting eye (his left into your right and vice versa). First, put the pinhead into the middle of the visual field and check that the patient sees it as bright red. Swap to the other eye and compare the perceived brightness of red reported by the patient for his two eyes. Loss of perceived redness in one eye (red desaturation) raises the possibility of a mild optic neuropathy. A patient who is already known to have poor acuity in one eye may have a central scotoma, in which case the pinhead will either not be seen in the centre of the field or will be perceived black. A small central scotoma can be defined by moving the pinhead outwards in four different directions until the patient sees its redness. Next, put the pinhead into each of the four quadrants of vision close to the centre and check that the patient sees it as bright red. This may detect a paracentral scotoma and is also a good way of detecting temporal field defects due to optic chiasm lesions such as pituitary tumours. Then finally, while ensuring that the patient maintains fixation into your eye, compare the periphery of his field with your own by moving the pin from outside the field in towards the centre at various points around the periphery, with the pin midway between you and the patient. The patient has to report not when he first sees the pin or your hand but when the pinhead colour changes from black to red.

The pupils

Examination of the pupils and their responses to light and accommodation provides information not only about specific neurological syndromes which affect the pupils, such as Adie's syndrome, but also information about the integrity of the anterior visual pathways (particularly the optic nerves), the brainstem and the efferent parasympathetic and sympathetic pathways to the pupillary sphincter and dilator muscles, respectively.

Pupil constriction is a parasympathetic function. The first-order neurons are in the Edinger-Westphal nucleus adjacent to the oculomotor nucleus in the midbrain. Axons travel in the oculomotor nerve to the ciliary ganglion in the orbit. Second-order neurons innervate the pupillary sphincter. Lesions of the Edinger-Westphal nucleus or the pupilloconstrictor nerve fibres in the oculomotor (third) cranial nerve or in the orbit lead to dilatation of the pupil (mydriasis) unless there is simultaneously a lesion of the sympathetic innervation of the pupil. In either case, there is a failure of constriction of the pupil to light. In general, compression of the third cranial nerve (classically by a posterior communicating artery aneurysm) affects the pupilloconstrictor fibres. A microvascular ischaemic lesion of the third nerve may spare the pupilloconstrictor fibres, giving rise to a pupil-sparing third nerve lesion. Microvascular lesions of the oculomotor nucleus may spare the Edinger–Westphal nucleus with the same result. A mid-sized unreactive pupil due to a lesion of both parasympathetic and sympathetic supplies is seen in aneurysms of the internal carotid artery within the cavernous sinus, along with other features of a cavernous sinus syndrome.

Pupil dilation is achieved by sympathetic innervation of pupillodilator muscle fibres. The first-order neurons are in the hypothalamus. They project down through the brainstem and cervical spinal cord to the ciliospinal centre in the lower cervical and upper thoracic spinal cord, from where second-order neurons project via the T1 nerve root and sympathetic chain to the superior cervical ganglion. Third-order axons run up the internal carotid artery as far as the cavernous sinus and from there through the orbit to the pupil. There is also sympathetic innervation of the levator palpebrae superioris muscle by the same route. A lesion of the sympathetic supply to the pupil at any point between the hypothalamus and the orbit will give rise to the two main features of Horner's syndrome: constriction of the pupil (which will still react to light by further constricting) and ptosis (drooping of the upper eyelid).

Examination of the pupils

First, in normal illumination, establish whether the pupils are of equal size. If they are not, bear in mind that there are two possibilities: either one is smaller than it should be or the other is bigger. Avoid jumping to the wrong conclusion.

Ideally, the reactions of the pupils to light should be tested in moderately low illumination. Use a bright torch, not an ophthalmoscope. Shine the light into one eye and observe the response of the pupil (the direct response), the normal response being constriction of the pupil which is sustained until the light is removed. Repeat the test, this time looking at the contralateral pupil, which will normally constrict (the consensual response). Then test the other eye. Next, test accommodation (constriction of the pupils when focusing on a near object). Ask the patient to look into the distance, then at your finger held at a distance and to keep looking as you advance your finger to a distance of about 20 cm from the patient's face. Advancing your finger in a wavy line allows you to check that the patient is looking at the finger. Observe the adduction of the eyes and the constriction of the pupils. Then ask the patient to look into the distance again.

Afferent pupillary defect

A patient with a severe lesion of the anterior visual system in one eye (an ophthalmological disorder or an optic nerve disorder such as severe optic neuritis or an ischaemic optic neuropathy) will have an afferent pupillary defect (i.e. a failure of constriction of either pupil to light shone into the affected eye). If the visual system on the other side is unaffected, light shone into the normal eye will lead to a normal direct pupillary response and there will also be a consensual response in the visually impaired eye, assuming the efferent pathway is intact.

Relative afferent pupillary defect

A patient with a mild lesion of the anterior visual apparatus on one side will exhibit a direct pupillary response to light, but it will be less vigorous than the consensual response to light shone into the other eye. In this situation, the swinging torch test may reveal a relative afferent pupillary defect. If a patient has a mild optic nerve lesion in the left eye, then acuity and colour vision may be only mildly impaired and the field normal. Shine the torch into the affected left eye and note the seemingly normal response.

After 2 seconds, move the torch briskly to shine into the normal right eye. The right pupil will already be constricted as a result of the consensual response. It will stay constricted and, if anything, will constrict a little further. After 2 seconds, move the torch briskly back to the left eye. Because of the subtle afferent defect, the signal strength of the input to the midbrain pupilloconstrictor (Edinger-Westphal) nuclei will be reduced, resulting in an apparently paradoxical dilation of the left pupil in spite of light being shone into it. If you keep swinging the torch back and forth from one eye to the other, the relative afferent pupillary defect will continue to be observed, although the defect is best seen within the first few attempts.

Afferent and relative afferent pupillary defects are important because they are objective. A person who gives the impression of having functional visual impairment in one eye, but who has an afferent pupillary defect, must have an organic problem. In contrast, a person who reports uniocular blindness and has normal pupillary responses to light will not be blind.

Efferent pupillary defect (part of a third cranial nerve lesion)

A lesion of the pupilloconstrictor nerve fibres in the oculomotor nerve will lead to dilation of the ipsilateral pupil (due to the unrestrained effect of the intact sympathetic supply). Further, there will be failure of constriction of the pupil to light, although the consensual response in the other eye will be preserved. Light shone into the contralateral eye will elicit a normal direct response but no consensual response.

Other common pupillary abnormalities of neurological relevance

- Simple (physiological) anisocoria (inequality of pupil size): this is common. The pupillary inequality is not marked and the reactions to light and accommodation are normal.
- Tonic pupil: this is seen in Holmes Adie syndrome, a relatively benign polyneuropathy comprising a lesion of the ciliary ganglion and a degree of loss of tendon reflexes. An acute Adie pupil is enlarged, does not react to light and there is a slow constriction to accommodation. Redilation of the pupil after accommodation is delayed such that, temporarily, the normal pupil may be larger than the affected one.
- Argyll Robertson pupils: these are small, irregular, unequal pupils which do not react to light but do to accommodation. They were seen in advanced syphilis. Without the irregularity but with the other features, diabetic small vessel disease is currently the most common cause.
- The pupils in coma: this is important but covered elsewhere (Ch. 9).

Fundoscopy

Fundoscopy is described in Chapter 20. The neurological examination focuses on papilloedema, optic atrophy, pigmentary retinal degeneration and vascular disease.

The oculomotor (III), trochlear (IV) and abducens (VI) nerves – eye movements

Abnormalities of eye movements may result from disorders of the cerebral hemispheres; brainstem; cerebellum; cranial nerves III, IV and VI; the neuromuscular junctions between oculomotor nerves and eye muscles; the eye muscles themselves and from lesions affecting the structure and contents of the orbits. Their importance in neurological and general physical examination is therefore evident.

The nucleus for the third cranial nerve is in the midbrain (Fig. 16.2). The nerve emerges ventrally (anteriorly), medial to the cerebral peduncle, passing forward through the cavernous sinus to the superior orbital fissure. In the orbit, the superior ramus supplies superior rectus and levator palpebrae superioris. The inferior ramus supplies inferior rectus, inferior oblique and medial rectus, and parasympathetic fibres from the inferior ramus pass to the ciliary ganglion and thence to the ciliary muscle and the pupil sphincter.

The fourth nerve nucleus lies just caudal to the third nerve nucleus in the brainstem. The nerve fibres of the fourth nerve decussate. The nerve starts on the dorsal aspect of the brainstem and passes around the brainstem through the cavernous sinus and

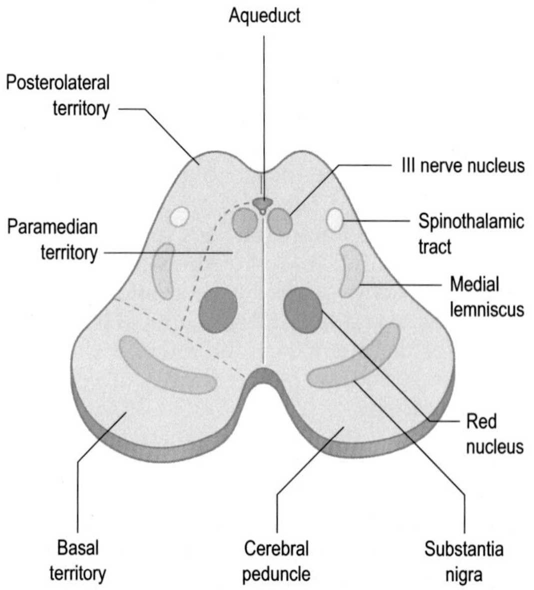

Figure 16.2 A diagram of the midbrain. Note the dorsally positioned third nerve nuclei. Vascular territories are shown on the left.

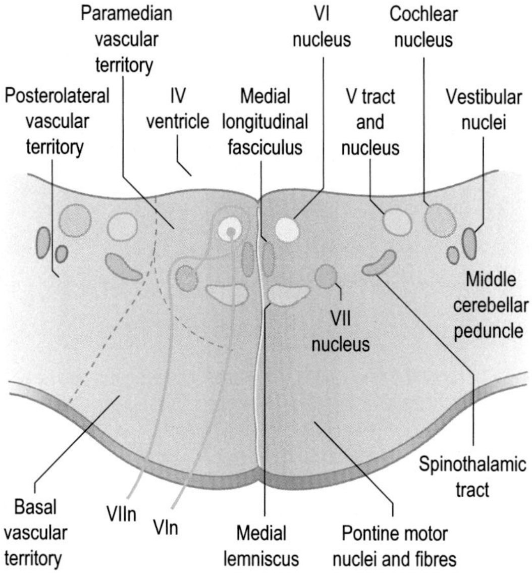

Figure 16.3 A diagram of the fifth, sixth and seventh nerve nuclei in the pons. Note how the nerve fibres of VII loop round the nucleus of VI.

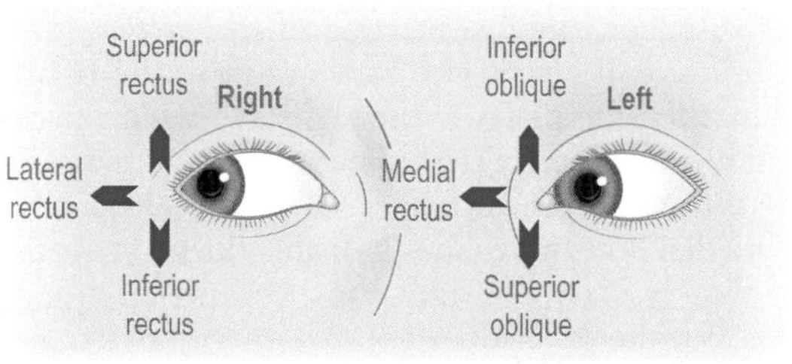

Figure 16.4 A diagram showing which muscles elevate and depress the abducted and adducted eye.

superior orbital fissure to the superior oblique muscle. Consequent upon the decussation of fibres, the right trochlear nucleus innervates the left superior oblique and vice versa.

The sixth nerve nucleus is beneath the floor of the fourth ventricle in the pons (Fig. 16.3). Nerve fibres run forward (ventrally) through the pons emerging at its lower border, then up the skull base and forward through the cavernous sinus to the superior orbital fissure and into the orbit to supply the lateral rectus muscle. The nerve is long, thin and very susceptible to dysfunction, most notably in the setting of raised intracranial pressure of any aetiology, which may give rise to either unilateral or bilateral sixth nerve lesions. This is referred to as a 'false localizing sign', since a focal mass lesion causing raised intracranial pressure may be remote from the sixth nerves and their nuclei or there may be no focal cause of the raised pressure at all (e.g. idiopathic intracranial hypertension).

Table 16.4 and Fig. 16.4 outline the actions of each eye muscle.

Table 16.4 Actions of the eye muscles

Nerve	Muscle	Action: With eye abducted	Action: With eye adducted
Abducens; VI	Lateral rectus	Abduction	Abduction
Oculomotor; III	Inferior rectus	Depression	Depression; extorsion
Oculomotor; III	Inferior oblique	Extorsion; elevation	Elevation
Oculomotor; III	Medial rectus	Adduction	Adduction
Oculomotor; III	Superior rectus	Elevation	Elevation; intorsion
Trochlear; IV	Superior oblique	Intorsion; depression	Depression

The eye is offset laterally in relation to the apex of the orbit which accounts for why the superior and inferior rectus muscles have only purely vertical actions when the eye is abducted. Adduction of the eye turns the superior and inferior oblique muscles into a pure depressor and elevator, respectively.

Terminology in eye movements

Horizontal movement of the eye outwards (laterally) is termed abduction and inwards (medially) is termed adduction. Vertical movement upwards is termed elevation and downwards is depression. The eye is also capable of diagonal movements (version) at any intermediate angle. Rotary movements are those in which the eye twists on its anterior–posterior axis. Intorsion is rotation such that the upper part of the eye moves medially and the lower part of the eye moves laterally. Extorsion is the opposite. Convergence refers to adduction of both eyes to fixate on a near object. Lateral rotation of the head causes reflex movement of the eyes in the opposite direction (adduction of one eye, abduction of the other). A squint (the eyes point in different directions) is described as convergent or divergent strabismus, depending on whether the eyes point towards or away from each other. Saccades are abrupt, rapid, small movements of both eyes, such as those needed to shift fixation from one object to another. Nystagmus denotes rhythmic oscillations of one or (more usually) both eyes. In pendular nystagmus, the movement is slow in both directions. In jerk nystagmus, there is a slow phase in one direction and a fast phase in the opposite direction. By convention, the direction of nystagmus is the direction of the fast phase, but the defect is in fact the slow phase and is either an abnormal deviation of the eyes or a failure of the eyes to maintain position, and the fast phase is a compensatory saccade aimed at restoring the correct position of the eyes. Some types of nystagmus are outlined below.

Examination of eye movements

As with every other component of examination, the detail in which the eye movements are examined

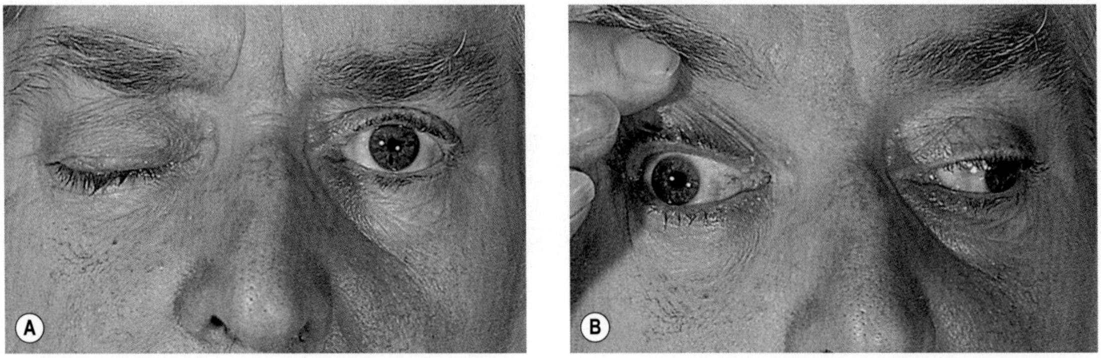

Figure 16.5 A severe right third nerve lesion with complete ptosis **(A)**. With the paralysed eyelid raised, paresis of adduction is seen on attempted left gaze **(B)**. In this patient the pupil is spared, as is commonly seen in ischaemic lesions but not in compressive lesions. The other features of a third nerve lesion are paresis of elevation of the eye and intorsion of the eye on attempting to look down, due to the action of the superior oblique muscle on an eye that cannot be adducted (reproduced from Forbes and Jackson, Color Atlas and Text of Clinical Medicine, Mosby, 2002).

depends on whether there are relevant symptoms and whether abnormal signs are likely to be present. Ask the patient to keep his head still (assist him by putting your left hand on his head to steady it) and then to look at your right index finger held directly in front of his eyes at about half a metre distance. In the primary position of gaze, look for any visible abnormality of the alignment of the two eyes (an affected patient may or may not complain of double vision) and any pendular or vestibular nystagmus (see below). Now move your finger to the right, then left, and then up and down. The pursuit eye movements which are elicited should precisely follow your finger at the appropriate constant velocity. Eye movements which are 'broken up' into a series of short saccades indicate a brainstem or cerebellar lesion affecting eye movement control. Patients with diplopia will usually experience their diplopia at some point (or at all times) during this simple test. However, in patients with a complaint of diplopia it is important not just to test vertical eye movements from the primary position of gaze but to test movements to the right and up and down and then to the left and up and down. During pursuit eye movement examination, gaze-evoked and vestibular nystagmus will be observable (see below). When looking for nystagmus, it is important not to get the patient to look too far in any direction since, at the extremes of gaze, nystagmus can be normal as the patient struggles to deviate his eyes beyond what is possible. Look for nystagmus at about 30° away from the primary position of gaze.

Diplopia testing

If a patient complains of double vision, first establish that it is true diplopia and not monocular diplopia. In patients who have obvious, easily visible paresis of movement of one or both eyes, the reason for diplopia is self-evident.

Diplopia develops with even very subtle misalignment of the eyes, which cannot be seen on simple inspection. In this situation, if the ophthalmoparesis affects just one eye, it is possible to work out which eye muscles are underactive by diplopia testing. The true image is that generated by the eye with normal movements. The false image is that generated by the eye with the paretic muscle or muscles. For example, if a patient develops double vision on looking to the right, with horizontal separation of the images, the false image will be the one further out to the right. This is true whether it is the right eye which does not abduct adequately (right lateral rectus weakness) or if it is the left eye which does not adduct adequately (left medial rectus weakness). If this does not seem immediately clear, consider the extreme case: one eye moves, the other does not. An image (an examiner's finger or a white pinhead) moves to the patient's right. The image remains in the middle of the field of the eye which moves but moves progressively to the right of the field of the eye which does not. The same rule applies in all directions of gaze. Diplopia is always maximal in the direction in which the weak muscle has its purest action (see Table 16.4).

The severity of the diplopia should be assessed in eight positions: looking to left and right, up and down, and obliquely up and down to the left and obliquely up and down to the right. To work out which muscle is underactive, where the diplopia is maximal, cover each eye in turn and get the patient to tell you which of the two images disappears. Inconsistent answers are common, however, and the assistance of an ophthalmologist or optometrist is frequently desirable. The features of lesions of the third, fourth and sixth cranial nerves are summarized in Table 16.5.

In assessing patients who have double vision, it is best first to establish which muscles appear to be weak and then try to decide what the nature of the problem is likely to be, taking into consideration all the physical signs. Thus, impairment of eye movements in one eye in combination with proptosis of that eye may occur because of mechanical restriction of eye movements by an intraorbital lesion. Weakness of

Table 16.5 The effects of lesions of the oculomotor (III), trochlear (IV) and abducens (VI) nerves

Affected nerve	Signs	Comment
Oculomotor*	Paresis of adduction (medial rectus)	The eye becomes abducted because of unopposed action of lateral rectus, and slightly depressed because of action of superior oblique
	Paresis of elevation (superior rectus and inferior oblique)	The pure depressor action of superior oblique cannot be tested because the eye cannot be adducted
		Intorsion of the eye on attempted down gaze indicates intact trochlear nerve and superior oblique function
	Paresis of depression (inferior rectus)	
	Ptosis due to paresis of levator palpebrae superioris	With complete ptosis, there is of course no diplopia
	Dilated, unreactive pupil	This feature is not present in pupil-sparing lesions (microvascular lesions of nucleus or nerve)
Trochlear	Paresis of superior oblique	Extorsion of the eye due to unopposed action of inferior oblique leads to diplopia such that a vertical line looks V-shaped
		The patient compensates with a head tilt to the side opposite the lesion, intact intorsion on that side tending to correct the diplopia
Abducens	Paresis of lateral rectus	Horizontal diplopia

*Figure 16.5 shows a patient with a severe oculomotor palsy.

Box 16.2 Cranial nerve involvement in lesions of the cavernous sinus and superior orbital fissure

1 Lesion of the cavernous sinus (e.g. internal carotid aneurysm, internal carotid artery dissection, meningioma):
   - potential involvement of cranial nerves III, IV, VI, V_1 (ophthalmic division), V_2 (maxillary division) and sympathetic pupillodilator nerve fibres
   - cavernous sinus thrombosis combines the above with proptosis, chemosis, papilloedema and visual failure
2 Lesion of the superior orbital fissure (e.g. Tolosa Hunt syndrome):
   - potential involvement of III, IV, VI and V_1 (ophthalmic division)
   - extension into the orbit may lead to involvement of the optic nerve

muscles in both eyes with different patterns of involvement of the muscles in the two eyes is likely to be due to a disorder of the muscles themselves (orbital myositis, thyroid eye disease) or due to ocular or generalized myasthenia. The pupils will not be involved. Bilateral, asymmetrical combinations of cranial nerve lesions are relatively uncommon (neoplastic infiltration, cranial polyneuritis). Bilateral sixth cranial nerve lesions are common, usually but not exclusively as a feature of raised intracranial pressure. Multiple oculomotor neuropathies in one eye direct attention to the superior orbital fissure and the cavernous sinus (see Box 16.2).

Horizontal gaze paresis; internuclear ophthalmoparesis

Neural control of voluntary lateral gaze to the right starts in the left cerebral hemisphere, such that a large left cerebral hemisphere lesion may be associated with failure of right gaze and a tendency for the eyes to deviate to the left (the side of the lesion). Output runs to the right paramedian pontine reticular formation (PPRF); hence, a right-sided pontine lesion may involve a right gaze paresis. Output from the right PPRF goes to the right sixth nerve nucleus, resulting in right eye abduction, and across, via the left medial longitudinal fasciculus (MLF), to the left third nerve nucleus, resulting in simultaneous left eye adduction. Attempted right gaze in the setting of a left MLF lesion results in abduction of the right eye but failure of adduction of the left eye – an internuclear ophthalmoparesis (INO) (see Fig. 16.6). Bilateral MLF lesions give rise to bilateral INO, in which case, with lateral gaze in either direction, only the abducting eye moves normally. Nystagmus is commonly seen in the abducting eye. The pathway for adducting both eyes for near vision is separate and sometimes in bilateral INO, preservation of adduction of the eyes for near vision (convergence) can be demonstrated, proving that the problem is not bilateral medial rectus weakness.

Vertical gaze pareses

The neural control of upgaze and downgaze is complex. Ultimately, output for upgaze is via components of the third nerve nucleus mainly to the superior rectus and inferior oblique muscles bilaterally. The output for downgaze is from the third and fourth nerve nuclei to the inferior rectus and superior oblique muscles, respectively. In general, defects of upgaze or downgaze localize rather poorly, but lesions such as pineal tumours which compress the midbrain and bilateral descending connections from the hemispheres often cause upgaze paresis. Rare midbrain ischaemic strokes due to occlusion of a perforating vessel from

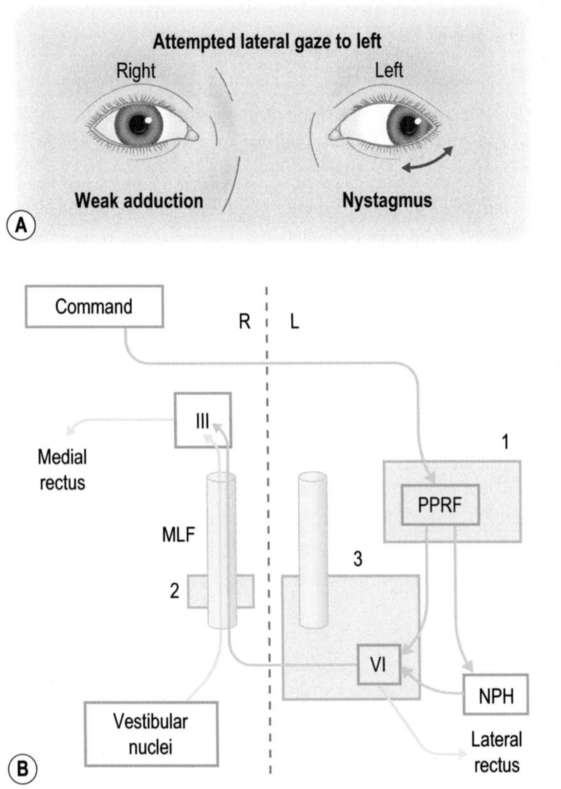

Figure 16.6 **(A)** A right internuclear ophthalmoparesis. **(B)** A diagram of the pathways for horizontal gaze. The command for left gaze originates in the right cerebral hemisphere. Descending nerve fibres decussate to reach the left pons. Lesion 1 produces a left horizontal gaze paresis. Lesion 2 produces a right internuclear ophthalmoparesis. Lesion 3 produces the 'one and a half' syndrome: a left gaze paresis and left internuclear ophthalmoparesis (failure of adduction of the left eye on right gaze) – only abduction of the right eye on right gaze remains. NPH, nucleus prepositus hypoglossi; MLF, medial longitudinal fasciculus; PPRF, paramedian pontine reticular formation.

the top of the basilar artery include downgaze paresis among the clinical manifestations.

Non-paralytic strabismus

Clinicians need to be able to recognize developmental non-paralytic strabismus. Decompensation of a long-standing squint may be a cause of acquired diplopia.

Testing saccadic eye movements

Getting a patient to follow a moving finger tests pursuit eye movements. It takes very little time to test saccadic eye movements and useful signs may be detected. First, simply ask the patient to keep his head still and look to the left, to the right, up and down. Then hold your hands up in front of the patient, one in the primary position of gaze, the other to the side, with palms facing the patient, fists closed. Ask the patient to keep his head still. Open the fist of the hand in front of the patient and ask him to look at it. Then close that fist and open the other and ask the patient to switch his gaze to the hand at the side. By alternating which hand is open you can get the patient to refixate briskly to and fro. Then check the other side. These manoeuvres test saccadic movements; in disease, saccades may be slowed or interrupted. A mild INO will be best seen during saccadic horizontal eye movements. Because detecting a mild INO requires observing a difference in the velocity of movement of the two eyes, it is difficult to appreciate if the examiner fixates on one or the other eye; perhaps, unintuitively, it is best to look at the bridge of the patient's nose to see the movement of the two eyes at the same time.

Supranuclear gaze pareses

Reflex eye movements related to head movements are generated and organized by vestibular, cerebellar and brainstem systems, whereas voluntary gaze is initiated in the cerebral hemispheres. A patient's gaze paresis is therefore supranuclear if reflex eye movements are intact. Take a patient with selective paresis of downgaze. If brisk backward rotation of the head (extension of the neck) produced reflex depression of both eyes, a supranuclear lesion would be inferred. In practice, this is often not easily achieved since the relatively common disorder giving supranuclear downgaze paresis is progressive supranuclear palsy, a condition in which there is also axial rigidity affecting neck movements.

Peripheral vestibular nystagmus

This occurs in lesions of the labyrinth or vestibular nerve. Normally there is tonic input to the brainstem vestibular nuclei from the periphery. Loss of this tonic input leads to deviation of the eyes towards the affected side (slow phase) with fast-phase nystagmus directed to the opposite side. In mild lesions, the nystagmus is only seen when the eyes look in the direction of the fast phase. In more severe lesions, the nystagmus is seen with the eyes in the primary position of gaze or even when looking away from the direction of the fast phase. Usually the nystagmus is of high frequency and relatively low amplitude.

Gaze paretic nystagmus

Gaze paretic nystagmus is a gaze-evoked nystagmus in which the eyes are not able to maintain a position away from their primary position, so the slow phase is a drift back to the primary position while the fast phase is in the direction of gaze. In the primary position, the eyes are still. The nystagmus may be of large amplitude and low frequency. Drug-induced nystagmus (alcohol, benzodiazepines, antiepileptic medication) is of this sort and is seen in all directions of gaze. Structural brainstem or cerebellar lesions may cause asymmetric gaze paretic nystagmus. In cerebellar hemisphere lesions, the nystagmus may be unidirectional with the fast phase towards the side of the lesion.

Upbeat nystagmus (fast phase upwards) may occur with lesions at various locations in the brainstem and with cerebellar vermis lesions. Downbeat nystagmus is characteristic of cervicomedullary junction lesions such as Chiari malformations but can also be seen with cerebellar degenerations.

Congenital nystagmus

The rule here is that the nystagmus is horizontal, even when the patient looks up or down. On left gaze, it is left beating, and on right gaze, it is right beating. There may be a null point at which the nystagmus is least conspicuous, but it is not necessarily in the primary position, and the eyes may not be completely still. Congenital nystagmus is damped by convergence.

Pendular nystagmus

This may be seen as a complication of congenital or acquired very poor vision. It is also seen in pontine lesions (e.g. multiple sclerosis).

The trigeminal (V) nerve

The trigeminal nerve is a mixed motor and sensory nerve. The nerve trunk emerges from the pons as sensory and motor roots.

Sensory component of the trigeminal nerve

The primary sensory neurons are in the trigeminal ganglion, just behind the cavernous sinus at the apex of the petrous bone. Central projections run in the trigeminal nerve into the pons. Fig. 16.7 shows the cutaneous distribution of the three divisions of the trigeminal nerve: ophthalmic (V_1), maxillary (V_2) and mandibular (V_3). These nerves also mediate general sensation inside the mouth and nose and proprioception. The ophthalmic nerve passes through the cavernous sinus and superior orbital fissure. The maxillary nerve also passes through the cavernous sinus but leaves the inside of the skull through the foramen rotundum. The mandibular nerve passes through the foramen ovale.

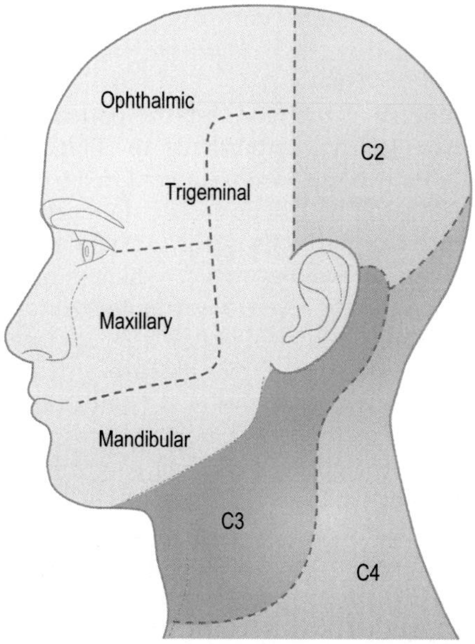

Figure 16.7 Areas of cutaneous innervation of the head and neck by the three divisions of the trigeminal nerve and the upper cervical nerve roots.

Afferents mediating touch sensation pass to the principal sensory nucleus of the trigeminal nerve in the pons. Pain and temperature afferents go into the spinal tract and pass caudally into the medulla and into the spinal nucleus of the trigeminal nerve, which extends down from the medulla as low as the upper cervical spinal cord. Thus, lesions in the medulla can give rise to dissociated sensory loss in trigeminal territory (loss of pinprick sensation with preserved light touch sensation).

Motor component of the trigeminal nerve

Motor nerve fibres from the motor nucleus in the pons run in the motor root of the trigeminal nerve, bypassing the trigeminal ganglion to enter the mandibular nerve. They supply the muscles of mastication: masseter, temporalis and the lateral pterygoids.

Trigeminal territory sensory loss

Patients with impaired sensation on one side of the face may have a trigeminal nerve lesion, a trigeminal nucleus lesion or a lesion of central trigeminal sensory pathways. Not uncommonly, unilateral facial sensory symptoms remain unexplained, which does not necessarily make them 'non-organic'. Much is made of distinguishing between patients whose distribution of sensory loss is anatomical and those in whom it is not. Sensory loss which ends at the jaw line and at the hairline would be regarded as non-anatomical but too much dogma may be unwise – patients are often not very careful reporters of exactly where their sensory symptoms are. Clearly defined symptoms of reduced sensation render examination almost redundant, but the area of hypoaesthesia can be delineated in the same way as sensory loss anywhere else using a pin and testing from a numb area outwards towards where sensation is normal.

The corneal reflex

A sensory stimulus applied to the cornea causes a reflex blink which cannot be suppressed; its absence on one side establishes unequivocally the presence of a trigeminal lesion. Patients with an anaesthetic cornea are at risk of corneal injury, so it is important to identify affected individuals by testing patients who very clearly have symptoms and other signs of a trigeminal lesion. It is also an important test in coma. The test is uncomfortable and should not be part of a 'routine' neurological examination. The presence of a normal corneal reflex does not mean that there is no lesion of the trigeminal nerve or its connections.

Explain to the patient what is going to happen. Ask him to look in such a direction that the eyes are wide open. Using the corner of a clean tissue, touch the centre of the patient's cornea, approaching from the side. The normal response is a brisk blink. Some use cotton wool, but there is a risk of strands getting stuck in the eye because of the blink. In coma, a drop of saline applied to the cornea is a good stimulus. Remember that if there is ipsilateral facial paralysis (e.g. Bell's palsy), the reflex will be absent on the affected side, but will be readily seen on the other side.

Testing the motor component of the trigeminal nerve

Look for wasting of the temporalis and masseter muscles. Feel for contraction of the masseter muscles when the patient clenches his jaw. Ask the patient to open his mouth; the lateral pterygoid muscles on each side draw the mandible forward, such that a severe lesion of the trigeminal nerve will lead to deviation of the jaw towards the side of the lesion due to weakness of the pterygoid muscles on the affected side. The pterygoid muscles may be further tested by asking the patient to push his open jaw sideways against your hand.

The facial (VII) nerve

The facial nerve is principally a motor nerve, supplying facial muscles on one side, but it also has small general somatic sensory and major gustatory sensory components, as well as important parasympathetic functions.

The facial nerve nucleus is in the caudal pons, lying ventrolateral to the sixth cranial nerve nucleus (see Fig. 16.3). It receives upper motor neuron input from both cerebral hemispheres. Lower motor neuron fibres from the facial nucleus first pass round the sixth nerve nucleus, then emerge from the pons to form the facial nerve. From here, it travels laterally, adjacent to the eighth cranial nerve, to the internal auditory meatus, thence to the facial canal which has a relatively long and tortuous course through the skull, emerging at the stylomastoid foramen. The nerve then passes forward into the parotid gland and divides into branches which supply all the facial muscles and the platysma muscle on one side. In the facial canal, a branch of the facial nerve supplies the stapedius muscle.

The nerve cell bodies of the sensory components of the facial nerve are in the geniculate ganglion in the facial canal. Gustatory sensory afferents from the anterior two-thirds of the tongue travel in the lingual nerve and then via the chorda tympani nerve to join the facial nerve in the facial canal. Central projections reach the medulla via the nervus intermedius between the facial and eighth cranial nerve.

The peripheral projections of the small general somatic sensory contribution innervate the tympanic membrane, external auditory meatus and tragus of the ear. This accounts for the herpetic vesicles seen in the ear in patients with the Ramsay Hunt syndrome of facial paralysis caused by herpes zoster affecting the facial nerve.

Secretomotor parasympathetic efferents leave the pontomedullary junction in the nervus intermedius which joins the facial nerve in the internal auditory meatus. Some of the parasympathetic nerves leave the facial nerve at the geniculate ganglion in the greater petrosal nerve, eventually mediating tear secretion from the lachrymal glands. Others leave via the chorda tympani nerve to reach salivary glands.

These complexities are relevant to clinical neurology because a facial nerve lesion, depending on its location, may be associated with loss of taste, hyperacusis (if the stapedius is paralysed) and, in chronic lesions, 'crocodile tears' (i.e. inappropriate tear production when salivary glands should be activated), attributed to aberrant reinnervation of salivary and lachrymal glands.

Facial weakness occurs because of muscle disorders (invariably bilateral weakness), myasthenia (invariably bilateral but may be asymmetric early on), polyneuropathies (e.g. Guillain-Barré syndrome or vasculitis, unilateral or bilateral), facial nerve or nuclear lesions (most commonly unilateral), motor neuronopathies (usually bilateral) or upper motor neuron disorders (usually unilateral, but occasionally bilateral).

A lower motor neuron lesion affecting the whole of the facial nerve nucleus or the whole of the facial nerve will cause weakness of all muscles of one side of the face. A unilateral upper motor neuron lesion, however, will cause weakness of the lower half of the face with sparing of the upper half of the face because there is bilateral representation of the upper half of the face in the motor cortex.

Testing the facial nerve

Look for asymmetry of the face. Ask the patient to raise his eyebrows (to look astonished), to blink and then to screw both eyes up, firmly closed. On a weak side, the eyelashes will be less buried by the eyelids. Attempt to raise the patient's eyebrows while his eyes are closed and screwed up; mild weakness may be detected. When there is severe lower motor neuron facial weakness, the patient will not be able to close the affected eye. Attempted eye closure will be accompanied by elevation of the eyes (Bell's phenomenon). Ask the patient to blow his cheeks out, to show his teeth (or gums) and then to grimace. Observe the patient's spontaneous smiles. (In some upper motor neuron disorders of facial muscle control, voluntary movement of the lower face is lost but smiling is relatively preserved.) Ask the patient to purse his lips together and attempt to open them using your fingers. These tests usually suffice to pick up facial weakness and to distinguish between upper and lower motor neuron disorders.

The cochlear and vestibular (VIII) nerves

These two nerves convey afferents from the cochlea and the vestibular apparatus, respectively, via the internal auditory meatus to the pontomedullary junction in close proximity to the facial nerve, reaching cochlear and vestibular nuclei in the brainstem. Acute sensorineural deafness and acute vestibular neuritis reflect separate pathologies selectively affecting each of these nerves.

Testing the cochlear and vestibular nerves

The assessment of deafness is covered in detail elsewhere (Ch. 21). At the bedside, a crude assessment of hearing can be achieved by rubbing your index finger and thumb together close to the patient's ear or by whispering numbers close to his ear, with the contralateral ear occluded. Rinne's test is good for distinguishing between conduction and sensorineural deafness, as long as you use the appropriate tuning fork (frequency 512 Hz – not the lower frequency tuning fork (128 Hz) used for testing vibration sense).

Conduction deafness is sometimes of neurological significance if an infective or neoplastic middle ear lesion has spread to affect middle or posterior cranial fossa structures.

Unilateral sensorineural deafness is an important feature of 'cerebellopontine angle lesions', such as acoustic neuroma or meningioma, along with variable combinations of facial weakness (facial nerve), facial sensory symptoms (trigeminal nerve), nystagmus (brainstem and vestibular nerve), ataxia (brainstem and cerebellum), and ultimately long tract signs (brainstem) and raised intracranial pressure.

Bilateral sensorineural deafness may be a feature of certain multisystem neurological disorders, particularly mitochondrial disorders.

Two important tests of vestibular function assess much of the vestibular system (the semicircular canals of the labyrinths, the vestibular nerves and the vestibular nuclei of the brainstem). These are the Dix-Hallpike test for positioning vertigo and nystagmus and the head thrust test. They should be performed in patients with vertigo.

The Dix-Hallpike test is described in Chapter 21. Far and away the commonest cause of positioning vertigo is the condition benign paroxysmal positioning vertigo, a labyrinthine disorder, and it is by far the commonest cause of an abnormal Dix-Hallpike test. Vestibular neuritis is usually associated with nystagmus that does not require a change in head position to elicit it, but in this condition vertigo and nystagmus are usually exacerbated by positioning tests. Brainstem disorders may also be the cause of positioning vertigo and nystagmus. Typically peripheral disorders are associated with a latent period between head movement and onset of vertigo and nystagmus, intense vertigo, and a reduction of the vertigo and nystagmus with repeated testing, whereas central positioning nystagmus may be associated with rather mild vertigo but nystagmus that does not diminish with repeated testing.

The head thrust test (head impulse test) detects a failure of the afferent component of the vestibulo-ocular reflex. In a normal individual, fixating on an object straight ahead, an abrupt rotation of the head to one side or the other will not disrupt ocular fixation. In a patient with an acute unilateral peripheral vestibulopathy (vestibular neuritis), a head thrust rotating the front of the head towards the side of the lesion will result in the eyes turning with the head momentarily and a noticeable saccade to bring the eyes back to restore fixation. This test is useful in distinguishing acute vertigo caused by vestibular neuritis from vertigo caused by a brainstem stroke or transient ischaemic attack. With the patient's gaze fixed on the examiner's nose, the examiner then abruptly turns the patient's head successively about 30° to the right and left.

The glossopharyngeal (IX) nerve

There are anatomical and functional relationships between the glossopharyngeal nerve, the vagus nerve and the cranial component of the accessory nerve. The nucleus ambiguus in the medulla (Fig. 16.8) contains the motor neurons which innervate striated muscle of the palate, pharynx, larynx and upper oesophagus, fibres running partly in the glossopharyngeal nerve, mainly in the vagus nerve and partly in the cranial portion of the accessory nerve. Situated more dorsally in the medulla, the dorsal motor nucleus of the vagus and the inferior salivatory nucleus (whose fibres join the glossopharyngeal nerve) contain preganglionic parasympathetic neurons which control

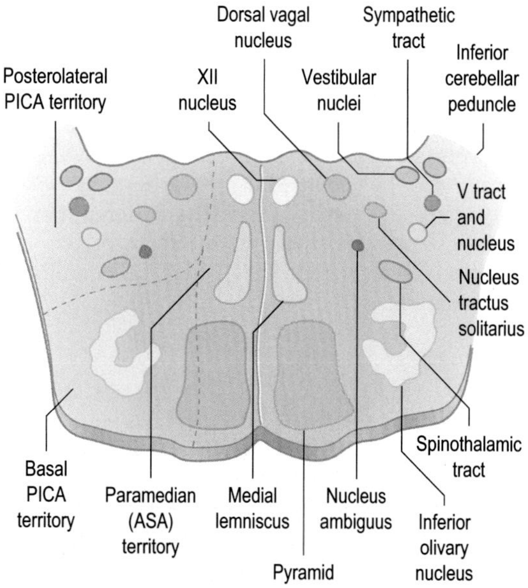

Figure 16.8 A diagram of cranial nerve nuclei and tracts in the medulla. Vascular territories are shown on the left. ASA, anterior spinal artery; PICA, posterior inferior cerebellar artery.

glands and smooth muscle. Special visceral afferents (i.e. taste fibres from the intermediate nerve and the glossopharyngeal nerve) enter the solitary tract to end in the nucleus of the solitary tract in the medulla. General somatic sensory afferents in the glossopharyngeal and vagus nerves join trigeminal sensory nuclei.

The glossopharyngeal nerve rootlets emerge from the medulla just rostral to those of the vagus nerve. The glossopharyngeal nerve leaves the skull via the jugular foramen. It mediates somatic sensation of the palate and pharynx and gustatory sensation from the posterior third of the tongue, has autonomic secretomotor fibres which reach the parotid gland, and supplies the stylopharyngeus muscle (which cannot be tested clinically).

Testing the glossopharyngeal nerve

The glossopharyngeal nerve is not tested in routine neurological examinations. If there are particular clinical indications to test it, such as a symptom of pharyngeal sensory impairment, pharyngeal neuropathic pain or a lesion of the vagus nerve, pharyngeal sensation can be tested using an orange stick to touch lightly the mucosa of the posterior pharyngeal wall. This requires tolerance and cooperation on the part of the patient. Some normal individuals will gag even at the approach of a tongue depressor or orange stick. In stuporous or comatose patients, testing the gag reflex may be useful. The afferent component of this reflex involves the glossopharyngeal nerves.

The vagus (X) nerve

The rootlets of the vagus emerge from the medulla just below those of the glossopharyngeal nerve. Both nerves leave the base of the skull through the jugular foramen. The vagus nerve passes down the neck adjacent to the internal carotid artery and internal jugular vein. Motor efferent fibres supply pharyngeal muscles. The superior laryngeal nerve supplies the cricopharyngeus muscle of the larynx and conveys sensation from the larynx. Lower down in the thorax, the recurrent laryngeal nerve passes back up the neck to supply the laryngeal muscles other than cricopharyngeus. The visceral afferent and efferent fibres of the vagus nerve downstream of the recurrent laryngeal nerves are not amenable to clinical neurological examination.

Testing the vagus nerve

A patient with a proximal unilateral lesion of the vagus nerve may complain of dysphagia and nasal regurgitation of swallowed fluids. There will be weakness of the muscles of the soft palate on the affected side. Attempted voluntary elevation of the soft palate (ask the patient to say 'Ahh', preferably fairly high pitched) reveals the weakness of elevation of the palate on the affected side, along with deviation of the uvula to the unaffected side, because of the unopposed action of the palatal muscles on that side. In addition, ipsilateral vocal cord paresis will lead to dysphonia. Bilateral lesions of the vagus nerves will invariably be associated with dysphagia. (Bilateral palatal weakness is not commonly due to bilateral vagus lesions but rather to more diffuse disorders such as polyneuropathy or myasthenia gravis.) The effects of bilateral lesions of innervation of the larynx vary depending on whether there is weakness mainly of vocal cord abduction or adduction or both. Bilateral abductor weakness puts the patient at risk of stridor and respiratory obstruction. Bilateral adductor weakness leads to dysphonia and inability to generate a normal explosive cough (the cough which the patient can manage is described as a bovine cough).

The accessory (XI) nerve

The cranial accessory nerve is formed of nerve fibres from the nucleus ambiguus and they soon leave the accessory nerve to rejoin their equivalents in the vagus nerve. The spinal accessory nerve consists of motor nerve fibres from the cervical spinal cord (C2-6); instead of leaving the spinal cord in spinal roots, they pass rostrally up into the medulla and emerge as the accessory nerve which, along with the glossopharyngeal and vagus nerves, passes through the jugular foramen. The spinal accessory nerve supplies the sternocleidomastoid muscle and the upper part of the trapezius muscle.

Testing the accessory nerve

The left sternocleidomastoid muscle contributes to rotation of the head to the right and vice versa. Weakness of the left sternocleidomastoid is therefore assessed by asking the patient to turn his head to the right with force, while the examiner opposes the rotation with the left hand, pushing carefully against the right side of the face. Failure of contraction of the muscle can be seen. Weakness of the upper part of trapezius is one of the causes of winging of the scapula, the other being weakness of serratus anterior due to a lesion of the long thoracic nerve (see p. 331). Scapular winging due to trapezius weakness is most commonly caused by a lesion of the accessory nerve in the posterior triangle of the neck, often iatrogenic related to surgical excision of a lymph node.

The hypoglossal (XII) nerve

The hypoglossal nucleus in the medulla contains motor neurons which innervate tongue muscles. The nerve leaves the lower medulla, passing through the hypoglossal canal to leave the base of the skull, then down and forward to reach the tongue.

Testing the hypoglossal nerve

A unilateral hypoglossal nerve lesion in the acute stage leads to weakness of tongue muscles on the affected side. Attempted protrusion of the tongue results in deviation of the tongue towards the weak

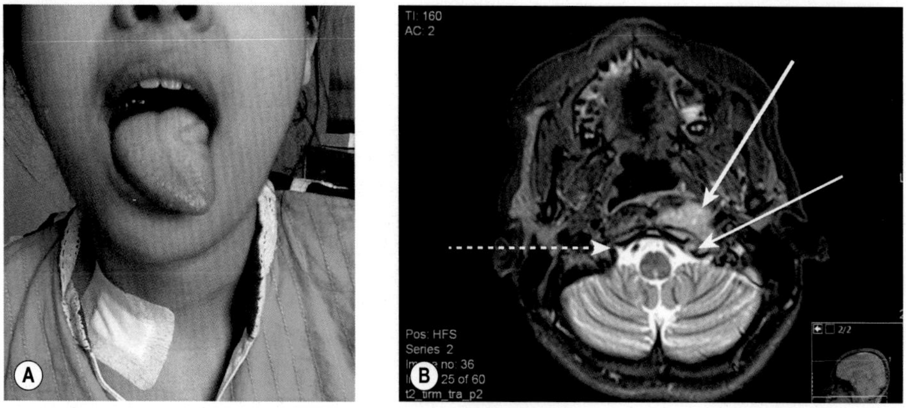

Figure 16.9 **(A)** The tongue of a patient with an acute left hypoglossal nerve lesion. She had noticed weight loss for 3 months and pain at the back of the neck on the left side for 1 month. She was afebrile and the only sign was the weak tongue. **(B)** A T2-weighted MRI scan at the base of the skull shows abnormal tissue (thick arrow) under the skull and infiltrating into the hypoglossal canal (thin arrow). The hypoglossal canal on the right side is normal (dotted arrow). MRI scans of the neck revealed lymphadenopathy (not shown). A fine needle aspirate from one of the nodes (hence the adhesive dressing seen in the photograph) was not diagnostic. An open lymph node biopsy confirmed the diagnosis of tuberculosis.

side (Fig. 16.9). A chronic lesion will be associated with visible muscle atrophy of the affected side of the tongue. Bilateral wasting and weakness of the tongue with fasciculation are usually due to the progressive bulbar atrophy of motor neuron disease.

Speech

Dysphonia is an abnormality of production of vocal sounds. Vocal cord paresis therefore causes dysphonia. Parkinson's disease may cause dysphonia and certainly hypophonia, a low-volume voice.

Dysarthria is an abnormality of articulation, for which neurological disease is an important cause. Those with a musical ear may be good at distinguishing spastic from cerebellar dysarthrias, but experienced neurologists sometimes get this wrong. The important thing is to detect mild dysarthria and look for other signs which will clarify its basis and to consider that a patient who has dysarthria may, more importantly, have dysphagia.

Spastic dysarthria

An upper motor neuron disorder affects the tongue, pharynx and facial muscles. Tongue movements are slow, the jaw jerk is brisk and facial stretch reflexes may be present. If part of a pseudobulbar palsy is due to diffuse small vessel cerebrovascular disease or motor neuron disease, there will be associated cognitive abnormalities and limb signs.

Cerebellar (ataxic) dysarthria

Look carefully for nystagmus and other eye movement disorders and for limb and gait ataxia.

Parkinsonism (hypokinetic dysarthria)

In parkinsonism there may be dysarthria and other disorders of speech and language such as acquired stutter as well as dysphonia.

Bulbar palsy (flaccid dysarthria)

Bulbar refers to the medulla oblongata, and bulbar palsy denotes any weakness of muscles supplied by the seventh to twelfth cranial nerves from the pons and medulla. Dysarthria and dysphagia are the main manifestations. Palatal weakness allows nasal escape of air during production of plosive sounds. There are many causes, ranging from muscle disorders, myasthenia gravis and polyneuropathies to lower motor neuronopathies. In myasthenia, fatigue may be evident, the dysarthria developing as the patient talks.

Severe upper motor neuron lesions such as strokes will produce dysarthria, and it may also be a feature of certain dysphasias.

Motor system

For the purposes of clinical neurological examination and interpretation of neurological signs, the anatomical considerations can be kept simple. The motor neurons whose axons terminate at neuromuscular junctions and which activate voluntary striated muscle contraction are situated in the anterior horns of the spinal cord grey matter and in motor cranial nerve nuclei. These are the lower motor neurons. Upper motor neurons are those situated in the cerebral cortex whose axons leave the cortex to control, directly or indirectly, the lower motor neurons. Some of these are in the somatotopically organized primary motor cortex (Fig. 16.10) in the precentral gyrus at the back of the frontal

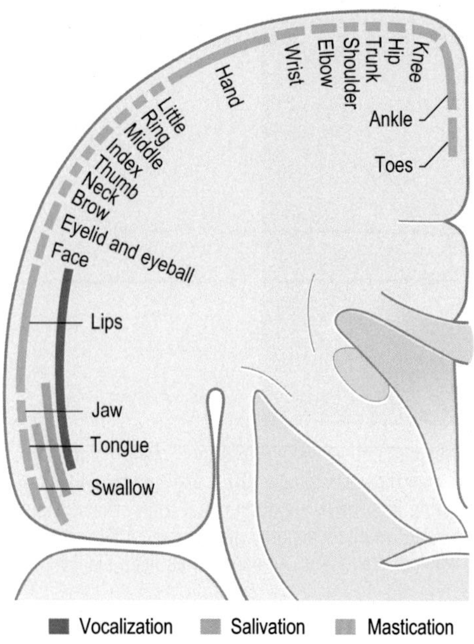

Figure 16.10 Somatotopic representation in the primary motor cortex.

lobe, but the distribution of upper motor neurons in the cortex is much wider than just the primary motor cortex and includes the supplementary motor area and premotor cortex in the frontal lobes. The cerebral control of posture and movement involves widely distributed cortical motor systems. Crucial also are circuits involving the basal ganglia and cerebellum. Output from the cortex is either direct to motor neurons via corticospinal and corticobulbar tracts or indirect via projections to the brainstem which has major influences by various pathways.

The corticobulbar and corticospinal tracts pass via the internal capsule and cerebral peduncle to the ventral pons. The corticobulbar tract projects to motor nuclei of cranial nerves V, VII, IX, X and XII bilaterally. The corticospinal tract continues in the medullary pyramid. The majority of corticospinal tract fibres decussate in the lower ventral medulla, passing into the lateral corticospinal tract of the spinal cord to innervate contralateral spinal motor neurons. These fibres control movements of the limbs. A minority of corticospinal tract fibres do not decussate but proceed straight on into the spinal cord in the anterior corticospinal tract to project to motor neurons bilaterally. They control axial muscles involved in posture.

Lower motor neurons in the brainstem send their axons directly into cranial nerves. Lower motor neurons in the spinal cord send their axons via ventral nerve roots into spinal nerves. Spinal nerves divide into dorsal and ventral rami. Dorsal rami innervate paraspinal muscles of the back. Ventral rami innervate the other muscles. The anatomy of the thoracic spinal nerves is relatively simple, directly reflecting embryological segmentation. The ventral rami supply intercostal and abdominal trunk muscles. Cervical, first thoracic, lumbar and sacral spinal nerve ventral rami pass into plexuses (cervical, brachial and lumbosacral) from which are formed named peripheral nerves which mainly supply the limbs. The muscles supplied by a spinal nerve collectively constitute a 'myotome'. (The cutaneous area supplied by a spinal nerve is a dermatome.)

The fundamental effect of a lower motor lesion is weakness (ultimately paralysis) of affected muscles with marked wasting. The effects of upper motor neuron lesions are more variable, depending on which descending pathways are affected. They are loss of dexterity, weakness and spasticity. An upper motor neuron lesion may cause mild weakness but, nevertheless, be incapacitating because of spasticity and impaired dexterity. On the other hand, a lesion restricted to cells in the primary motor cortex itself causes weakness without spasticity. With upper motor neuron lesions, muscle wasting is much less marked and occurs late.

Motor system examination

The examination technique for formal assessment of the motor system depends very much on the circumstances. For instance, a follow-up outpatient assessment to gauge the response to treatment of a patient with myasthenia gravis, polymyositis or even chronic idiopathic demyelinating polyneuropathy may be effectively achieved in the consultation room without recourse to the examination couch. Here, it is assumed that the patient is presenting for a diagnosis; this requires complete exposure of limbs, shoulders, trunk and buttocks, and careful assessment of muscle power of a large number of muscles or muscle groups.

Inspection

Start by looking at the muscles of the limbs and trunk. Pathological hypertrophy of muscle is rare. Pseudohypertrophy is also uncommon. It is seen mainly in the calf muscles of individuals with certain muscular dystrophies. It is termed 'pseudohypertrophy' because it is associated with weakness, and pathologically there is degeneration of muscle with replacement of muscle tissue by fat.

Wasting of muscle is a common sign of disease, but does not always have a neurological basis. With disuse, muscles atrophy, sometimes quite fast. Generally disuse atrophy is fairly mild. Power is preserved if it can be tested (e.g. quadriceps wasting in someone with severe knee arthritis). Cachexia involves diffuse muscle wasting, but usually power is surprisingly good. Thyrotoxicosis leads to diffuse muscle wasting and ultimately there is weakness (thyrotoxic myopathy). Many myopathic disorders give rise to wasting, and the pattern of wasting (proximal, distal, symmetrical, asymmetrical and selective, e.g. finger flexor muscles in the forearm in inclusion body myositis) helps diagnostically. Wasting is an important sign of peripheral nerve disease which affects motor nerve fibres. It is denervated muscle which wastes markedly, indicating motor nerve terminal or axon or nerve cell body loss. Focal motor nerve demyelination with conduction block but without denervation causes weakness, but there may be little or no wasting. In mononeuropathies, the wasting only affects muscles supplied by the affected nerve. Sometimes an ulnar neuropathy or median nerve lesion at the wrist or a common peroneal nerve lesion can be correctly diagnosed with reasonable confidence just by observing the pattern of wasting. In mononeuropathies, plexopathies and radiculopathies, wasted muscles will be weak. Motor and mixed motor and sensory polyneuropathies also cause wasting, most commonly distally and symmetrically. Disorders of motor nerve cell bodies lead to loss of associated axons and wasting. Thus, a range of pathologies of the spinal cord cause wasting, including processes which affect just motor nerve cell bodies, such as motor neuron disease, hereditary motor neuronopathies (spinal muscular atrophies) and poliomyelitis, and structural spinal cord disorders such as syringomyelia. Many elderly patients appear to have wasting of the small muscles of the hand, but if the strength is normal, there is probably actually no muscle wasting.

Fasciculations are spontaneous contractions of the muscle fibres of individual motor units within a muscle at rest, seen as twitches within a muscle. While widespread fasciculations are rather characteristic of amyotrophic lateral sclerosis, they are not always seen in that condition, and they may be seen in peripheral neuropathies and radiculopathies and in normal individuals who are not fully at rest. They may also be an isolated, benign abnormality. Fasciculations restricted to the calf muscles are common in normal individuals.

Pes cavus (Fig. 16.11) with clawing of the toes may be idiopathic or an indication of long-standing imbalance of muscle power in the feet (mainly weakness of intrinsic foot muscles), caused commonly by Charcot-Marie-Tooth disease but also by other hereditary or congenital disorders of peripheral nerve or spinal cord. Contractures of joints can be a consequence of muscle disease, peripheral neuropathy or CNS disease. Scoliosis is common in neurofibromatosis, but may be a complication of other neurological disorders such as syringomyelia and Friedreich's ataxia.

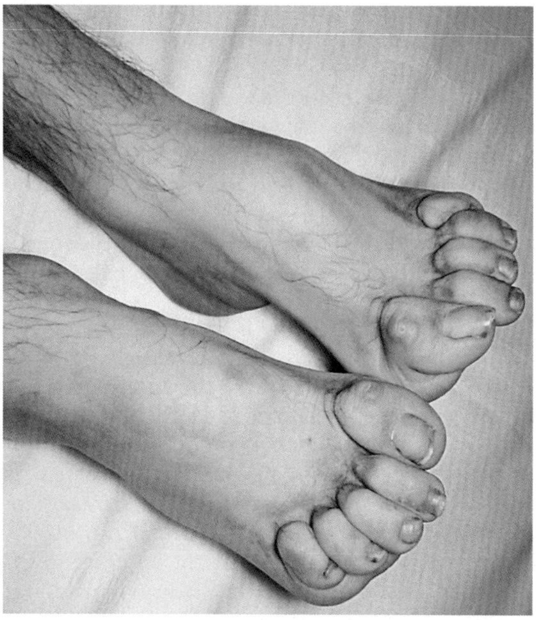

Figure 16.11 Pes cavus, with clawing of the toes in a patient with familial neuropathy. This patient had Refsum's disease and the peripheral nerves were slightly enlarged.

Assessment of muscle tone

Some people can relax their muscles extremely well, whereas others tense up during an examination, sometimes making for difficulty in assessing tone. Generally, in adult neurological practice, apparent hypotonia is not very diagnostically useful. The two common and important forms of pathological increase in muscle tone are spasticity, reflecting an upper motor neuron disorder (imprecisely designated 'pyramidal' because the corticospinal tracts constitute the medullary pyramids) and the 'extrapyramidal' rigidity of parkinsonism.

Spasticity

Spastic hypertonia in the upper limbs affects flexor muscles more than extensor muscles. This may give rise to a characteristic posture of the limb which is flexed at the elbow, wrist and fingers. There will be more resistance to passive extension of these joints than to passive flexion. The resistance increases in proportion to the speed of stretch of affected muscles until it suddenly reduces (so-called clasp-knife rigidity). Accordingly, detecting spasticity is best achieved by fairly fast and vigorous movements of the patient's limb to stretch relevant muscles. Hold the patient's elbow and hand and extend the elbow briskly, from a fully flexed to a fully extended position. Similar considerations apply at the wrist and fingers. A spastic arm will also have increased tone in pronator muscles. Brisk passive supination of the forearm will elicit clasp-knife rigidity felt as a 'pronator catch'.

In the leg, spasticity typically affects adductors and extensors more than flexors. With spinal cord lesions, the spasticity is often bilateral (a spastic paraparesis). Mild bilateral adductor spasticity can be detected with the patient lying supine on a couch or bed. Pick up one leg and abduct it. In doing so, adduction of the contralateral leg will be observed. Mild spasticity in quadriceps can be detected by asking the patient to relax. Then briskly flex his hip by lifting the leg behind the knee. In a normal limb, this will lead to flexion of the knee by gravity of the lower leg. The ankle will remain on the couch, being dragged proximally. If there is spasticity, however, the lower leg will be lifted off the bed briefly before falling back down. Spasticity at the ankle causes plantarflexion. Brisk passive dorsiflexion of the ankle, best done with the knee partially flexed, elicits the spasticity in the form of clonus – a succession of involuntary brief contractions of the calf muscles. Clonus may range from a few beats to sustained clonus in which there are repetitive calf muscle contractions until pressure on the sole of the foot is removed.

Parkinsonian extrapyramidal rigidity

Parkinsonian extrapyramidal rigidity takes two forms: either an increase in muscle tone affecting any movement of any muscle groups (so-called lead-pipe rigidity) or rigidity which is modified by tremor (so-called cogwheel rigidity, in which a high-frequency intermittency in the severity of the resistance to movement is felt). Mild parkinsonian rigidity is sometimes absent when the patient is relaxed but may be induced by getting the patient to use the arm contralateral to the arm being assessed (activated rigidity). Passive flexion and extension of the wrist or a rotatory movement of the hand at the wrist are good manoeuvres to pick up parkinsonian rigidity. Test first with the contralateral arm at rest. Then, if appropriate, test again, this time for activated rigidity, with the patient moving his opposite arm up and down with the fist clenched. In early Parkinson's disease (PD), rigidity will be detected in a limb or the limbs of one side and, although the signs remain asymmetric throughout, in advanced PD rigidity will affect all the limbs and the neck and trunk. Extrapyramidal neck rigidity affects movements of the neck in all directions. This contrasts with the neck stiffness of meningitis (see Chapter 9) in which neck flexion is stiff, restricted and painful, while rotation is relatively supple.

Paratonia (Gegenhalten)

This is seen in patients with fairly advanced dementia. Whichever way you attempt to move the patient's limb, he puts up active resistance.

Testing muscle power

This is a skill which requires considerable practice in order to learn how to encourage patients to cooperate fully and demonstrate the full amount of power they have at their disposal and to be able to make correct judgements about the presence of weakness. With few exceptions, isometric contraction (in which a muscle exerts a force but does not change in length) is tested by the examiner opposing the action of the patient's muscle(s). Clearly the average healthy young doctor will be stronger than a child or a frail elderly person but otherwise normal person, so judgement has to be applied. Conversely some patients will be stronger than the examiner. It is important to be thinking about the patterns of muscle weakness which are likely to be found in different kinds of disease processes and to look for and register the evolving pattern of weakness as you go along.

A common problem is non-organic weakness. This may reflect malingering or a conversion disorder, but sometimes just indicates that the patient is keen to impress on you that there is something the matter. In non-organic weakness, intermittency of effort is apparent, with variability of power produced from second to second, often with a prominent tendency abruptly to give way or withhold effort. In contrast, the muscle of a patient with organic weakness exerting as much force as he can will give in a smooth, continuous way, not a jerky, fluctuating way. Non-organic paralysis is often quite easy to diagnose because of inconsistencies in the patient's capabilities. For instance, a patient may walk into the consulting room normally, mount the examination couch unaided but be unable to lift a leg into the air because of apparent paralysis of hip flexion. The non-organic nature of unilateral hip extension weakness may be established by Hoover's sign. A patient appears to have paralysis of hip extension. Keep a hand under the affected leg and ask the patient to flex the opposite hip against the resistance of your other arm. In doing so, the patient will unwittingly activate the previously paralysed hip extensors.

Clinical methods of recording the severity of muscle weakness have considerable shortcomings, but in neurological practice it is desirable to chart muscle strength in order to document progression or recovery and to gauge the effectiveness of therapeutic interventions. The Medical Research Council scale is widely used (Box 16.3), but a problem with this scale is that the vast majority of muscle weakness one will encounter is grade 4. It also performs badly for fingers and toes where gravity has scarcely any influence, so that grades 1, 2 and 3 are more or less identical. Many clinicians find a scale of normal power, mild, moderate and severe weakness and paralysis is practical for everyday use. Accurate quantitative myometry ought to be a way forward but has hardly entered routine clinical practice.

There is not the space here to describe in detail the testing of all the important individual muscles and muscle groups. Tables 16.6 and 16.7 represent a summary of commonly tested muscles and their actions, but a number of specific points are important:

- There are two tests in which muscle strength is routinely tested isotonically (i.e. the muscle shortens while lifting a constant load) as opposed to isometrically. Abdominal trunk muscles are tested by asking the patient to sit up from lying flat with his arms folded on his chest. Standing up from a sitting position or rising from a crouched position are good tests of hip and knee extension and spine extension muscles and are useful in testing patients with myopathies. Normally these actions can be accomplished without use of the arms. Weak patients often have to resort to using their arms

Box 16.3 The Medical Research Council scale for grading muscle strength

- Grade 0: no contraction
- Grade 1: flicker or trace of contraction
- Grade 2: active movement with gravity eliminated
- Grade 3: active movement against gravity
- Grade 4: active movement against gravity and resistance
- Grade 5: normal power

Commonly Grade 4 is divided into 4–, 4 and 4+, denoting severe, moderate and mild weakness, and some use 5– to signify minimal weakness.

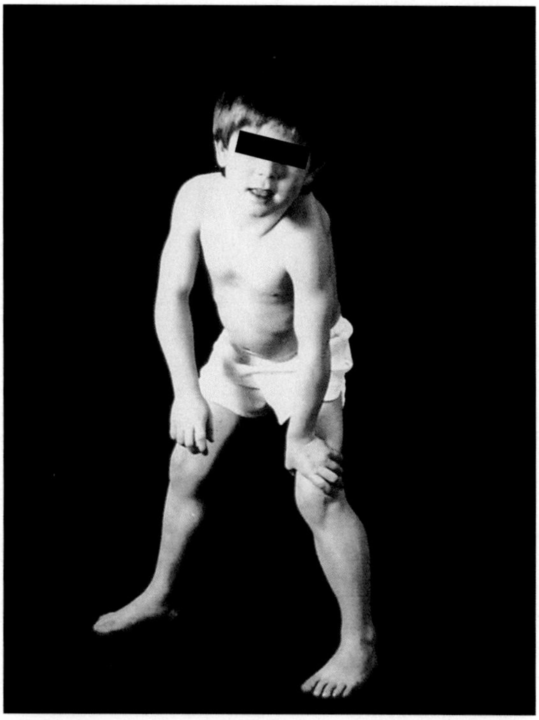

Figure 16.12 Duchenne muscular dystrophy (Xp21 dystrophy). There is pseudohypertrophy of the weak muscles (e.g. the calves and deltoids). The child is 'climbing up himself' with legs widely placed as he gets up from the sitting position to the standing position. This is Gowers' sign.

to push themselves up, either using surrounding furniture or, failing that, pushing themselves up with their arms on their own legs (Gowers' sign; Fig. 16.12).

- Testing neck flexion and extension is important in myopathies, in myasthenia gravis and in motor neuron disease.
- Deltoids, spinati, the pectoralis major muscles, hip abductors and hip adductors can be tested bilaterally simultaneously, but all other muscles must be tested in each limb separately.
- People sometimes test ulnar nerve-supplied small hand muscles by squeezing together the abducted index and small fingers (first dorsal interosseous and abductor digiti minimi muscles). It is better to test these two muscles individually.
- Mild weakness of calf muscles (gastrocnemii and soleus) is difficult to detect on a couch. A good technique is to get the patient to walk around on 'tiptoes'. The ankle sags in a leg affected by mild plantarflexion weakness.
- Rather than thinking solely about the myotomes supplying the relevant muscles, it is better simultaneously to be thinking, 'Is this the pattern of weakness one sees in upper motor neuron disorders (monoparesis, hemiparesis, paraparesis, tetraparesis); is this the weakness of a polyneuropathy (usually distal symmetrical weakness except in demyelinating polyneuropathies which give substantial proximal weakness as well); is the weakness best explained by a nerve root lesion or lesions; is the weakness best explained by a lesion of an individual nerve or by a number of nerves or by a plexus lesion; is the pattern of weakness due to a muscle disorder (often proximal symmetrical weakness)?'

Cerebellar system

The anatomy of the cerebellum is complex; it receives afferents of virtually every kind and its efferents connect to virtually every part of the brain and spinal cord. Important afferents include those from the motor cortex, visual cortex, vestibular nuclei and spinal cord. Vestibular afferents connect to the flocculonodular lobe. Lesions here cause disequilibrium and gait ataxia. Spinocerebellar tracts go mainly to the vermis, in the midline of the cerebellum. Lesions here cause truncal and gait ataxia. Each cerebellar hemisphere receives a major input from the contralateral cerebral cortex via pontine nuclei and the middle cerebellar peduncles. The major output from the cerebellum is via the superior cerebellar peduncles. Fibres from the cerebellar hemispheres cross to the contralateral red nucleus and thalamus, thence to spinal cord and basal ganglia and cerebral hemispheres. Thus, whereas cerebral cortex lesions affect contralateral limbs, cerebellar hemisphere lesions cause incoordination of ipsilateral limbs.

Incoordination, ataxia and tremor are the main effects of cerebellar lesions. Given the widespread afferent and efferent connections of the cerebellum, it is clear that lesions outside the cerebellum itself may have clinical manifestations which closely resemble those of cerebellar disease, and this needs to be borne in mind when examining patients. Thus, gait ataxia may be seen with cerebral, brainstem or spinal cord disorders, and tremor and ataxia can be manifestations of brainstem lesions.

Table 16.6 Muscles of the upper limbs which are commonly examined (P is patient; E is examiner)

Action	Muscle	Nerve, nerve roots	Method	Comment
Shoulder				
Abduction	Supraspinatus	Suprascapular, C5, C6	P attempts to abduct arms from chest; E resists	
External rotation	Infraspinatus	Suprascapular, C5, C6	P holds upper arms down, forearms forward and attempts to externally rotate upper arms; E resists	
Abduction, extension	Deltoid	Axillary, C5, C6	Arms abducted; E pushes down	
Adduction of arms with shoulder flexed	Pectoralis major	Pectoral nerves, C5, C6, C7, C8	P: arms stretched forward horizontal; P pushes fists together; E resists	
Lateral and forward movement and fixation of the scapula	Serratus anterior	Long thoracic, C5, C6, C7	P pushes arm forward against resistance	Serratus weakness causes winging of the scapula, noticed more with the arm forward* Trapezius weakness is the other major cause of scapula winging, noticed more with the arm abducted Instability of the shoulder caused by either is disabling
Elbow				
Flexion	Biceps	Musculocutaneous, C5, C6	E holds P's distal forearm and shoulder; P pulls; E resists	
Flexion	Brachioradialis	Radial, C5, C6	P flexes elbow with forearm midway between pronation and supination; E resists	The muscle is not the major flexor, but can be seen and palpated Weak, therefore less visible, with a radial nerve lesion Weak and wasted in certain dystrophies
Extension	Triceps	Radial, C6, C7	E holds P's distal forearm and shoulder; P pushes; E resists	
Wrist				
Extension, abduction	Extensor carpi radialis longus (ECRL)	Radial, C6, C7	P makes a fist and extends wrist against resistance	
Extension, adduction	Extensor carpi ulnaris (ECU)	Posterior interosseous, C7, C8	P makes a fist and extends wrist against resistance	If ECU is weak and ECRL is not, on wrist extension there is radial deviation (abduction) of the wrist
Flexion, abduction	Flexor carpi radialis (FCR)	Median, C6, C7	P flexes supinated wrist up against resistance, fingers relaxed	Adduction (ulnar deviation) occurs if FCR is weak and FCU is not
Flexion, adduction	Flexor carpi ulnaris (FCU)	Ulnar, C7, C8, T1	P flexes supinated wrist up against resistance, fingers relaxed	Abduction (radial deviation) occurs if FCU is weak and FCR is not
Fingers				
Extension	Extensor digitorum communis	Posterior interosseous, C7, C8	Hand prone, P extends fingers against resistance	

Continued

Table 16.6 Continued

Action	Muscle	Nerve, nerve roots	Method	Comment
Flexion	Flexor digitorum profundus (FDP)	F2, F3: anterior interosseous, C7, C8, T1 F4, F5: ulnar, C7, C8, T1	P has back of hand on a flat surface; E holds middle phalanx down; P flexes distal phalanx against resistance	Finger flexion is achieved by FDP and flexor digitorum superficialis The latter flexes the proximal interphalangeal (IP) joints and secondarily the metacarpophalangeal joints FDP flexes the distal IP joints, and secondarily the other two Testing grip (all flexors together) is useful, for instance in a patient with a hemiparesis Testing each component of FDP individually is useful in anterior interosseous and ulnar nerve lesions
Thumb abduction	Abductor pollicis brevis (APB)	Median, C8, T1	P has palm flat and sticks thumb up in the air and keeps it there while E attempts to push it towards the index finger	APB can be seen and palpated and its strength can be tested (abductor pollicis longus has a different action, being more of an extensor, so action of APB can reliably be assessed more or less in isolation)
Abduction of the index finger	First dorsal interosseous muscle (1st DIO)	Ulnar, C8, T1	P spreads fingers; E attempts to adduct P's index finger; P resists	1st DIO can be seen and palpated and its strength tested You can pit the strength of your 1st DIO against that of the patient
Abduction of fifth finger	Abductor digiti minimi	Ulnar, C8, T1	P spreads fingers; E attempts to adduct P's fifth finger; P resists	Usually not much added value over 1st DIO, except in a lesion of the deep palmar branch of ulnar nerve when ADM will be strong but 1st DIO weak

F2, index finger; F3, middle finger; F4, fourth finger; F5, fifth finger.

Table 16.7 Muscles of the lower limbs which are commonly examined (P is patient; E is examiner)

Action	Muscle	Nerve(s), nerve roots	Method	Comment
Hip				
Flexion	Iliopsoas	Lumbar plexus, femoral, L1, L2, L3	P flexes hip to 90° and flexes knee; E attempts to extend hip; P resists Can be done with P lying or sitting If sitting, stabilize P at shoulder	
Extension	Gluteus maximus	Inferior gluteal, L5, S1, S2	P lies on back; E attempts to lift the leg, lifting distal femur If P really tries, pelvis will lift off bed	Method described is quick, but to inspect or palpate the muscles, P needs to lie prone
Adduction	Adductor magnus, longus and brevis	Obturator, L2, L3, L4	P squeezes legs together; E tries to prise them apart	
Abduction	Gluteus medius, gluteus minimus	Superior gluteal L4, L5, S1	P tries to separate legs; E pushes them together	

Table 16.7 Continued

Action	Muscle	Nerve(s), nerve roots	Method	Comment
Knee				
Extension	Quadriceps femoris	Femoral, L2, L3, L4	P lying down, flexes knee to 90°; E puts left arm under knee; P extends knee (raises lower leg up into the air, not along the bed*); E resists with right hand Can also test knee extension with P sitting, legs dangling	*P could extend knee pushing heel down bed or couch against resistance even with very weak quads by using hip extension
Flexion	Hamstrings	Sciatic, L4, L5, S1, S2	P pulls heel towards bottom; E applies resistance, one hand behind ankle, the other at the front of the knee	If signs at the ankle and foot do not distinguish an L5 lesion from a common peroneal nerve lesion, look carefully for weakness here
Ankle				
Dorsiflexion	Tibialis anterior (TA)	Deep peroneal, L4, L5	P dorsiflexes ankle fully; E attempts to plantarflex (extend) ankle	Another way of testing ankle dorsiflexion is to get P to walk around on his heels
Inversion	Tibialis posterior (TP)	Tibial, L5, S1	P inverts foot against resistance Foot must be fully plantarflexed or otherwise TA contributes to inversion	Clear weakness of TP helps to distinguish an L5 radiculopathy from a common peroneal nerve lesion
Eversion	Peroneus longus and brevis	Superficial peroneal, L5, S1	P everts foot against resistance	
Plantarflexion	Medial and lateral gastrocnemius; soleus	Tibial, L5, S1, S2	P uses E's hand as an accelerator or clutch pedal; E resists	Mild weakness is best appreciated by having P walk around on tiptoes Muscle bulk on the two sides is best compared with P standing
Toes				
Big toe extension	Extensor hallucis longus	Deep peroneal, L5, S1	P extends great toe against resistance	This may be the only weakness detectable in a mild L5 radiculopathy
Extension of the other toes	Extensor digitorum longus and brevis (EDL and EDB)	Deep peroneal, L5, S1	P extends toes against resistance	EDB wastes in individuals with weak feet due to polyneuropathy but may remain bulky in those with myopathy
Flexion	Flexor digitorum longus; flexor hallucis longus	Tibial, L5, S1	P flexes toes against resistance	The long toe flexors flex the distal interphalangeal joints primarily Intrinsic foot muscles (plantar nerves) flex the toes at the metatarsophalangeal (MTP) joints Weakness of them leads to extension of the toes at the MTP joints and flexion more distally, seen in association with pes cavus*

*see Fig. 16.11

Examination of limb coordination

The finger-nose test

A mild cerebellar lesion gives rise to no limb signs at rest, but movements of affected limbs may be accompanied by action tremor. Actions are clumsy and inaccurate. Coordination of the arm is tested by the finger-nose test. Hold up an index finger in front of the patient. Ask him to touch it with the tip of his index finger, then with the same finger to touch his nose, and then ask him to carry on, touching alternately your finger and his nose. Some make the test a bit more difficult by moving the finger from place to place, but this adds little. More important is to make sure that the patient has to stretch a little to reach the finger, so that coordination is seen over the full range of movement of the arm. The observed action tremor is of fairly low tremor frequency, sometimes of quite large amplitude, and it becomes more marked in amplitude as the patient's finger approaches the target (his nose or your finger). This gives rise to the term 'intention tremor'.

In more severe cerebellar lesions, there will be postural as well as action tremor. In the extreme, the postural and action tremors are incapacitating. In such circumstances, the finger-nose test is inappropriate, being dangerous to the patient, whose finger might poke an eye or any other part of his face.

Dysdiadochokinesis

Ask the patient to tap his fingers rapidly on the back of his other hand. Then get him to repeat the test, this time turning the tapping hand so that the tapping is alternately done with the palmar and the dorsal sides of the fingers. Each tap should be on the same spot, not adjacent parts of the back of the hand.

Irregularity and clumsiness indicate an ipsilateral cerebellar hemisphere disturbance. Dysdiadochokinesis is not very specific; impairment is also seen in pyramidal and extrapyramidal disorders as well.

The heel-shin test

The heel-shin test assesses lower limb coordination. The patient lies on a couch or bed. Ask him first to lift one leg into the air, then to put the heel of that leg on to the shin of the other leg just below the knee and run the heel down the front of the shin on to the dorsum of the foot. Cerebellar dysfunction is revealed as tremor when the patient attempts to place his heel at the top of the shin and as an inability accurately to run the heel down the shin.

In testing cerebellar function, allowance has to be made for any weakness, particularly spastic weakness which by itself causes a certain amount of incoordination. Furthermore, it is essential to test proprioception, because proprioceptive loss can give rise to signs which look just like cerebellar incoordination (sensory ataxia).

Reflexes

The jaw jerk, tendon reflexes, abdominal reflexes and plantar reflexes comprise the major commonly tested reflexes.

The jaw jerk and tendon reflexes

The jaw jerk and tendon reflexes are monosynaptic stretch reflexes. Sudden stretching of a muscle by striking its tendon sends an impulse from muscle spindle afferents which synapse directly with motor neurons, leading to reflex contraction of that muscle. The reflexes provide information about both the motor system and the sensory system. Abnormally brisk reflexes contribute to the clinical picture of an upper motor neuron disorder. Absence of reflexes occurs in disorders of sensory afferents from muscle spindles in a wide range of sensory polyneuropathies, radiculopathies and mononeuropathies. Motor neuropathies and eventually myopathies may entail areflexia, but areflexia more commonly reflects a sensory rather than a motor system disorder. The other important cause of widespread areflexia, which can cause considerable confusion, is a spinal cord lesion which is extensive up and down the cord. In this situation, interruption of afferents to motor neurons in the anterior horns or damage to the motor neurons themselves prevent the reflexes from occurring. Examples include syringomyelia, extensive myelitis, spinal cord infarction and extensive intramedullary spinal cord tumours.

Pathologically brisk reflexes below a particular myotome level raise the possibility of a spinal cord lesion between the lowest normal reflex level and the highest abnormal reflex level. Remember that a focal spinal cord lesion will interrupt the pathway of any reflex at that level. Thus, the combination of loss of a reflex at a particular level and abnormally brisk reflexes subserved by levels below points strongly to a focal spinal cord lesion. One of the limitations of these analyses is the restricted number of reflexes that can be examined. The biceps reflex is at C5 or C6 level and there is no reflex that corresponds to C4 or higher except for the jaw jerk. If all the reflexes are pathologically brisk but the jaw jerk is not, there may be a high cervical spinal cord lesion. Normal upper-limb power and reflexes and a spastic paraparesis with pathologically brisk lower-limb reflexes may indicate a thoracic spinal cord lesion, but there are no tendon reflexes between C8 (finger reflexes) and adductor reflexes (L2 or L3) to localize the lesion more precisely. A pathologically brisk jaw jerk in a patient with a spastic tetraparesis points to the site of the causative pathology being in the cerebral hemispheres (e.g. diffuse small vessel cerebrovascular disease, amyotrophic lateral sclerosis or hydrocephalus) rather than in the cervical spinal cord.

Testing the jaw jerk

Ask the patient to let his jaw hang down in a relaxed manner with the mouth slightly open. Place your index finger across his chin. Strike it lightly with a tendon hammer; reflex contraction of both masseters is the response. Sometimes an extremely brisk jaw jerk is accompanied by clonus.

Testing the tendon reflexes

Eliciting tendon reflexes is not completely straightforward and requires practice. The aim is to ensure that the tendon of the relevant muscle being tested is briskly and effectively struck. Accordingly, sufficient force must be delivered. For the biceps reflex, place your own finger over the tendon and strike your finger. Similarly the brachioradialis reflex can be elicited by applying the tendon hammer to your own fingers positioned just above the wrist on the lateral aspect of the radius bone. The other standard reflexes (triceps, knee (quadriceps) and ankle (gastrocnemii and soleus)) involve directly striking the tendon with the tendon hammer. The standard tendon reflexes examined are summarized in Table 16.8.

The range of briskness of normal reflexes is very variable both between and within individuals, so it is important not to jump to conclusions about the presence of upper motor neuron lesions or polyneuropathies just on the basis of reflexes alone. Normal individuals who have absent reflexes tested in the standard way will usually have reflexes if they are brought out by reinforcement. To reinforce lower limb reflexes, ask the patient to put his hands together with the fingers interlocked. Then get ready to elicit the reflex, ask the patient to squeeze with his hands and then directly test the reflex. Upper limb reflexes can also be reinforced. Ask the patient to squeeze firmly something held in the hand contralateral to the limb in which the reflexes are to be tested (e.g. the barrel of a standard ophthalmoscope).

Abdominal reflexes

The stimulus is a light stroke of the abdominal skin using an orange stick. The normal response is contraction of abdominal wall muscles in the region where the stimulus is delivered, noted as movement of the umbilicus towards the region where the response is positive. The reflex is absent in spinal lesions above

Table 16.8 Frequently examined tendon reflexes

Reflex	Nerve	Nerve root(s)	Technique	Comment*
Biceps	Musculocutaneous	C5, C6	Elbow flexed 90°, arm relaxed Strike your finger or thumb located over the tendon	Reduced or absent in radiculopathy or focal cord pathology at C5–C6 cord level
Brachioradialis	Radial	C5, C6	Elbow flexed 90°, arm relaxed Strike your finger over the distal radius	Mainly of interest when it is inverted (see text)
Triceps	Radial	C6, C7	Elbow flexed 90°, arm relaxed Strike the tendon directly, just above the ulna at the back of the elbow	Reduced or absent in high radial nerve lesion, radiculopathy or focal cord pathology at C6–C7 level
Finger	Median and ulnar	C8	Have the patient's hand supine on a flat surface Put your index finger across the middle phalanges, which will be slightly flexed Strike your finger so as to abruptly stretch the finger flexors	Mainly of interest when abnormally brisk Hoffman's reflex is a variant
Adductor	Obturator	L2, L3	Separate the legs Apply fingers to medial thigh just above knee Strike fingers	Result is adduction of both legs when there is a spastic paraparesis Retained adductor reflex with absent knee reflex suggests a femoral neuropathy rather than plexopathy or radiculopathy
Knee	Femoral	L3, L4	Knee flexed 45-90°, supported and relaxed Strike the patellar tendon, just below the patella	Reduced in radiculopathy, lumbar plexopathy or femoral neuropathy
Ankle	Tibial branch of sciatic	S1	Patient externally rotates hip and flexes knee Hold the foot distally Strike the Achilles tendon	Absence may be the only sign other than restricted straight leg raising in S1 radiculopathy due to L5/S1 disc prolapse

*The remarks are made with reference to common abnormalities, not every possible one.

the level at which the reflex is being tested, and the reflexes are sometimes absent at a very early stage in multiple sclerosis. With symptoms or signs of a sensory level on the abdomen, the reflexes may be absent below the sensory level and retained above.

Testing the abdominal reflexes

The patient should be supine, relaxed, with the abdomen fully exposed. Start the stroke of the orange stick right round in the flank, drawing it to the midline. Test all four quadrants of the abdomen.

The plantar reflex

Except in neonates and infants, the normal response to uncomfortable or painful cutaneous stimulation of the sole of the foot includes plantarflexion of the toes. In addition there may be flexion withdrawal of the limb, comprised of dorsiflexion of the ankle and flexion of the knee and hip, which can be suppressed voluntarily. A remarkably reliable feature of an upper motor neuron lesion (anywhere in the spinal cord above L5 cord level or in the brain) affecting the leg being tested is the extensor plantar response (the Babinski reflex). The minimum extensor response is extension of the great toe only and it is the key feature to look for. In addition there may be fanning of the other toes and in the thigh contraction of tensor fascia lata. A marked response to plantar stimulation in a paralysed patient includes involuntary dorsiflexion of the ankle, flexion of the knee and flexion of the hip. If you are dealing with a patient who clearly has spasticity of the leg, a pyramidal distribution of weakness, pathologically brisk reflexes and ankle clonus, it hardly matters what the plantar response is. Occasionally, however, a patient has weakness without spasticity or hyperreflexia and the evidence that there is a CNS disorder hinges on the plantar reflex. Conversely, agitated individuals may have increased tone and very brisk reflexes but the flexor plantar reflex responses reassure one that there is no neurological problem.

A patient with lower motor neuron paralysis of toe extension cannot have a conventional extensor response regardless of the severity of any upper motor neuron disorder he may also have. A small number of malingerers learn to produce extensor responses.

Testing the plantar reflex

The ideal instrument to use is an orange stick (Fig. 16.13). Hold the patient's foot. Apply the orange stick to the sole of the foot on the lateral border just in front of the heel. Draw it forward towards the base of the fifth toe. This may suffice. Some continue round across the ball of the foot. It is best to press fairly firmly, warning the patient that this is not a pleasant test. Try to do the test effectively once or twice, not a large number of times. If you remain in doubt as to whether a response is extensor or not, then later, when testing pinprick sensation, test the dorsum of the toe in question. Involuntary extension of the toe towards the pin is an extensor response.

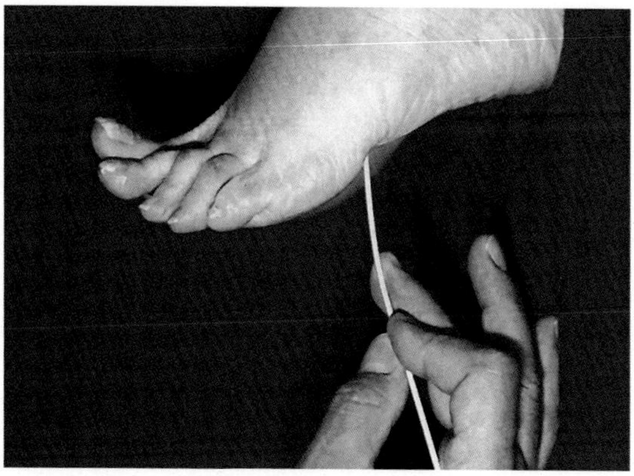

Figure 16.13 The plantar response. A firm, stroking stimulus to the outer edge of the sole of the foot evokes dorsiflexion (extension) of the large toe and fanning of the other toes.

Primitive reflexes

Certain reflexes found in neonates and infants can no longer be elicited once the cerebrum matures sufficiently, but in the setting of acquired disorders of one or both frontal lobes of the brain, they reappear and are useful as evidence of frontal lobe dysfunction.

The grasp reflex

Placement of the index and middle fingers into the palm of a normal adult will elicit no response, but a patient with a grasp reflex will, to a greater or lesser extent, grip the fingers. With a strong grasp reflex it will be possible to pull the arm or indeed the whole patient forward without having given any instruction to the patient. A unilateral grasp reflex indicates a contralateral frontal lobe lesion, for instance a tumour or a stroke. Bilateral grasp reflexes are usually due to diffuse disorders such as fronto-temporal lobar degenerations or advanced Alzheimer's disease, diffuse small vessel cerebrovascular disease or hydrocephalus. The sign is important when there is a paucity of other signs. An inert, mute individual could be depressed, but the presence of grasp reflexes would alert one to the likelihood of organic disease.

The pout reflex

A gentle tap on the lips of the patient causes reflex pouting of the lips. This also reflects bilateral frontal pathology. It can be elicited using the head of a tendon hammer held covered by a tissue for hygiene.

Movement disorders

This is a large field encompassing a whole range of abnormalities of posture, locomotor function and movement, with a spectrum from the very common to the distinctly rare. Both hypokinesia and hyperkinesia are abnormal, and the most common important disease in this sphere, Parkinson's disease, combines both, with akinesia, bradykinesia, dystonia, tremor and dyskinesia (the latter usually drug induced).

Tremor

Tremor by itself is a common reason for neurological referral. Tremor that has not hitherto been noticed by the patient or his doctors may contribute to neurological diagnosis. Getting a tremor diagnosis wrong is rarely serious, but giving patients incorrect diagnoses or prognoses is unsatisfactory and may lead to futile and inappropriate treatments or deprive a patient of worthwhile treatment.

The common tremor disorders include enhanced physiological tremor, essential tremor, parkinsonian tremor, dystonic tremor, cerebellar ('intention') tremor, drug-induced tremor and psychogenic tremor (Table 16.9). Combinations of tremor and myoclonus are seen in encephalopathies, mainly in hospitalized patients.

The classical tremor of Parkinson's disease (PD) is called a rest tremor (a slight contradiction in terms), and it is not always easy to diagnose. The patient's limb shakes when it is relaxed and doing nothing. Getting a patient into a position which allows his arms completely to relax in a chair may be difficult; beware you are not simply observing the postural tremor of a patient with essential tremor. In fact, you can quite often establish the presence of rest tremor as well from the history as from examination: 'When relaxed on a comfortable sofa watching television, does your arm start to shake?', 'Do any of your limbs shake when you are lying in bed?' Rest tremor may be observed in a relaxed patient sitting in a chair or lying on a couch. Furthermore, if a patient is walking and the fingers of one hand are shaking (and the arm is not swinging), it is likely to be the rest tremor of PD. PD tremor is seen most commonly in the fingers, wrist and forearm. It may also affect a foot. Classically, when a PD patient with upper limb rest tremor holds his hands out in front of him, his tremor stops for 10-20 seconds, whereafter a postural tremor may become evident. PD tremor is almost invariably asymmetric, starting in one limb and remaining more marked on that side throughout.

Essential tremor is not present at rest. It is noted with maintained postures and during movement. It mainly affects upper limbs. It is usually not markedly asymmetric. The action tremor may be examined during the finger-nose test and may also be assessed by tasks such as drawing a spiral or a wavy line between two straight lines or while writing, and these can be documented in case records. Jaw and lip tremor can be seen in PD and essential tremor patients.

Even with all the other aspects of examination at one's disposal (rigidity, bradykinesia/akinesia, posture, gait), distinguishing PD and essential tremor is

Table 16.9 Common forms of tremor

Tremor variety	Comment
Physiological	Normal
Enhanced physiological	Normal in a stressful enough situation A constitutionally anxious person may have this and psychogenic tremor
Thyrotoxicosis	Perhaps a variant of enhanced physiological tremor
Drug induced	The mechanisms here are various: some drugs may also cause ataxia, some parkinsonism, some polyneuropathy
Essential	Sporadic or familial Called benign, but severe cases are disabling Mainly upper limbs, but severe cases can affect legs too (see text)
Parkinsonism	Mainly idiopathic Parkinson's disease (see text), but sometimes parkinsonian tremor is seen in other forms of parkinsonism Wilson's disease must be excluded in young people with tremor
Dystonic	More jerky and irregular than essential tremor, particularly with jerks occurring in one direction Features of dystonia are also seen Often a neck tremor
Cerebellar	See text
In association with polyneuropathy	Some patients with Charcot-Marie-Tooth disease Some patients with chronic idiopathic demyelinating polyneuropathy
Psychogenic	Typically exaggerated in clinic Variable Settles when patient distracted from shaking Patient cannot maintain the same frequency of tremor when performing a repetitive task with the contralateral limb at a different frequency unless it is a harmonic

sometimes difficult. Where there is uncertainty, withholding judgement and reviewing after an interval is often helpful.

Parkinson's disease

The main motor features of PD are summarized in Box 16.4. Rigidity and tremor have been discussed above. Posture and gait are discussed below.

Impaired facial expression and generalized bradykinesia or akinesia are observations, but bradykinesia can also be tested formally; elements of the Unified Parkinson's Disease Rating Scale can be readily incorporated into routine clinical practice (see Box 16.5). Postural stability is tested by the pull test, done after testing gait.

Box 16.4 Cardinal motor features of Parkinson's disease

- Tremor
- Akinesia, bradykinesia
- Rigidity
- Abnormalities of posture
- Impairment of postural control and balance
- Abnormalities of gait
- Dysphonia, dysarthria, stammer

Box 16.5 Tests for bradykinesia in Parkinson's disease

1 Finger tapping:
 – ask the patient to tap repeatedly with his index finger on his thumb. The amplitude of each movement should be as large as possible and the speed should be as fast as possible. Test one side, then the other, not both together.

2 Hand movements:
 – ask the patient repeatedly to fully open his fist and fully close it, again with maximum amplitude and speed. Test one side, then the other, not both together.

In these two tests, in PD there is slowness and progressive reduction of amplitude of the movement, sometimes such that the movement ceases altogether. Asymmetry is the rule.

3 Pronation-supination movements of the arms:
 – ask the patient to hold both arms out, and repeatedly to pronate and supinate them, with maximum amplitude and speed. Test both arms together.

In this test, asymmetry with impaired amplitude on the more affected side is readily observed.

4 Leg agility:
 – ask the patient to stamp his heel rapidly and repeatedly on the ground, lifting his whole leg at least 3 inches (8 cm) each time. Test each leg separately.

The pull test

The patient stands with his feet side by side. Stand behind the patient with one foot slightly behind the other. Explain that, without warning, you are going to pull the patient abruptly backwards by his shoulders. The patient's task is not to fall over. He is allowed to step backwards in order to maintain his balance. Be prepared to catch the patient should he topple. A normal individual either remains upright even without moving his feet or does so by taking a single step backwards. 'Retropulsion' refers to the patient taking a number of small paces backwards, either succeeding or failing to reposition his centre of gravity; this is parkinsonian and abnormal. Some patients will simply fall backwards without taking any paces at all.

Other movement disorders (hyperkinetic movement disorders)

Generally hyperkinetic movement disorders are identified simply by history and by observation rather than any other component of examination. They are summarized in Table 16.10.

Sensation

The cell bodies of primary sensory neurons are in dorsal root ganglia and equivalent ganglia on cranial nerves (particularly the trigeminal ganglion). Their peripheral axons convey sensory information from sensory end organs in skin, muscle spindles and tendons and other tissues. Their central axons project into the spinal cord or brainstem. Large-diameter myelinated axons transmit proprioception, vibration and touch. Small diameter myelinated and unmyelinated axons transmit pain and temperature. The centrally projecting axons for proprioception and vibration sense enter the spinal cord and turn immediately to head rostrally in the posterior (dorsal) columns ipsilaterally, to synapse in the gracile and cuneate nuclei at the cervicomedullary junction. Axons from these nuclei cross in the medulla and proceed to the thalamus. In contrast, axons for pain and temperature, having entered the spinal cord, synapse in the dorsal horns. The axons of second-order sensory neurons cross over to the contralateral anteriorly (ventrally) situated spinothalamic tracts and run rostrally all the way to the thalamus. Touch sensation travels by both routes. Sensory pathways from the trigeminal sensory nuclei cross in the brainstem to project to the contralateral thalamus. From the thalamus, third-order neurons project via the posterior limb of the internal capsule to the primary sensory cortex in the parietal lobe, which is somatotopically organized (Fig. 16.14), akin to the primary motor cortex.

The anatomical separation of different modalities of sensation in the spinal cord accounts for dissociation

Table 16.10 Common kinds of movement disorders

Movement disorder	Characteristics
Parkinsonism	See text
Dystonia	Abnormal muscle contractions which may be sustained or repetitive, also involving co-contraction of antagonist muscles, leading to an abnormal posture, with or without jerks or tremor Associated pain and disability Can be focal, segmental, axial or generalized A wide range of causes In adults, idiopathic cervical dystonia is common
Chorea and athetosis (choreoathetosis)	Chorea denotes irregular, brief, jerky, unrepetitive, unintentional movements, affecting differing parts randomly (unilateral in hemichorea) In mild cases, the patient just looks fidgety Many causes including metabolic, drug induced, autoimmune, neurodegenerative Athetosis denotes slower, more writhing movements than chorea The two often coexist, particularly in levodopa-induced dyskinesia
Ballism	Not very common Usually hemiballism due to an ischaemic stroke affecting the subthalamic nucleus The movements are violent with flinging of the limbs
Myoclonus	Sudden shock-like jerks of limbs or trunk Can reflect cortical, brainstem or rarely spinal cord pathology or an encephalopathy Epileptic myoclonus is fairly common
Asterixis	Negative myoclonus. A sudden brief loss of tone. Particularly associated with hepatic encephalopathy
Tardive dyskinesia	A complication of dopamine antagonist neuroleptic medication Abnormal movements may affect any body part, but usually mainly affect the face, lips, jaw and tongue
Tic	Usually fairly small twitchy movements made semivoluntarily by a patient Preceding urge to make the movement, and brief relief having done so Often affect the face (blinks, grimaces, twitches of the nose), neck, shoulders An individual may have one or several different tics

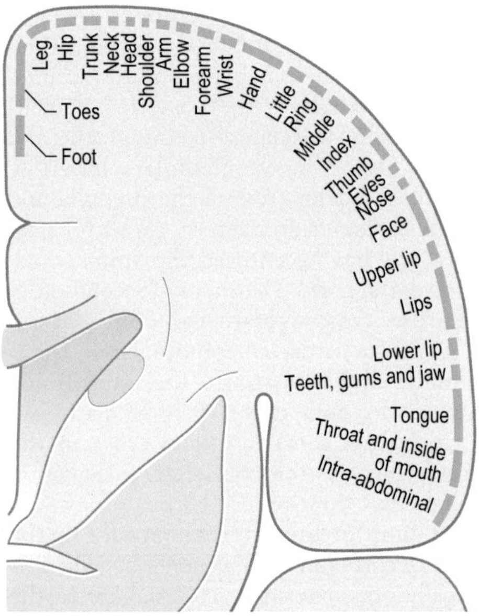

Figure 16.14 Somatotopic representation in the primary sensory cortex.

of sensory loss in spinal cord lesions which affect one side of the spinal cord or which affect either the anterior or posterior cord (see below).

With regard to the peripheral nervous system, cutaneous nerve fibres from dorsal root ganglia get to their end organs via spinal nerves, plexuses and peripheral nerves. A lesion of an individual peripheral nerve or a plexus lesion or a spinal nerve or nerve root lesion gives rise to loss of cutaneous sensation in a particular distribution which is diagnostically very helpful (see Figs 16.15 and 16.16 and Table 16.3). The cutaneous area supplied by a spinal nerve is called a dermatome. Loss of cutaneous sensation restricted to one dermatome indicates a spinal nerve or nerve root lesion. Loss of cutaneous sensation in all the dermatomes on both sides of the body below a particular level indicates a spinal cord lesion.

Cutaneous sensory examination

By the time sensation is examined, it may be apparent from the history and the clinical examination thus far what the diagnosis is and consequently what needs to be looked for during sensory testing. This is important because, in general, sensory testing needs to be goal directed; otherwise it tends to be fruitless

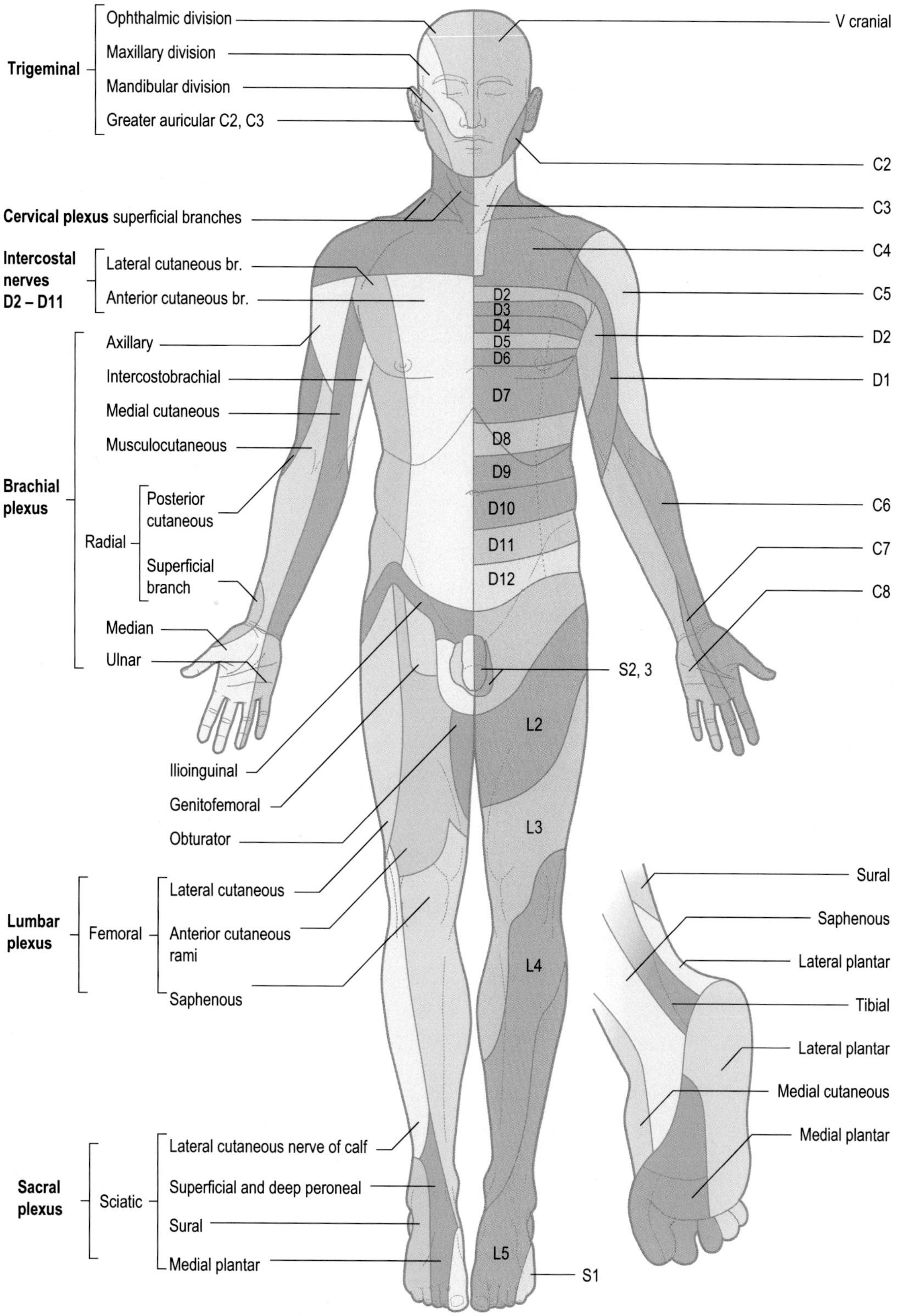

Figure 16.15 Anterior view to show the segmental innervation of the skin, i.e. the dermatomes (left) and the peripheral nerve supply (right).

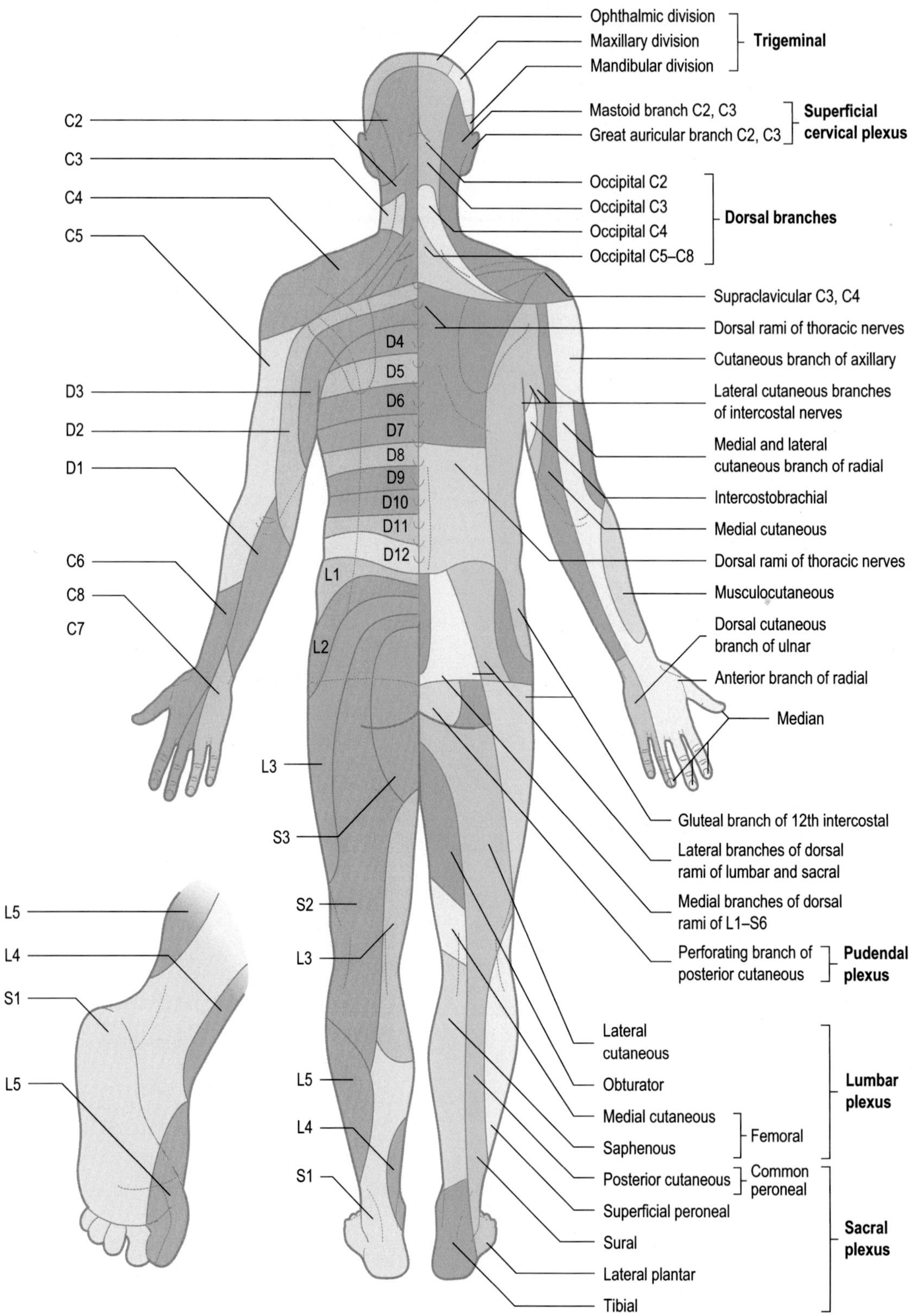

Figure 16.16 Posterior view to show the segmental innervation of the skin, i.e. the dermatomes (left) and the peripheral nerve supply (right).

or misleading. If a patient gives a very clear description of impaired sensation in the distribution of, for example, the ulnar nerve, diagnostically it makes little difference whether he can or cannot feel sharp pinpricks in the area of his symptoms. The symptoms still suggest an ulnar neuropathy either way. With very few exceptions (the corneal reflex would be one), all sensory tests are subjective – in other words the examiner relies on what the patient reports. Patients with no sensory symptoms may have signs suggesting impaired cutaneous sensation; in that situation, the examiner has to exercise judgement as to whether they are of significance.

Disorganized sensory testing tends to confuse both patient and examiner. With cutaneous sensory testing, the goal is to see whether any hypoaesthesia conforms to a meaningful pattern (see Table 16.13 and Figs 16.15 and 16.16). Defining an area of hypoaesthesia is almost invariably better achieved by starting testing within the area of hypoaesthesia and moving the stimulus out into areas where sensation is normally perceived.

One of the less satisfactory modalities of sensation to test is light touch. It is often done by dabbing the skin lightly with a piece of cotton wool, but there may be differences between touching the skin and stroking it. Tickle is a different modality; moving hairs on hairy skin is different again. In the context of spinal cord pathology, an abnormality of light touch sensation will not differentiate a posterior column lesion from one affecting the spinothalamic tracts. When testing light touch sensation, it can be helpful to ask the patient to close his eyes and then to report when he perceives the touches because some patients with anaesthesia will report that they feel touches when they see them being applied. Touch/pressure can be somewhat more rigorously assessed using a 10-gram monofilament to apply a standard quantity of pressure, and this can be useful as a screening test in situations where a patient is at risk of development of sensory peripheral neuropathy (e.g. diabetes).

Pinprick testing is more informative diagnostically and useful in mononeuropathies, polyneuropathies, radiculopathies and spinal cord lesions as well as brainstem and cerebral hemisphere lesions. It is, however, totally subjective. The patient reports whether the pinprick has a sharp, slightly painful quality or whether it is merely felt as a blunt touch. Testing can be done with the patient looking. In some clinical situations, it is worth testing pinprick sensation even when a patient has no sensory symptoms. A patient with a spastic monoparesis of one leg could have a brain or spinal cord lesion, but impaired pinprick sensation in the contralateral leg would strongly suggest a spinal cord lesion (Brown-Séquard lesion, see below). A patient with a slowly progressive spastic paraparesis or tetraparesis might have a neurodegenerative disorder, but the finding of a clear-cut sensory level on the trunk or neck would strongly suggest a structural spinal cord lesion.

Perception of heat and cold can be tested but in routine clinical practice adds little. A patient with impaired thermal sensation caused by a cerebral or spinal cord disorder will have impaired pinprick sensation in the same distribution. Impaired thermal sensation in patients with small fibre polyneuropathies is best assessed in a neurophysiology laboratory, but it does not contribute greatly to making the diagnosis.

Vibration sense

Patients do not complain of impaired vibration sense, but finding it on examination is a useful sign of either a polyneuropathy or a spinal cord lesion. Vibration sensation is conveyed in large-diameter sensory neurons, the central projections of which run in the posterior columns of the spinal cord.

Testing vibration sense

Set a low-frequency tuning fork vibrating noiselessly by striking it against the heel of your hand. Then apply the base of the tuning fork to bony parts of the limbs and ask the patient to report whether he feels the vibrations. Start distally and work proximally if necessary. In the upper limb, start on a distal phalanx. If the patient has absence of vibration sense there, then test the wrist and, if necessary, the elbow. In the lower limb, test the distal phalanx of the big toe and then the medial malleolus and top of the tibia, if necessary. If you suspect you are getting false-positive answers from the patient, ask him to close his eyes and then randomly apply the tuning fork either vibrating or not vibrating to his limb; the patient reports whether it is or is not vibrating.

Proprioception

Impaired proprioception occurs in large-fibre sensory (or sensory and motor) polyneuropathies, spinal cord lesions affecting the posterior columns and in lesions at higher levels including lesions of the sensory cortex. Proprioceptive loss is the basis of sensory ataxia. Patients with polyneuropathies which cause severe proprioceptive loss have gait and limb ataxia which looks very much like cerebellar ataxia. There are several clinical tests or signs which address proprioception: joint position sense (more strictly joint movement sense), pseudoathetosis and Romberg's test.

Testing joint position sense

Joint position testing does require the patient to look away or have his eyes closed. With the thumb and index finger of one hand, hold each side of the middle phalanx of the patient's middle finger. With your other hand, grasp the sides of the distal phalanx. Explain to the patient that he is to say which way his finger moves, that it will only go up or down and that the movements up or down will be random.

Move the distal phalanx either up or down through a small angle – the patient should be able to perceive as small a movement as you will be able to make. Make sure each movement is random, not just up, down, up, down, etc. If the patient fails to understand the test or to concentrate, do it first with him looking at the joint being tested. If joint position sense is impaired at the distal interphalangeal joint, move more proximally to the metacarpophalangeal joint and, if necessary, to the wrist or elbow, employing bigger angles of movement. The same applies in the foot and leg: start with the interphalangeal joint of the big toe and, if necessary, the ankle or knee. The normal threshold for perception of joint movement in the toe is larger than in the finger.

Pseudoathetosis

Patients with impaired joint position sense in their fingers may exhibit so-called pseudoathetosis: outstretched fingers drift up or down or to the side when the patient has his eyes closed. This is because, proprioception having failed, vision is the only means by which the patient knows where his fingers are and can keep them in one place (Fig. 16.17).

Romberg's test

Ask the patient to stand with his feet together side by side. Having established that his balance is satisfactory with his eyes open, ask him to close his eyes, having reassured him that nothing untoward will happen. If he loses balance with his eyes closed, the test is positive. You need to be prepared to catch the patient if he shows signs of toppling. Sometimes this kind of proprioceptive loss is evident in the clinical history – the patient comments on loss of balance in the dark or when he closes his eyes to wash his face.

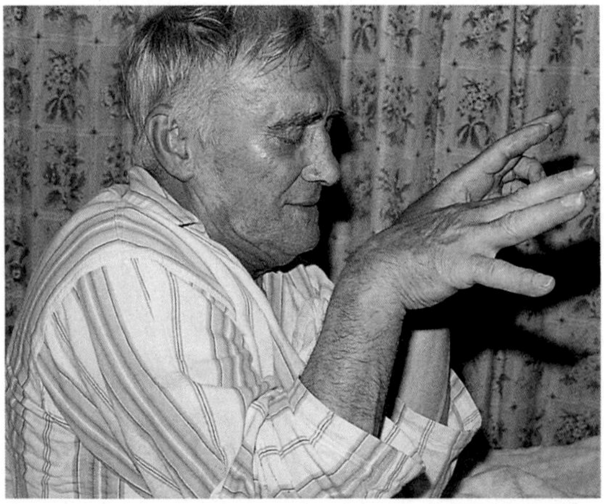

Figure 16.17 Paraneoplastic sensory neuropathy due to small cell carcinoma of the lung. With the eyes closed, the patient's outstretched arms become flexed and abnormal postures develop in the fingers.

Cortical sensory loss

Cerebral hemisphere lesions may disrupt sensory afferents or the primary sensory cortex in such a way as to give rise to very straightforward sensory loss affecting the usually tested modalities. In the same way that occipital lesions may give rise either to visual loss or to disorders of visual interpretation, parietal lesions can cause sensory impairment without anaesthesia. One such disorder is sensory inattention which is akin to visual inattention. A patient may feel sensory stimuli in limbs on the affected side, so does not have a hemianaesthesia, but sensory stimuli presented simultaneously on both sides are registered by the patient only on the normal side.

In tactile agnosia, a patient has no difficulty naming an item shown to him, but with his eyes closed and the item put into his hand, he is unable to work out by its size, consistency and texture what it is. Similarly a patient may be unable to distinguish different very familiar coins by feel alone. Dysgraphaesthesia is another form of cortical sensory impairment. Use an orange stick or a pen with the cap on. Write numbers on the patient's palm, clarifying with him which way up they are going to be. With eyes open, the patient will cope with 2, 3, 6, 1, etc. but will not recognize the numbers with his eyes closed.

Clearly it is only valid to test these sorts of cortical sensory impairments in patients who do not have a hemianaesthesia.

Testing sensory inattention

This is done with the patient's eyes closed. Randomly touch lightly his right or left hand (or foot) or both together, getting him to report each time whether he feels the touch on the right or left or on both sides. A patient who has right-left disorientation can still do this test, indicating which side or sides were touched by a finger movement. The lesion responsible for sensory inattention may be in the parietal cortex or in the subcortical white matter.

Stretch tests

In patients with pain radiating into a leg as a result of a painful compressive radiculopathy, usually due to intervertebral disc prolapse, stretching the sciatic or femoral nerve may worsen the pain or bring it on. Straight leg raising with the patient lying on his back (see also Chapter 15) stretches the sciatic nerve and therefore the nerve roots which form it, and the test is most commonly positive in L4/L5 and L5/S1 disc protrusions causing L5 and S1 root lesions, respectively. The femoral nerve stretch test is performed with the patient lying on his front. The knee is flexed fully on to the back of the thigh and the thigh is raised, extending the hip. Pain provoked in the anterior thigh points to a L2/L3 or L3/L4 disc lesion (L3 or L4 root lesion, respectively). As with so many other tests, stretch tests are not specific. They can be positive in patients with painful inflammatory or infiltrative polyradiculopathies and false positives are not uncommon in patients with a lot of back pain but no neurological disorder.

Posture and gait

In the outpatient setting, a patient's gait will inevitably be observed, although it may well be desirable to inspect it in some detail, perhaps by taking him out into a corridor. In hospitalized patients, it is easy to neglect to test gait if the patient is encountered in his bed. Mobility is so fundamental that gait must be considered and assessed in every appropriate patient and does not take long to do.

First, simply observe the patient standing. Look for abnormalities of posture. Established PD gives a kyphotic posture (Fig. 16.18). Neck extension weakness causes forward flexion of the neck; in extreme cases, a state of drop head is apparent. Axial dystonia may be observed. Muscular dystrophy may be associated with hyperlordosis. Check the patient's balance and do Romberg's test (see above). Then ask the patient to walk a short distance, turn round and walk back again. Mild gait ataxia can be brought out by getting the patient to walk heel to toe. If relevant, test for retropulsion (the pull test; see p. 338).

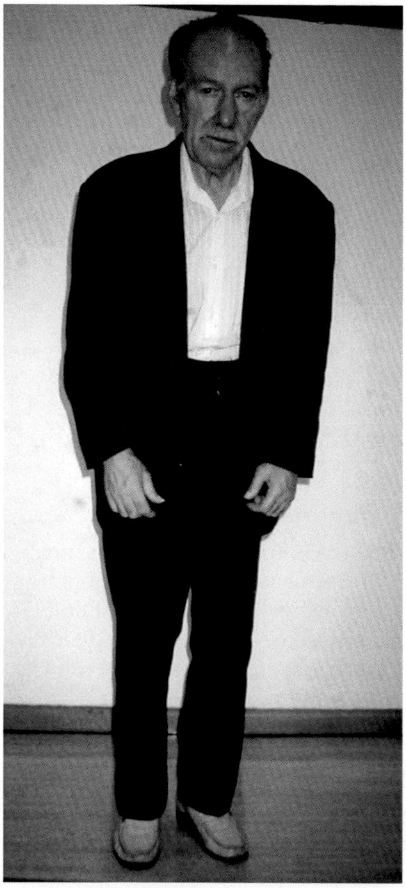

Figure 16.18 Parkinson's disease, showing the typical rigid, flexed posture involving the trunk and limbs. The face is impassive.

Table 16.11 provides a summary of important kinds of neurological gait disorders. Sometimes it can be difficult to be certain that a patient with a frontal gait disorder does not also have PD. Patients with severe osteoarthritis of the hips sometimes have a gait disorder which looks deceptively like a myopathic gait. Finally, as in other domains, a functional gait disorder does not necessarily mean that there is no organic disease.

Patterns of motor and sensory signs

Formulating the nature of the neurological problem and its localization on the basis of the signs requires a combination of basic anatomical knowledge and pattern recognition. It is important to be able to recognize the limitations of information the physical signs convey in terms of localization. A patient with gait ataxia and extensor plantar reflexes and no other signs could have a lesion in the thoracic or cervical spinal cord or in the cerebellum with early brainstem compression, or it could be a diffuse cerebral process such as small vessel cerebrovascular disease or hydrocephalus. It may also be that two different lesions account for the two manifestations. Conversely, dysfunction affecting several different systems does not necessarily imply a multifocal disorder: diplopia, nystagmus, dysarthria, ataxia, upper motor neuron signs in the limbs, widespread sensory loss and impairment of bladder control might be caused by multiple sclerosis, but a single brainstem lesion could equally account for all of the symptoms and signs.

In the following section, patterns of motor signs and patterns of sensory signs are outlined separately – and, of course, the examiner encounters them sequentially, but for many syndromes it is the characteristic combination of motor and sensory features that allows accurate diagnosis.

Patterns of motor signs

Diagnosing lesions of individual motor or motor and sensory peripheral nerves requires knowledge of which muscles are supplied by which nerve; the same considerations apply to nerve root lesions. Plexus lesions can be difficult, particularly if patchy and multifocal, but can sometimes be diagnosed confidently on clinical grounds simply from the anatomy. For example, a patient with a combination of what appears to be a radial nerve lesion and an axillary nerve lesion will have a lesion affecting the posterior cord of the brachial plexus.

Distal symmetrical weakness in the limbs would be typical for a generalized motor polyneuropathy. The same pattern can be seen in distal myopathies and some spinal muscular atrophies (hereditary motor neuronopathies), neither being common.

Table 16.11 Common gait disorders

Gait	Characteristics
Myopathic (proximal, symmetrical myopathy)	Hyperlordosis (axial and pelvic muscle weakness) Waddling gait (weak gluteus medius muscles, among others, bilaterally)
High stepping or 'steppage'	A consequence of foot drop (unilateral or bilateral) – common peroneal nerve lesion, motor polyneuropathy, e.g. Charcot-Marie-Tooth disease, distal myopathy The leg has to be lifted abnormally high to make a step With mild ankle dorsiflexion weakness, the foot slaps onto the ground as weight is transferred on to the heel
Ataxic	Midline cerebellar lesion (cerebellar vermis): wide-based unsteady gait with irregular sized paces and potential to topple in any direction; there may be little or no limb incoordination Cerebellar hemisphere lesion: the patient veers towards the side of the lesion; there is ipsilateral limb incoordination Sensory ataxia: there may be limb and gait incoordination
Hemiparetic	The spastic arm is held adducted at the shoulder with the elbow flexed and the forearm in front of the chest with flexion at the wrist and fingers Swinging of the affected arm is reduced The spastic leg is stiff with impaired knee flexion and ankle dorsiflexion, with abduction of the leg to bring the plantarflexed foot round and forward when taking a step (circumduction)
Spastic (paraparesis; tetraparesis)	Bilateral spastic legs Bilateral circumduction, such that the leading leg may end up adducted in front of the trailing leg – hence a 'scissor gait'
Parkinsonian	Kyphotic posture Start hesitation Initially small paces, which may get bigger Acceleration of rate of steps once walking initiated ('festinant gait') Reduced or absent arm swing unilaterally or bilaterally May suddenly get stuck, e.g. in a doorway Increased number of paces to turn round Improvement of gait with visual cues on the ground
Frontal gait disorder This term has a number of mainly less satisfactory synonyms, including gait apraxia, lower body parkinsonism, atherosclerotic or vascular parkinsonism, marche à petits pas	Gait ignition failure Start hesitation Small paces (but no acceleration) Unsteadiness Improvement of gait with visual cues on the ground Prominent swinging of the arms Ability to use the legs to make cycling movements on a bed or in a chair, yet inability to use legs to walk

Demyelinating polyneuropathies (Guillain-Barré syndrome (GBS) being the most important) give rise to proximal as well as distal weakness, short nerves being as susceptible to conduction block as long ones. Hence, the presentation of GBS may be with exclusively 'proximal' and life-threatening weakness of muscles of swallowing and breathing.

Mainly proximal, symmetrical limb weakness should prompt consideration of myopathy, particularly polymyositis and dermatomyositis, and muscle disease secondary to metabolic or drug-induced disorders such as steroid myopathy, thyrotoxic myopathy and osteomalacic myopathy. Test getting out of a chair or rising from a crouch. The different muscular dystrophies tend to have particular patterns of muscle involvement which may help diagnostically.

Patients who have weakness and no sensory symptoms or signs and no upper motor neuron signs usually have muscle disorders or neuromuscular junction disorders (such as myasthenia gravis (MG), Lambert Eaton myasthenic syndrome or botulism). Typically, MG affects the eyelids, eye muscles, face, jaw, muscles of swallowing and breathing and axial and proximal limb muscles, but atypical cases occur.

Upper motor neuron disorders affecting the leg

The lesion may be in the spinal cord or brain. Weakness affects the flexor muscles more than extensor muscles; hence the abnormal findings are of weakness in hip flexion (iliopsoas), knee flexion (hamstrings) and ankle dorsiflexion (tibialis anterior). Spasticity usually predominates in the hip adductors and the extensor muscles of the leg and foot (gluteus maximus, quadriceps and calf muscles). These circumstances account for the characteristics of the hemiparetic and paraparetic gait (see Table 16.11).

Upper motor neuron disorders affecting the arm and hand

Here the typical pattern is almost the opposite of that in the leg: weakness mainly affects deltoid and the extensors of the arm and hand – elbow extension (triceps), wrist extensors and finger extensors. Spasticity is mainly in the flexors (biceps and brachialis, wrist flexors and finger flexors) and in forearm pronators. Thus, the typical posture of the arm in an ambulant patient with a hemiparesis is adduction at the shoulder, flexion at the elbow, pronation of the forearm and flexion of the wrist and fingers.

The distribution of weakness in upper motor neuron lesions of the limbs is often referred to as 'pyramidal', a useful but not completely accurate term. Table 16.12 summarizes where in the CNS lesions need to be to produce the various categories of upper motor neuron lesions.

Patterns of sensory loss (Table 16.13)

The diagnosis of lesions of individual sensory peripheral nerves or the sensory component of mixed nerves requires knowledge of anatomy, in this case the area of cutaneous sensation mediated by the nerve in question (see Table 16.13 and Figs 16.15 and 16.16). In lesions affecting mixed nerves, sensory symptoms with or without signs commonly precede motor symptoms and signs. Thus, a clear description by a patient of sensory loss in ulnar nerve distribution provides compelling evidence for an ulnar neuropathy even if there are no signs. The right combination of motor and sensory signs allows the diagnosis of a mononeuropathy to be made. Nerve conduction studies and electromyography may contribute to the assessment of the nature of the lesion (precise location, extent of conduction block, extent of axonal damage, subclinical involvement of other nerves, presence of an underlying subclinical polyneuropathy) but are not necessary for making the diagnosis if there are clear-cut signs.

Familiarity with the areas of cutaneous sensation mediated by nerve roots (dermatomes – see Figs 16.15 and 16.16) is important for two reasons. First, it enables lesions of individual nerve roots to be diagnosed. Second, the level of a spinal cord lesion can be ascertained to some extent (see below).

Distal cutaneous sensory loss (touch, pinprick) in all four limbs, often in a 'glove and stocking' distribution, usually indicates a sensory polyneuropathy. Vibration sense and joint position sense may also be affected, and loss of reflexes, particularly the ankle reflexes, provides strong clinical support for a diagnosis of sensory polyneuropathy. Cervical spinal cord lesions sometimes produce quite widespread sensory symptoms in both

Table 16.12 Localization of upper motor neuron lesions

Pattern of weakness	Site of lesion
Spastic monoparesis	Cerebral hemisphere Arm (and face) – MCA territory Leg – ACA territory Brown-Séquard syndrome in thoracic cord gives a monoparesis of the ipsilateral leg
Spastic paraparesis	Thoracic spinal cord lesion (i.e. above lumbar cord, but below cervical cord) A parasagittal meningioma in the falx between the cerebral hemispheres affecting the motor cortex for the leg bilaterally is a much quoted but rare cause of a paraparesis
Spastic hemiparesis	A large hemisphere lesion, e.g. MCA territory stroke, but the arm will be worse affected than the leg A lesion of the internal capsule (Pure motor hemiplegia is a lacunar syndrome) A brainstem lesion affecting the corticospinal tract on one side Brown-Séquard syndrome in the high cervical spinal cord
Spastic tetraparesis	High cervical spinal cord lesion, e.g. C3/C4 disc Diffuse bilateral cerebral hemisphere disease affecting motor pathways bilaterally, e.g. small vessel cerebrovascular disease Hydrocephalus Brainstem disease affecting the corticospinal tracts bilaterally, e.g. basilar artery territory stroke (which causes locked-in syndrome)
'Cortical hand'	A small lesion in the primary motor cortex subserving the hand Weakness and difficulty using the hand but little or no spasticity
'Cortical foot'	A small lesion in the primary motor cortex subserving the foot Weakness and difficulty using the foot but little or no spasticity

ACA, anterior cerebral artery; MCA, middle cerebral artery.

Table 16.13 Patterns of sensory loss

Clinical sensory findings	Site of lesion
Hemianaesthesia (all modalities) Incomplete, e.g. face and arm Complete	Parietal cortex or subcortical white matter (corona radiata) Thalamus or internal capsule Pure sensory stroke is a lacunar syndrome
Crossed sensory deficit: loss of cutaneous sensation on one side of the face and loss of spinothalamic tract-mediated sensation on the other side of the body	Lateral medullary syndrome: lesion of spinal tract and nucleus of trigeminal ipsilateral to the facial sensory loss, and of crossed spinothalamic tract
Cape or half-cape distribution of dissociated suspended sensory loss (spinothalamic, with an upper and a lower level) with preserved proprioception and vibration sense	Central cord lesion: syringomyelia (and syringobulbia if there is no upper level but the sensory loss affects the face)
Loss of all modalities below a dermatomal level on legs (rare), trunk or neck	Transverse spinal cord lesion affecting posterior columns and spinothalamic tracts Cord compression by tumour, cord trauma, severe myelitis
As above but with sacral sparing of cutaneous sensory loss	A severe intramedullary spinal cord lesion, e.g. tumour, bleed, but with sparing of the outermost spinothalamic fibres which come from sacral dermatomes
Brown-Séquard syndrome: loss of spinothalamic sensation on one side, with a level, and loss of vibration and proprioception in affected limbs on the other side	Hemisection of the spinal cord: involvement of the posterior columns (uncrossed) and spinothalamic tract (crossed) on one side The lesion is on the side with the proprioceptive loss Cord compression (tumour, disc), myelitis (e.g. multiple sclerosis), cord trauma
Anterior spinal artery syndrome	Infarction affecting the anterior (ventral) thoracic spinal cord Involvement of spinothalamic tracts bilaterally Posterior columns spared If the infarction extends down to the lumbar spinal cord, the lower limb reflexes are lost Otherwise they become brisk because of the paraplegia caused by bilateral corticospinal tract involvement
Radicular distribution of cutaneous sensory loss	Radiculopathy One of the clinical problems is that the distribution for nerve roots and individual peripheral nerves can be similar, e.g. C5 and axillary nerve, L4 and saphenous, L5 and common peroneal
Extensive sensory loss in one limb, not accounted for by a nerve root or a peripheral nerve	Consider a plexopathy (brachial or lumbar) The motor features are likely to predominate
Sensory loss in the distribution of individual sensory or sensory and motor nerves	Mononeuropathy Entrapment neuropathies of mixed nerves may present with sensory features only, or with motor and sensory features, which makes clinical diagnosis easier For some nerves, you have to rely solely on clinical acumen – the nerve is not amenable to neurophysiological investigation, e.g. lateral cutaneous nerve of the thigh
Distal sensory loss in limbs	Polyneuropathy – classically 'glove and stocking' but may be much less marked (toes only) or much more marked, only sparing the back close to the spine Multifocal polyneuropathies have features of a multiplicity of mononeuropathies

hands which might make one think of peripheral nerve pathology, but the motor signs in the legs and possibly autonomic manifestations (sexual dysfunction, impaired bladder and bowel control) ought to clarify the situation. However, rarely, cervical spinal cord lesions can also give rise to distal lower limb sensory symptoms which can be misleading.

Spinal cord and cauda equina lesions

The characteristic sensory disturbance associated with compression of the cauda equina or spinal cord is one of loss of all modalities of sensation below the level of the compression. If the compression is of the cauda equina (e.g. a big central posterior intervertebral disc prolapse), all nerve roots below and possibly at the level of the lesion will be affected, including the buttocks and perineum. A severe spinal cord lesion (often compression, but any process which functionally transects the cord at one site) will result in a sensory level on the trunk (abdomen and back, or chest, including the arms if the lesion is between C5 and T1 spinal cord level) or on the neck. Knowledge of the anatomy of the dermatomes allows the spinal cord level (not the same as the spinal column level) to be determined. In spinal cord lesions of mild to moderate severity, the sensory level (which is less dense than in severe lesions) is some distance below the spinal cord level of the lesion. As the lesion evolves, the patient develops progressively worse sensory symptoms, first perceived at a level well below that of the lesion but which then extend up towards the level of the lesion. This process may not have been completed at the time the patient is evaluated and can sometimes lead to the wrong part of the spinal cord being imaged.

Brown-Séquard syndrome

Brown-Séquard syndrome refers to the signs resulting from a focal lesion affecting the right or left half of the spinal cord, such as an intramedullary inflammatory or an extramedullary compressive lesion. Disruption of the descending corticospinal tract on the affected side results in an ipsilateral upper motor neuron disorder below the level of the lesion (commonly in one leg but a high cervical lesion would affect the arm as well). Involvement of the posterior columns on the affected side results in ipsilateral loss of vibration sense and joint position sense in the leg or arm and leg below the lesion. The spinothalamic tracts on the side of the lesion are affected, but sensory input into the spinothalamic tracts comes from pain and temperature afferents on the opposite side which cross over on entering the spinal cord, so loss of pinprick and temperature sensation occurs below the level of the lesion on the opposite side (Fig. 16.19). Some patients with mild lesions comment that while it is one leg which drags and feels weak and stiff, it is the other leg which has impaired sensation.

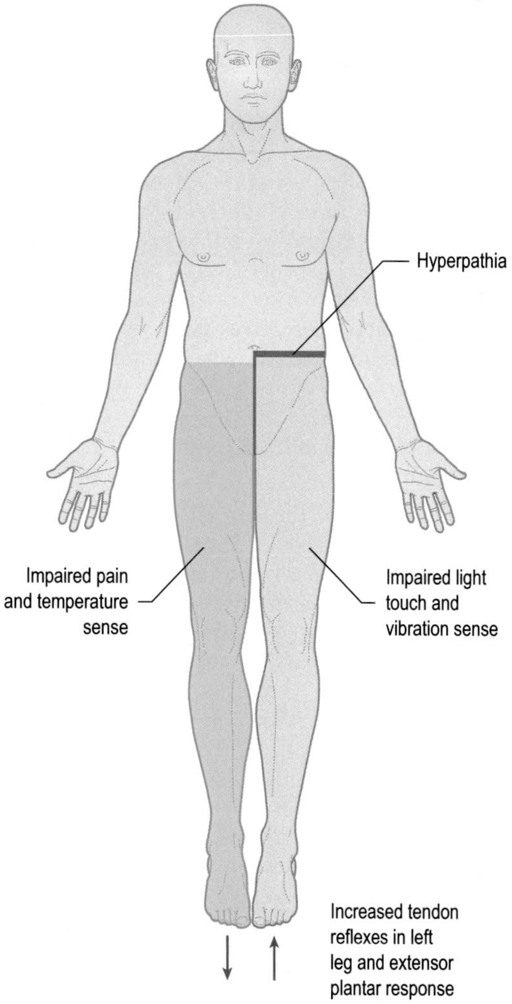

Figure 16.19 Brown-Séquard syndrome. Note the distribution of corticospinal, posterior column and lateral spinothalamic tract signs. The cord lesion is on the left side.

Central spinal cord lesion (especially syringomyelia)

A syrinx is a pathological tube-shaped cavity in the spinal cord, usually cervical and extending down into the thoracic area. It expands the spinal cord, but ascending and descending long tracts are unimpaired except in extreme cases. Anterior horn cells are damaged, leading to the motor manifestations of wasting and weakness of muscles in the arms and hands. Tendon reflex pathways are affected leading to upper limb reflex loss. There may be abnormalities of autonomic control of blood vessels and sweating in affected limbs. Most remarkable, however, are the patterns of sensory impairment. The classical findings are described by two adjectives: the sensory loss is *dissociated*; and a sensory level is found which is *suspended*. Dissociated sensory loss denotes loss of pain and temperature sensation with preservation of vibration and proprioception. The central cord lesion interrupts the sensory afferents which cross the middle of the spinal cord from dorsal roots on one side to spinothalamic tracts on the other side. Sensory afferents proceeding directly from dorsal roots into posterior columns are unaffected. Spinothalamic afferents which have already crossed below the lower limit of the lesion are also unaffected. This dictates that the loss of pinprick sensation will have an upper level corresponding approximately to the top of the syrinx, but there will also be a lower level, usually on the trunk, so the sensory loss is suspended by comparison with the situation in lesions affecting the spinothalamic tracts themselves (such as complete transverse cord lesions, the Brown-Séquard lesion or anterior spinal artery territory spinal cord infarction).

Anterior spinal artery territory spinal cord infarction

A major component of the arterial supply to much of the cord, particularly the thoracic spinal cord, comes from the anterior spinal artery, which receives its main blood supply via the artery of Adamkiewicz from the thoracic aorta. Spinal cord infarction is uncommon; when it occurs, it is usually the thoracic cord which is affected. Occlusion of the artery of Adamkiewicz may be atherosclerotic, arteritic or consequent upon dissection of the aorta. The result is infarction of the anterior (ventral) half of the spinal cord over a variable length. The corticospinal tracts are involved bilaterally, resulting in abrupt-onset paraplegia. The major autonomic manifestations are loss of bladder and bowel control. The spinothalamic tracts are affected on both sides of the cord. Thus, there is dense loss of pinprick sensation with a sensory level on the trunk. The striking feature, in a numb paraplegic individual, is preservation of sensation mediated by the posterior columns – intact vibration and joint position sense in the toes and feet.

Patterns of sensory loss in lesions of the medulla

In the midbrain, pons and medulla, so many nuclei and nerve tracts are found in such restricted anatomical confines that inevitably the clinical manifestations resulting from small lesions in different parts vary substantially. Considering sensation in isolation, a lesion of the lateral medulla on one side may affect the spinothalamic tract on that side conveying pain sensation from the contralateral side of the body and, at the same time, affect the spinal tract and nucleus of the trigeminal nerve, which mediates pain on the ipsilateral side of the face.

Hemianaesthesia

A lesion affecting the sensory afferent pathways rostral to the principal sensory nucleus of the trigeminal nerve in the pons (i.e. in the midbrain, diencephalon, thalamus or internal capsule) will result in a hemianaesthesia: loss of sensation on the whole of one side of the body including the head and face. A large lesion, such as a middle cerebral artery territory ischaemic stroke affecting the whole of the primary sensory cortex, will have the same effect. Smaller lesions in sensory cortex will affect sensation (all modalities) in only part of one side of the body.

Cognitive function

There is a risk in neurological examination that cognition may be neglected. It is a useful simplification to divide domains of cognition into those which are distributed and those which are localized. The anatomical substrates of distributed cognitive functions are bilateral and widespread in the brain. An implication is that a single focal neurological lesion will have little perceptible impact on that function. In contrast, a focal lesion in a particular place will have a major effect on a localized cognitive function.

The two major syndromes of cognitive impairment, which may be accompanied by no neurological signs, are dementia and delirium. They are covered in Chapter 7. In this section, emphasis is placed on cognitive deficits which, to some extent, have localizing value and which may be seen in patients with focal cerebral lesions as well as those with more generalized neurodegenerative disorders.

Amnesia

Memory is a distributed cognitive function. Dense amnesia requires bilateral hemisphere lesions, but those lesions may be very focal – bilateral thalamic infarction or damage to the mamillothalamic tracts in Wernicke's encephalopathy can cause devastating amnesia – and the anatomy of memory in each hemisphere is localized and well defined. Furthermore, unilateral lesions, such as a posterior cerebral artery occlusion causing temporal lobe infarction, do have discernible effects on memory. Normal episodic memory (memory of events which have been personally experienced) depends on integrity of the hippocampi and entorhinal cortex in the temporal lobes, the fornices, the thalami and the mamillary bodies. Anterior temporal lobes subserve semantic memory (memory for facts, learning and general knowledge). Verbal memory is dependent on the left temporal lobe, visual memory on the right temporal lobe. Some important causes of amnesia are listed in Table 16.14. Amnesia emerges mainly from the history taken from an informant rather than from the patient. Episodic memory may be assessed by testing recall of a name and address that the patient has registered and by testing the patient's recall of events from his past, both recent and distant.

Dysphasia

Dysphasia or aphasia is an acquired disorder of language function. The auditory processing of language involves the superior temporal gyri bilaterally. The

Table 16.14 Some causes of amnesia

Cause	Comment
Acute	
Transient global amnesia	The name describes well what happens; the pathology remains obscure; imaging indicates a hippocampal process
Transient epileptic amnesia	Here amnesia is the seizure
Epilepsy more generally	Temporal lobe seizures may involve amnesia; postictal amnesia follows any generalized convulsion
Closed head injury	Concussion involves retrograde and anterograde post-traumatic amnesia
Drugs: benzodiazepines, alcohol	Amnesia can occur without significant impairment of alertness
Chronic	
Hippocampal damage	
Herpes simplex encephalitis	Bilateral temporal lobe damage
Limbic encephalitis	Bilateral temporal lobe damage
Cerebral anoxia	
Temporal lobectomy with a lesion in the other temporal lobe	Should not happen in modern practice because of improvements in preoperative assessment
Bilateral posterior cerebral artery territory infarction	
Closed head injury	Bilateral temporal lobe damage is common
Early Alzheimer's disease	Later there are other prominent cognitive deficits as well
Diencephalic damage	
Korsakoff's syndrome	This is what results from untreated Wernicke's encephalopathy, due to thiamine deficiency
Third ventricular tumours and cysts	Potentially affecting the fornices and thalami bilaterally
Bilateral thalamic infarction	Either two separate events or, if the bilateral paramedian thalamosubthalamic arteries of Percheron branch from one common vessel (a not uncommon variant), one stroke
Subarachnoid haemorrhage from anterior communicating artery aneurysm	

The list on the left is adapted from John R. Hodges 1994 Cognitive Assessment for Clinicians, Oxford University Press.

meaning of words requires the dominant temporal lobe. The planning of speech production occurs in the dominant frontal lobe (including Broca's area in the inferior frontal lobe). The motor control of speech production depends on the sensorimotor cortex bilaterally. In routine practice, four major parameters of language can be used to assess dysphasia: fluency, comprehension, repetition and naming skills. Naming skills are affected in all forms of dysphasia. Dominant frontal lobe lesions are likely to give rise to a non-fluent dysphasia characterized by effortful speech and a poverty of language but with comprehension intact, while lesions in Wernicke's area (posterior superior dominant temporal lobe) result in impairment of comprehension but with fluent speech that conveys rather little meaning. Global aphasia occurs as a result of large dominant hemisphere lesions of the frontal, temporal and parietal lobe. Dysphasia is often associated with dyslexia and dysgraphia. A severe comprehension deficit as a result of dysphasia makes it challenging to assess other aspects of cognition although they may be intact. The most common cause of dysphasia is dominant hemisphere stroke, but any appropriately placed focal lesion may cause dysphasia, and it is an important feature of neurodegenerative dementias.

Apraxia

This term refers to an inability to do things in spite of having intact motor and sensory systems. Dressing apraxia, an inability to put on items of clothing, particularly jackets and gowns, is seen in patients with non-dominant parietal lesions. Visuospatial disabilities and neglect contribute to this form of apraxia. Constructional apraxia likewise reflects impaired visuospatial function. The main form of motor apraxia (ideomotor apraxia) manifests as difficulty using instruments and tools (toothbrush, scissors, etc.) in spite of knowing what the device in question is. Other manifestations of ideomotor apraxia include inability to carry out actions such as waving goodbye or saluting, inability to mime actions (e.g. using a comb to comb one's hair, hammering a nail) and to copy finger and hand positions demonstrated by the examiner. This form of apraxia usually occurs in dominant parietal lesions. An apraxic individual may be unable to make a cup of tea, but agnosia (see below) might give rise to the same inability. Furthermore, a test for apraxia which requires a sequence of actions probes comprehension, memory and executive skills as well as praxis. Patients with dominant inferior frontal lobe lesions may have apraxia affecting the use of lips, tongue and mouth, often in association with a non-fluent dysphasia. Gait apraxia is covered in Table 16.11.

Agnosia

Agnosia is a failure of recognition. A simple classification is by the sensory modality affected: visual, auditory, tactile, olfactory. There is overlap between tactile agnosia and cortical sensory loss. Visual agnosia (potentially the most severely disabling agnosia) reflects visuoperceptual impairment due to occipitoparietal and occipitotemporal lesions which are often bilateral and may be associated with a visual field defect but basic visual function in the preserved field is intact. A patient with visual agnosia may not recognize a watch until it is put into his hand but would answer correctly the question 'What do you wear on your wrist and use to tell the time?' Prosopagnosia is an inability to recognize familiar faces (though parts of the face are correctly identified, and the patient may be able to match correctly two different photographs of the face he cannot recognize). Bilateral occipitotemporal lesions underlie prosopagnosia.

Neglect phenomena

A lesion in either hemisphere may lead to a form of neglect affecting the opposite side, but neglect is much more commonly seen when the lesion is in the right cerebral hemisphere, affecting the left side. Usually the lesion is large, such as a stroke. Different forms of neglect may have different localizations. Parietal lobe involvement is often prominent. A patient with neglect of personal space may pay no attention to the affected side of the body, in the extreme even denying that the affected side belongs to him. Denial of a hemiplegia is anosognosia; unconcern about a hemiplegia is anosodiaphoria. Neglect of extrapersonal space leads to failure to eat the food off one side of a plate, failure to complete one side of a drawing, failure to read the left side of a text, even failure to write the first part of a word. Sensory and visual inattention are forms of neglect.

Localizing the neurological lesion

Having taken a history and undertaken a neurological and relevant general medical examination, it is important to decide where the likely lesion is and, ideally, its likely nature (e.g. vascular, inflammatory, degenerative, neoplastic). This can often seem bewildering for students and doctors in training. In addition to those points made above regarding the identification of muscle disorders, neuromuscular junction disorders, mononeuropathies, polyneuropathies, radiculopathies and spinal cord disorders, the following are some helpful principles regarding brainstem, cerebellar and cerebral hemisphere lesions.

If a patient has a hemiparesis and a hemianaesthesia on the same side, the lesion has to be above the decussation of the corticospinal tracts in the medulla. The lesion is most likely to be in the contralateral cerebral hemisphere but could also be in the brainstem.

The range of possible manifestations of brainstem lesions is extensive, but a good general rule is that a cranial nerve lesion (III, V, VI, VII, VIII, X or XII) on one side and long tract signs on the other side of the body indicate a brainstem lesion. The long tract signs may be motor, sensory or both. A brainstem lesion has to be considered if there are bilateral long tract signs and the lesion is above neck level. Nystagmus and long-tract signs indicate a brainstem lesion. Vertical gaze paresis of acute onset and internuclear ophthalmoparesis are indicators of midbrain and pontine lesions, respectively. Extensive brainstem lesions affecting the reticular formation will cause coma. A basilar artery thrombosis may spare the dorsal brainstem such that consciousness is preserved but the devastating consequence is the locked-in syndrome.

Cerebellar lesions should be suspected with combinations of gait ataxia, limb ataxia, dysarthria and nystagmus. Ataxia by itself is rather non-localizing, being a feature of polyneuropathy and spinal cord, cerebellar, brainstem and cerebral hemisphere disease. Remember that anyone who is vertiginous will be ataxic until the vertigo settles, so ataxia in combination with vertigo may be due to a peripheral vestibular rather than a neurological disorder. Cerebellar mass lesions readily compress the brainstem which complicates the signs and, moreover, brainstem compression readily causes hydrocephalus.

Common manifestations in large unilateral cerebral hemisphere lesions include contralateral hemianopia, horizontal gaze paresis, hemiparesis and hemianaesthesia together with cognitive impairment (dysphasia in dominant hemisphere lesions, neglect and visuospatial problems in non-dominant). A frontal lobe lesion affecting prefrontal structures may give rise to behavioural and cognitive deficits only. Anterior cerebral artery territory ischaemic strokes cause spastic paresis in the contralateral leg. Middle cerebral artery territory ischaemic strokes cause all of the features of large unilateral hemisphere lesions. The hemiparesis is maximal in the face and arm. Posterior cerebral artery territory ischaemic strokes cause hemianopia because of occipital lobe infarction and cause cognitive deficits due to involvement of the temporal lobe.

The clinical manifestations of hydrocephalus depend on how acutely it develops. Acute hydrocephalus causes headache, papilloedema, drowsiness and coma. In the setting of established hydrocephalus, acute exacerbations cause hydrocephalic attacks, which may manifest with abrupt headache, paralysis, drop attacks and coma. In some cases, however, hydrocephalus occurs with hardly any raised pressure at all. In such cases, the manifestations are cognitive impairment, ataxia, urinary incontinence, upgaze paresis and extensor plantar reflexes. Hydrocephalus is a common cause of bilateral long-tract (corticospinal tract) signs of cerebral origin. The other is diffuse or multifocal bilateral white matter disease, which may be ischaemic or inflammatory. Large supratentorial mass lesions ultimately cause bilateral long tract signs, pupillary changes and impending coma due to brain herniation.

Investigations

It is crucial for investigations in neurological practice to be focused and directed on the basis of the clinical findings. Imaging, cerebrospinal fluid (CSF) examination and neurophysiological investigations may all play a role in diagnosis.

Imaging

Headache

A discussion about which patients with headache should be imaged is beyond the scope of this chapter, but a number of points are worth noting:

- Migraine, tension-type headaches, medication overuse headaches and post-traumatic headaches can be diagnosed with a high degree of accuracy without scans.
- Normal scans undoubtedly reassure worried patients with headaches, but incidental abnormalities found on scans risk perpetuating worry.
- Normal scans do not cure headaches (though a proportion of patients who know their scan is normal do not attend their follow-up appointment).
- Patients with serious intracranial disorders rarely just have headache.
- Occasionally migraine really is 'symptomatic', i.e. caused by a structural intracranial disorder.

Computed tomography (CT) remains a good investigation for headache in the emergency setting, to image large tumours, particularly supratentorial tumours, abscesses, brain swelling, hydrocephalus and haemorrhage, particularly subarachnoid haemorrhage. However, the radiation dose is the equivalent of 200 chest X-rays so, if available, magnetic resonance imaging (MRI) is preferable, especially in an elective setting.

Epilepsy

The investigation of choice for late-onset epilepsy is a MRI head scan; the information required is whether there is an identifiable structural cause for the epilepsy. Electroencephalography (EEG) in this situation is less useful. In the paediatric/adolescent age group, imaging is usually normal but the EEG may well be informative (see below).

Stroke

Imaging is central to the investigation of stroke and transient ischaemic attacks. The advent of thrombolysis and the possibility of other forms of emergency treatment of ischaemic stroke mandates extremely rapid but accurate diagnosis of stroke and of stroke severity. CT, including CT angiography, and MRI both contribute.

Focal central nervous system lesions

All focal CNS lesions will require imaging. Usually MRI is preferable to CT, but the choice may be dependent on local resources. It is crucial, by means of the clinical methods outlined above, to decide where the focal lesion is, so as to image the appropriate part of the nervous system. This is particularly true of spinal imaging.

Multiple sclerosis

All patients presenting for the first time with manifestations of multiple sclerosis (often but not always the first attack) must have a MRI head scan, and imaging of the spinal cord may be necessary.

Cognitive impairment

As a rule all patients with cognitive impairment should have structural imaging of the brain. Metabolic imaging contributes and molecular imaging (e.g. of amyloid) will soon become a clinical tool.

Peripheral nervous system

MRI is the investigation for radiculopathies. MRI also has a role in the investigation of plexus lesions but imaging of the brachial plexus remains problematic. The vast majority of compressive mononeuropathies are not imaged, but consideration should be given to imaging (MRI, ultrasound) in certain progressive and severe mononeuropathies to look for tumours and cysts.

Muscle diseases

MRI has a role in the investigation of muscle disorders, contributing to the assessment of some patients with dystrophies or inflammatory muscle disease, particularly in guiding the decision as to which muscle to biopsy.

Electroencephalography

Electrodes applied to the patient's scalp pick up small changes of electrical potential which, after amplification, are recorded on paper or displayed on a video monitor and recorded electronically. The main use of EEG is in diagnosing the nature of the epilepsy in young patients (particularly in distinguishing generalized from focal epilepsies), but it has significant limitations since, in the majority of cases, what is recorded is an interictal EEG which may or may not show diagnostically useful abnormalities. EEG is a poor test in individuals who have undiagnosed attacks of symptoms which might be epilepsy. Video telemetry is invaluable in clarifying whether attacks are epileptic or non-epileptic, the main limitation being that the attack frequency has to be high enough to make it likely that attacks will be recorded.

EEG may be a useful investigation in encephalopathic states where the clinical picture may be one of delirium. Here, EEG can identify non-convulsive status epilepticus or point to a diagnosis of encephalitis as opposed to a toxic or metabolic encephalopathy. It has a supportive role in diagnosing Creutzfeldt-Jakob disease.

Nerve conduction studies and electromyography

Sensory nerve conduction studies (NCS) are achieved by stimulating electrically a purely sensory nerve percutaneously and recording, usually by surface electrodes, the resulting sensory action potentials (SAPs) in the relevant nerve either more proximally or distally. The SAP amplitude and conduction velocity are measured. Motor NCS require stimulation of a motor or mixed nerve, recording the resulting motor action potentials from a muscle supplied by the nerve, again usually with surface electrodes. Stimulation of the nerve at two different sites allows calculation of the conduction velocity between the two sites. Electromyography (EMG) entails recording electrical activity generated by muscle fibres and motor units (groups of muscle fibres supplied by a single motor neuron) at rest and during contraction, using a needle electrode inserted into the muscle. Different abnormalities of EMG arise in denervation, disorders of neuromuscular transmission and disorders of muscle itself. NCS contributes to the diagnosis of many but not all entrapment neuropathies. It has to be anatomically possible to stimulate and record from the nerve proximal to the entrapment site. In patients with clear physical signs, NCSs are not needed to make the correct clinical diagnosis but may help in the assessment of severity and prognosis. Every patient who is going to have surgical decompression of an entrapped peripheral nerve should have an NCS. NCS is invaluable in confirming the suspected diagnosis of nerve entrapment when there are no definite signs, a common circumstance in carpal tunnel syndrome.

NCS and EMG may contribute to the assessment of plexopathies and radiculopathies though, in the latter, the combination of careful clinical evaluation and imaging should suffice. NCS and EMG help to confirm a diagnosis of polyneuropathy and provide information about the nature of polyneuropathies (axonal, demyelinating, multifocal, small fibre). NCS and EMG are helpful in suspected disorders of neuromuscular junctions. EMG helps in the diagnosis of myopathy and is an important test for patients with undiagnosed weakness.

Cerebrospinal fluid examination

CSF is usually obtained by lumbar puncture (LP), which is uncomfortable, invasive and attended by a number of potential complications, the most common one being post-lumbar puncture headache. There is a risk of death from brain herniation when LP is undertaken in a patient with raised intracranial pressure due to a mass lesion or obstructive hydrocephalus. Papilloedema, any grade of impaired level of consciousness or any focal neurological signs mandate brain imaging before consideration of LP and it is contraindicated in patients with mass lesions and obstructive hydrocephalus. However, it is an essential investigation in patients with papilloedema due to suspected raised intracranial pressure who have a normal good quality MRI, to pursue the possibility of idiopathic intracranial hypertension and to exclude low-grade chronic meningitis, as well as to treat the raised pressure. Pressure measurement as well as CSF analysis will be required.

Meningitis

The single circumstance in which LP is an emergency investigation is CNS infection, particularly meningitis. There is controversy as to whether CSF examination in meningitis is really necessary or at least whether the risk is worth taking. In adult neurology, the consensus remains that CSF should be obtained if possible but that, in cases of suspected pyogenic bacterial meningitis, there must be no delay in starting antibiotic treatment pending cranial imaging. Thus, if there is no contraindication to LP, it should be performed expeditiously immediately after clinical assessment and obtaining blood cultures, in order to provide a microbiological diagnosis. If cranial imaging is necessary, treatment should start directly after clinical assessment and blood cultures. CSF obtained after imaging has shown that LP is expected to be safe may still be diagnostic even some hours after treatment has started.

CSF examination is important, sometimes critical, in diagnosis of all forms of infective meningitis: bacterial, tuberculous, yeast, fungal and viral. The key parameters are the white cell count, the types of white cells (polymorphonuclear neutrophil white cells, lymphocytes), the CSF glucose concentration (low in bacterial meningitis) which must be compared with a simultaneous blood glucose concentration, microscopy for microorganisms (Gram stain, tuberculosis stain, India ink preparation for cryptococci), DNA analysis for viral and bacterial DNA (using polymerase chain reaction (PCR) techniques) and appropriate microbiological culture. The CSF protein concentration is of some importance and the CSF lactate concentration may be helpful.

CSF analysis is also urgent in encephalitis, which will be treated as herpes simplex encephalitis until CSF PCR tests for herpes simplex virus have proved negative. CSF examination in myelitis will follow imaging.

In all other situations, CSF examination is not so urgent, even if it is still essential. In low-grade meningitis which is suspected to be due to tuberculosis, to maximize the chance of identifying and culturing mycobacteria send up to three CSF samples on consecutive days before starting treatment.

Subarachnoid haemorrhage

In suspected subarachnoid haemorrhage with cranial imaging that does not show evidence of blood in the subarachnoid space, CSF must be examined. It is important to wait until 12 hours after the suspected bleed so that red blood cells will have lysed and haemoglobin will have undergone metabolism to oxyhaemoglobin and bilirubin, which can be detected by spectroscopy or seen with the naked eye as xanthochromia. Failure to allow time for xanthochromia to develop makes it impossible to distinguish a traumatic CSF tap from bloodstained CSF due to subarachnoid haemorrhage.

CNS inflammatory disorders

CSF lymphocytosis is usually a feature of conditions such as CNS vasculitis, neurosarcoidosis, Behçet's disease and sometimes systemic lupus erythematosus.

With regard to multiple sclerosis (MS), if the clinical features and MRI appearances are typical (particularly in a young patient), CSF examination may not be necessary. It remains important if scans do not fulfil diagnostic criteria or if there is ambiguity as to whether scan lesions are inflammatory or ischaemic, or reflect some other pathology. CSF protein electrophoresis to detect oligoclonal IgG immunoglobulins is the most sensitive test to provide evidence of chronic inflammatory CNS demyelination. Occasionally in suspected MS results of CSF examination are incompatible with a diagnosis of MS because of either a very high cell count or a very high protein concentration, mandating a revision of the diagnosis.

Guillain-Barré syndrome

A high CSF protein concentration without a high cell count is characteristic of Guillain-Barré syndrome (GBS), but this takes time to develop so will not be found if the CSF is examined early in the course of the condition. Every patient with GBS should have CSF looked at in order to make sure that the patient does not have a rapidly progressive polyradiculopathy due to diffuse neoplastic leptomeningeal infiltration. Accordingly, when the LP is done, care should be taken to order cytology as well as a cell count, blood and CSF glucose concentration, protein concentration and, if appropriate, culture.

Neoplastic leptomeningeal infiltration

Neoplastic leptomeningeal infiltration, either by a haematological malignancy (leukaemia, lymphoma) or metastatic carcinoma (lung, breast, others) may present as a cranial neuropathy or spinal polyradiculopathy or with headache, encephalopathy or hydrocephalus. High-protein and low-glucose concentrations in CSF are typical but not diagnostic. The presence of malignant cells in the CSF is diagnostic, but they are not always seen. Sending serial samples on consecutive days (up to three) increases the chance of a positive result.

Urogenital system 17

John Peters, James Green and Lina Hijazi

The diagnostic process in nephrology and urology

Nephrology and urology systems are more dependent than most on laboratory, histopathology and imaging techniques to complete the diagnostic process, but the basic principles and requirements of clinical assessment often lead towards an area of diagnosis which directs subsequent laboratory and other technically oriented investigations. Diseases of the kidney and urinary tract manifest a somewhat restricted array of symptoms and signs, but almost all patients can be categorized as having a well-defined renal or urological syndrome, and keeping these in mind informs the clinical diagnostic process. There are many areas of overlap between clinical and pathological processes within a single syndrome, and in general it is not helpful to create artificial distinctions between the two. Once the syndrome has been established, further details of assessment and management objectives become clearer. It is important to emphasize that a number of these syndromes were first described many years ago. They have stood the test of time principally because of their pragmatic value and relative ease of recognition on the basis of clinical assessment and quite simple tests.

Symptoms of renal and urological disease

Pain

Pain arising from the urinary tract is a common symptom that is often due to obstruction, infection or tumour. Renal pain is usually felt in the flank or the loin. When renal pain arises from ureteric obstruction (e.g. a stone), discomfort may additionally radiate to the iliac fossa, the testicle or the labia, the pattern depending to a certain extent on the level of the obstruction. Patients with polycystic kidney disease may suffer chronic flank pain. Exacerbations occur with cyst infection and haemorrhage.

Acute bladder outflow obstruction presents with severe suprapubic pain. However, pain in the suprapubic region and perineum most commonly arises from lower urinary tract infection due to cystitis or urethritis. Such pain is frequently accompanied by dysuria, frequency or strangury (painful micturition). These symptoms comprise the syndrome of cystitis. It is nearly always associated with urinary abnormalities on urine stick testing (protein, blood and leukocytes). In men, this pain may be associated with severe perineal or rectal discomfort, in which case prostatitis is suggested.

In young children with urinary tract infection and cystitis, the symptoms may be much less obvious, but cystitis should be suspected in any child who cries on micturating. Pain from the kidneys, if it results from acute infection or abscess, may occasionally reflect tracking of pus upwards to the diaphragm, causing diaphragmatic pain, or in the retroperitoneal space to the psoas muscle, leading to pain when the muscle is stretched on passive hip extension. Glomerulonephritis is usually painless. Kidney tumours may cause a dull persistent flank pain.

Haematuria

Blood in the urine can be present with or without pain and may be continuous or intermittent. If visible to the naked eye, it is termed macroscopic or visible haematuria; if detected only by stick tests or microscopy, it is called microscopic haematuria. Haematuria as a result of parenchymal renal disease is usually:

- continuous
- painless
- microscopic (occasionally macroscopic).

Haematuria arising from renal tumours is likely to be:

- intermittent
- associated with renal pain
- macroscopic.

Bleeding from bladder tumours is often intermittent, with associated local symptoms suggesting cystitis.

It is important to decide early in the diagnostic process whether the haematuria originates from the kidneys or elsewhere in the urinary tract (Box 17.1). This decision affects the order in which investigations should be conducted. For example, continuous painless

Box 17.1 Causes of haematuria

Systemic

- Purpura
- Sickle cell trait
- Bleeding disorders, including anticoagulant drugs

Renal

- Infarct/papillary necrosis
- Trauma
- Tuberculosis
- Stones
- Renal pelvis transitional cell carcinoma, and other renal tumours:
  - Wilms' tumour (in children)
- Acute glomerulonephritis

Postrenal

- Ureteric stones
- Ureteric neoplasms
- Bladder tumours (transitional cell carcinoma)
- Bladder tuberculosis and bilharziasis
- Radiation cystitis
- Drug-induced cystitis, e.g. cyclophosphamide
- Prostatic enlargement
- Urethral neoplasms
- Bacterial cystitis

microscopic haematuria with associated proteinuria in a young man or woman is most likely to be the result of glomerulonephritis or other renal pathology. However, haematuria in an older person with risk factors for urothelial malignancy (smoking) is more likely to be caused by a bladder or ureteric tumour and merits a cystoscopy early in the investigative process. It is important to remember that the commonest cause of dipstick haematuria in women is contamination from menstrual blood.

Oliguria/anuria

Oliguria is the passage of less than 500 ml of urine per day. Anuria is the complete absence of urine flow. A reduction in urinary flow rate to the point of oliguria may be physiological, as in a patient whose fluid intake is low. Physiological reduction of urinary flow rate implies that the glomerular filtration rate (GFR) remains normal, and that the kidney is avidly retaining sodium and water. If inadequate fluid intake leads to a significant reduction in the extracellular fluid compartment, the resulting decrease in renal blood flow leads to oliguria and reduction of the GFR. Oliguria arising in this fashion is termed prerenal and is clearly pathological. Renal oliguria implies the presence of intrinsic renal disease, whereas postrenal oliguria results from mechanical obstruction at any level, from the collecting system in the kidney to the urethra. Anuria and oliguria may be signs of renal failure.

Polyuria

Polyuria implies no more than a high urinary flow rate. There will always be an associated increase in the frequency of micturition (frequency) and often nocturia as well. Polyuria results from excessive water intake (e.g. psychogenic polydipsia or beer drinking), from an osmotic diuresis (glucose as in diabetes mellitus, urea as in chronic renal failure and sodium chloride as in diuretic use) and finally from abnormal renal tubular water handling, as seen in cranial diabetes insipidus (inadequate secretion of antidiuretic hormone) or nephrogenic diabetes insipidus (renal resistance to antidiuretic hormone).

Frequency of micturition

Increased frequency of micturition results from polyuria, a reduction in functional bladder capacity or bladder/urethral irritation. The commonest cause of polyuria is excessive fluid intake, whereas reduced functional bladder capacity is seen most frequently in patients with prostatic hypertrophy and bladder outlet obstruction. Lower urinary tract infection (cystitis) causes bladder irritation and an increase in urinary frequency. Some patients with neurological diseases, in particular multiple sclerosis, also have frequency of micturition. The detrusor muscle of the bladder contracts at an inappropriately low bladder volume, resulting in a low functional bladder capacity.

Nocturia

The term nocturia implies the need to empty the bladder during the hours of sleep. In health, there is a substantial diurnal variation in urinary flow rate: a night-time reduction in urine flow, together with adequate functional bladder capacity, serves to obviate the need for night-time micturition. Thus polyuria of any cause, or any cause of reduction of functional bladder capacity, may lead to nocturia. In addition, failure of the urine concentrating ability of the kidneys, as occurs in renal impairment and sickle cell disease, will also lead to nocturia. Obviously, diuretics taken in the evening and at night will lead to this symptom.

Dysuria

Dysuria is a specific form of discomfort arising from the urinary tract in which there is pain immediately before, during or after micturition. The urine is often described as 'burning' or 'scalding', and there is usually associated frequency of micturition and decreased functional bladder capacity. Infection and neoplasia in the bladder or urethra are the most important causes. An extreme form of dysuria, strangury, implies an unpleasant and painful desire to void when the bladder is empty or nearly so.

Urgency of micturition, incontinence and enuresis

Urgency is the loss of the normal ability to postpone micturition beyond the time when the desire to pass urine is initially perceived. Incontinence is the involuntary passage of urine. In extreme cases, urgency may lead to urge incontinence, in which the desire to void cannot be voluntarily inhibited. Stress incontinence, on the other hand, is leakage of urine associated with straining or coughing, often due to weakened pelvic floor muscles. The term enuresis is usually used to describe nocturnal enuresis, or bed wetting.

Slow stream, hesitancy and terminal dribbling

The triad of slow stream, hesitancy and terminal dribbling is most frequently seen in elderly men with prostatic hypertrophy. Here the bladder outlet is partially obstructed by the enlarging prostate gland, with the result that the maximum achievable urinary flow rate during micturition is reduced. There is often difficulty in initiating micturition (hesitancy) and in completing micturition in a 'clean stop' fashion (terminal dribbling). The symptoms are nearly always associated with frequency of micturition and nocturia, the result of a low functional bladder capacity. In more advanced cases, there may be progressive bladder enlargement, with eventual overflow incontinence and continuous or intermittent dribbling of urine.

Urethral discharge

Urethral discharge is usually noticed only by men and always requires further investigation. There may be associated symptoms of urethral irritation and the underlying pathology is likely to be urethritis, which is often infective and sexually transmitted (see later in this chapter).

Physical signs in renal and urological disease

These physical signs fall into three principal groups:

1. Local signs related to the specific pathology, for example an enlarged palpable tender kidney in renal carcinoma, an obstructed kidney or a palpably enlarged bladder in a patient with acute or chronic retention.
2. Symptoms of disturbance of renal salt and water handling, with resulting clinical evidence of extracellular fluid volume expansion or contraction.
3. Signs of failure of the kidney's normal excretory and metabolic functions.

In many renal patients, particularly those with advanced chronic renal failure and uraemia, signs from all three of the above categories may be present.

General features

Patients with chronic renal failure look unwell. The skin is pallid, the complexion sallow and a slightly yellowish hue is often evident. The mucous membranes are pale, reflecting the associated normochromic, normocytic anaemia. There may be bruises, purpura and scratch marks due to uraemic pruritus, and also an underlying disorder of platelet function and capillary fragility. The nails often appear pale and opaque (leuconychia) in the nephrotic syndrome and sometimes in chronic renal failure. Intercurrent episodes of severe illness in the past may have led to the appearance of Beau's lines, which appear as transverse ridges across the nails. Splinter haemorrhages in the nail beds point to underlying vasculitis, which may be the cause of the renal failure or be indicative of endocarditis; there may be an associated purpuric rash (Fig. 17.1). When blood urea is very high, a uraemic frost may be seen on any part of the body and appears as a white powder; it is formed from crystalline urea deposited on the skin via the sweat. The onset of chronic renal failure in childhood is associated with impaired growth, causing short stature. Severe bony deformity (Fig. 17.2) may be evident in some cases, particularly in children, who may develop rickets. Advanced uraemia is also associated with metabolic flap, a coarse tremor which is best seen at the wrists when in the dorsiflexed position. It is similar to the metabolic flap seen in patients with advanced liver disease or respiratory failure. The presence of metabolic acidosis leads to increased ventilation with an increased tidal volume, known as Kussmaul respiration.

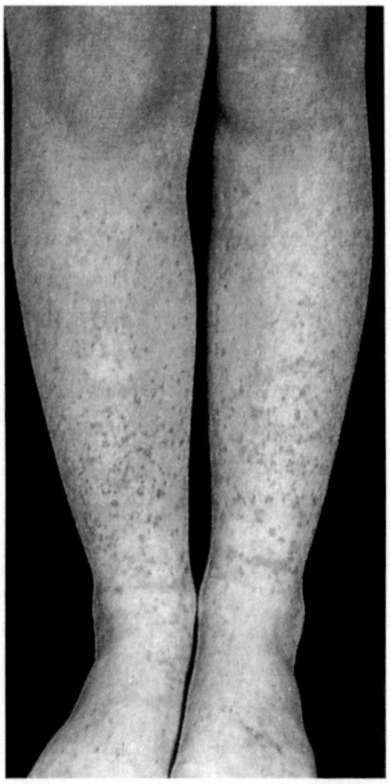

Figure 17.1 Purpura in Henoch–Schönlein disease.

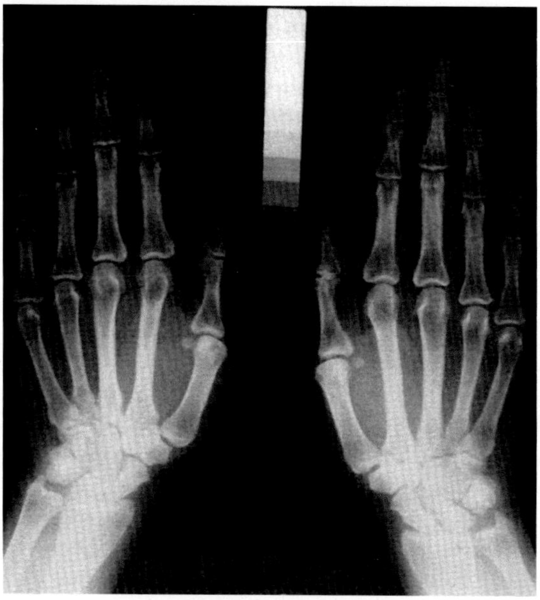

Figure 17.2 X-ray of the hands of a patient with chronic renal failure and secondary hyperparathyroidism, showing renal osteodystrophy. There is a loss of density of the tips of the digits (acro-osteolysis) with loss of density on either side of the interphalangeal joints and subperiosteal bone resorption. The latter is best seen in the middle phalanges of the index and middle fingers.

The circulation in the renal patient

Of crucial importance here is the correct assessment of the patient's fluid volume status. It is important to define whether the patient is euvolaemic, hypovolaemic or hypervolaemic. This is a bedside assessment that, with practice, can usually be made correctly.

Hypervolaemia is associated with some or all of the following:

- Hypertension
- Elevation of the jugular venous pressure
- Peripheral oedema at the ankles or sacrum
- Basal crackles on lung auscultation
- Ascites
- Pleural effusion

In patients with nephrotic syndrome (see below), oedema and salt and water retention are caused by reduced plasma oncotic pressure. Oedema with expansion of the extracellular fluid is often accompanied by hypertension and, particularly if the cardiac reserve is poor, may progress to pulmonary oedema and other manifestations of heart failure. The presence of oedema itself, however, can coexist with intravascular volume depletion, especially in patients with nephrotic syndrome.

The diagnosis of hypovolaemia requires the absence of any signs of hypervolaemia. The hypovolaemic patient may have the following:

- Low blood pressure, often exaggerated in the upright position – postural hypotension
- Sinus tachycardia (exaggerated in the upright position)
- Low pulse pressure (exaggerated in the upright position)
- Flat neck veins even when almost supine

Poor skin turgor, 'sunken eyes' and dry mucous membranes are often cited as signs of volume depletion, but these are generally unreliable features.

Abdominal palpation

The detection of the kidneys in the abdominal examination is described in Chapter 14. In slim people with relaxed abdominal muscles, it is sometimes possible to feel a normal right kidney (the right kidney is situated slightly lower than the left at the level of T12-L3). More often a palpable kidney can only be felt because it is enlarged, as in hydronephrosis, multiple cysts (polycystic kidney disease) or tumour (generally unilateral). A distended bladder is identified in the lower abdomen by a combination of palpation and percussion. Rectal examination is an important part of the clinical assessment of the renal patient: bimanual palpation of the bladder is a more reliable way of assessing bladder enlargement than is simple per abdominal examination. In men, rectal examination also allows evaluation of the prostate gland, both for benign enlargement and for the detection of malignant change suggested by hard irregularity of the gland and absence of the central groove.

Auscultation

Uraemic pericarditis and pleurisy may be suggested by pericardial and pleural friction rubs, respectively. Their presence points to either advanced uraemia or a multisystem inflammatory disorder such as systemic lupus erythematosus (SLE), which may have both renal and extrarenal manifestations. Added heart sounds (S3 and S4) suggest, respectively, volume expansion and incipient heart failure, and ventricular hypertrophy, often as a consequence of hypertension. The presence of vascular bruits and/or impairment of the major arterial pulses is an important finding, raising the possibility of renal vascular disease, which may underlie hypertension and/or renal failure if bilateral.

The eye in uraemia

Corneal calcification (limbic calcification) occurs in patients with long-standing hyperparathyroidism with elevation of blood calcium and phosphorus concentrations (see Ch. 18). The presence of limbic calcification should not be confused with a corneal arcus (arcus senilis), which is a broader band at the edge of the cornea and merges with the sclera. Corneal arcus is usually most marked in the superior and inferior positions, whereas limbic calcification is seen medially and laterally or circumferentially. Retinal changes are extremely important in uraemic patients, many of whom have hypertension and/or diabetes. Renal dysfunction in the absence of diabetic retinopathy cannot be attributed to diabetic nephropathy in patients with type 1 diabetes. In type 2 diabetes, however, diabetic nephropathy is present in many patients without any diabetic eye changes. Patients with renal disease as part of systemic vasculitis may have manifestations of the latter in the retinae, with haemorrhages and exudates. Patients with chronic renal failure are at greatly increased risk of a range of vascular complications affecting both the macrovasculature and the microvasculature. In the retinae, thrombosis of the central retinal artery or its branches, or of the central retinal vein and its branches, is an important manifestation of this. The presence of Kayser-Fleischer rings may help confirm a diagnosis of Wilson's disease.

The renal and urological syndromes

Renal and urological syndromes are listed in Table 17.1. Some are exclusively renal, others exclusively urological, and some fall into both areas. The effects of renal failure on other organ systems are listed in Box 17.2.

Acute renal failure

Acute renal failure is the abrupt onset of declining renal function occurring over a period of hours or days, usually (but not always) accompanied by a marked reduction or cessation of the urinary flow rate. Central to the diagnosis, however, is a rapid decline in the GFR, leading to nitrogen retention and usually to sodium and water retention as well. An exception is the patient in whom the decline of GFR is not accompanied by reduction of urine flow, so-called non-oliguric acute renal failure. The outlook depends on the cause. Many are reversible spontaneously (repair of ischaemic injury as in tubular necrosis) or as a result of therapy (removal of stone or other cause of obstruction).

Table 17.1 Renal and urological syndromes

Renal	Renal and urological	Urological
Chronic renal failure Acute nephritic syndrome Nephrotic syndrome Renal hypertension Tubular syndromes	Acute renal failure Asymptomatic urinary abnormality Recurrent visible haematuria	Urinary tract infection Urinary tract obstruction Renal and urinary tract stone

Chronic renal failure

Chronic renal failure implies that the GFR has been reduced for a considerable period and that the reduction is largely or completely irreversible. It can result from almost any form of renal parenchymal disease, chronic renal ischaemia or unrelieved urinary obstruction. If renal impairment is severe, there may be clinical manifestations of uraemia. These are usually evident when the GFR has fallen to one-third of

Box 17.2 Effects of renal failure on other organ systems

Disturbances of water and electrolyte balance

- Breathlessness due to salt and water overload
- Deep sighing breathing (Kussmaul respiration) due to acidosis
- Weakness and postural fainting due to hypotension caused by salt and water depletion
- Lethargy and weakness from hypokalaemia

Disturbances of the haematological system

- Lethargy and breathlessness associated with anaemia owing to impaired production of erythropoietin by the kidneys
- Defective coagulation and excessive bruising (advanced renal failure)
- Haemorrhage from the gastrointestinal tract or lungs

Disturbances of the cardiovascular system

- Cardiac failure or angina associated with fluid overload, hypertension, anaemia and impaired ventricular function (uraemic cardiomyopathy)
- Precordial chest pain due to pericarditis
- Cardiac arrhythmias associated with left ventricular hypertrophy and hyperkalaemia/hypokalaemia

Disturbances of the respiratory system

- Breathlessness and haemoptysis from fluid overload
- Chest pain due to pleurisy

Disturbances of the musculoskeletal system

- Muscular weakness and bone pain due to impairment of vitamin D activation and to excessive parathyroid gland activity
- Acute pain due to gout

Disturbances of the nervous system

- Hypertensive stroke and encephalopathy
- Clouding of consciousness, fits and coma in advanced renal failure
- Impaired sensation or paraesthesia in the feet, due to peripheral neuropathy in long-standing uraemia
- Impaired higher mental/intellectual function
- Entrapment neuropathies

Disturbances of the eyes

- Pain from conjunctivitis caused by local deposits of calcium
- Visual blurring from hypertensive retinal damage or retinal vascular disease

normal or less. The implication of the term chronic renal failure is that the timescale of onset and progression is rarely shorter than a few months and often much longer. A further and crucial implication is an irreversible reduction in the number of functioning nephrons with no prospect of significant recovery. These patients manifest a number of symptoms that are not attributable to specific pathophysiological changes. Lethargy, poor concentration, irritability and failure of higher mental functions and ability to handle tasks are all commonly reported. In advanced cases, there may be confusion, fits and stupor. These are preterminal, but reversible if steps are taken to remove the excess uraemic toxins by dialysis. Nausea, vomiting and diarrhoea are also common in advanced uraemia and likewise improve following restoration of normal kidney function or treatment with dialysis or transplantation.

The acute nephritic syndrome

As in acute renal failure, the acute nephritic syndrome implies a fairly brisk onset (days, weeks or months) of reduction in GFR and retention of nitrogenous waste and usually salt and water also. Oliguria is, therefore, common. The underlying pathology is an acute glomerulonephritis which, as well as causing the functional abnormalities described above, also results in florid abnormalities of the urine. Haematuria (macroscopic or microscopic), proteinuria and tubular casts are often present. Many of the causes of acute nephritis are associated with functional abnormalities of the immune system which may be detected by laboratory tests and which may also manifest with disease in other organs, for example the skin, joints or eyes, as in SLE, Henoch-Schönlein purpura (see Fig. 17.1) and systemic vasculitis.

The nephrotic syndrome

Nephrotic syndrome is defined somewhat imprecisely as the presence of heavy proteinuria (usually >3 g/day, compared with normal of <150 mg/day), hypoalbuminaemia, hypercholesterolaemia and oedema. It is not generally very helpful to attempt a more precise definition because the clinical response to a given level of proteinuria shows considerable variability from patient to patient. It is, however, unusual for nephrotic syndrome to occur when the proteinuria is <2 g/day, and conversely some patients are able to maintain a normal or near-normal serum albumin concentration despite very heavy proteinuria in excess of 6 g/day.

Proteinuria of this magnitude implies glomerular pathology and may coexist with a significant reduction in GFR. Thus, a number of the pathological entities capable of causing nephrotic syndrome may also present as acute nephritic syndrome or the syndrome of chronic renal failure in other patients.

Asymptomatic urinary abnormality

Asymptomatic urinary abnormality is the presentation that arises in the patient who presents for a routine medical examination, often in the context of an employment or life insurance health check or at a screening visit to a primary care practitioner (PCP) or general practitioner (GP). Urine testing leads to the unexpected finding of proteinuria, haematuria or pyuria in an otherwise healthy patient. Further assessment may reveal the coexistence of other renal syndromes, but nevertheless it is worth maintaining the operational definition 'asymptomatic urinary abnormality' because this is such a frequent presentation in clinical practice. It should not be forgotten that this syndrome may not only reflect disease of the kidneys, as it can also be a manifestation of malignancy anywhere in the urinary tract, infection or stone (if asymptomatic).

Recurrent visible haematuria

Recurrent visible haematuria implies intermittent, or in some cases continuous, bleeding into the urinary tract to a degree sufficient to alter the macroscopic appearance of the urine. Depending on the circumstances of the bleeding, the urine may be a rusty-brown colour, lightly tinged with red blood or more heavily bloodstained. The source of the bleeding may be anywhere in the urinary tract, from the glomeruli at the top to the urethra at the bottom. Important causes are certain types of glomerulonephritis, renal tumours and infections (particularly tuberculosis), and tumours of the urinary tract transitional cell epithelium (urothelium) anywhere from the renal pelves to the bladder and urethra.

Urinary tract infection

The normal urinary tract is sterile except at its extreme distal end. Infection in the urinary tract leads to a range of symptoms and signs that reflect the location and severity of the infection. By far the most frequent site is the bladder, and the local symptoms reflect bladder irritation, with frequency of micturition, low functional bladder capacity and dysuria. The presence of urinary tract infection is defined importantly by the presence of a significant number of infecting organisms in the urine. A working definition of a proven urine infection would be the detection of more than 10^5 colony-forming units/ml urine in a carefully collected mid-stream specimen of urine (MSU). For less common infections, this definition may not be appropriate. For example, in tuberculosis of the urinary tract, the number of organisms being excreted may be extremely low, and formal identification on the basis of urine culture is sometimes difficult or impossible.

Sterile pyuria can be caused by a treated infection, parasites such as schistosomiasis, TB, bladder stones, inflammation or a tumour.

Urinary tract obstruction

Urinary tract obstruction syndrome may conveniently be divided into lower and upper tract obstruction. Lower urinary tract obstruction is defined by residual urine in the bladder after micturition or in more extreme forms by urinary retention with inability to empty the bladder at all. The most common causes relate to prostatic hypertrophy (benign hyperplasia or carcinoma), and a characteristic array of symptoms and signs arises (frequency, nocturia, poor stream, hesitancy, terminal dribbling). All of these are a consequence of low functional bladder capacity, an inability to empty the bladder completely and impairment of the urinary flow rate.

The presence of upper urinary tract obstruction is established in most cases by the demonstration of a dilated renal collecting system (renal pelvis and/or calyces), often seen to be proximal to a specific obstructing lesion. These features may be demonstrated by a number of imaging techniques, including ultrasound and intravenous urography (IVU) as well as cross-sectional imaging techniques such as computed tomography (CT) scanning. Upper and lower urinary tract obstruction may coexist, most frequently when the lower urinary tract obstruction is severe and/or of long standing, and leading to progressive dilatation of the upper urinary tract with consequent renal damage. It is important to remember that unilateral renal obstruction should not result in a rise in the serum creatinine. Therefore, if the creatinine is elevated, there is also dysfunction of the contralateral kidney.

It is important to remember that an infected and obstructed urinary system is considered an emergency and potentially life threatening.

Renal and urinary tract stones

The operational definition of renal and urinary tract stones is largely observational, depending on the demonstration of one or more stones in any part of the urinary tract. Resulting symptoms and signs depend on the location of the stone(s) and on size. For example, small stones in the kidneys are frequently asymptomatic, or they may lead to subtle urinary abnormalities, presenting initially with asymptomatic urinary abnormality. Larger stones in the kidneys frequently lead to renal pain, whereas stones in the ureter are particularly likely to cause acute obstruction and very severe ureteric and renal pain. Bladder stones are usually associated with symptoms suggestive of cystitis with frequency, haematuria and pain all common, and often associated with urinary tract infection.

Renal hypertension

By far the most common cause of sustained blood pressure elevation is essential hypertension. However, in a minority of patients with raised blood pressure, renal disease will be found to be the cause, and the likelihood of this is greatly increased in patients with coexisting renal disease of any kind. Hypertension may be one of the presenting features of virtually any disease of the renal parenchyma, including all forms of glomerulonephritis, many forms of tubulointerstitial disease, renal vascular disease, renal stone disease and obstruction. Renal tumours and renal infections may occasionally present with hypertension, which in some cases can be the only presenting feature. Thus, in any patient with newly identified hypertension, the possibility of underlying renal disease should be considered. Conversely, the exclusion of renal disease as a cause of hypertension is generally straightforward, comprising the absence of symptoms and signs of renal disease, the absence of urinary abnormalities on simple stick testing and the presence of a normal GFR as judged by serum creatinine concentration or other surrogate measurement for GFR.

Renal tubular syndromes

The majority of patients with parenchymal renal disease or obstructive renal damage manifest disordered tubular function, although in only a few of these are the tubular defects responsible for specific clinical manifestations. Tubular syndromes arising in this context are generally unobtrusive and are certainly common. Much less common is the patient in whom the tubular defect dominates the clinical picture. These defects may be inherited or acquired, and are seen mainly in children. They usually require careful laboratory testing to characterize them fully. Proximal tubular abnormalities include renal phosphate wasting, aminoaciduria (of these, cystinuria with cystine stone formation is the most important) and renal tubular acidosis leading to chronic metabolic acidosis. Distal tubular defects are also associated with metabolic acidosis and with disturbances of potassium metabolism, sodium-losing nephropathy and nephrogenic diabetes insipidus, with resulting failure, respectively, of salt and water conservation.

Laboratory assessment and imaging of the kidneys and urinary tract: assessment of structure and function

The urine

The urine should be tested as part of every general medical examination and not just in patients with known renal or urinary tract disease. Not only may the testing lead to the discovery of hitherto unsuspected diseases, such as diabetes or renal disease, but also documentation of normal urine often provides a very useful historical reference point in the event of the later development of renal disease or urinary abnormalities. The urine specimen should be passed into a clean container without additives. Testing should normally be conducted as soon as possible, and if delayed more than 2 hours, the urine should be refrigerated (not frozen) and returned to room temperature before testing. For microbiological assessment, it is essential to minimize the chances of contamination. This is best done by placing a sterile container in the path of the urine stream once voiding has commenced (i.e. a mid-stream specimen).

Quantity

Normal adults in temperate climates usually pass between 750 and 2500 ml of urine every 24 hours. The minimum daily urine output compatible with normal renal excretory function varies from person to person and also with other factors such as diet. Abnormally low urine output (oliguria or anuria) implies that the flow rate is below the minimum required to allow excretion of the daily solute load (usually <500 ml/day in an adult). Polyuria is an imprecise term implying no more than the passage of a large volume of urine but implying nothing about the reasons for this.

Colour

Urochrome and uroerythrin are pigments that contribute to the natural yellow tinge of urine. Darkening occurs on staining as a result of oxidation of urobilinogen to coloured urobilin. The colour of urine is also heavily influenced by the urinary flow rate, with high flow leading to dilute urine and hence a pale colour. Bile pigments in excess will colour the urine brown, with a characteristic yellow froth on shaking. Small to moderate quantities of blood impart a smoky appearance, with larger amounts leading to progressive brown or, in the case of brisk bleeding, bright red discoloration. Free haemoglobin from intravascular haemolysis (e.g. in severe malaria – blackwater fever) produces a darker red colour, verging on black in severe cases. Myoglobin may appear in the urine after acute muscle necrosis (rhabdomyolysis), causing a brown-red discoloration. Certain drugs discolour the urine (e.g. rifampicin (red), anthraquinone purgatives such as senna (orange), nitrofurantoin (brown) and methyldopa (grey)). Urine is normally transparent when freshly passed and still warm but may be cloudy if there are large numbers of red blood cells or leukocytes or if phosphates have precipitated in significant amounts.

Specific gravity and osmolality

Specific gravity and osmolality measurements yield similar information and, in the absence of significant glycosuria, are functions of the urinary concentrations of sodium, chloride and urea. The range of specific gravity is 1.001-1.035, which is equivalent to 50-1350 mOsmol/kg water (Fig. 17.3). The presence of renal insufficiency leads to a reduction in the range of osmolality that the kidneys can generate and, in advanced renal disease, the osmolality becomes relatively fixed at about 300 mOsmol/kg water, close to that of the glomerular filtrate (Fig. 17.4). This is termed isosthenuria, and because the urine concentration cannot be varied, predisposes the patient to sodium and water overload if intake is high, and to salt and water depletion if intake is low.

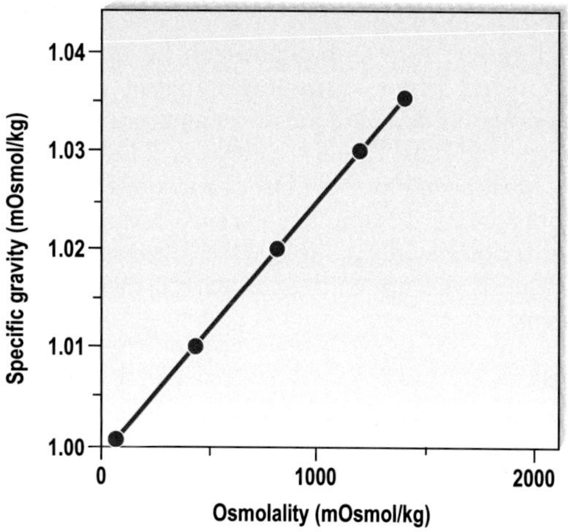

Figure 17.3 Relationship between specific gravity and osmolality.

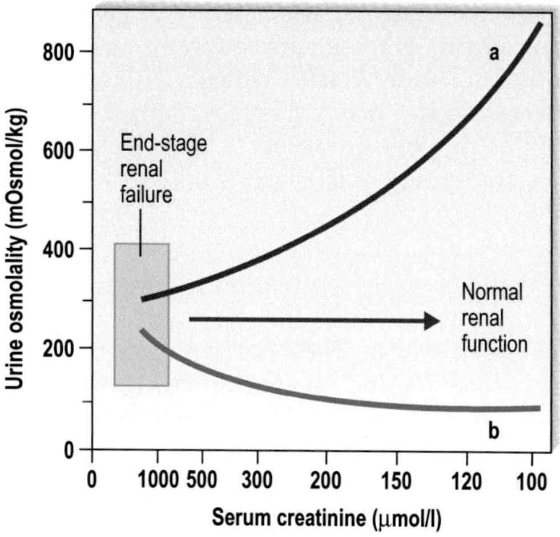

Figure 17.4 Relationship between renal concentration and diluting capacity, and serum creatinine concentration. The serum creatinine is plotted on a logarithmic scale. This therefore represents linear changes in GFR, such as might occur in progressive renal failure. End-stage renal failure is shown on the left, and normal renal function on the right. Curve (a) represents maximum concentrating capacity, e.g. in water deprivation, when the normal kidney can maintain the serum creatinine in the normal range by increasing urine osmolality. In renal failure, the urine cannot be concentrated and the serum creatinine rises. Curve (b) represents the maximum diluting capacity, e.g. after the ingestion of large volumes of water. The normal kidney excretes urine of low osmolality. In end-stage renal failure, urine osmolality cannot be reduced and the water load is not adequately handled. There is also isosthenuria, i.e. the urine tends towards an iso-osmolar state (specific gravity 1.010).

pH

The pH varies from 4 to 8 and can be measured crudely using paper strips impregnated with an indicator. If more accurate measurements are needed, as in suspected renal tubular acidosis, a pH electrode is used. Most people pass acid urine most of the time, exceptions being in some vegetarians, certain types of renal tubular acidosis, rapid water diuresis, metabolic alkalosis and urine infection with urea-splitting organisms.

Glucose

Glucose oxidase-impregnated dipsticks provide a quick and semiquantitative test for glucose in urine. By far the commonest causes of abnormal glycosuria are elevation of the plasma glucose to a point where the tubular reabsorptive capacity for glucose is exceeded (usually seen in people with diabetes) and during pregnancy, in which glycosuria occurs with normal plasma glucose concentrations. Very rarely, tubular transport defects may be associated with glycosuria at normal plasma glucose concentrations, and more frequently, but less predictably, patients with acquired chronic renal diseases may exhibit glycosuria at normal plasma glucose concentrations. Collectively these disorders are termed renal glycosuria.

Protein

The normal daily urine protein output is <150 mg. Dipsticks reactive to urine albumin provide a simple semiquantitative test. They are sensitive to 200-300 mg protein/l and have almost completely superseded the more cumbersome sulfosalicylic acid test. The urinary protein excretion rate generally rises in the upright posture and with activity and, in some normal individuals, this may lead to apparently abnormal proteinuria on spot urine specimens in ambulant patients and even in 24-hour urine collections (orthostatic proteinuria). Measurement of protein in an early-morning urine specimen, however, reveals no protein, and this serves to distinguish abnormal proteinuria from orthostatic proteinuria. A further refinement is the specific measurement of urine albumin, which is increasingly used, which should be <20 mg/day. Albumin excretion in the range 20-200 mg/day is termed microalbuminuria. Although this range is frequently too low to be detectable by stick testing, it is an important finding, particularly in diabetics in whom it predicts the later onset of overt diabetic nephropathy. The albumin:creatinine (ACR) and protein:creatinine (PCR) ratios are useful surrogate markers for proteinuria and are increasingly used instead of the 24-hour urine collection for quantification of protein excretion (Table 17.2).

The diagnostic implications of proteinuria depend greatly on its magnitude (Table 17.3). Heavy proteinuria (>1.5 g/day) is nearly always glomerular in origin, and albumin predominates over larger proteins such as globulins. Other proteins, rarely measured, arise from the renal tubules and include Tamm-Horsfall protein, retinol-binding protein and nephrocalcin, the latter helping to prevent the formation of urinary stones. It is worth noting that urine light chains may not be detected by some routine laboratory urine protein assays and have to be sought separately.

Microscopy

Microscopy (see Figs 17.5-17.8) is performed after slow spinning (at not more than 1000 *g*) of a fresh urine specimen for approximately 2 minutes. The pellet is resuspended in 0.5 ml of urine and examined unstained on a microscope slide under a coverslip. Important findings include leukocytes (suggestive of infection), red blood cells and various types of tubular casts. The presence of tubular casts is indicative of parenchymal renal disease. They may be red cell casts or white cell casts in which Tamm-Horsfall protein

Table 17.2 Relationship between ACR, PCR and 24-hour urine protein excretion

	ACR (mg/mmol)	PCR (mg/mmol)	24-hour urine protein (g/day)
Microalbuminuria	3-30		
Proteinuria	>30	>50	>0.5

Table 17.3 Proteinuria

Mild (<500 mg/day)	Moderate (up to 3 g/day)	Heavy (>3 g/day)
Benign hypertensive nephrosclerosis	Chronic pyelonephritis	Acute glomerulonephritis
Obstructive nephropathy	Acute tubular necrosis	Chronic glomerulonephritis
Prerenal uraemia	Acute glomerulonephritis	Diabetic nephropathy
Renal tumour	Chronic glomerulonephritis	Pre-eclampsia
Fever	Obstructive nephropathy	Myeloma
Tubulointerstitial nephropathy	Accelerated phase hypertension	All causes of nephrotic syndrome
Chronic pyelonephritis	Orthostatic proteinuria	
Early diabetic nephropathy	Urinary tract infection	
Orthostatic proteinuria		

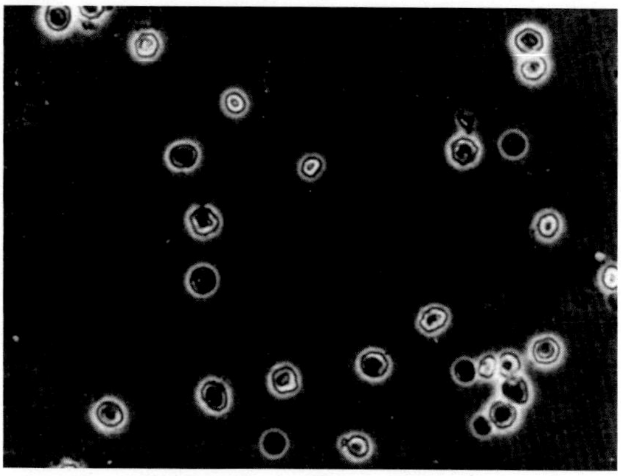

Figure 17.5 Erythrocytes in urinary sediment.

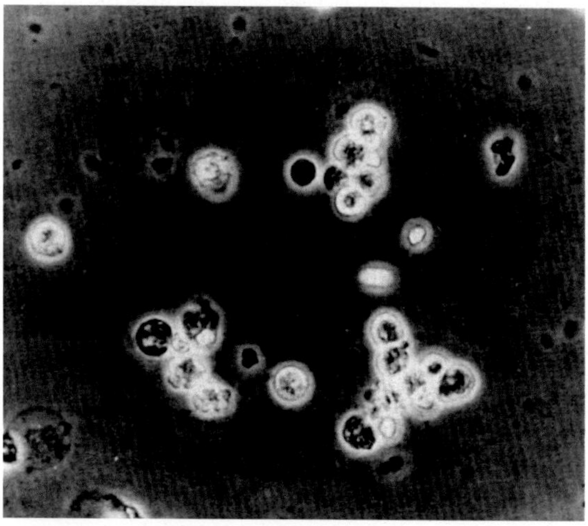

Figure 17.6 Leukocytes in urinary sediment.

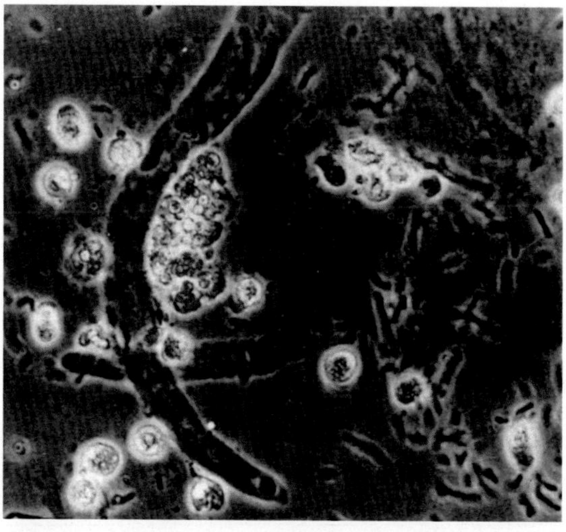

Figure 17.7 Hyaline casts, leukocytes and bacteria in urinary sediment. (Reproduced with permission from Spencer ES, Petersen I 1971 Hand Atlas of Urinary Sediment. Munksgaard, Copenhagen.)

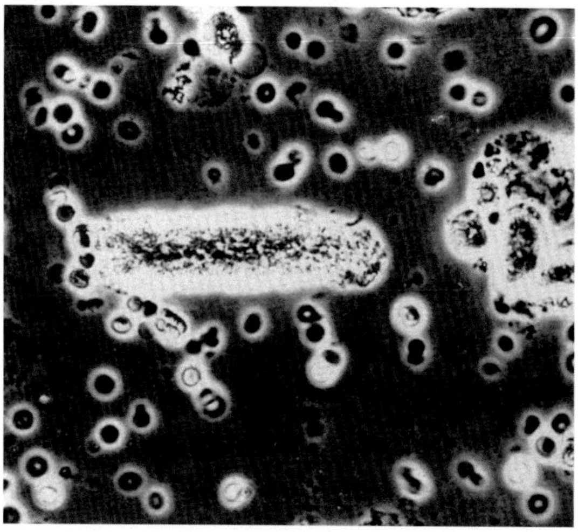

Figure 17.8 Granular casts in urinary sediment.

matrix has solidified and is studded with red or white blood cells. Granular casts probably represent degenerate cellular casts and have a grainy appearance. Hyaline casts contain no elements or debris and may be seen in small numbers in normal urine. It is usual to express the number of cells or casts seen per high-power field. The presence of red cell casts should alert one to the possibility of an aggressive glomerulonephritis. Red cell morphology may be a useful indicator as to the source of bleeding. Red cells with a normal outline usually, but not always, arise from the renal collecting system or from a point downstream of that, whereas red cells arising from the glomeruli are often distorted, probably as a result of movement through the glomeruli or osmotic insults during passage down the renal tubule.

Microbiological examination of the urine

Mid-stream urine specimens are normally satisfactory but are always contaminated to a certain extent during passage to the exterior. Extensive studies have shown that the finding of more than 10^5 bacteria per ml in a mid-stream specimen is usually associated with active urinary infection, especially when accompanied by leukocytes. Occasionally, to avoid contamination, urine is taken directly from the bladder for diagnostic purposes via suprapubic aspiration.

Measurement of the glomerular filtration rate

Accurate assessment of the GFR requires measurement in blood alone or blood and urine of a compound that is filtered freely at the glomerulus and neither reabsorbed nor secreted by the tubules (Table 17.4). Inulin is the best agent but involves a continuous infusion of inulin and measurements of inulin concentration in plasma and urine. This is a laborious investigation that is generally confined to research and is not routinely available. A number of surrogates for the inulin clearance method exist, however, and

Table 17.4 Measurement of the glomerular filtration rate	
Method	**Comments**
Plasma urea	Poor surrogate: – variable production rate – variable excretion rate
Plasma creatinine	Better than urea Poor discrimination at near-normal GFR
Calculated GFR	Useful surrogate of creatinine clearance
Creatinine clearance	Reasonable surrogate but depends on accurate timed urine collection (usually 24 hours)
^{51}Cr-EDTA	The best surrogate in clinical practice Expensive
Insulin clearance	Near-perfect measurement of GFR but: – needs continuous infusion – difficult urine and plasma assays – research studies only: not suited to clinical practice

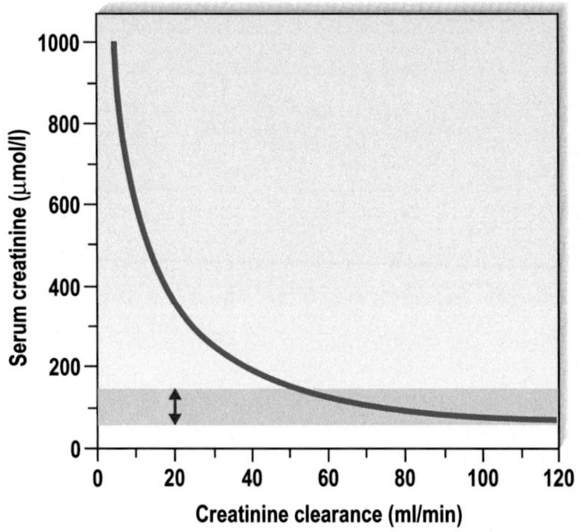

Figure 17.9 Relationship between creatinine clearance and plasma creatinine concentrations. The normal range of serum creatinine concentration can be maintained only when the renal creatinine clearance is greater than about 60 ml/min. The red area represents the normal range of creatinine concentration.

Table 17.5 Estimation of GFR formulae	
Cockcroft and Gault	Male GFR = [1.23 × weight (kg) × (140 – age)]/creatinine
	Female GFR = [1.03 × weight (kg) × (140 – age)]/creatinine
Modification of Diet in Renal Disease	GFR = 186 × Pcr – 1.154 × age – 0.203 × 1.212 (if black) × 0.742 (if female)

Pcr, plasma creatinine in mg/dl.

details of these are given in Table 17.4. The most frequently used surrogates, and also the crudest ones, are the plasma urea and plasma creatinine concentrations. Both compounds are produced endogenously (at an inconstant rate in the case of urea) and excreted by glomerular filtration. Neither is particularly accurate when used to establish the absolute level of glomerular filtration in an individual patient, although the plasma creatinine concentration is certainly very useful when used to follow changes in an individual patient's renal function, especially when the GFR is significantly reduced (Fig. 17.9). Creatinine clearance is more precise but requires a 24-hour urine collection with measurements of plasma creatinine concentration and urine creatinine excretion rate. The clearance is then calculated using the simple formula UV/P where U equals the urinary concentration of creatinine, V the urinary flow rate (usually expressed in ml/min) and P equals the plasma creatinine concentration. This formula can be applied to urea or to any other compound subject to renal excretion. Only those compounds that are freely filtered at the glomerulus and neither secreted nor reabsorbed by the renal tubules are suitable for GFR measurement.

The use of mathematical formulae to estimate GFR has been gaining in popularity, as most of these calculations require simple information such as the age, sex, weight and serum creatinine to derive an estimated GFR (Table 17.5). Precise measures of GFR used in clinical practice depend on measurement of the excretion of certain administered compounds. The most commonly used is ^{51}Cr-EDTA, which gives a relatively easy and reproducible measure of GFR. It should be remembered that the GFR peaks at 20-25 years of age and at about 120 ml/min and declines steadily thereafter at a rate of approximately 1 ml/min/year. Appreciation of this age-related change in GFR is important in clinical practice, particularly when prescribing drugs to the elderly.

Measurement of renal tubular function

The two tests most frequently utilized are:

1 Tests of renal concentrating ability when investigating possible causes of polyuria.
2 Tests of renal acidification in patients with metabolic acidosis and possible underlying renal tubular acidosis.

Renal concentrating ability involves treating the patient in a way that should lead to the production of a concentrated urine. Water deprivation is the most common provocation, and after 12 hours the urine osmolality should be at least 750 mmol/kg (specific gravity 1.020). Failure to concentrate the urine in these circumstances indicates either impairment of vasopressin output (pituitary diabetes insipidus) or resistance of the renal tubules to the action of vasopressin (nephrogenic diabetes insipidus). These two possibilities may be distinguished by measuring the urine osmolality after an injection of vasopressin (or an analogue) when the urine osmolality should increase to at least 750 mmol/kg.

Renal tubular acidification can be assumed to be adequate if the pH of a random specimen of urine is below 5.5. Urine pH >5.5 in the presence of metabolic acidosis usually indicates renal tubular acidosis. If the patient is only minimally acidotic and the urine pH is >5.5, a provocative test, in which ammonium chloride is given at a dose of 0.1 g/kg body weight to provide an acid load and an acute mild metabolic acidosis, can be performed. The pH should fall to <5.4 if acidification is normal.

Assessment of the urine in the stone-forming patient

Assessment of urine in a stone-forming patient involves measurement of the important constituents of stone whose outputs may be abnormally increased and also measurement of at least one of the natural inhibitors of stone formation. Ideally this should be combined with analysis of the stone itself. The tests that should be undertaken in all stone patients are:

- Plasma calcium, phosphate, alkaline phosphatase, urea, urate, creatinine and electrolytes.
- 24-hour urine collection for simultaneous measurement of:
  - calcium
  - uric acid
  - oxalate
  - citrate
  - creatinine
  - sodium.
- Nitroprusside test for cystine.

The identification of increased excretion rates of calcium, uric acid, oxalate or cystine indicates a strong predisposition to recurrent stone formation. Conversely, citrate is a natural inhibitor of stone formation, and a low urine citrate is associated with increased stone risk. All patients who make radiopaque stones should be screened for cystinuria using the nitroprusside test. If hypercalciuria or hypercalcaemia are noted, then the parathyroid and serum angiotensin-converting enzyme should also be measured.

Kidney biopsy

Kidney biopsy, in which one or two small cores of renal cortex are removed using a needle-biopsy technique, is performed in patients in whom diffuse renal parenchymal disease is suspected. However, not everyone with renal parenchymal disease requires a biopsy. The procedure is invasive and carries a small but definite risk of serious complications. It is therefore important to define the indications and contraindications carefully. The risk of the procedure can be minimized by the following preconditions:

- A cooperative patient
- Prior knowledge of the position and size of both kidneys (usually provided by ultrasound)
- A solitary functioning kidney should only be biopsied if the diagnostic yield is deemed to be crucial or to exclude malignancy
- Absence of a bleeding disorder
- Availability of blood for transfusion in the event of haemorrhage
- An appropriate indication

Kidney biopsy is often the only way to distinguish the various forms of glomerulonephritis, both from one another and from tubulointerstitial diseases of the kidney.

Imaging of the urinary tract

Plain radiographs

In many people, one or both of the kidneys can be seen outlined by perirenal fat on plain abdominal films or nephrotomograms. The information gleaned is limited, although certain types of renal stone or other calcifications may be identified.

Ultrasound

Ultrasound provides good images of the renal parenchyma and collecting system, and in nearly all patients gives a reliable estimate of renal size as well as identifies discrete lesions within the parenchyma, hydronephrosis and stone. Doppler studies often permit assessment of blood flow in the main renal arteries and in the larger intrarenal branches. The resistive index, measured by Doppler ultrasound, indicates the degree of chronic intrarenal ischaemic injury. Although the upper ureter can be seen quite well in most patients, the lower ureter is not adequately visualized. Ultrasound examination of the bladder is also extremely useful, allowing calculation of the bladder capacity when full and also after micturition (emptying should be virtually complete), as well as visualization of the bladder wall and lesions projecting into the bladder itself (e.g. tumours). It can be combined with a measurement of urinary flow rate along with post micturition residual to assess the efficiency of micturition and bladder emptying in patients with lower urinary tract symptoms (LUTS) or incontinence.

Intravenous urography

Intravenous urography (IVU) involves the intravenous injection of organic iodine compounds that are excreted and concentrated radiographically. It is an extremely good technique for examining the renal collecting system, the ureters and the bladder, but gives less information than ultrasound about the renal parenchyma (Fig. 17.10). Imaging by IVU depends on renal function. This is useful in that it gives a crude

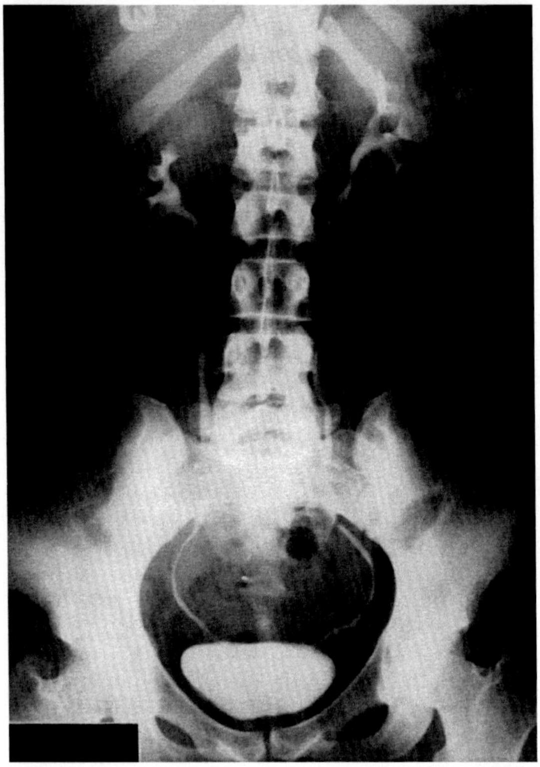

Figure 17.10 Normal excretion urogram. In this film, taken 15 minutes after intravenous injection of the iodine-based contrast medium, the calyces of both kidneys, the ureters and the bladder can be seen.

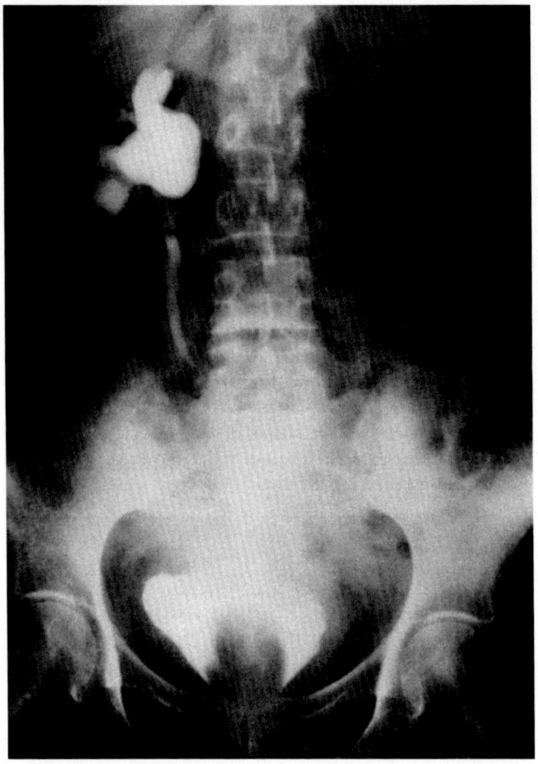

Figure 17.11 Excretion urogram. In this film, made 30 minutes after injection of contrast, the left kidney fails to excrete a detectable concentration of contrast (non-functioning left kidney) and the right kidney shows dilated, hydronephrotic calyces. The right ureter is partially obstructed at the level of the body of the fifth lumbar vertebra. The circular lucency in the bladder is the dilated balloon of a Foley catheter.

measure of the symmetry, or otherwise, of excretory capacity, but it also means that the image quality is poor in patients with renal insufficiency in whom the GFR is low (Fig. 17.11).

Antegrade and retrograde urography

In antegrade and retrograde urography X-ray contrast material is instilled directly into the urinary tract via a percutaneous needle (antegrade) or a ureteric catheter inserted via a cystoscope (retrograde). These tests are invasive and are most often used in the evaluation of patients with clear obstruction of the urinary tract.

Cystography

In cystography, the bladder is filled with contrast medium via a urethral catheter and X-rays are taken before, during and after micturition. The test indicates the completeness of bladder emptying, and also whether or not urine refluxes up the ureters during micturition. This also is an invasive test, the principal risk being the introduction of infection. Urodynamics (the measurement of pressure and urine flow) may be included in more detailed studies of bladder function.

Radionuclide studies

Diethylenetriamine penta-acetic acid (^{99}Tc-DTPA) is used to investigate the excretory function of each kidney selectively (Fig. 17.12). The test is very useful for the assessment of symmetry of function, delayed onset of excretion (as may happen in renal artery stenosis) and retention of excreted isotope (as seen in the presence of obstruction). ^{99}Tc-DMSA (dimercaptosuccinic acid) is a similar technique used to show the gross renal morphology. MAG3 (mercaptoacetyltriglycine) renogram can assess comparative function and demonstrate upper urinary tract obstruction.

Computed tomography and magnetic resonance imaging

Computed tomography scanning of the kidneys sometimes complements the information gained from ultrasound and certainly yields important information about the surrounding structures in the retroperitoneum (Fig. 17.13). It is particularly useful in patients

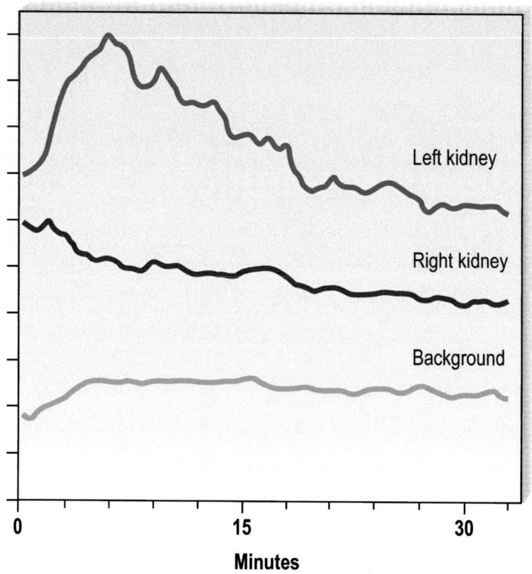

Figure 17.12 Radioisotope excretion (ordinate) during the 30 minutes after intravenous injection in a patient with right renal artery stenosis and hypertension. The left kidney achieves more rapid excretion of isotope. The malfunctioning right kidney was the cause of the patient's hypertension.

with ureteric obstruction from, for example, retroperitoneal malignancy or retroperitoneal fibrosis. Spiral CT is becoming the investigation of choice for renal calculi as well. Triple-phase CT is used to discriminate malignant renal tumours from benign ones. In some cases, more information is obtained using magnetic resonance imaging (MRI). Caution has to be exercised, however, if gadolinium is required, as its use has been associated with nephrogenic systemic fibrosis in patients with renal disease. Current data suggest an increased risk of this condition in patients with a GFR below 30 ml/min.

Arteriography and venography

Arteriography and venography are both invasive and are used in selected patients in whom detailed evaluation of the renal blood supply (arterial or venous) is required. The commonest indication is the patient with hypertension and/or renal insufficiency in whom renal artery stenosis is suspected. In the context of renal insufficiency, contrast-induced deterioration of function is often see, but can usually be minimized by adequate prehydration and the use of non-ionic contrast agents. MRI can be used to generate images of the major renal vasculature. Although the images are generally not as good as those from conventional arteriography, the technique has the advantage of avoiding contrast nephropathy and of being non-invasive. CT imaging may also be used in this way but still requires some contrast.

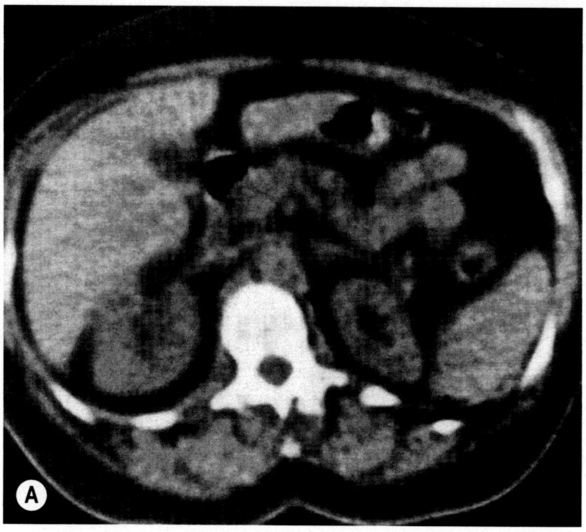

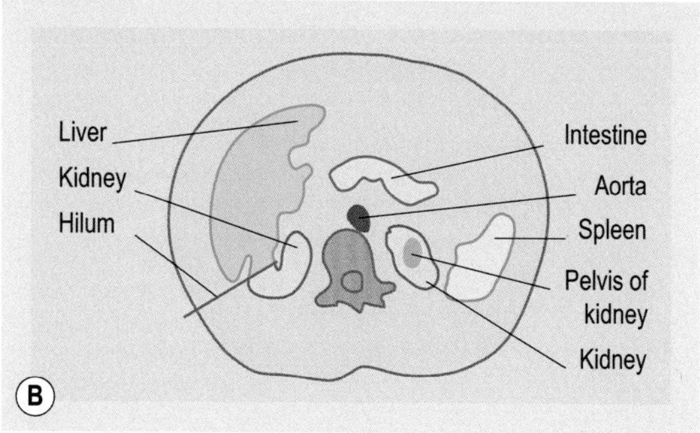

Figure 17.13 **(A)** CT scan with **(B)** drawing showing normal kidneys.

Sexually transmitted infections

Introduction

In this section we will cover the main principles of sexually transmitted infection (STI) management including history, examination and infection management as well as important and common non-infective conditions that can affect the genitals and mimic STI.

There are two main principles in the management of STI. First, an infected patient implies that at least one other person is also infected. Anyone who has had sexual contact with the index patient could be infected; this includes monogamous partners, babies and victims of sexual assault and abuse. Thus, treating a patient in isolation will not control the spread of these infections. Second, a patient may harbour more than one sexually transmitted infection (Box 17.3). Many infections are asymptomatic, acquired months or even years previously. Stigma and shame are often associated with STI and patients are often uncomfortable or embarrassed to give their sexual history or a history of genitourinary symptoms. Therefore, maintaining confidentiality is key.

Box 17.3 Sexually transmitted/microbial agents in the genital tract (diseases)

Bacteria

- *Treponema pallidum* (syphilis)
- *Neisseria gonorrhoeae* (gonorrhoea)
- *Chlamydia trachomatis* of D-K serovars (non-gonococcal urethritis)
- *Chlamydia trachomatis* of LGV 1-3 serovars (lymphogranuloma venereum)
- *Haemophilus ducreyi* (chancroid)
- *Mycoplasma genitalium* (non-gonococcal urethritis)
- *Klebsiella granulomatis* (donovanosis/granuloma inguinale)
- *Gardnerella vaginalis*, anaerobes, e.g. *Mobiluncus*, *Bacteroides*, *Atopobium vaginae*, bacterial vaginosis-associated bacteria 1-3, *Leptotrichia*, *Sneathia* species (bacterial vaginosis)
- *Shigella* species (shigellosis)
- *Salmonella* species (salmonellosis)

Viruses

- Herpes simplex virus types 1 and 2 (genital herpes)
- Human papilloma virus (genital warts)
- *Molluscum contagiosum* virus (molluscum contagiosum)
- Human immunodeficiency virus (AIDS and related diseases)
- Hepatitis A, B, C and delta viruses
- Cytomegalovirus

Fungal

- *Candida albicans* (thrush/moniliasis/candidiasis/candidosis)

Ectoparasites

- *Phthirus pubis* (pediculosis pubis)
- *Sarcoptes scabiei* (scabies)

Protozoa

- *Trichomonas vaginalis* (trichomoniasis)
- *Entamoeba histolytica* (amoebiasis)
- *Giardia lamblia* (giardiasis)

Nematodes

- *Enterobius vermicularis* (enterobiasis)

History taking and examination must be carried out in private, confidentially and using non-judgemental attitude and language.

Diagnosis is achieved by taking a good history (Box 17.4) and examination and performing the relevant laboratory tests. Effective treatment and partner notification/contact tracing should be instituted promptly. In children under 16 years of age, ensure they are able to understand the clinical process (follow the Fraser's guidelines in the UK) and that any child safeguarding issues are managed appropriately (via children safeguarding team).

Box 17.4 History in sexually transmitted infection

- Urethral discharge
- Dysuria
- Urinary frequency
- Vaginal discharge
- Dyspareunia
- Genital ulcer
- Painful scrotal swelling
- Pubic genital itch
- Genital rash
- Anorectal symptoms

History

Taking a sexual history has many similarities with that of any other medical history in that the clinician needs to ask about systemic symptoms, past medical history, medication and allergies, etc. There are also some very basic differences, including that the presenting history is commonly genital symptoms and the questions are about a very private part of peoples' lives. Therefore, its important that thorough histories of presenting complaint and sexual activity are taken. A non-judgemental tone and attitude are essential to allow the patient to give an accurate history. Starting with neutral questions such as presenting complaint and past medical history allows the clinician to establish a rapport with the patient

Sexual history includes taking details of when the sexual activity took place, the gender of the partner(s) and sexual activity itself (e.g. vaginal, oral, anal sex;

mutual masturbation; use of sex toys, etc), whether the patient was the active or receptive partner for these activities or both and whether any barrier protection (condom) was used. These questions need to be asked for each of their sexual partners. The time frame the sexual history usually covers is the last 3 months unless the infection has a much longer incubation period/ asymptomatic phase, e.g. late latent syphilis or HIV.

The type of sexual practice will dictate the sites from which to take tests. Familiarity with the colloquial words for common sexual practices is useful to allow the patient to use his own words when giving the sexual history. 'Straight sex' indicates heterosexual (penovaginal) intercourse, oroanal intercourse ('rimming') more commonly in men who have sex with men, insertive or receptive brachioanal intercourse ('fisting') and, rarely, urinating onto each other ('watersports') or using faeces during intercourse ('scat'). 'Bare backing' is unprotected anal intercourse; 'cottaging' is sexual intercourse in public places.

Sex 'toys' or 'dildos' (artificial penises) are objects inserted into the rectum or vagina. 'Fisting' and 'toys' may cause injury presenting as an acute abdomen. 'Bondage', in which the person is tied up during sex, may be associated with masochism (sexual gratification through the infliction of pain on another). This should be considered if superficial injuries are present without an obvious cause.

The partners' sexual health risks should be assessed as much as possible; asking if the partner has any genitourinary symptoms or STI, is from a high-risk country for HIV infection or is an injecting drug user, etc will help assess the risks of the patient of any STI.

Sexually transmitted infections can have extragenital manifestations, making a systematic review relevant in some cases. Examples include unilateral kerato-conjunctivitis with gonococcal, chlamydial and herpes infections and bilateral kerato-conjunctivitis in Reiter's disease, joint involvement in gonorrhoea, syphilis and Reiter's disease, lower abdominal pain with PID and right upper quadrant pain with Fitzhugh-Curtis syndrome.

With increasing awareness of STI and HIV, a significant number of patients attend for asymptomatic sexual health screens. This presents a good opportunity to educate the patient around safe sex, STI prevention and effective contraception to prevent unplanned pregnancies.

Presenting symptoms

Male

The most common symptoms men complain of are urethral discharge, dysuria, frequency and testicular pain. The important aspects would be the duration and timing of the symptoms. It is important to exclude other conditions that can have the same symptoms but are not STI; e.g. skin inflammation causing dysuria or physiological prostatic secretions seen as early morning urethral discharge. Ensure that the discharge is from the urethra and not from under the foreskin and that the urinary frequency is not secondary to urinary tract infection or physiological conditions such as irritable bladder syndrome or anxiety.

Common STI can be complicated by epididymo-orchitis presenting with scrotal swelling and pain. It is important to exclude testicular torsion and hernia strangulation which are surgical emergencies.

Acute epididymo-orchitis in those under 35 years old is likely due to gonococcal or chlamydial infection and in those over 40 to a bacterial urinary tract infection such as caused by *Escherichia coli*. Testicular pain is not a common presentation of testicular cancer.

Erectile dysfunction and loss of libido are common presentations that can be a significant cause of anxiety for the patient. These are not normally secondary to an STI and tend to be due to other factors including psychological, e.g. anxiety and stress or general medical conditions, e.g. diabetes.

Female

The most common symptoms women complain of are vaginal discharge or a change in the vagina discharge and dyspareunia. The history should include duration and timing of symptoms as well as a menstrual and basic obstetric history, including contraception, to ascertain risk of pregnancy.

Many women have a physiological discharge that is not offensive or itchy and is normal for them. This physiological discharge may increase in pregnancy or during sexual arousal.

The presence of an offensive odour may indicate bacterial vaginosis or *Trichomonas vaginalis* or a retained foreign body, e.g. tampons.

The commonest cause of an itchy discharge is candidal infection (thrush) or a physiological discharge in the presence of an itchy dermatitis, e.g. eczema or lichen sclerosus.

Common STI causes of vaginal discharge include gonococcal, chlamydial or herpetic infections of the cervix (Fig. 17.14).

Dyspareunia is pain during sexual intercourse. Pain can be deep or superficial. Deep dyspareunia is usually caused by pelvic pathology including pelvic inflammatory disease (PID), endometritis and ovarian pathology. PID is treated with antibiotics and the other conditions are managed by the gynaecology team.

Superficial dyspareunia caused by vulvitis must be differentiated from vulvodynia, which is localized vulval tenderness or pain not always associated with sexual intercourse and can be multifactorial in origin. Women with vulvodynia may need management from the multidisciplinary team including specialist psychology and physiotherapy input.

Both male and female patients

There are some presentations that are common to both sexes including anogenital ulceration (also known

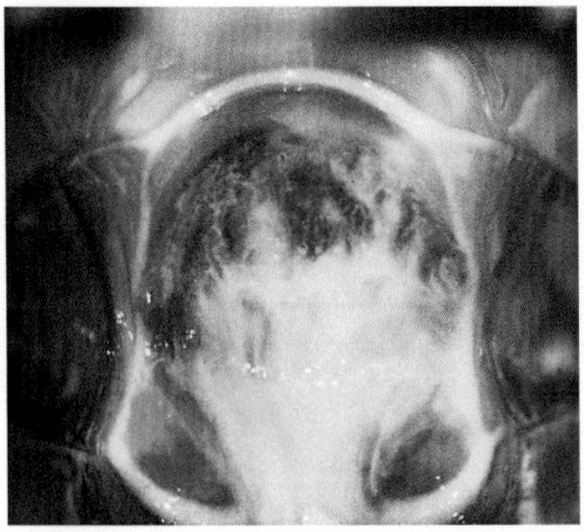

Figure 17.14 Mucopurulent cervicitis caused by *Chlamydia trachomatis.*

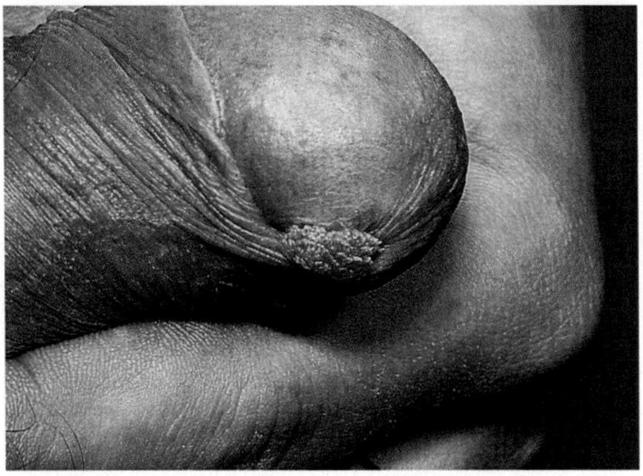

Figure 17.16 Genital wart on the frenum of the penis.

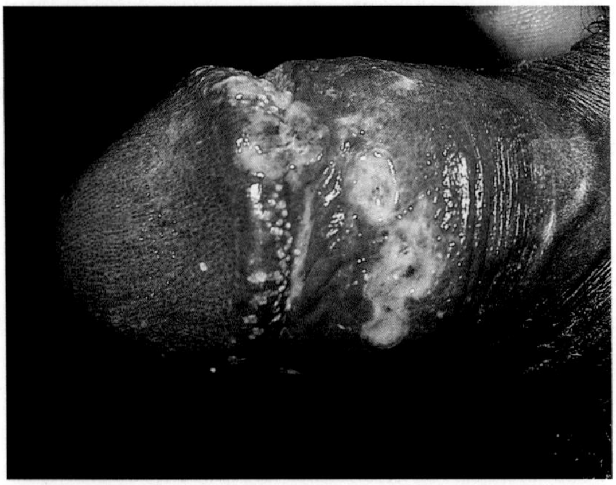

Figure 17.15 Acute ulcers of primary genital herpes. Both herpes simplex virus types I and II can cause genital herpes.

as sores), pubic or genital itch, lumps and anorectal symptoms.

In general, anogenital ulceration is due to herpes (Fig. 17.15) or syphilis unless proven otherwise.

Painful anogenital ulcerations, especially if recurrent, are most commonly due to herpes simplex infections. Other causes include trauma, chancroid and Behcet's disease.

Painless ulcers are most commonly due to syphilis infection, though occasionally syphilitic chancres can be painful when a secondary bacterial infection is present.

If the infection is acquired in a tropical country, then chancroid, lymphogranuloma venereum and donovanosis should also be considered.

In recent years lymphogranuloma venereum has become endemic in MSM but is more likely to present as a proctitis rather than an ulcer.

Pubic and genital itch is usually due to pediculosis pubis, scabies or other inflammatory genital conditions, such as allergic dermatitis, but may be psychological or be due to lichen simplex.

Similar symptoms in sexual or household contacts indicate that an STI is more likely.

'Crabs' and nits on the hair shaft may be seen in patients with pediculosis pubis, allowing the appropriate treatment to be given quickly.

Itching secondary to scabies tends to be more generalized except for the face. Intradigital burrows and genital nodules may be seen in these cases, aiding the diagnosis.

If a genital rash is present, then dermatological conditions need to be considered. The most common conditions are eczema, psoriasis, lichen sclerosus, lichen simplex or a contact dermatitis

Lumps are a common presentation of genital warts (Fig. 17.16) or molluscum contagiosum but also of normal skin variants including penile pearly papules and epidermal cysts.

Anorectal symptoms include pain, soreness, itching, rectal discharge, change in bowel habit and other symptoms of proctitis. This may be the early presentation of a gastrointestinal or systemic condition such as Crohn's disease or ulcerative colitis. It may also be an infective proctitis resulting from herpes simplex, gonococcal, chlamydia D-K serovar or lymphogranuloma venereum infection. A careful history including details of sexual activity (especial unprotected anal sex) and other systematic symptoms is important.

Anal itch (pruritus ani) may be secondary to rectal discharge, anal warts, perianal dermatitis or poor anal hygiene. If the itch is worse at night, then threadworm infestation should be considered.

Special groups

Men who have sex with men (MSM)

MSM are at higher risk of a number of STI including rectal infections (associated with receptive anal intercourse), HIV and viral hepatitides especially hepatitis B and C. These risks are increased when recreational drugs are used (via the nasal, oral, rectal and intravenous routes) to enhance the sexual experience (chemsex). With this in mind, the history taken should include history of chemsex, route the drugs were administered as well as previous testing for these viral infections and previous vaccination for hepatitis A and B.

Additional investigations may be needed from MSM including Gram-stained smears from the rectum and cultures from the rectum and throat to exclude gonorrhoea. In cases of proctitis, cultures or NAAT for herpes simplex and *Chlamydia trachomatis* of both D-K and LGV serovars may be indicated.

MSM with diarrhoea should have their stools examined for giardia, amoebas, shigella and salmonella and, if HIV infection is suspected, other causes of HIV-related diarrhoea should be looked for.

Screening for blood-borne viruses (HIV, Hep B, Hep C) and syphilis is important, with prompt treatment or vaccination as appropriate.

Very recently, there has been convincing evidence concerning the efficacy of post-exposure prophylaxis (PEP) and pre-exposure prophylaxis (PrEP) for HIV in this high-risk group. At the time of this writing, post-exposure prophylaxis is funded in the UK whilst pre-exposure prophylaxis is not, although funding has been approved in other countries in the developed world. The presence of these strategies could have very significant impact on the course of the HIV epidemic in the next few years.

Sex workers

Sex workers are a vulnerable group of people who are at higher risk of STI. Taking a thorough history is important and the sites screened would be dependent on the history elicited. Hepatitis screening and vaccination is indicated. Support to enable them to better negotiate safe sex and increasing awareness around safe sex practices and drug and alcohol dependence should be provided.

Young people

STI are more common in young people, as are unplanned pregnancies. Tests indicated are dependent on the history elicited. Support and information around safe sex practices, drug and alcohol dependence and contraception should be provided.

Its important to ensure that the young person understands what is being said and done in the clinical setting (i.e. Fraser competent) and is safe and not at any risk of coercion either at home or in the school environment. It is essential that children (under 18 years) are screened using an appropriate child safeguarding questionnaire. Any concerns raised should be discussed with the appropriate safeguarding team.

Genital examination

It is essential when performing genital examination that the patient understands and consents to the examination and that it takes place in a private well-lit room. Gloves should always be worn. Chaperones

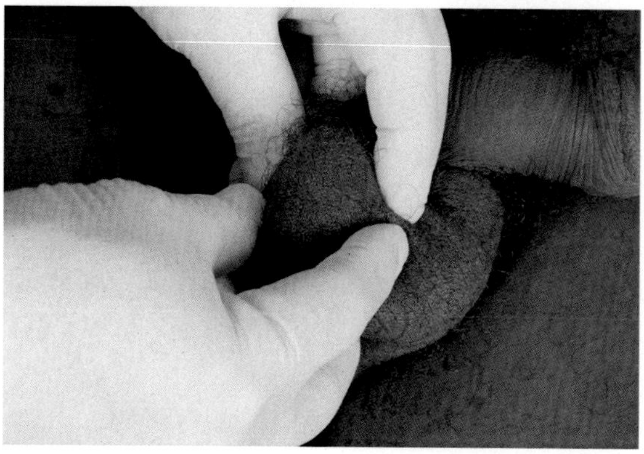

Figure 17.17 Palpation of the testis. Gloves should be worn.

should be offered, especially when female patients are being examined by male clinicians.

The examination should be systematic covering the whole of the genital area. The clinician should note any skin changes, colour, epidermal markings, fissures, ulcers, masses, tender areas, the presence of any discharge and its characteristics, e.g. frothy, purulent, clear etc. and any piercings or any other abnormalities seen.

Male examination

All the areas need to be examined, the skin (including perineum and perianal areas), pubis and inguinal areas (for lymphadenopathy), scrotum (including testis (Fig. 17.17), epididymis), penis (shaft, prepuce, glans and meatus). Anal, prostate and natal cleft examination including proctoscopy may be indicated by the history elicited.

Female examination

All the areas need to be examined, including the skin (including the perineum and perianal areas), pubis, inguinal areas (for lymphadenopathy), labia majora, labia minora and vulva. Then speculum examination should be done to examine the vagina and cervix. Further bimanual examination of the pelvis, anal and natal cleft examination including proctoscopy may be indicated by the history elicited.

Tests and further management

With improving technology there has been a paradigm shift in STI testing. Nucleic acid amplification tests (NAAT) and point-of-care tests (POCT) with improved sensitivities and specificities have meant better and quicker diagnosis and therefore improved management of STI and partner notification, even in the most resource-poor areas of the world.

Currently we use a combination of microscopy, NAAT and antibody testing to perform a full sexual health screen. Point-of-care testing is also used, mainly for HIV. The two-glass test is now obsolete.

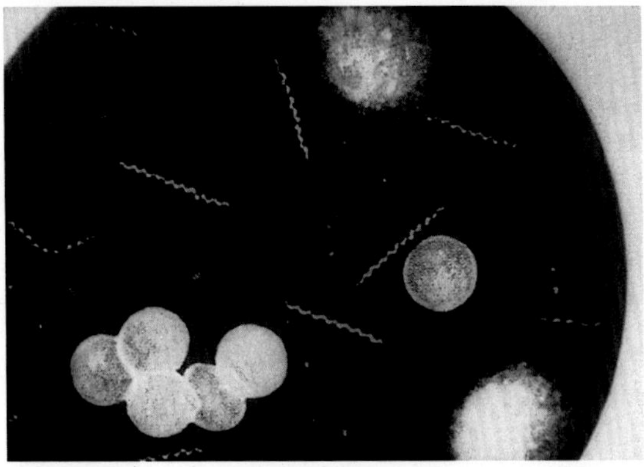

Figure 17.18 *Treponema pallidum* seen under the dark-field microscope. The spiral-like treponemes can be seen, together with red blood cells.

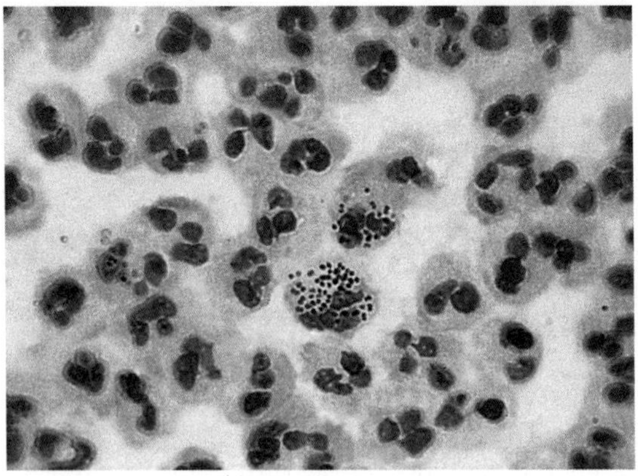

Figure 17.19 Gram-stained smear showing Gram-negative intracellular diplococci typical of *Neisseria gonorrhoeae*.

Box 17.5 Procedure for Gram staining

- Fix the smear on the slide by passing it through a flame twice
- Stain with 2% crystal violet for 30 seconds, then wash with tap water
- Stain with Gram's iodine for a further 30 seconds and wash with water
- Decolorize with acetone for a few seconds
- Wash with water and counterstain with 1% safranin for 10 seconds
- After a final wash with water, dry by pressing between filter paper

Near patient diagnosis, in the form of microscopy, is still important in patients with a discharge or a painless ulcer. To perform microscopy a sample of the discharge needs to be obtained using a loop or swab and smeared onto the slide, either dry or wet. The dry slide is Gram-stained for examination; the wet slide is not stained prior to examination.

Dark ground microscopy is used to diagnose primary syphilis chancre (Fig. 17.18).

Gram staining

The Gram-staining procedure is outlined in Box 17.5.

Urethral sample

If the patient has passed urine just before the test, the urethral smear may show no polymorphonuclear leukocytes because the urine will have washed out the accumulated urethral material. In such cases, the patient should be asked to re-attend for another urethral swab after having held urine for at least 2 hours. Gram-negative intracellular diplococci, which appear as opposing bean-shaped cocci within polymorphonuclear leukocytes under the microscope (Fig. 17.19), suggest gonococcal urethritis. The presence of five or more polymorphonuclear leukocytes per high-power field (×1000 magnification) with a negative test for gonococci indicates non-gonococcal urethritis (Box 17.6). The most common cause of non-gonococcal urethritis is *Chlamydia trachomatis*.

Box 17.6 Causes of non-gonococcal urethritis

Sexually transmitted diseases

- *Chlamydia trachomatis* D-K serovars (approximately 30%)
- *Mycoplasma genitalium* (approximately 30%)
- Unknown (up to 50%)
- *Trichomonas vaginalis*
- *Ureaplasma urealyticum*
- Herpes simplex virus
- Intrameatal warts
- Meatal chancre

Non-sexually transmitted diseases

- Bacterial urinary tract infection
- Tuberculosis
- Urethral stricture
- Stevens-Johnson syndrome
- Benign mucous membrane pemphigoid
- Chemical
- Trauma
- Others

A wet preparation, made by mixing urethral material using a loop with a drop of normal saline on a slide, can be examined by bright- or dark-field illumination for trichomonas, which appear as ovoid protozoa with beating flagellae and in jerky motion.

Vaginal sample

A vaginal sample is taken to look for the spores and pseudomycelia of thrush and for the absence of lactobacilli and the presence of mixed flora and 'clue cells' (Ison-Hay criteria), which are indicative of bacterial vaginosis. 'Clue cells' are vaginal epithelial cells covered with *Gardnerella vaginalis*, which are Gram-variable but mainly Gram-negative coccobacilli.

pH

A vaginal pH >4.5 using a litmus paper or strip is present in bacterial vaginosis and trichomoniasis.

Nucleic acid amplification testing

There are many different platforms for testing for infections using nucleic acid testing. There is a range of turnaround times and specimen delivery systems that allow samples to be taken from different sites (pharynx, urine, vagina, cervix and anal canal) and tested even if there is a long transport time. These advances have meant that testing hard-to-reach groups is more practical and the results more reliable.

NAAT is the mainstay of screening for *Neisseria gonorrhoea, Chlamydia trachomatis* and herpes simplex infections. Anyone found to be gonorrhoea positive on screen then needs samples sent for culture to ascertain antibiotic sensitivities. Recent studies have shown that self-taken vaginal samples are more sensitive and specific than cervical nucleic acid testing in women.

Worldwide nucleic acid testing is also used for screening for *Trichomonas vaginalis* and *Treponema pallidum* infections.

Culture

Culture is still used for STI testing, mainly in cases when the patient has a positive nucleic acid amplification test for gonorrhoea. The other time would be for speciation and sensitivity testing in patients with recurrent candidal infections.

Antibody testing

Antibody testing is the main screening method for the blood-borne viruses and *Treponema palladium* infections. These can be either by formal blood test or point-of-care testing. The advantages of point-of-care testing are being less invasive (finger prick or saliva testing), quick results (5-20 min). Any positive results need to be confirmed by formal blood test.

Serological tests for syphilis

There are two groups of serological tests for syphilis:

1. Non-specific/cardiolipin:
   - anticardiolipin antibody, such as Venereal Disease Research Laboratories (VDRL) and rapid plasma reagin (RPR).
2. Specific antitreponemal antibody tests:
   - treponemal enzyme immunoassay (EIA)
   - *T. pallidum* particle agglutination (TPPA)
   - *T. pallidum* haemagglutination (TPHA)
   - *T. pallidum* line immunoassay (LIA)
   - fluorescent treponemal antibody absorption (FTA-abs).

The titre of the non-specific tests indicates disease activity and is useful for following up patients, particularly those who have been treated for primary, secondary or early latent syphilis, when the test should become negative or sustain a greater than two-fold dilution or four-fold decrease in antibody titre within 6-12 months. After successful treatment of all stages of syphilis, the specific tests usually remain positive whereas the VDRL or RPR test may slowly revert to negative, but commonly remains positive in lower titre in late syphilis. A greater than two-fold dilution or four-fold increase in antibody titre following treatment indicates recrudescence or reinfection.

All patients should be screened for syphilis with serological tests using the treponemal EIA, TPPA or TPHA or combination of the VDRL/RPR and TPHA/TPPA. A positive EIA is confirmed with TPPA or TPHA (and vice versa) and a VDRL/RPR performed to assess activity. If syphilis is endemic, these tests should be repeated after 3 months if initial tests are negative. If primary syphilis is suspected, the EIA-IgM or FTA-abs IgM test is also performed, as this can be the first serological test to be positive, although any one or combination of treponemal tests may be positive. In babies with suspected congenital syphilis, the EIA-IgM or FTA-abs tests using an IgM conjugate should be requested because of passive transfer of maternal IgG antibodies across the placenta. Positive serological results must be confirmed by a second set of tests, but treatment should be started immediately in early infectious syphilis or in pregnant women while awaiting confirmation.

Endemic treponematoses, such as yaws, bejel and pinta, may result in positive serological tests for syphilis. It is not possible to differentiate the treponematoses by serological tests. Patients may recall having such infection, or there may be a history of being brought up in the countryside in endemic areas, with evidence of signs of such infection such as 'tissue-paper' scarring of the shins in yaws, which may suggest non-venereal treponematoses. However, there may be coinfection with syphilis, and it would be prudent to treat all positive treponemal serology as for syphilis.

Tropical infections

Tropical infections include donovanosis, lymphogranuloma venereum and chancroid.

The diagnosis of donovanosis is based upon the demonstration of Donovan bodies, which stain in a bipolar fashion giving a 'safety pin' appearance within the cytoplasm of mononuclear cells in a Giemsa-stained tissue smear. Tissue is obtained by infiltrating the edge of the ulcer with 1% lidocaine and removing a small piece from the edge, which is then smeared onto a glass slide or crushed between two glass slides. If chancroid or lymphogranuloma venereum is suspected, culture or NAAT for *Haemophilus ducreyi* and *Chlamydia trachomatis* of the lymphogranuloma venereum serovars, respectively, may be indicated using material obtained from the ulcer or bubo.

Further management

The diagnosis should be explained to the patient, antimicrobial treatment given according to current guidelines, partner notification done and advice given on risk reduction strategies for the future.

In the United Kingdom the British Association for Sexual Health and HIV (BASHH) guidelines are used. These can be found at www.bashh.org.

HIV infection

The worldwide spread of HIV infection has resulted in a dramatic lowering of life expectancy in some countries, especially in Africa. HIV infection is categorized as A, B and C (Box 17.7), based broadly on the clinical evolution of the immunodeficiency state that leads to the development of the acquired immune deficiency syndrome (AIDS), on average some 8-15 years after infection if untreated.

- Acute primary illness – with fever, malaise, lymphadenopathy, muscle pain and sore throat, often with an erythematous, maculopapular rash and headache. Night sweats, weight loss,

Box 17.7 Centre for Disease Control (CDC) HIV clinical categories

Category A: asymptomatic

- Acute infection
- Persistent generalized lymphadenopathy

Category B: symptomatic infection excluding category A

- Bacteria:
  - bacillary angiomatosis
  - listeriosis
- Candidiasis – oropharyngeal, vulvovaginal (persistent or resistant to therapy)
- Viral:
  - herpes zoster (≥2 episodes or >1 dermatome)
  - oral hairy leukoplakia
- Constitutional symptoms: fever (>38.5°C), diarrhoea >1 month
- Other:
  - cervical dysplasia – moderate or severe
  - idiopathic thrombocytopenic purpura
  - pelvic inflammatory disease
  - peripheral neuropathy

Category C: AIDS-defining illness

- Bacteria:
  - *Mycobacterium tuberculosis* – pulmonary, extrapulmonary
  - *Mycobacterium avium* complex, *M. kansasii* or other mycobacterial infection – disseminated or extrapulmonary disease
  - pneumonia – recurrent (≥2 episodes in 12 months)
  - *Salmonella* septicaemia, recurrent (non-typhoid)
- Fungal:
  - candidiasis – oesophagus, trachea, bronchi, lungs
  - coccidioidomycosis – disseminated or extrapulmonary
  - cryptococcosis – extrapulmonary
  - histoplasmosis – disseminated or extrapulmonary
  - *Pneumocystis jiroveci* pneumonia
- Helminth: strongyloidosis – extraintestinal
- Protozoal:
  - cryptosporidiosis – chronic intestinal (>1 month)
  - isosporiasis – chronic intestinal (>1 month)
  - toxoplasmosis of brain
- Viral:
  - cytomegalovirus infection (other than liver, spleen or lymph node)
  - HIV encephalopathy
  - wasting syndrome (involuntary weight loss >10% of baseline weight) associated with chronic diarrhoea (≥2 loose stools per day ≥1 month) or chronic weakness and documented fever ≥1 month
  - herpes simplex – chronic ulcers >1 month, bronchitis, pneumonitis, oesophagitis
  - progressive multifocal leukoencephalopathy
- Tumours:
  - cervical carcinoma, invasive
  - Kaposi's sarcoma
  - lymphoma – Burkitt's, immunoblastic or primary nervous system

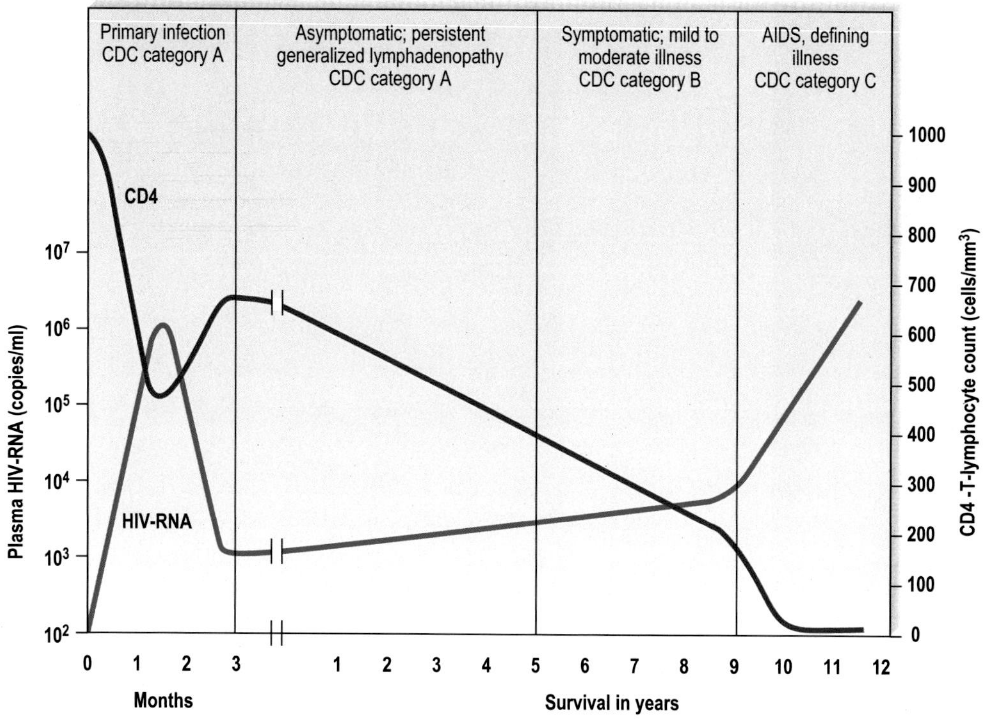

Figure 17.20 The clinical categories associated with untreated HIV infection and survival can be loosely correlated with the plasma HIV-RNA and circulating CD4 T-lymphocyte count. Treatment with antiretrovirals and prophylaxis for opportunistic infections increases survival and can prevent or delay the progression to AIDS.

diarrhoea, meningism, neuropathy and oral thrush may occur. There is HIV viraemia and severe immunosuppression, indicated by a high plasma HIV-RNA and a low CD4 T-lymphocyte count.

- Asymptomatic phase (category A) – following the acute infection (primary HIV or acute seroconversion infection), the patient may be asymptomatic, or there may be persistent lymphadenopathy; the HIV-RNA decreases and the CD4 T-lymphocyte count increases and stabilizes (Fig. 17.20) to a baseline level.
- Symptomatic phase (category B).
- AIDS-defining illnesses (category C) – especially opportunistic infections such as tuberculosis and *Pneumocystis jiroveci* pneumonia, and neoplasms such as Kaposi's sarcoma (Fig. 17.20) and lymphoma.

Assessment of the patient with HIV infection should cover the extent of the disease and its complications. Multisystem involvement is common, and in each system there may be multiple causes. Examination of the mouth and the skin may provide clues that a patient is immunosuppressed. Common chest infections include tuberculosis, *Pneumocystis* and other bacterial pneumonias. Common cerebral lesions include toxoplasmosis, tuberculoma, other bacterial or fungal abscesses and lymphoma. Diarrhoea may be caused by HIV, drug treatment or opportunistic infections. Antiretroviral drug therapy may itself cause serious complications (Fig. 17.21).

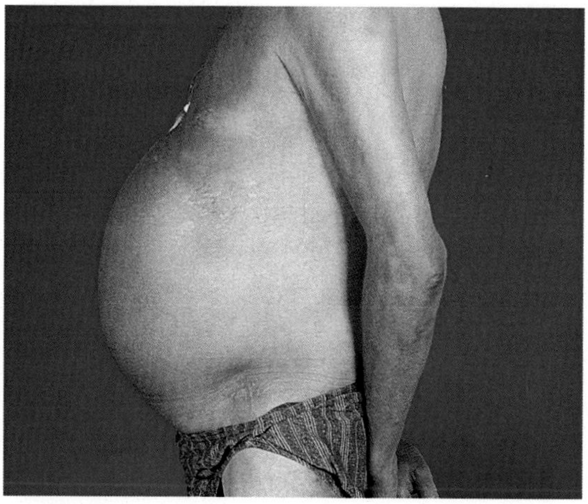

Figure 17.21 Lipodystrophy with abdominal adiposity and thin arm resulting from protease inhibitor treatment. Hyperlipidaemia and insulin resistance may be present.

In the United Kingdom up to 25% of those with HIV are unaware they have the infection and this percentage could be higher in other parts of the world. Late diagnosis, with CD4 counts below 200, are not uncommon. Multiple organ involvement and complex symptomatology is not uncommon, making systemic examination crucial.

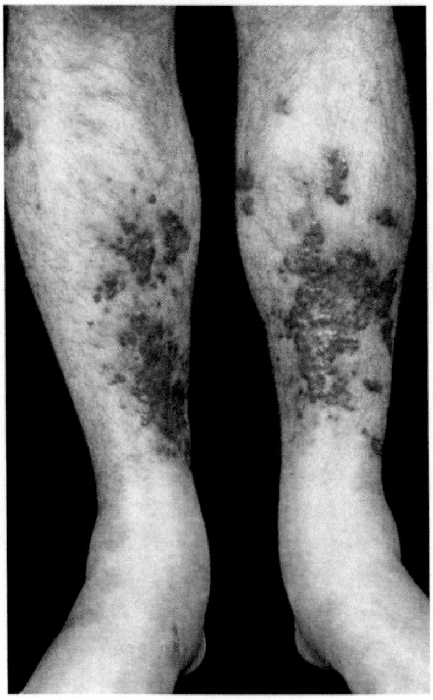

Figure 17.22 Kaposi's sarcoma of the lower legs with ankle oedema in a patient with AIDS.

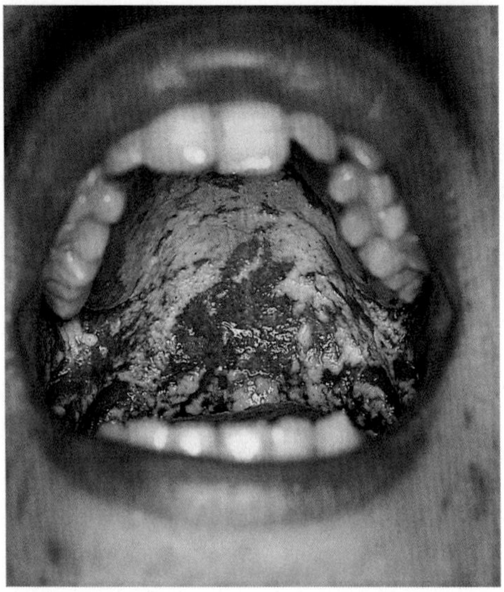

Figure 17.23 White plaques of oral candidiasis (which can be scraped off to reveal an erythematous base) in an HIV-positive patient.

Signs commonly seen in late HIV infection

- Kaposi's sarcoma Fig. 17.22
- oropharyngeal thrush Fig. 17.23

Blood tests done to assess an HIV-positive patient

- HIV viral load – to measure viral activity. This value should decrease to below the level of detection with effective treatment.
- CD4 count – to assess the patient's immune status. At CD4 counts below 200 the risk of AIDS-defining conditions is increased significantly. The CD4 count normally increases once the patient starts effective treatment.

Very recently there has been a consensus around the timing of HIV treatment initiation. The current guidelines say that HIV treatment with highly active antiretroviral therapy should be offered to anyone who is HIV positive and willing to take the lifelong medication. The exact combination offered will depend on the HIV genotype and resistance test results, HLA B5701 status, patient lifestyle factors and of course the affordability of these medications.

Mother-to-child transmission

Mother-to-child transmission can be kept at very low levels (<2%) by the appropriate medical interventions being put into place. These include treating the mother with highly active antiretroviral medication so that her viral load is undetectable at the time of delivery, ensuring the appropriate obstetric care is in place, giving the mother the appropriate advice around breast feeding and ensuring the baby gets the appropriate post-exposure prophylaxis.

As maternal HIV IgG crosses the placenta, the baby will need to be tested using HIV viral PCR to ensure that they are and remain HIV negative. The last test normally occurs when the baby is about 18 months old.

Further detailed guidelines are found at www.BHIVA.org.uk.

Endocrine and metabolic disorders

18

Tahseen A. Chowdhury and William M. Drake

Introduction

The endocrine system comprises the classic endocrine organs:

- Hypothalamus/pituitary
- Thyroid
- Parathyroid
- Adrenal
- Pancreatic islet cells
- Gonads

The mode of presentation of endocrine disorders does not fit neatly into a system-based model, the symptoms rarely being specific to a particular system. Frequently, endocrine disease is suggested by a constellation of non-specific symptoms.

The endocrine history

As in other systems, the history consists of presenting symptoms, the history of the development of the illness and the family history.

Presenting symptoms

There are a number of symptom complexes that particularly suggest endocrine disease.

Thirst and polyuria

Excessive thirst (polydipsia) and increased urine output (polyuria) are the most important presenting symptoms of diabetes mellitus; these are discussed in detail below. Polydipsia and polyuria may also be due to impairment of renal concentrating capacity as a result of a deficiency of antidiuretic hormone (cranial diabetes insipidus) or a failure of antidiuretic hormone action (nephrogenic diabetes insipidus). The latter may be inherited or may occur secondary to impairment of antidiuretic hormone action by hypercalcaemia or hypokalaemia. Sometimes apparent polydipsia and polyuria may be due to increased fluid intake, which at its most extreme may be vastly excessive (psychogenic polydipsia). The distinction between psychogenic polydipsia and diabetes insipidus is important. Generally, nocturnal polyuria is not a feature of psychogenic polydipsia, but this is not an absolute distinction and further investigation of urine concentrating capacity is usually required.

Weight loss

Loss of weight is a feature of decreased food intake or increased metabolic rate. Sometimes both factors may operate to reduce body weight, as in the cachexia of malignant disease. Thyroid overactivity (hyperthyroidism) is nearly always associated with a combination of unintentional or effortless weight loss and increased appetite, although occasionally the latter may be stimulated more than the former so that there is a paradoxical increase in weight. Weight loss is rarely the sole presenting symptom of hyperthyroidism and other clinical features often predominate, particularly in younger patients (Box 18.1). In the elderly, however, hyperthyroidism may be occult or may simulate the gradual weight loss of malignant disease. Cardiac arrhythmias are a frequent feature in the elderly. Anorexia nervosa, a psychogenic disorder characterized by a long history of low body weight in the absence of other features of ill health, must be considered, especially in young women. Any form of weight loss may be associated with amenorrhoea.

Other endocrine conditions in which weight loss is a major feature are listed in Box 18.2.

Weight gain or redistribution

An increase in body weight (Box 18.3) is a predictable result of a reduction in metabolic rate. Weight gain is therefore a common feature of primary hypothyroidism. However, obesity is rarely a consequence of specific endocrine dysfunction, an exception being the very rare phenomenon of leptin deficiency. In the majority of patients, 'simple obesity' is due to a long-standing imbalance between energy intake and expenditure; it frequently begins in childhood and is often present in more than one family member. Glucocorticoid hormone excess (Cushing's syndrome) results in an increase in body fat predominantly involving abdominal, omental and interscapular fat (truncal obesity), with paradoxical thinning of the limbs due to muscle atrophy.

Box 18.1 Clinical features of hyperthyroidism

- Tachycardia
- Atrial fibrillation/heart failure
- Eye signs
- Lid lag
- Lid retraction
- Exophthalmos (Graves' disease)
- Sweating
- Thyroid gland enlargement and bruit (Graves' disease)
- Fine distal tremor
- Thinning of hair
- Proximal weakness; cannot rise from squat
- Chorea

Box 18.2 Endocrine and metabolic diseases in which weight loss is a clinical feature

- Hyperthyroidism
- Type 1 diabetes mellitus
- Hypopituitarism
- Adrenocortical failure (Addison's disease)
- Anorexia nervosa

Box 18.3 Conditions in which increased body weight is a feature

- Simple obesity: energy intake/expenditure imbalance
- Primary hypothyroidism
- Cushing's syndrome
- Hypothalamic lesions
- Leptin deficiency

Box 18.4 Conditions in which metabolic myopathy is a feature

Painless

- Hyperthyroidism
- Cushing's syndrome, including iatrogenic steroid myopathy
- Acromegaly

Painful

- Vitamin D deficiency
- Osteomalacia
- Hypothyroidism

Muscle weakness

Symptomatic muscular weakness not due to neurological disease is a feature of several metabolic disorders, including thyrotoxicosis, Cushing's syndrome and vitamin D deficiency. In all these conditions, the metabolic myopathy (Box 18.4) causes symmetrical proximal weakness, mainly involving the shoulder and hip girdle musculature. There is usually associated muscle wasting. The major symptom is difficulty in climbing stairs, boarding a bus or rising from a sitting position. Most patients with hyperthyroidism have proximal weakness. This may be subclinical; it is best demonstrated by asking the patient to rise from the squatting position. The proximal myopathy of vitamin D deficiency is often painful, in contrast to other causes. The differential diagnosis of painful proximal muscular weakness includes polymyositis and polymyalgia rheumatica, as well as spinal root or plexus disease.

Box 18.5 Conditions in which temperature intolerance is a feature

- Intolerance to cold: hypothyroidism
- Intolerance to heat: hyperthyroidism

Box 18.6 Clinical features of hypothyroidism

- Weight gain
- Sallow complexion and dry skin
- Thinning of scalp and lateral eyebrow hair
- Cold intolerance
- Deepened, gruff voice
- Slow physical and mental activity
- Unsteadiness and slightly slurred speech
- Tingling in toes and fingers
- Aching muscles with cramp
- Mild proximal weakness
- Slow pulse and shortness of breath

Cold intolerance

An abnormal sensation of cold, out of proportion to that experienced by other individuals, may indicate underlying hypothyroidism (Boxes 18.5 and 18.6). This symptom differs from the localized vasomotor symptoms in the hands found in Raynaud's phenomenon and is rather non-specific, especially in the elderly.

Heat intolerance

The increased metabolic rate of thyrotoxicosis may be associated with heat intolerance in which, at its most extreme, the patient is comfortable at an ambient temperature that others find unpleasantly cold. This is an important symptom, highly specific for thyroid overactivity, which may partly explain some of the seasonal variation in presentation of the condition.

Increased sweating

Hyperhidrosis (excessive sweating) may be a constitutional abnormality, characterized by onset in childhood or adolescence and sometimes by a family history. A recent increase in sweat secretion, on the other hand, may be an early indication of thyroid overactivity. Paroxysmal sweating is a common feature of anxiety. Increased catecholamine secretion from a phaeochromocytoma of the adrenal medulla is a rare cause of hyperhidrosis. Intermittent sweating after meals (gustatory hyperhidrosis) may occur in patients with autonomic dysfunction. Growth hormone excess (acromegaly) also increases sweating, perhaps because of hypertrophy of the sweat glands, and this feature can be used to assess the activity of the disease in the clinic. Increased sweating should be distinguished from flushing that occurs physiologically at the time of the natural menopause. Flushing may be a presenting feature of serotonin-secreting carcinoid tumours of the gut and usually indicates extensive disease with hepatic metastases.

Tremor

A fine rapid resting tremor is one of the cardinal clinical features of thyrotoxicosis. This must be distinguished from the coarser and more irregular tremor of anxiety, which is usually associated with a cool peripheral skin temperature, in contrast to the warm skin of the thyrotoxic patient. Tremor due to neurological disease is greater in amplitude, slower in rate, and may be present at rest, as in Parkinson's disease, or on movement, as in cerebellar tremor. It therefore rarely simulates thyrotoxic tremor. Essential tremor is not so rapid as thyrotoxic tremor, is variable and is worse in certain postures. It often involves the head and neck.

Palpitations

Palpitations are a heightened, unpleasant awareness of the heart beat. They may be a feature of thyrotoxicosis but are more likely to be due to anxiety. Awareness of the heartbeat while lying down is normal. Other causes of rapid heart rate include paroxysmal tachyarrhythmias. The sensation of intermittent forceful cardiac contraction, sometimes described by the patient as a missed beat, is often due to a compensatory pause following an ectopic beat and is usually a normal phenomenon.

Postural unsteadiness

Dizziness, or a sensation of faintness on standing, should prompt measurement of lying and standing blood pressure. Postural hypotension, a fall of diastolic blood pressure on standing, occurs with reduced blood volume. In the absence of obvious bleeding or gastrointestinal fluid loss, adrenal insufficiency should be considered. Postural hypotension is frequently due to autonomic neuropathy, especially in long-standing diabetes mellitus. It is also a common complication of any drug therapy for essential hypertension. The drug history is particularly important in the elderly patient with dizziness.

Visual disturbance

Several endocrine conditions may cause visual symptoms. Decreased visual acuity may be due to space-occupying lesions compressing the optic nerve. For example, severe dysthyroid eye disease and orbital or retro-orbital tumours may present in this way. Bitemporal hemianopia (bilateral loss of part or all of the temporal fields of vision), often asymmetrical or incongruous, is a major feature of suprasellar extension of pituitary adenomas compressing the optic chiasm but may occur in other tumours in this location. Double vision (diplopia) on lateral or upward gaze often results from medial or lateral rectus muscle tethering in dysthyroid eye disease. Apparent magnification of vision (macropsia) can occur in hypoglycaemia.

Fasting symptoms

Tachycardia, sweating and tremor occurring intermittently, especially when fasting, are suggestive of hypoglycaemia. These symptoms resemble those associated with the increased sympathetic drive found in states of fear or with excess secretion of noradrenaline (norepinephrine), as in phaeochromocytoma. In severe persistent hypoglycaemia, these symptoms may progress to decreased consciousness. This is a serious emergency implying neuroglycopenia sufficient to impair brain function. Spontaneous or fasting hypoglycaemia can be due to the following:

- Autonomous insulin production due to an insulinoma
- Glucocorticoid deficiency, with or without thyroxine and growth hormone deficiency (e.g. primary adrenal failure or hypopituitarism)
- Inappropriate insulin or excessive sulphonylurea drug administration in a diabetic patient
- Rarer causes of hypoglycaemia, for example hepatic failure and rapidly growing malignant lesions, especially thoracic or retroperitoneal mesothelial tumours secreting proinsulin-like growth factor II

Cramps and 'pins and needles'

Intermittent cramps and 'pins and needles' (paraesthesiae), especially if bilateral, can be due to a decreased level of circulating ionized calcium. This may occur in hypoparathyroidism or be associated with a fall in the ionized component of serum calcium because of an increased extracellular pH (alkalosis). The latter may occur with any alkalosis but is particularly well recognized in hyperventilatory states (respiratory alkalosis) and hypokalaemia (metabolic alkalosis). Refractory cramping symptoms after correction of hypocalcaemia can be due to an associated hypomagnesaemia. However, the differential diagnosis of paraesthesiae in the hands includes median nerve compression at the wrist (carpal tunnel syndrome), a syndrome that is usually accompanied by typical sensory and motor disturbance suggestive of a lesion in the median nerve (see Ch. 16).

Nausea

This is a rare symptom of endocrine disease. It is an important presenting feature of adrenal insufficiency, in which typically it is maximal in the morning and may be associated with vomiting. Similar symptoms may occur with severe hypercalcaemia and may be the sole manifestation of this condition. These two conditions should be considered early in the differential diagnosis of a patient presenting with upper gastrointestinal symptoms in the absence of demonstrable structural disease. Occasionally, thyrotoxicosis may present with nausea and vomiting, although looseness of stools is the more common gastrointestinal manifestation of this condition.

Dysphagia

Difficulty in swallowing is an unusual manifestation of endocrine disease but may be the presenting feature of multinodular thyroid enlargement with retrosternal extension. Smaller goitres only rarely result in dysphagia. Severe hyperthyroidism with generalized weakness may be associated with a reversible myopathy of the pharyngeal musculature and consequent dysphagia.

Neck pain and swelling

Superficial discomfort in the neck may lead to the incidental finding of thyroid enlargement. Modest degrees of thyroid enlargement are very common, whereas pain arising from the thyroid is comparatively unusual. The most common cause of local discomfort and tenderness in the neck is inflammatory lymphadenopathy. Severe tenderness of the thyroid itself, especially when accompanied by fever and signs of thyrotoxicosis, suggests a diagnosis of viral subacute thyroiditis (de Quervain's thyroiditis). Occasionally, autoimmune thyroiditis may give rise to pain and tenderness, which mimics a viral thyroiditis but is less severe. The sudden onset of localized pain and swelling in the thyroid is indicative of bleeding into a pre-existing thyroid nodule and is a recognized complication of multinodular goitre. The symptoms are self-limiting. Painless enlargement of the thyroid gland (goitre) presents either with pressure effects, resulting in dysphagia progressing to tracheal compression and stridor, or cosmetic disturbance. The underlying cause of thyroid enlargement is often difficult to establish. The family history and subsequent investigation may point to autoimmune thyroiditis or dyshormonogenesis. A history of rapid enlargement of the gland, especially in an elderly patient, suggests an anaplastic thyroid carcinoma. Coexisting severe diarrhoea points towards a diagnosis of medullary carcinoma of the thyroid. In the differential diagnosis, goitrogenic drugs, for example lithium, should be considered, as should residence in an iodine-deficient area. Previous exposure to neck irradiation or to radioactive iodine in childhood may also be important.

Impotence

Reduced erectile potency may be a consequence of primary abnormalities, such as the following:

- Decreased blood supply to the penis (e.g. atherosclerosis)
- Neural dysfunction (e.g. autonomic neuropathy complicating diabetes)
- Testosterone deficiency (e.g. hypopituitarism and primary testicular failure)
- Hyperprolactinaemia
- Drug therapy (e.g. certain antihypertensives)
- Psychological factors
- A combination of several causes

It is often difficult to distinguish with certainty between impotence due to organic factors and that which is psychological, although total erectile failure and the absence of nocturnal and morning erections suggest a physical cause. Impotence in a diabetic patient should not be assumed to be inevitably due to autonomic neuropathy, and other causes should be considered. Most importantly, it should be recognized that male impotence is often complicated by a psychological disturbance, which may serve to exacerbate the problem.

Gynaecomastia

Gynaecomastia refers to a smooth, firm, mobile, often tender disc of breast tissue under the areola in the male. It should be distinguished from the soft, fatty enlargement often seen in obesity. Mild gynaecomastia (sometimes unilateral or asymmetrical) frequently occurs as a temporary phenomenon in normal puberty and may persist for several years or sometimes indefinitely. In adults, gynaecomastia may result from:

- excess oestrogen stimulation
- reduction in circulating androgen
- antagonism of androgen action
- androgen insensitivity (Box 18.7).

Clinical assessment of the patient with gynaecomastia should therefore include an enquiry about any change in libido and examination of thyroid

Box 18.7 Causes of gynaecomastia

Increased oestrogen/testosterone ratio

- Chronic liver disease
- Thyrotoxicosis
- Phenytoin therapy

Androgen receptor antagonists

- Spironolactone, digoxin

Inherited androgen receptor defects

- Testicular feminization syndrome

Testosterone deficiency or oestrogen excess

- Primary and secondary hypogonadism
- Tumour production of human chorionic gonadotrophin (hCG)
- Oestrogen production by Leydig cell tumour of testis

Congenital and hereditary

- X-linked spinal muscular atrophy (Kennedy syndrome)
- Klinefelter's syndrome (karyotype XXY)

status, the genitalia, the muscles and for stigmata of chronic liver disease.

Amenorrhoea

The term amenorrhoea describes absence of menstrual periods (menses). Perhaps the most common cause of failure of onset of menses (primary amenorrhoea) is physiological delay of puberty, a diagnosis that can only be made with certainty in retrospect. Important pathological causes include:

- hypothalamic–pituitary dysfunction (e.g. due to tumours)
- ovarian failure (e.g. failure of normal ovarian development or cytotoxic chemotherapy)
- thyroid dysfunction
- defects in lower genital tract development.

Important diagnostic pointers in the history include symptoms suggestive of thyroid disease, or any visual disability that might indicate compression of the optic chiasm by a hypothalamic or pituitary tumour. Secondary amenorrhoea (cessation of previously established menses) has similar causes. In addition, marked weight loss may lead to amenorrhoea, as in anorexia nervosa or inflammatory bowel disease. Amenorrhoea or oligomenorrhoea (infrequent scanty periods) may occur in women subject to excessively rigorous physical training programmes. Normal pregnancy is the most common cause of secondary amenorrhoea.

Galactorrhoea

Occasionally, physiological lactation may persist after breastfeeding has ceased. Inappropriate lactation is usually bilateral. There are a number of causes, which include the following:

- Prolactin-secreting tumours of the pituitary gland
- Idiopathic galactorrhoea, in which there is an apparent increased sensitivity to normal levels of serum prolactin
- Hyperprolactinaemia due to hypothyroidism
- Hyperprolactinaemia due to dopamine antagonist drugs
- Hyperprolactinaemia due to lactotroph disinhibiting lesions of the hypothalamopituitary region

Inappropriate secretion of breast milk should therefore always prompt enquiry for symptoms referable to the thyroid and pituitary glands, and a thorough drug history should be taken. Even with very high prolactin levels, galactorrhoea is rare in men.

Excess hair growth

An increase in the growth of facial and body hair in adult females is a relatively common symptom and may be due to increased circulating androgens. However, it is most commonly a normal, constitutional characteristic. Pathological causes of hirsutism include:

- polycystic ovary syndrome
- late presentation of congenital adrenal hyperplasia
- androgen-secreting ovarian or adrenal tumours.

The history is vital in the clinical assessment. If the symptoms commenced shortly after the menarche, then a tumour source of androgen is unlikely. A regular menstrual cycle is good evidence against severe androgen excess but does not exclude polycystic ovary syndrome. Increased libido suggests substantially increased androgen secretion, which may be either ovarian or neoplastic in origin.

Bowel disturbance

Constipation and abdominal distension may be features of hypothyroidism, hypercalcaemia or panhypopituitarism. Diarrhoea may occur as part of autonomic neuropathy involving the gut in diabetes mellitus. Peptic ulceration may occur in Zollinger–Ellison syndrome, in which gastrin-secreting tumours of the gut result in increased gastric acid secretion.

Skin changes

Pallor often occurs in primary testicular failure and in panhypopituitarism. Excessive pigmentation occurs in adrenocorticotrophic hormone (ACTH)-dependent Cushing's syndrome, and increased sebum production causing greasy skin and acne on the face and shoulders may occur in all causes of glucocorticoid excess. In carcinoid tumours of the gut or lung, increased humoral secretion results in a violaceous cyanosis-like skin discoloration. A variegate, patchy rash is a feature of porphyria, an inherited abnormality of haem metabolism. In primary hypoadrenalism, there is increased pigmentation of the conjunctival membrane beneath the eyelids and of the inside of the mouth, the axillae and the palmar skin creases. In hypothyroidism, the skin appears dry, pale, sallow or even slightly yellow, scalp hair is coarse and lateral eyebrow hair is thinned. In hyperthyroidism, the skin is dry and hot but often not flushed. In hypocalcaemia, the nails are friable. In uraemia, the skin is pale or yellow and slightly pigmented, and in terminal uraemia, a 'uraemic frost' may appear on the skin.

Vitiligo, a patchy depigmentation of the skin, is common in association with many autoimmune disorders, particularly autoimmune hypothyroidism and vitamin B_{12} deficiency.

Family history

The family background in endocrine or metabolic disease may be particularly useful in the evaluation of several of the more common disorders. It is also particularly important in the assessment of less common inherited disorders of metabolism.

Thyroid disease

Autoimmune hypothyroidism and hyperthyroidism frequently show familial aggregation. Dyshormonogenetic goitre is also often inherited. A family history of organ-specific autoimmune disease (e.g. pernicious anaemia, vitiligo, Addison's disease) may also point to an autoimmune aetiology of thyroid disease.

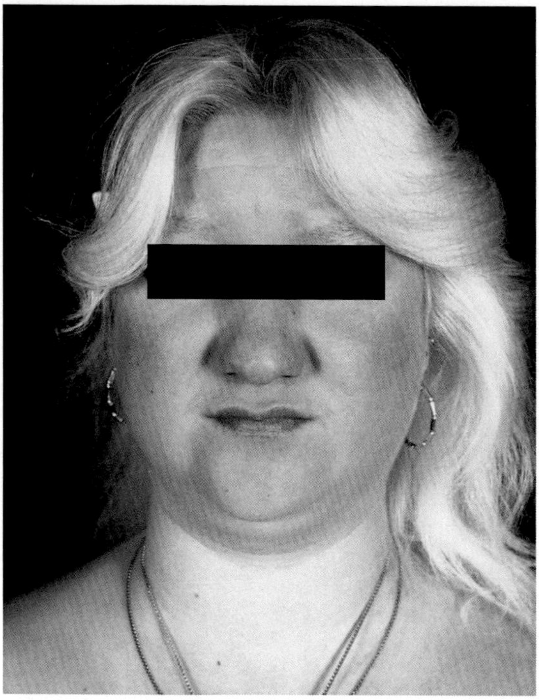

Figure 18.1 Typical facial appearance of Cushing's syndrome. Note the increased fat deposition and the plethoric appearance. The patient presented with a 2-year history of secondary infertility, easy bruising and central adiposity.

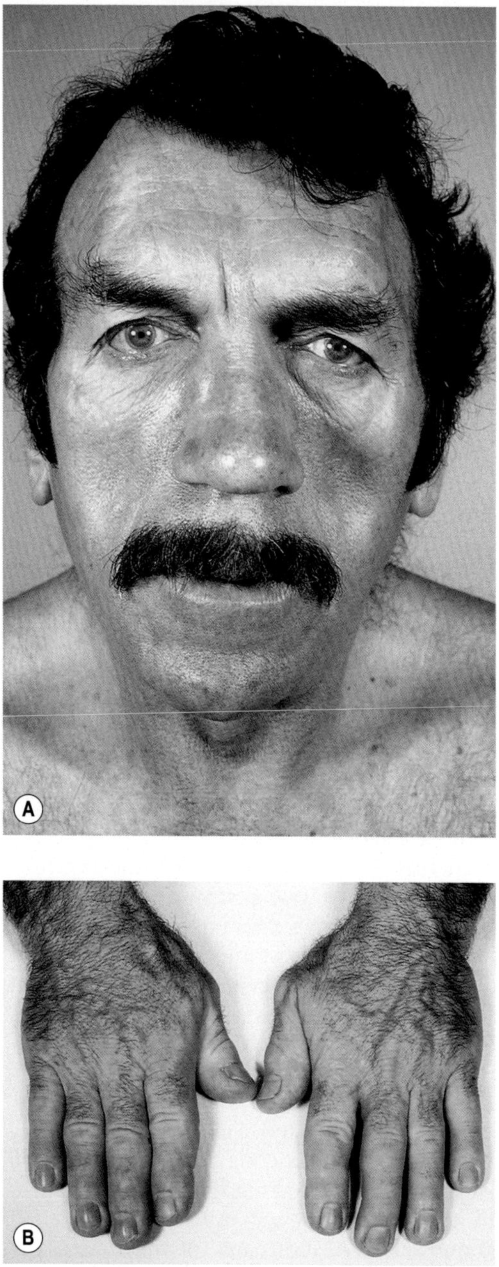

Figure 18.2 The facial **(A)** and hand **(B)** appearance of acromegaly. There is overgrowth of the facial skeleton, coarsening of features and an increase in soft tissues, most obvious in the hands. The patient had a 4-year history of excessive sweating, increased shoe size, frontal headache and 'pins and needles in fingers'.

Renal calculi

Primary hyperparathyroidism, an important cause of renal stones, may be familial, occurring either as an isolated disorder or as a part of the syndrome of multiple endocrine neoplasia (type I).

The examination

General assessment

This should begin with observing the general appearance of the patient. Start by assessing the state of nutrition and by measuring weight and height. Calculate the body mass index (BMI). The distribution of fat should be noted. Deposition of fat in the intra-abdominal, thyrocervical and interscapular regions with relative sparing of the limbs (truncal obesity) is characteristic of Cushing's syndrome and is accompanied by a typical moon-faced plethoric appearance (Fig. 18.1) because of a combination of increased subcutaneous fat and thinning of the skin.

Patients with growth hormone hypersecretion resulting from somatotroph pituitary adenomas also demonstrate a classic facial appearance, with increased fullness and coarsening of soft tissues, including the lips and tongue which, in patients with long-standing disease, may be accompanied by overgrowth of the zygoma, orbital ridges and mandible (prognathism) (Fig. 18.2). Acromegaly in young people occurring before epiphyseal fusion causes abnormally tall stature (gigantism). Increased adiposity in a child who is growing poorly suggests the possibility of growth hormone deficiency, hypothyroidism or, rarely, Cushing's syndrome. Simple obesity is associated with normal or increased linear growth velocity.

The skeletal proportions should be noted: a long-limbed appearance may indicate delayed epiphyseal fusion due to hypogonadism (eunuchoidism) or the

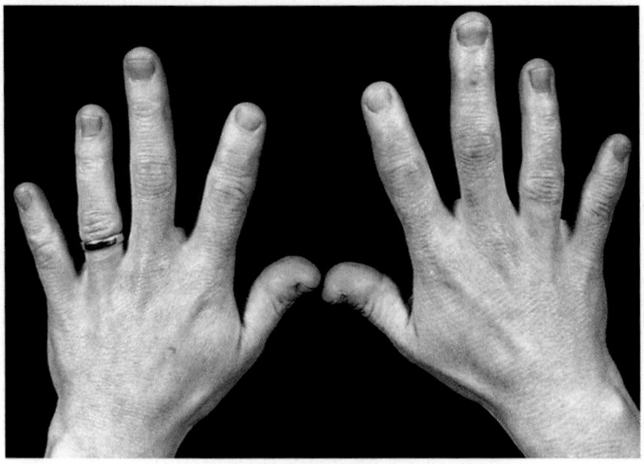

Figure 18.3 The hands in pseudohypoparathyroidism. Note the characteristic shortening of the fourth and fifth metacarpals.

connective tissue abnormality Marfan syndrome. A eunuchoid body habitus is confirmed by demonstrating that the leg length (top of symphysis pubis to ground) exceeds the sitting height or that the span exceeds the total height. Shortening of the limbs occurs with a variety of skeletal dysplasias.

The cytogenetic disorder Turner syndrome (karyotype 45XO), which is characterized by gonadal dysgenesis and the variable presence of other visceral abnormalities, has a typical phenotypic appearance, including short stature, failure of secondary sexual development, decreased or absent secondary sexual hair, an increase in the normal angulation between the humerus and the lower arm, a low posterior hairline and an exaggerated fold of skin between the neck and shoulder. It is most important that accurate wall-mounted stadiometers be used in the assessment of normal growth and its possible disorders.

The hands should be carefully examined for evidence of finger clubbing which, among other things, may be a rare manifestation of thyrotoxic Graves' disease (thyroid acropachy). Palmar erythema may also be found in thyrotoxicosis of any cause as well as in patients with chronic liver disease or rheumatoid arthritis, and in pregnancy.

A unique selective shortening of the fourth and fifth metacarpals may be found as the major somatic manifestation of a group of recessively inherited disorders of parathormone action (pseudohypoparathyroidism; Fig. 18.3).

The skin

Pigmentation, especially buccal, circumoral or palmar, may indicate the increased secretion of ACTH that occurs with adrenal failure (Addison's disease; Fig. 18.4); patches of depigmentation, or vitiligo (Fig. 18.5), may also be found in Addison's disease or other organ-specific autoimmune disorders. Violaceous striae, arising as a result of stretching of thin skin with exposure of the dermal capillary circulation, suggest the possibility of glucocorticoid excess (Fig. 18.6), and abnormal dryness of the skin and coarseness

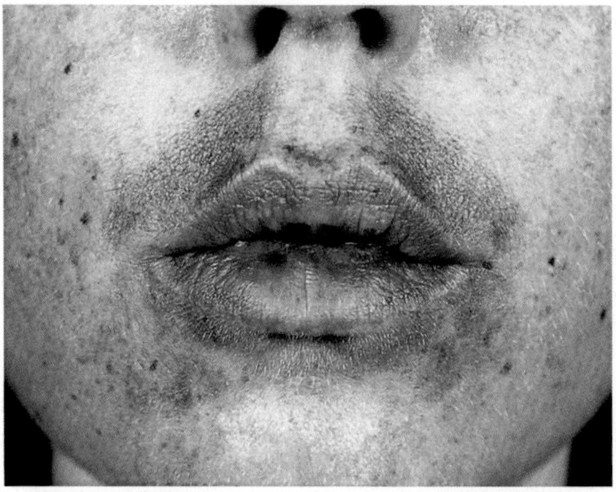

Figure 18.4 Circumoral pigmentation in a patient with hypersecretion of ACTH.

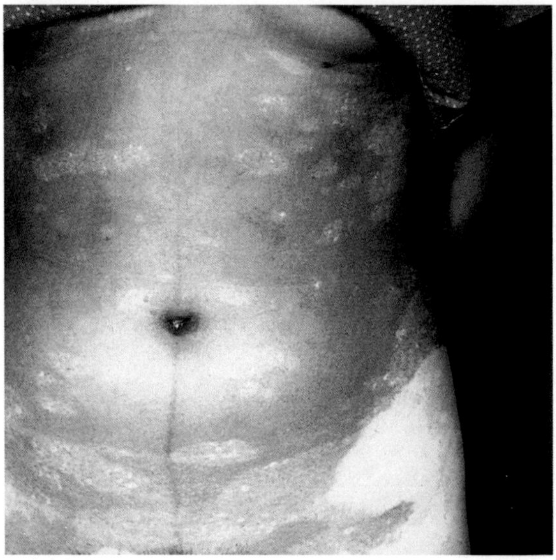

Figure 18.5 Extensive areas of depigmentation (vitiligo) in a patient with organ-specific autoimmune disease.

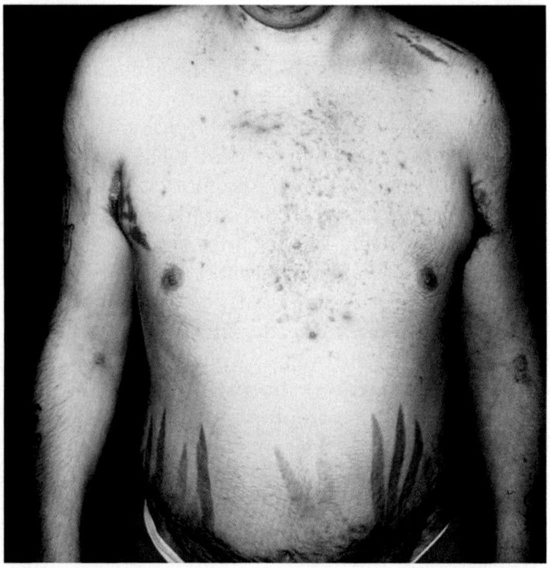

Figure 18.6 Violaceous striae typical of Cushing's syndrome.

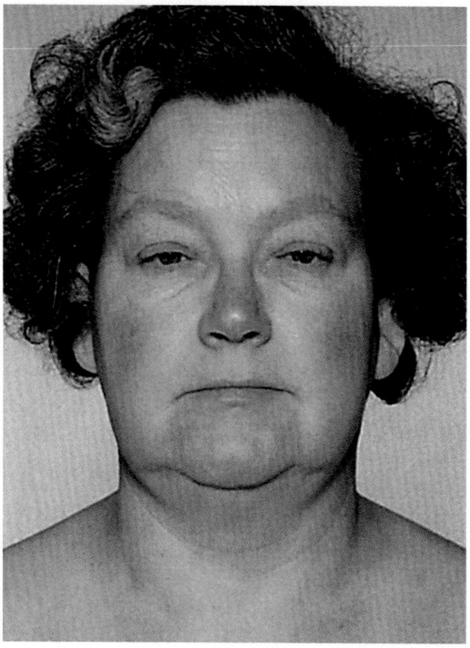

Figure 18.7 The facial appearance of hypothyroidism. The patient demonstrates periorbital puffiness and coarsening of scalp hair. (Figure 14.18 in Jarvis C: Physical examination & health assessment, ed 4, Philadelphia, 2004, Saunders, p 295.)

of the hair are found in hypothyroidism (Fig. 18.7). Localized thickening of the dermis due to mucopolysaccharide and inflammatory cell deposition, particularly on the anterior aspects of the legs when it is known as pretibial myxoedema, is one of the classic but relatively rare extrathyroidal manifestations of Graves' disease.

In females, dermatological examination should also include attention to any abnormality of hair distribution, either excess hair growth in an androgen-dependent distribution (hirsutism) or hair loss in a male pattern, both of which may indicate increased circulating androgen and should prompt examination for evidence of virilization (see below).

The thyroid

The anatomical landmarks relevant to inspection and palpation of the thyroid are shown in Fig. 18.8. Immediately inferior to the thyroid cartilage (with its superior notch) is the cricoid cartilage, with the thyroid isthmus lying just below in the midline. The right and left lobes of the thyroid curve posterolaterally around the trachea and oesophagus and are partially covered by the sternomastoid muscles. The attachment of the thyroid to the pretracheal fascia dictates that it moves superiorly on swallowing; absence of this movement raises the possibility of an infiltrative thyroid carcinoma. Remember that the right lobe is slightly larger than the left; hence, diffuse thyroid enlargement, as in Graves' disease, is often apparently asymmetrical. There are several methods for examining the thyroid, but a suggested routine is as follows.

With the patient's neck slightly extended, inspect the area below the cricoid cartilage. Ask him to take a sip of water, extend the neck again and swallow. Watch for the superior movement of the gland, carefully noting its contour and any asymmetry.

Thyroid palpation is best carried out from behind, with the patient's neck slightly extended, but not so much that the neck musculature is tightened. This may feel awkward initially, but with time and practice it will become more comfortable. Have a glass of water available throughout the examination so the patient may take repeated sips and swallow as necessary. Position both hands to encircle the neck (Fig. 18.8A) with the fingers slightly flexed, such that the tips of the index fingers lie just below the cricoid in order to palpate the isthmus. Now rotate the fingers down and slightly laterally in order to feel the lateral lobes, including the inferior border (Fig. 18.8B). The anterior surface of each lobe should be no larger than the terminal phalanx of the patient's thumb.

The following points should be addressed:

- Is the thyroid diffusely enlarged, as in thyroid stimulating hormone (TSH)-mediated or autoimmune enlargement (Fig. 18.8D)? If so, is it soft (e.g. dyshormogenesis, diffuse goitre of puberty) or firm/hard (e.g. autoimmune thyroiditis). In general, the firmer the texture of an enlarged thyroid, the more likely is the pathology to be autoimmune.
- Are there two or more identifiable nodules (Fig. 18.8E, Fig. 18.9) and, if so, is the patient thyrotoxic and does the gland extend downward behind the sternum? (If the gland is partially or completely retrosternal, the inferior border may not be palpable or palpable only on swallowing.) Most multinodular goitres are benign, but a history of neck irradiation, enlarged cervical lymph nodes or progressive enlargement of one of the nodules raises the suspicion of malignancy.
- Is the palpable abnormality a single focal nodule (Fig. 18.8F), suggesting a cyst, adenoma or carcinoma? Rapid growth, hard texture, lack of movement on swallowing (see above), enlarged regional lymphadenopathy, male gender and a history of neck irradiation all increase the probability of malignancy.
- Is the goitre firm and asymmetrical?
- Are there features of local pressure effects or local infiltration (e.g. dysphonia from recurrent laryngeal involvement)?
- Are there weight loss and debility? These suggest anaplastic carcinoma or lymphoma.
- Is there a bruit, indicating increased blood supply? This is frequently found in untreated Graves' disease but should not be confused with a transmitted bruit from the carotid.

The cardiovascular system

Particular attention should be paid to any postural drop in blood pressure. This may indicate a depleted extracellular fluid volume, for example in patients with adrenal insufficiency, or autonomic dysfunction, the commonest cause of which is diabetes mellitus. Additional indicators of the latter include failure of reflex bradycardia during the Valsalva manoeuvre and loss of beat-to-beat variation in cardiac cycle length, as determined by electrocardiography. A hyperdynamic circulation, sinus tachycardia or atrial fibrillation may be found in thyrotoxicosis; this may progress to cardiac decompensation and cardiac failure.

The breasts and genitalia

A detailed description of growth and pubertal development is beyond the scope of this chapter. In brief, however, in the average adolescent female, pubertal

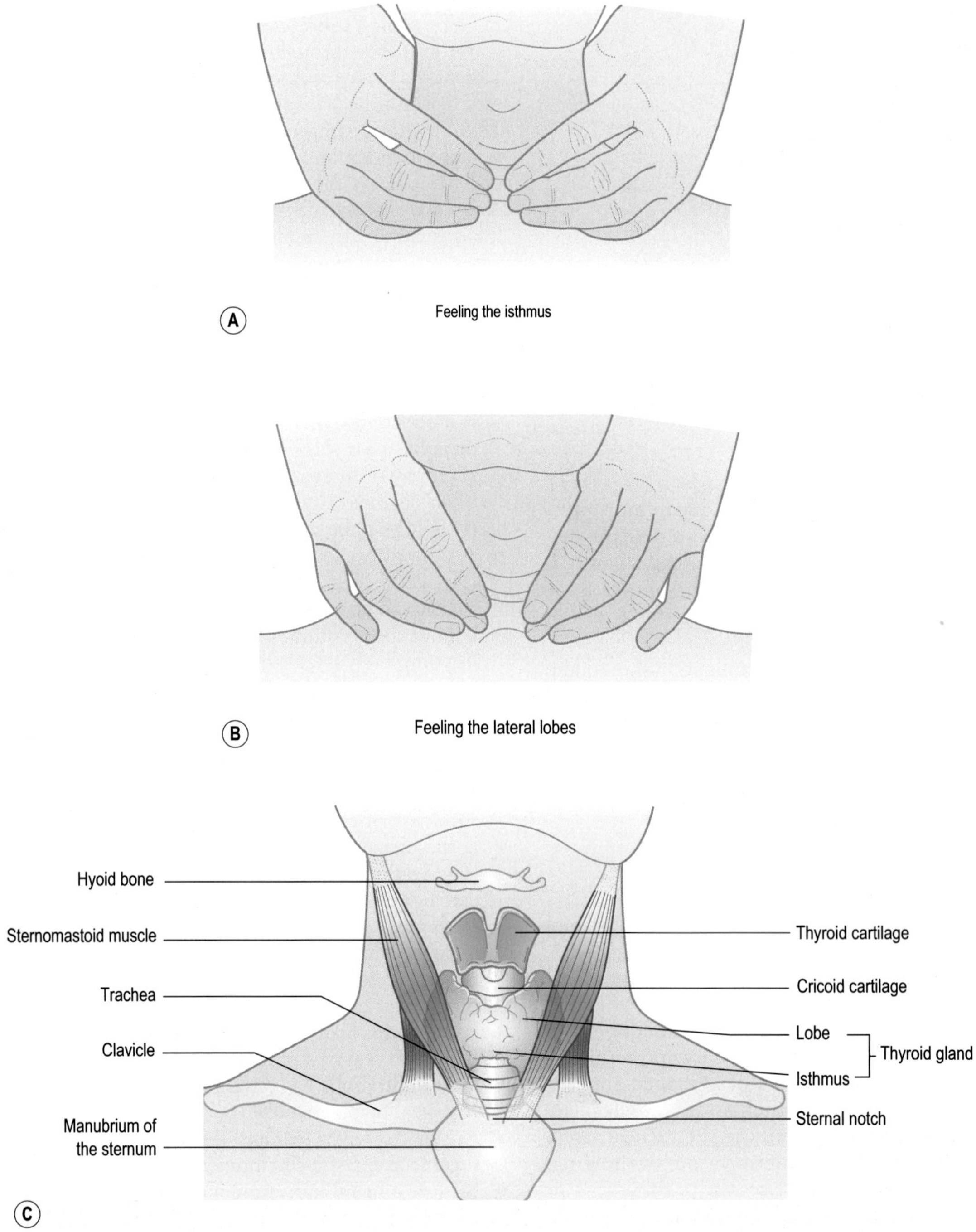

Figure 18.8 Examination of the thyroid. **(A)** Feeling the isthmus; **(B)** feeling the lateral lobes; **(C)** anatomical landmarks;

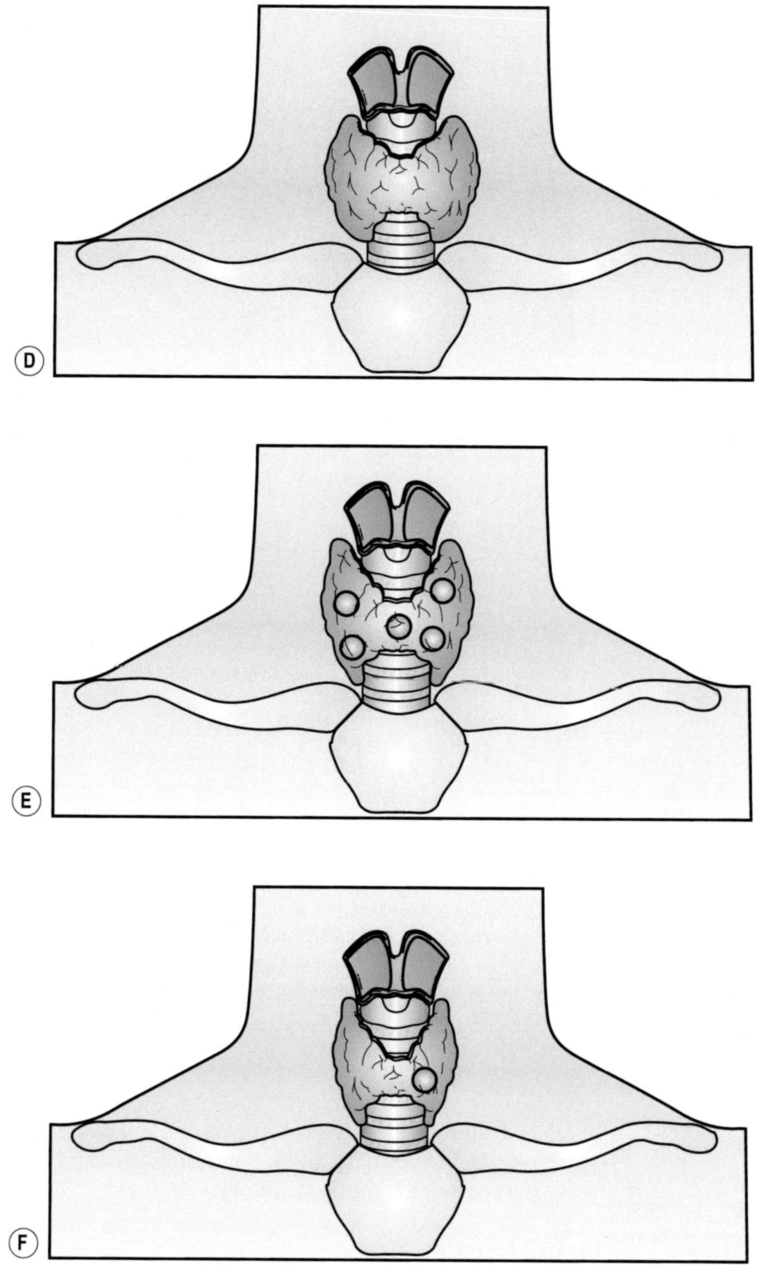

Figure 18.8, cont'd **(D)** diffuse enlargement; **(E)** multinodular goitre; **(F)** single nodule.

development usually commences between the ages of 10 and 11 and takes 3 to 4 years to complete. A growth spurt starts about 1 year before breast development, peak height velocity is reached on average 1 year later, and menarche follows in an average of 1 year. In males, pubertal development usually commences between the ages of 11 and 12, takes approximately 3 years to complete and has a characteristic sequence of adrenarche (onset of adrenal androgen secretion with appearance of secondary sexual hair), testicular development, beginning of pubic hair, beginning of growth spurt and peak height velocity.

The breasts should be examined for mass lesions and, if suggested by the history, for galactorrhoea. In the adolescent female, physiological breast enlargement provides a precise index of pubertal status and signals the onset of the pubertal growth spurt (Tanner stage 3 breast development). Onset of menses (menarche) is a relatively late pubertal event at which point pubertal breast development is virtually complete. In males, any tendency to gynaecomastia should be noted (Fig. 18.10). This may range from minor degrees of subareolar glandular enlargement to substantial breast prominence; breast enlargement associated with generalized adiposity should not be confused with true gynaecomastia.

Genital examination in the male should document testicular volume. This is particularly important in

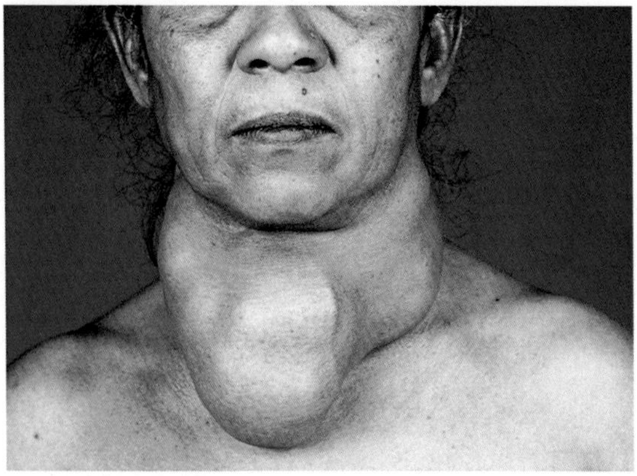

Figure 18.9 A large multinodular goitre. Note the asymmetrical growth of the nodules.

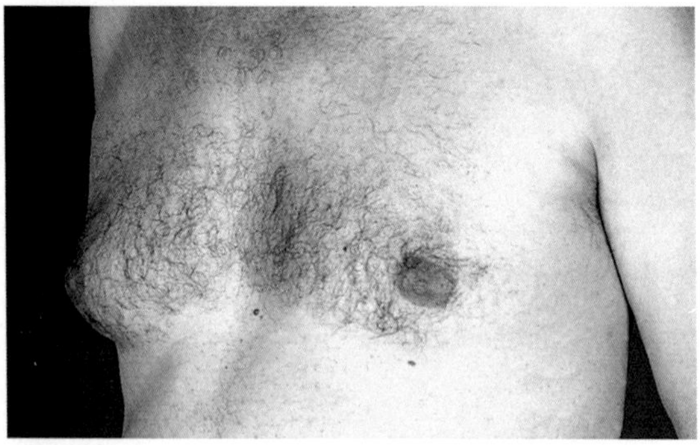

Figure 18.10 Gynaecomastia. There is enlargement of both breasts in this man.

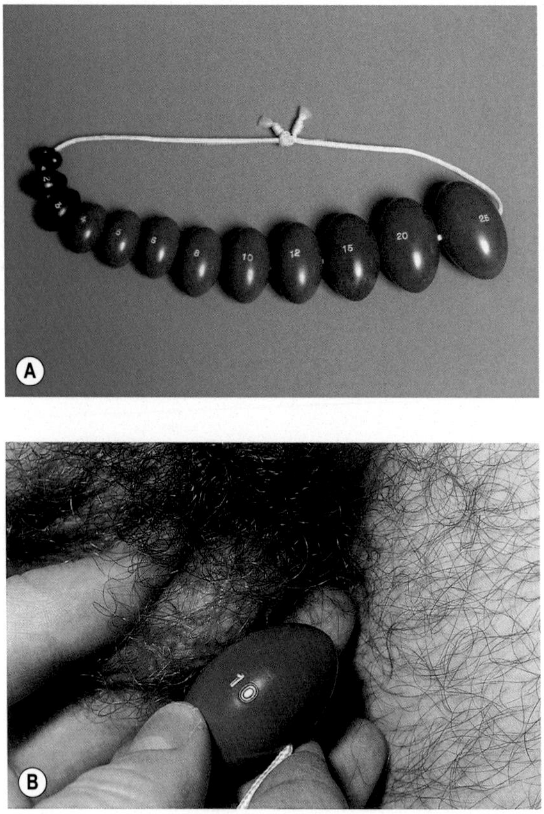

Figure 18.11 Prader orchidometer. **(A)** Testicular volume (in ml) may be estimated by comparison with calibrated ellipsoids. **(B)** Gently grip the testis in one hand and compare its volume (including the scrotal skin, but excluding the epididymis) with that of the ellipsoids. The patient shown has a reduced testicular volume of 8 ml, due to Klinefelter's syndrome; the normal secondary sexual hair is due to the provision of exogenous testosterone.

the assessment of pubertal development, for which volume should be measured by comparison with calibrated ovoids (Prader orchidometer; Fig. 18.11). Prepubertal testicular volume is less than 4 ml; increased volume implies pubertal gonadotrophin stimulation. Onset of the pubertal growth spurt in boys is associated with a testicular volume of 10 ml and normal adult testicular volume is in the range of 15 to 25 ml. In the assessment of normal puberty, it is important to establish that growth velocity and gonadal changes (testicular volume or breast stage) are concordant, since a discordance of puberty proceeding ahead of growth implies an abnormal source of sex steroid (e.g. androgen-secreting tumours or congenital adrenal hyperplasia). Testicular atrophy in the adult male indicates hypogonadism, due to primary testicular failure, hypothalamopituitary dysfunction or chronic liver disease. Tumours of Leydig cells are usually palpable and should be sought in any patient with gynaecomastia.

Examination of the external genitalia in the female is important when androgen hypersecretion is suspected. Enlargement of the clitoris is a feature of excess androgen secretion.

Ambiguity of the external genitalia is indicative of fetal androgen excess in the karyotypic female and of testosterone or dihydrotestosterone deficiency or resistance in the male; these conditions are rare and require specialized investigation.

The eyes

The hypercalcaemic patient should be carefully examined for corneal calcification, evident as a narrow band on the medial or lateral border of the cornea (Fig. 18.12); this usually indicates long-standing hypercalcaemia and a diagnosis of primary hyperparathyroidism.

In patients with thyroid disease, the presence of exophthalmos (proptosis) should be noted. This may be unilateral or bilateral and may be associated with apparent ophthalmoplegia due to tethering of the extraocular muscles, particularly the medial and inferior rectus muscles, such that diplopia occurs on upward or lateral gaze (dysthyroid eye disease; Fig. 18.13). These ocular signs are especially important in the diagnosis of autoimmune thyroid disease (Graves' disease). It must be remembered that

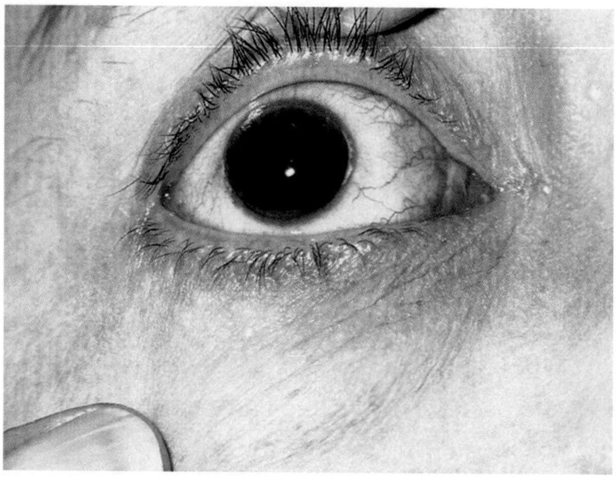

Figure 18.12 Corneal calcification (band keratopathy) in a patient with long-standing hyperparathyroidism.

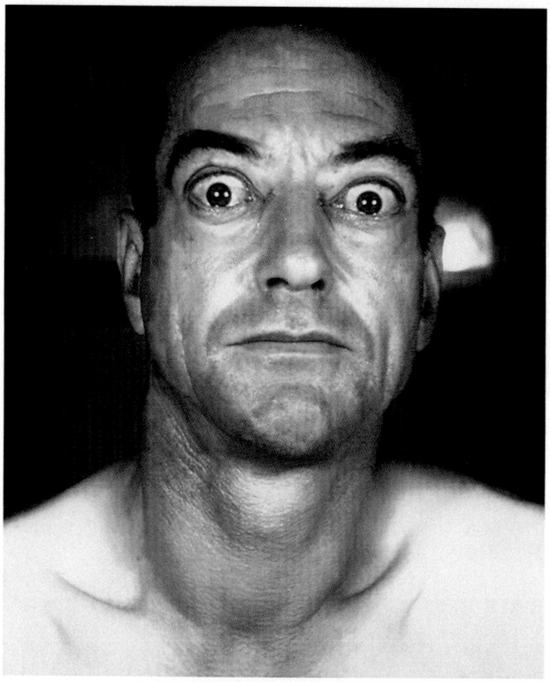

Figure 18.13 Lid retraction and proptosis in a patient with thyrotoxic Graves' disease. In this patient, there had been a 6-month history of effortless weight loss, tremulousness, shortness of breath on exertion and palpitations.

unilateral proptosis may also occur with an orbital tumour. Lid retraction, evident as a wide-eyed staring expression, and lid lag, in which depression of the upper lid lags behind the eye in a downward gaze, are due to increased activity of the sympathetic innervation of levator palpebri superioris and are not specific to Graves' disease. Any degree of corneal exposure due to failure of complete lid apposition should be documented.

Visual acuity should be measured both with and without a pinhole to correct for any refractive error. Reduced acuity may be a feature of optic nerve compression in severe dysthyroid eye disease or of asymmetrical pressure on the optic chiasm due to hypothalamopituitary space-occupying lesions. In the latter, assessment of the visual fields may reveal a bitemporal hemianopia; this is frequently incomplete and incongruous, reflecting the asymmetrical growth of the tumour. A detailed description of the visual pathways and examination of the visual fields is given in Chapter 16. In the context of suspected pituitary/peripituitary disease, use of a red object (e.g. a hat pin) is preferable to finger movements as this provides a more sensitive marker of early visual pathway compression. Examination of the optic discs with the ophthalmoscope may show papilloedema, indicating recent onset of optic nerve compression, or pallor, indicating neural atrophy resulting from long-standing pressure. In the context of a pituitary mass lesion, pallor of the optic discs suggests that full visual recovery is improbable.

The nervous system

In thyrotoxicosis, examination of the nervous system reveals a rapid fine tremor. Proximal weakness with or without wasting of the shoulder and hip girdle musculature (proximal myopathy) is a typical feature of thyrotoxicosis, glucocorticoid excess and vitamin D deficiency. Osteomalacic myopathy is often associated with myalgia.

Hypocalcaemia is associated with increased neural excitability, which may be demonstrated by gentle percussion over the proximal part of the facial nerve (as it exits from the parotid gland). The test is positive if this manoeuvre evokes involuntary facial muscular twitching (Chvostek's sign).

Tendon reflexes will be abnormally brisk in thyrotoxic patients and may show a slow relaxation phase in hypothyroidism. Both hypothyroidism and acromegaly may give rise to nerve entrapment syndromes, particularly of the median nerve at the wrist (carpal tunnel syndrome).

Investigation

The investigation of endocrine and metabolic disorders usually involves (a) the measurement of electrolytes, minerals, metabolites or hormones in plasma and (b) isotopic, ultrasonographic, radiological or magnetic resonance (MR) imaging of specific endocrine glands. In investigating endocrine disease, one is usually interested in whether a specific gland is overactive or underactive. These questions may be answered by basal hormone measurements, for example serum free thyroxine and thyroid-stimulating hormone in thyrotoxicosis and hypothyroidism, but in many instances the lack of a clear distinction between basal hyposecretion, normal secretion and hypersecretion necessitates the use of stimulation and suppression tests.

Endocrine stimulation tests

Endocrine stimulation tests are designed to demonstrate how much hormone a gland can secrete in response to a near-maximal stimulus. Examples include the following:

- Insulin tolerance testing, in which carefully controlled insulin-induced hypoglycaemia stimulates hypothalamopituitary secretion measured by serum growth hormone, cortisol and prolactin
- Tetracosactrin testing, in which an injection of a synthetic ACTH analogue is used to assess adrenocortical reserve
- Oral glucose tolerance test, which is an indirect test of insulin secretion and action as determined by the rise and subsequent fall in the plasma glucose level following an oral glucose load

Endocrine suppression tests

Endocrine suppression tests indicate whether a physiological feedback mechanism is intact or if secretion of the hormone in question has become at least partly autonomous. For example, the suppression of plasma cortisol by the synthetic glucocorticoid dexamethasone is incomplete in Cushing's syndrome, and suppression of serum growth hormone by an oral glucose load fails to occur in acromegaly.

Endocrine imaging

Plain X-ray imaging is of limited value in the investigation of endocrine disorders. However, lateral and anteroposterior views of the pituitary fossa can be useful in demonstrating abnormal calcification in the fossa or gross expansion and erosion of the fossa due to large intrasellar or suprasellar tumours. Plain abdominal radiology may show renal calcification (nephrocalcinosis; Fig. 18.14) in patients with long-standing hypercalcaemia or renal tubular acidosis.

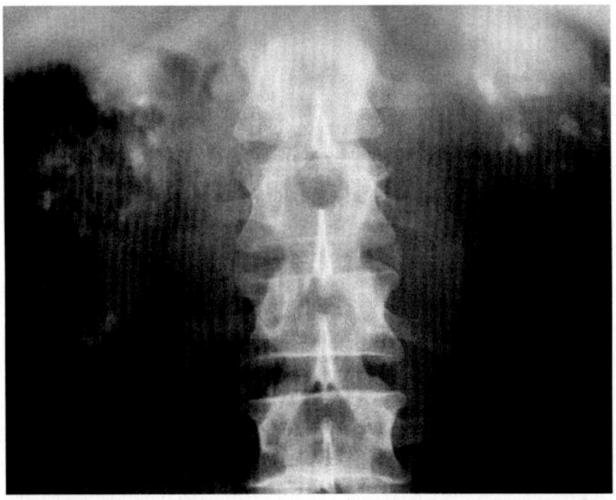

Figure 18.14 Widespread renal calcification typical of nephrocalcinosis in a patient with long-standing hyperparathyroidism.

Computed tomography (CT) imaging is useful in assessing the pituitary, adrenal glands (Fig. 18.15) and thorax. However, MR imaging of the pituitary (Fig. 18.16) offers definite advantages over CT in terms of improved precision in detecting small intrasellar tumours and better definition of the lateral border of the pituitary and the cavernous sinus.

Isotopic imaging is particularly useful for demonstrating autonomous function within endocrine tumours. This technique is applicable to the thyroid gland (radiolabelled pertechnetate; Fig. 18.17), the adrenal medulla (radiolabelled metaiodobenzylguanidine) and parathyroids (combined radiolabelled sesta methoxy-isobutyl-isonitrile (MIBI) and pertechnetate differential scanning).

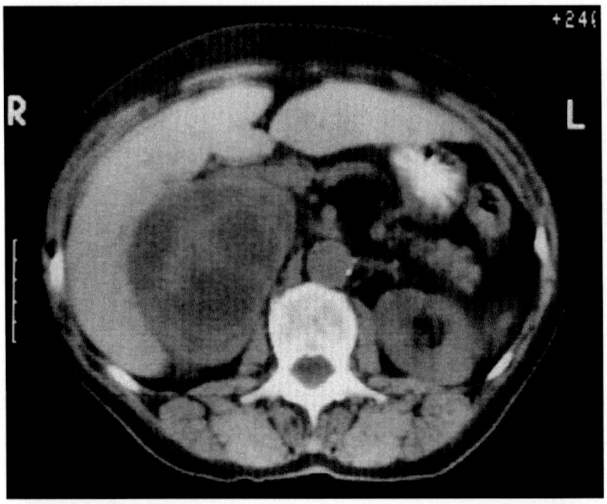

Figure 18.15 Axial CT scan of the abdomen in a patient with a right adrenal medullary phaeochromocytoma. Note the extensive tumour mass, with areas of hypodensity indicating episodes of partial tumour infarction.

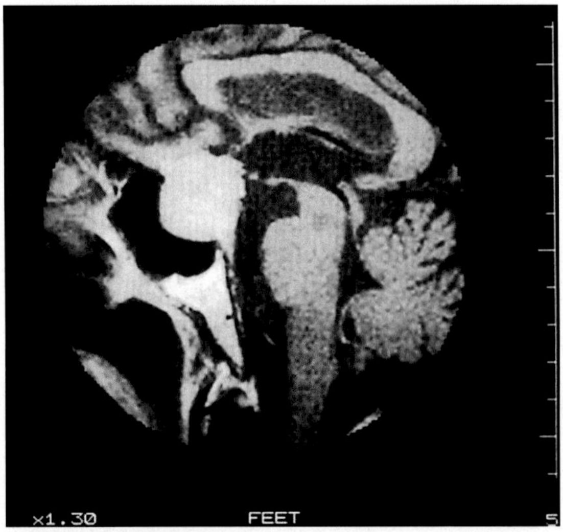

Figure 18.16 Magnetic resonance imaging (sagittal view) of the pituitary, demonstrating a large pituitary adenoma with suprasellar extension.

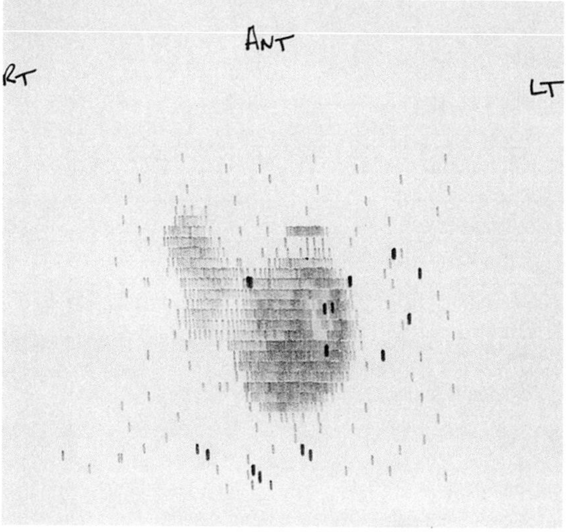

Figure 18.17 Technetium-labelled isotope scan of the thyroid in a patient with a focal thyroid nodule. Note the focal area of uptake corresponding to the palpable lesion, with surrounding inactivity indicating autonomous function within the nodule.

Diabetes mellitus

Diabetes is a Greek word meaning 'a passer through; a siphon', and mellitus derives from the Greek word for 'sweet'. The Greeks named it thus due to the excessive amounts of urine produced by sufferers which attracted insects because of its glucose content. The ancient Chinese tested for diabetes by observing whether ants were attracted to a person's urine.

Diabetes mellitus is the most common metabolic disorder encountered in clinical practice. It is strongly linked to obesity. Diabetes mellitus is characterized by abnormal carbohydrate and lipid homoeostasis, leading to elevation in plasma glucose, or hyperglycaemia, and abnormality of serum lipids, or dyslipidaemia. Glucose homoeostasis is modulated mainly by the release of insulin from the islet cells (β cells) of the pancreas. Diabetes develops as a result of a variable combination of absolute insulin deficiency as a result of pancreatic islet cell dysfunction and tissue insulin resistance due to reduced cellular responsiveness to insulin.

The World Health Organization (WHO) has developed a classification of diabetes mellitus based on its pathogenesis (Box 18.8). Type 1 is characterized by absolute insulin deficiency due to autoimmune-mediated pancreatic islet cell destruction. In contrast, type 2 diabetes is associated with a variable degree of tissue insulin resistance, leading – at least in the early stages – to high plasma insulin levels then subsequently to relative insulin deficiency as pancreatic islet cell function fails to overcome this resistance. The diagnostic criteria for disorders of glucose metabolism are shown in Box 18.9. Note that glycosuria itself (glucose in the urine) is not a reliable diagnostic test for diabetes mellitus.

Presenting symptoms of diabetes

Many people with type 2 diabetes may be asymptomatic at diagnosis, for example by routine screening of blood or urine, when there may be only mildly increased levels of hyperglycaemia. Once diagnosed, however, many patients do admit to some long-standing, often mild symptoms. Acute metabolic decompensation, leading to marked hyperglycaemia, occurs infrequently.

In contrast, type 1 diabetes is often abrupt in onset, and characterized by severe hyperglycaemia with acute life-threatening decompensation (diabetic ketoacidosis).

The cardinal symptoms of diabetes mellitus are unintentional (effortless) weight loss, polyuria and polydipsia, and their presence should always result in an immediate test for blood glucose and urine for ketones.

Polyuria, polydipsia and nocturia

Acute hyperglycaemia causes increased urine excretion (polyuria) and, as a result, excessive thirst and water ingestion (polydipsia). These presenting symptoms of diabetes mellitus are also termed osmotic symptoms. Raised plasma glucose leads to increased renal tubular delivery of glucose, which then exceeds the resorptive capacity of the renal tubule, leading to glycosuria. Therefore, despite hyperglycaemia, people with an increased renal threshold for glucose may have no osmotic symptoms. Conversely, people with a low renal threshold for glucose may have glycosuria despite being normoglycaemic. It is for this reason that glycosuria is an unreliable feature in the diagnosis of diabetes mellitus. Nocturia is also common in patients presenting with osmotic symptoms of diabetes, and enquiry regarding the frequency of passing urine at night can be helpful in evaluating symptoms.

Weight loss and lethargy

Loss of more than 5% of total body weight should be considered clinically important in a subject not deliberately attempting to lose weight. Weight loss is a common presenting symptom in people with type 1 diabetes and occasionally in type 2 diabetes with marked hyperglycaemia. Loss of weight in diabetes is predominantly due to renal glucose loss as a result of lack of insulin to enable cellular uptake of glucose. The weight loss usually occurs despite a normal appetite and dietary intake. This is in contrast to the weight loss of malignant disease, which is usually associated with reduced appetite and oral intake.

Lethargy and fatigue are also common presenting symptoms of diabetes mellitus, particularly type 2,

Box 18.8 The World Health Organization classification of diabetes mellitus

Type	Common subtypes/pathogenesis	Treatment
Type 1	Destruction of pancreatic islet cells leading to insulin deficiency	Insulin
Type 2	Ranges from predominantly insulin resistance with relative insulin deficiency (often associated with obesity) to predominantly insulin deficiency	Diet/oral hypoglycaemic agents/insulin
Other types		
Genetic defects of β-cell function	Diabetes associated with glucokinase, hepatic nuclear factor (HNF) 1α, HNF1β, HNF4α, Neurod1 and insulin promotor factor mutations (all previously grouped under maturity-onset diabetes of the young (MODY)) Mitochondrial diabetes	Tablets or insulin, depending upon genetic defect
Genetic defects of insulin action	Insulin-resistance syndromes (type A insulin resistance, leprechaunism, Rabson-Mendenhall syndrome lipoatrophic diabetes)	Insulin-sensitizing agents and insulin
Diseases of the exocrine pancreas	Fibrocalculous pancreatic diabetes, pancreatitis, trauma/pancreatectomy, neoplasia, cystic fibrosis, haemochromatosis, others	Frequently insulin required
Endocrinopathies	Cushing's syndrome, acromegaly, phaeochromocytoma, glucagonoma, hyperthyroidism, somatostatinoma, others	Treatment of underlying cause
Drug- or chemical-induced	Glucocorticoids, α-adrenergic agonists, β-adrenergic agonists, thiazides, interferon-α therapy	Avoid
Uncommon forms of immune-mediated diabetes	Insulin autoimmune syndrome (antibodies to insulin), anti-insulin receptor antibodies, 'stiff man' syndrome	Variable
Other genetic syndromes associated with diabetes	Down's, Friedreich's ataxia, Huntington's chorea, Klinefelter's, Lawrence-Moon-Biedl, myotonic dystrophy, porphyria, Prader-Willi, Turner's, Wolfram's	Variable
Gestational diabetes		Diet/insulin

Box 18.9 World Health Organization Criteria for diagnosis of diabetes mellitus

	Fasting plasma glucose (mmol/l)		2-hour plasma glucose (mmol/l)	Random plasma glucose (mmol/l)	Glycated haemoglobin (mmol/mol [%])
Diabetes mellitus	≥7.0	or	≥11.1	≥11.1	>48 [6.5] (if asymptomtic should be repeated)
Impaired glucose tolerance (IGT)	<7.0	and	Between 7.8 and 11.0	–	42-47 [6.1-6.4] – pre-diabetes
Impaired fasting glucose (IFG)	Between 6.1 and 6.9	and	<7.8	–	

where the symptoms may have been present for some time.

Skin problems

Dermatological manifestations of diabetes are common at diagnosis, especially in patients with poor glycaemic control. Skin infections, such as staphylococcal infection leading to boils, carbuncles or abscesses, which are often recurrent, may occur. Severe infection itself can lead to hyperglycaemia, and a new diagnosis of diabetes should be reconsidered once the acute infection has cleared.

Oral and genital candidiasis can also be presenting features of diabetes mellitus. The presence of the characteristic white plaques on the tongue and oropharynx in a previously healthy person not on antibiotic therapy should alert the physician to the possibility of diabetes mellitus, although other conditions leading to immune paresis, such as HIV infection or haematological malignancy, can also lead to candidiasis. Genital candidiasis in women leads to a thick white discharge and vaginal soreness. Similarly, in men it can lead to a severe balanitis (inflammation of the glans penis). Always check the blood glucose in people with recurrent candidiasis.

Visual disturbance

Hyperglycaemia can lead to blurred vision, owing to osmotic changes within the aqueous humour of the lens of the eye. This can also occur when chronic hyperglycaemia is treated, causing further osmotic shifts in the lens. The symptom usually settles once normoglycaemia is achieved.

Other important aspects of a diabetic history

Family history

A history of diabetes in first-degree relatives is a potent risk factor for diabetes. Type 2 diabetes appears to have a stronger genetic component than type 1, with around a third of patients having a positive family history compared to around 10% of type 1 diabetic patients.

A family history of premature cardiovascular disease is also important. Patients with diabetes are at risk of cardiovascular disease, and this risk is increased when there is a family history of vascular disease in fathers or brothers aged less than 55 years, or mothers or sisters aged less than 65.

Diet and lifestyle history

The cornerstone of management of diabetes is lifestyle; accordingly, periodic reassessment is important. Regularity of meals, the quality and quantity of foods eaten and the frequency of snacks should be known. Enquire about the following:

- Regularity of meals – three meals a day is ideal.
- Content of fatty/greasy foods – particularly discourage saturated (animal) fats, as this type of fat is linked to heart disease.
- Content of fruit and vegetables – at least five portions a day are recommended.
- Content of sugar and sugary foods – avoid carbonated drinks, cakes, sweets and biscuits.
- Content of salt – a high salt intake can lead to hypertension.
- Alcohol intake – a maximum of two units of alcohol per day for a woman and three units per day for a man.

The smoking history is of paramount importance, as smoking with diabetes is strongly linked to cardiovascular disease. Occupational history may be important, because if insulin therapy is required, this may have an impact on legal requirements for driving. Assess physical activity to ascertain whether increased activity may improve glycaemia and weight. At least 30 minutes of moderate exercise per day, for example brisk walking, is recommended.

Assessment of other cardiovascular risk factors

Cardiovascular risk is greatly increased in people with diabetes, and additional cardiovascular risk factors multiply the risk. Thus, any history of hypertension, hyperlipidaemia or previous vascular disease (cerebro-, cardio- or peripheral vascular) should be noted. Take a full medication history, including the use of antiplatelet, antihypertensive and lipid-lowering drugs.

Home glucose testing

In a patient previously diagnosed with diabetes, assess his self-monitoring of glucose. This will enable a reasonable judgement of glycaemic control. Self-monitoring can be done by home capillary blood testing or by urine testing for glycosuria.

Insulin injections

In patients taking insulin, it is important to ascertain whether the patient self-injects, the delivery device used (disposable pen, cartridge pen or syringe/vial), the sites chosen and whether they experience any problems.

Symptoms of complications of diabetes

Chronic complications of diabetes mellitus can be usefully subdivided into large blood vessels (macrovascular), small blood vessels (microvascular) and others (Box 18.10).

Symptoms of macrovascular disease

The features of ischaemic heart disease are described elsewhere (see Ch. 13). People with diabetes have fewer, less severe symptomatic chest pains, possibly due to autonomic neuropathy leading to reduced deep pain sensation – so-called 'silent ischaemia'. Thus, the only symptom of ischaemic heart disease in a diabetic subject may be breathlessness.

Peripheral vascular disease presents with claudication. In addition, in patients with diabetes, a combination of peripheral neuropathy and peripheral vascular disease can lead to foot ulceration, particularly at sites of pressure (Fig. 18.18).

Cerebrovascular disease in diabetic patients can present with any stroke syndrome (Ch. 16). Transient ischaemic attacks are common.

Symptoms of microvascular disease

Diabetic retinopathy is frequently asymptomatic until it causes significant visual loss, which may be acute in onset (e.g. because of a sudden retinal haemorrhage) or insidious (e.g. because of cataract or maculopathy). Diabetic nephropathy is similarly asymptomatic until renal dysfunction becomes so severe that uraemia

Box 18.10	Chronic complications of diabetes	
Macrovascular	Coronary heart disease Peripheral vascular disease Cerebrovascular disease	
Microvascular	Retinopathy	Non-proliferative (mild, moderate and severe) Proliferative Maculopathy
	Neuropathy	Peripheral sensory neuropathy Autonomic neuropathy Mononeuropathy Proximal motor neuropathy
	Nephropathy	
Other	Dermatological	Diabetic dermopathy Necrobiosis lipoidica diabeticorum Bullosis diabeticorum Granuloma annulare Acanthosis nigricans
	Rheumatological	Diabetic cheiroarthropathy Flexor tendinopathy Adhesive capsulitis Diabetic osteoarthropathy Charcot neuroarthropathy Diffuse idiopathic skeletal hyperostosis
	Hepatic	Non-alcoholic steatohepatitis

ensues (see Ch. 17). Uraemic symptoms include fatigue, breathlessness and tachypnoea, pleuritic chest pain due to pericarditis and pruritus. Heavy proteinuria may lead to the development of a nephrotic syndrome.

In contrast, diabetic neuropathy can manifest in a number of ways. Chronic peripheral sensory neuropathy is the commonest form, affecting around 5% of patients with diabetes. This can present with symptoms varying from numbness, a feeling of 'walking on cotton wool' and paraesthesiae (pins and needles) to burning, sharp and shooting pains. The latter is a

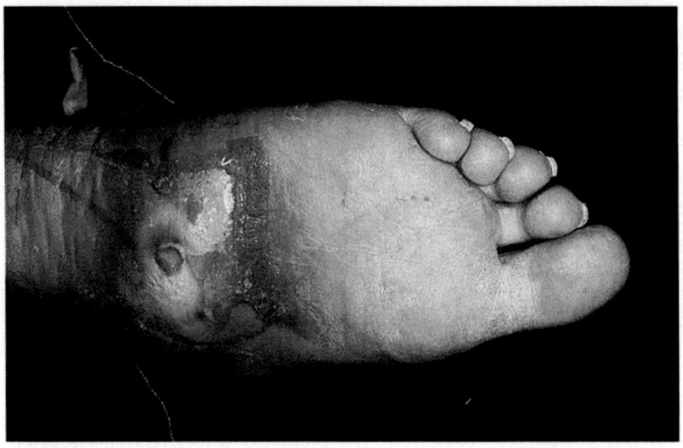

Figure 18.18 Diabetic neuropathic ulcer in a patient with Charcot neuroarthropathy.

feature of selective involvement of small pain fibres. Typically the symptoms start distally and spread up in a stocking distribution and are characteristically worse at night, frequently leading to insomnia.

Proximal motor neuropathy (diabetic amyotrophy or femoral neuropathy) is uncommon but is seen predominantly in middle-aged men with type 2 diabetes. The condition is characterized by severe, deep pain and paraesthesiae in the upper anterior thigh, followed by weakness and wasting of the quadriceps muscle. The condition is often unilateral, generally short-lived (around 3 months) and usually resolves spontaneously. Associated weight loss and cachexia are common.

Mononeuropathies, particularly affecting the median nerve of the hand (carpal tunnel syndrome; see Ch. 16), are common in patients with diabetes. This frequently presents with paraesthesiae and numbness in the median nerve distribution of the hand (lateral two-and-half digits) and is again worse at night. Similar symptoms may occur in the foot (tarsal tunnel syndrome). Cranial mononeuropathies are rare, but palsies of cranial nerves III, VI and VII are seen in patients with diabetes, leading to blurred or double vision due to ophthalmoplegia or a lower motor neuron facial palsy (Ch. 16). The pupillomotor fibres are usually spared in diabetic third-nerve palsy.

Diabetes can cause autonomic neuropathy, the symptoms of which can be very troublesome. They include impotence, gustatory sweating (severe facial sweating on tasting food), urinary retention or incontinence, dizziness or syncope due to postural hypotension, constipation or diarrhoea (so-called diabetic diarrhoea) and recurrent nausea and vomiting due to diabetic gastroparesis.

Hypoglycaemia

Treatment of diabetes is aimed at reducing symptoms and reducing the risk of diabetic complications. In attempting to reduce hyperglycaemia using oral hypoglycaemic tablets or insulin therapy, the patient with diabetes is at risk of hypoglycaemia.

Physiological responses to hypoglycaemia start at a plasma glucose of around 3.8 mmol/l, with the release of counter-regulatory hormones such as glucagon or adrenaline (epinephrine). Symptoms of hypoglycaemia normally occur at around this level because of sympathetic overactivation. Such symptoms include sweating, palpitations, hunger, agitation or blurred vision, and most patients recognize them as hypoglycaemia and are able to treat themselves rapidly. A further drop in plasma glucose leads to neuroglycopenic symptoms, in which cerebral glucose is low, leading to impaired intellectual activity or diminished psychomotor skills. Further drops in glucose levels can lead to severe agitation, confusion, coma and epileptiform seizures. The symptoms of hypoglycaemia can be distressing and have a significant adverse impact on quality of life. Loss of awareness of hypoglycaemia is sometimes a problem in diabetic patients with autonomic neuropathy, and in insulin-treated diabetes this can lead to unexpected hypoglycaemia. Patients at risk should be warned against driving motor vehicles and taught the early symptoms of hypoglycaemia in order to raise their awareness of this potentially serious complication of therapy.

Box 18.11 The diabetic annual review

History

- Patient concerns
- Events – life and medical
- Glucose diary (urine or blood)
- Current treatment
- Hypoglycaemia
- Driving
- Pregnancy/contraception in women
- Impotence
- Symptoms of coronary heart disease or peripheral vascular disease
- Smoking habit

Examination

- Weight/Body Mass Index
- Blood pressure – erect and supine
- Injection sites
- Urinalysis
- Eye examination
- Foot examination

Tests

- Renal function, liver function
- Glycated haemoglobin (HbA_{1c})
- Lipids
- Urine for albumin excretion

Examination of the diabetic patient

General assessment

Patients with diabetes can present with acute metabolic decompensation, leading to diabetic ketoacidosis (DKA), hyperosmolar hyperglycaemic syndrome (HHS) or, in treated patients, hypoglycaemia. Thus, it is mandatory for all patients presenting with coma or reduced conscious level to have their blood glucose checked immediately.

Characteristically, the cardinal symptoms of severe polyuria, polydipsia and weight loss will have been present for some time prior to coma; such symptoms should never be ignored in a diabetic person. Patients with acute hyperglycaemic crises are frequently severely dehydrated, with hypotension (including postural hypotension), tachycardia, dry mucous membranes and reduced skin turgor. Other signs of DKA include rapid deep sighing respiration (Kussmaul breathing – a respiratory compensation for metabolic acidosis) and ketones on the breath (a sweet odour reminiscent of nail polish remover). Diabetic ketoacidosis can occasionally present with symptoms of an acute abdomen.

In the non-acute setting, it is desirable for all patients with diabetes to undergo a full medical assessment once a year – the so-called diabetic annual review (Box 18.11).

Skin, nails and hands

Dermatological manifestations of diabetes are common. Fungal nail infections, particularly of the feet, are common, as are dermatophyte infections of the skin of the feet (tinea pedis). Staphylococcal skin infections leading to pustules, abscesses or carbuncles can also be seen. Other skins lesions seen in diabetes include necrobiosis lipoidica diabeticorum (Fig. 18.19). This is a rare complication of diabetes, predominantly seen in young women aged 15-40 years. This presents as a painless red macule, usually over the anterior shin, which then heals with scarring to form a yellowish/brown lesion. The condition can be unsightly, and little effective treatment is available. Vitiligo is seen in a small number of patients with type 1 diabetes, reflecting its autoimmune nature.

Diabetic dermopathy is characterized by brown macules on the lower legs that heal to form atrophic, shiny white scars. A further skin lesion seen in patients with diabetes is granuloma annulare, pale, shiny rings and nodules usually seen on the hands (Fig. 18.20). Bullosis diabeticorum is a rare manifestation, characterized by tense blistering, mainly on the feet. Acanthosis nigricans is characterized by a dark velvety appearance in the axillae or neck of people with insulin resistance (Fig. 18.21) and frequently accompanies type 2 diabetes but may occur in people with insulin resistance in the absence of diabetes.

Diabetic patients treated with insulin should have their injection sites examined for signs of lipohypertrophy (a physiological response to insulin injected near fat cells) (Fig. 18.22) or lipoatrophy (an allergic response to non-human insulins – now rarely seen) (Fig. 18.23).

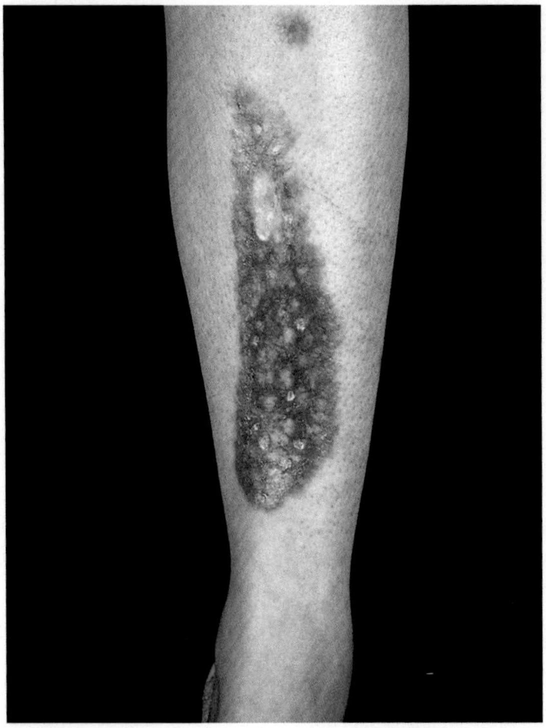

Figure 18.19 Necrobiosis lipoidica diabeticorum.

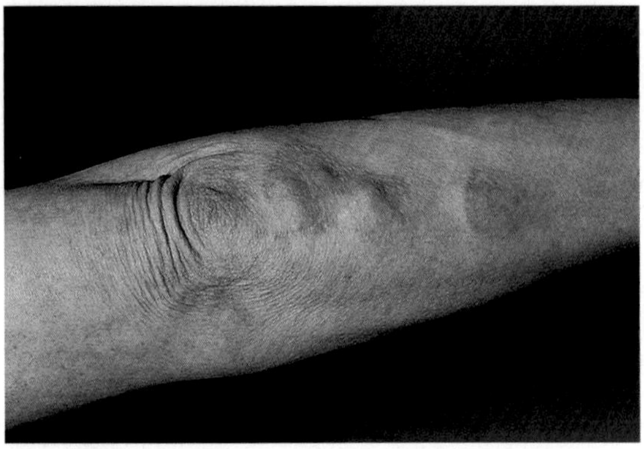

Figure 18.20 Granuloma annulare. (Courtesy of Dr David Peterson.)

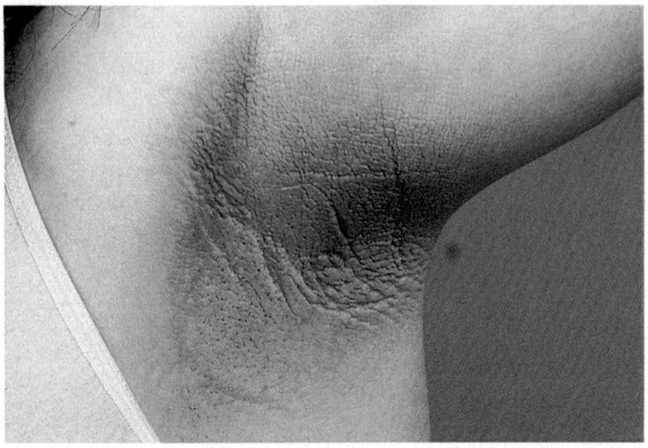

Figure 18.21 Acanthosis nigricans.

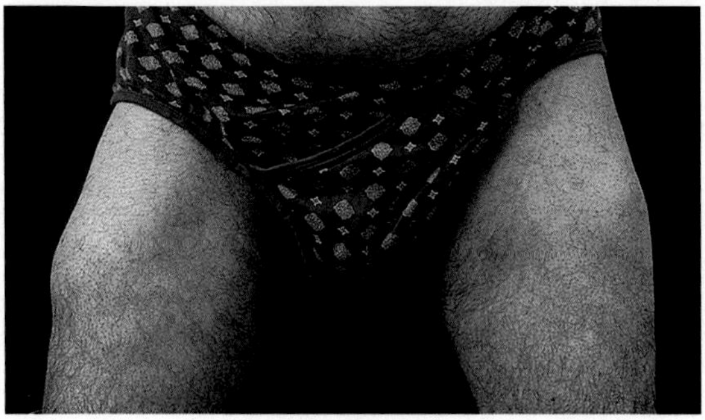

Figure 18.22 Lipohypertrophy. (Courtesy of Dr David Peterson.)

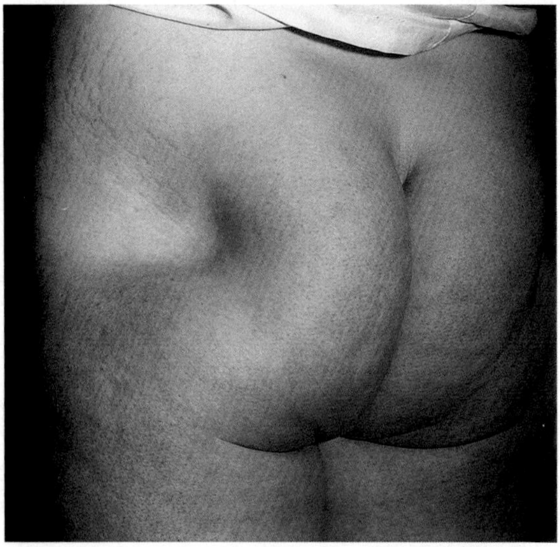

Figure 18.23 Lipoatrophy. (Courtesy of Dr David Peterson.)

Diabetic cheiroarthropathy, or 'stiff hand syndrome' or 'limited joint mobility', is seen in some patients with long-standing diabetes. It is characterized by skin thickening and sclerosis of the tendon sheaths, leading to reduced joint mobility and the characteristic prayer sign (Fig. 18.24). Examination of the hands for signs of carpal tunnel syndrome (Ch. 16) is important if the patient has suggestive symptoms. Thus, the presence of Tinel's sign (Fig. 18.25) and Phalen's sign (Fig. 18.26) should be sought. Thenar eminence wasting may also be seen.

Eyes

Examination of the eyes is mandatory in patients with diabetes. External examination may indicate signs of dyslipidaemia (corneal arcus and xanthelasmata; Fig. 18.27). A reduced pupillary response to light may indicate autonomic neuropathy. Visual acuity should be assessed yearly with a Snellen chart, and unexplained loss of acuity should be investigated. Funduscopy should be undertaken with pharmacological dilatation

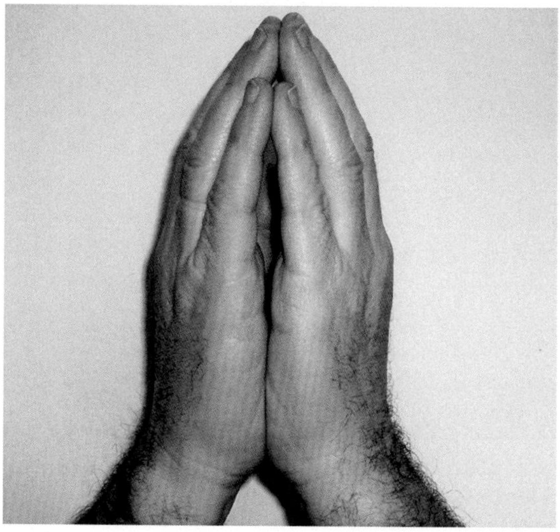

Figure 18.24 The prayer sign in diabetic cheiroarthropathy.

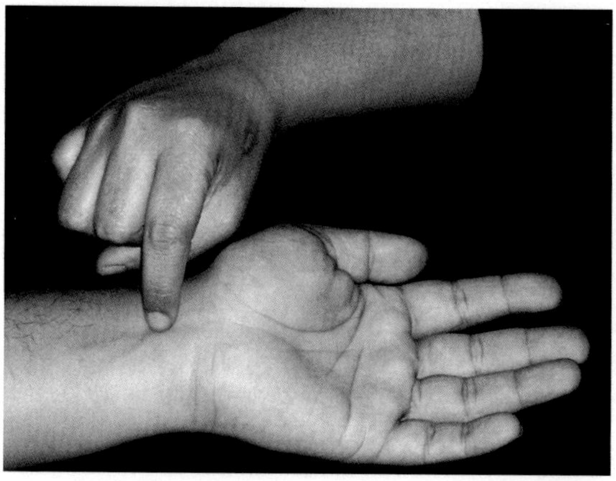

Figure 18.25 Tinel's sign in carpal tunnel syndrome: tapping on the median nerve at the wrist induces pain in the median nerve distribution.

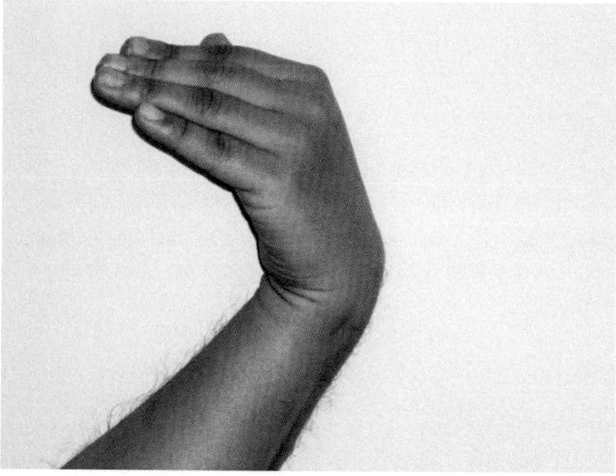

Figure 18.26 Phalen's sign in carpal tunnel syndrome: hyperflexion of the wrist leads to pain in the median nerve distribution.

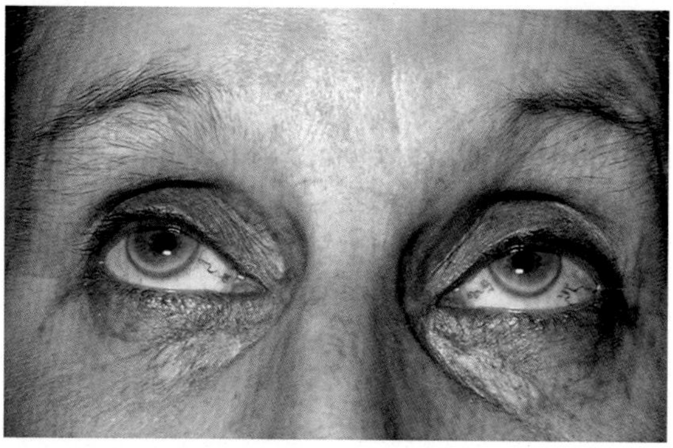

Figure 18.27 Corneal arcus and xanthelasmata in a patient with diabetic dyslipidaemia.

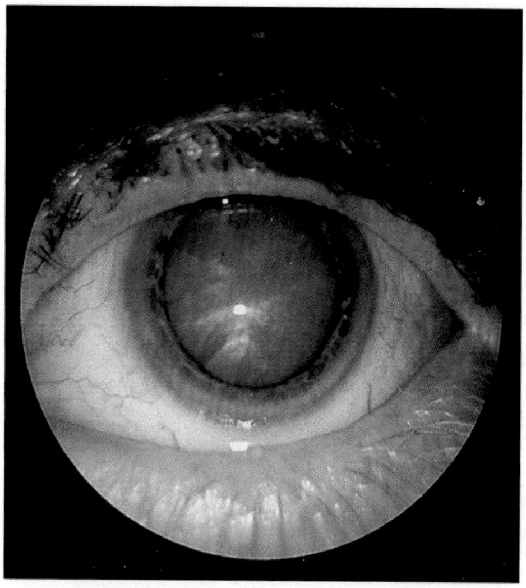

Figure 18.28 Diabetic cataract.

of the pupils in order to obtain an adequate view. Loss of the red reflex on fundoscopy may indicate cataract formation, and the lens should be assessed for opacities (Fig. 18.28). The vitreous and retina should be examined carefully, starting from the optic disc and radiating into each quadrant of the eye. The macula is examined last, as this can be quite uncomfortable for the patient. The use of green light may aid the detection of microaneurysms. Ideally, all patients with diabetes should have annual fundal photography. A classification of diabetic retinopathy is shown in Box 18.12 (and see Figs 18.29-18.33).

Cardiovascular system

Examination of the heart and vasculature is important in patients with diabetes. Palpation of peripheral pulses, especially of the feet, is extremely important, as is auscultation of the carotid and femoral arteries to detect bruits. Blood pressure should be measured frequently in patients with diabetes to detect hypertension (classed at >140/80 mmHg in patients with

Box 18.12 Characteristic features of diabetic retinopathy

Non-proliferative retinopathy

- Microaneurysms
- Dot hacmorrhages
- Hard exudates (lipid deposits) not involving the macula

Mild

- <5 microaneurysms
- Haemorrhages and/or exudates

Moderate

- Extensive (>5) blot haemorrhages and/or microaneurysms and/or cotton wool spots (retinal ischaemia)
- Venous beading
- Looping or reduplication
- Intraretinal microvascular anomaly (IRMA)

Severe

- Intraretinal deep blocked haemorrhages in four quadrants
- Venous beading in two quadrants
- Severe IRMA in one quadrant

Proliferative retinopathy

- New vessels on disc (NVD) or elsewhere (NVE)

Maculopathy

- Any retinopathy 1 disc diameter around the macula
- Focal or exudative maculopathy
- Diffuse
- Ischaemic

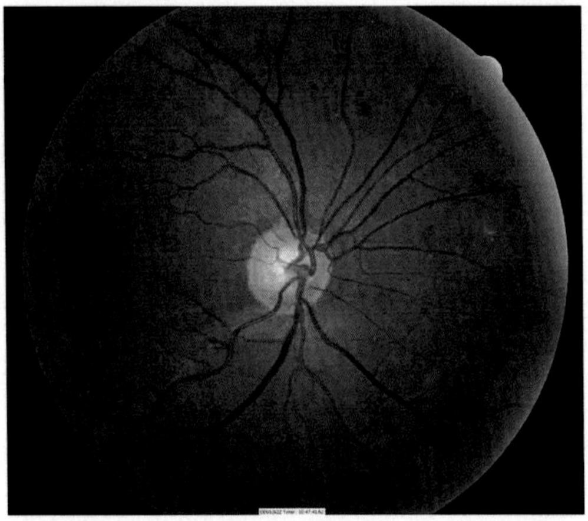

Figure 18.29 Background retinopathy (dot haemorrhages and microaneurysms) in the inferior nasal region. (Courtesy of Dr Paul Dodson.)

diabetes) or postural hypotension (drop in systolic BP >20 mmHg on standing). A resting tachycardia, loss of sinus arrhythmia (reflex bradycardia on expiration) and loss of reflex bradycardia during a Valsalva manoeuvre can indicate autonomic neuropathy, although these are best assessed by electrocardiography (ECG).

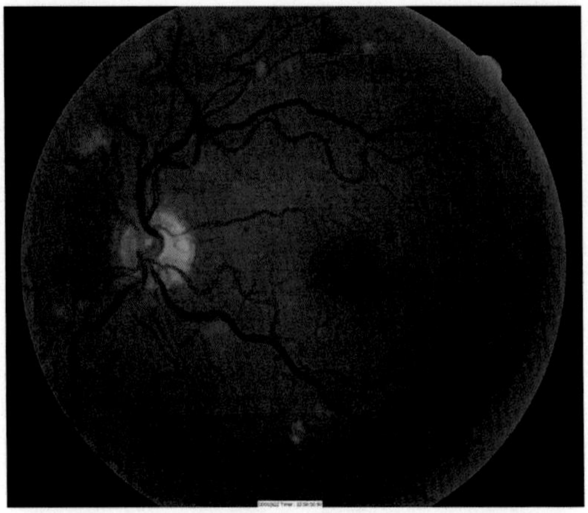

Figure 18.30 Preproliferative changes with multiple dot and blot haemorrhages and cotton wool spots. (Courtesy of Dr Paul Dodson.)

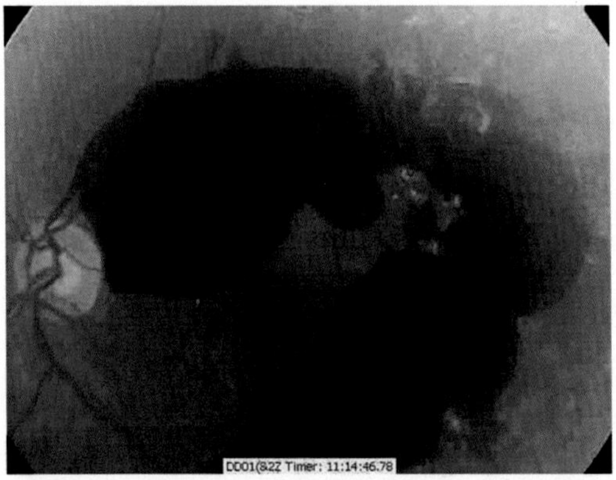

Figure 18.31 Retinal haemorrhage due to new vessel formation in severe proliferative retinopathy. (Courtesy of Dr Paul Dodson.)

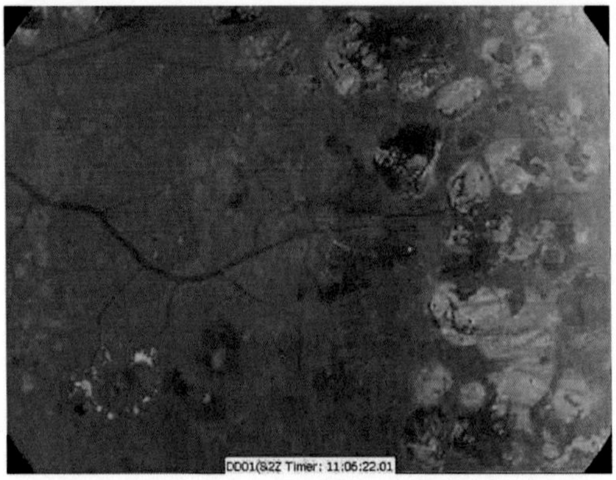

Figure 18.32 New vessel formation and laser photocoagulation burns in severe proliferative retinopathy. (Courtesy of Dr Paul Dodson.)

Feet

The feet of patients with diabetes should be examined at least once a year. Signs of deformity, callus (a sign of excessive pressure at this site), fungal infection especially between the toes, nail care and ulceration should be carefully assessed. Peripheral pulses and

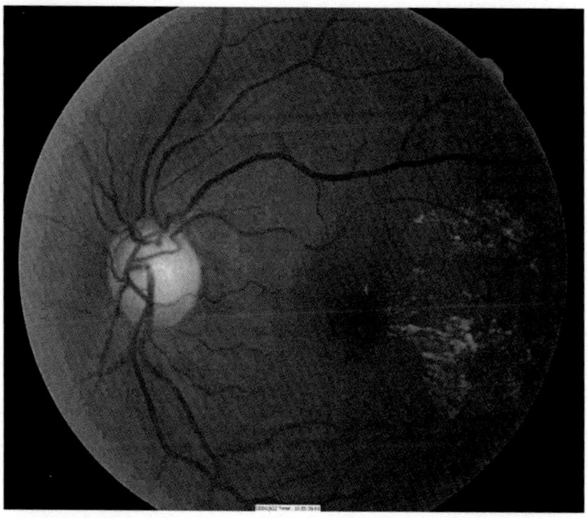

Figure 18.33 Exudative diabetic maculopathy. (Courtesy of Dr Paul Dodson.)

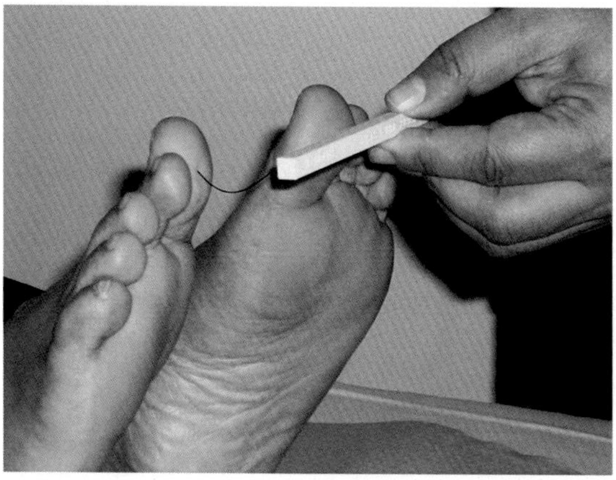

Figure 18.34 Testing for neuropathy using a Semmes Weinstein monofilament giving standard 10 g of fine touch.

nail-fold refill should be assessed for signs of peripheral vascular disease. Nerve function should be assessed by testing vibration sense at the great toe, medial malleolus and knee, and testing fine touch on the toes, metatarsal heads, heels and dorsum of the feet with a 10-g monofilament (Semmes Weinstein monofilament) (Fig. 18.34). Loss of ankle jerks is also a sign of early diabetic peripheral sensory neuropathy.

A complication of diabetic peripheral neuropathy is the neuropathic joint – Charcot neuroarthropathy (see Fig. 18.18). This usually affects the ankle and presents with a painless, swollen, hot red joint, sometimes with a history of minor local trauma. The natural history is of progressive deformity until the process settles, usually over a few months. Untreated, the joint develops severe deformity, which then puts the foot at high risk of ulceration, infection and amputation. Treatment is with immobilization in a plaster-cast boot and intravenous bisphosphonates.

Diabetic patients with signs of peripheral vascular disease or peripheral neuropathy, even if asymptomatic, should be classified as at high risk for ulceration and be given careful education on foot care by a podiatrist.

Investigation

Diagnosis of diabetes is based on a fasting plasma glucose, oral glucose tolerance test (OGTT) or Glycated Haemoglobin (HbA_{1c}) using the WHO criteria (see Box 18.9). Although clinically it is relatively simple to distinguish between type 1 and type 2 diabetes, occasionally the diagnosis is not clear, especially in younger-onset type 2 diabetes without a family history. In these circumstances, the use of immunological tests such as anti-islet cell (ICA) or antiglutamic acid decarboxylase (GAD) antibody may be helpful. Positivity of either is a good indicator of autoimmune islet cell destruction (and hence probable type 1 diabetes), insulin deficiency and a subsequent requirement for insulin therapy.

In acute hyperglycaemic decompensation of diabetes, urgent investigations are required, including a laboratory glucose estimation, assessment of renal function (urea and electrolytes), urinalysis testing for ketones and glucose, and arterial blood gas assessment to determine pH and bicarbonate level. A search for precipitating causes should be undertaken, including a chest radiograph, ECG, white cell count and, in younger women, a pregnancy test.

In order to reduce the risk of chronic complications, it is important to ensure a full biochemical assessment is undertaken yearly as part of an annual diabetic review. Renal and liver function should be checked, along with assessment of urine albumin excretion. Glycaemic control can be assessed using the HbA_{1c}, which is well correlated to prevailing glycaemic control over the preceding 10-12 weeks. Glycaemic targets are individualized according to the patient's age, comorbidities, risk of hypoglycaemia and his own preferences. An HbA_{1c} less than 53 mmol/mol (7.0%) is generally deemed to show acceptable glycaemic control. Lipid profile (cholesterol, triglycerides, low-density lipoprotein (LDL) cholesterol and high-density lipoprotein (HDL) cholesterol) should be checked yearly.

Lipid disorders

The two circulating lipids, cholesterol and triglyceride, are transported within lipoproteins in the circulation. The apolipoproteins over the surface of these molecules enable their recognition by cells in organs such as the liver. Lipid disorders are common and contribute significantly to the burden of cardiovascular disease. Primary lipid disorders are usually inherited, whereas secondary disorders are acquired as a result of other medical disorders, such as thyroid disease, diabetes, liver disease, nephrotic syndrome or alcohol excess.

History

Lipid disorders rarely cause significant symptoms, unless the patient presents with an acute feature such as acute pancreatitis or myocardial infarction. Thus, any previous history of vascular disease or acute abdominal pain should be sought. Acute pancreatitis is a rare complication of severe hypertriglyceridaemia and presents with acute, severe, generalized abdominal pain. Although alcohol and cholelithiasis are the commonest causes of acute pancreatitis, hypertriglyceridaemia is a well-recognized and easily overlooked cause of the condition, and any patient presenting with acute pancreatitis should have his serum lipids checked.

In the assessment of patients with lipid disorders, it is important to enquire about symptoms of ischaemic heart disease (chest pain history, admissions for ischaemic heart disease and any cardiological/cardiothoracic interventions), peripheral vascular disease (intermittent claudication) and cerebrovascular disease (transient ischaemic attacks, amaurosis fugax and strokes). Other cardiovascular risk factors should also be assessed. The smoking history is very important and a family history of premature vascular disease (under the age of 55 years) should be carefully sought. In familial hypercholesterolaemia, half of men and a fifth of women die before the age of 60 from coronary heart disease. Possible symptoms of secondary causes should also be assessed. Thus, symptoms of hypothyroidism (above), diabetes (above), renal failure or nephrotic syndrome (Ch. 17) and liver disease (Ch. 14) should be sought. Alcohol intake and dietary history should also be assessed.

Examination

The diagnostic hallmark of familial hypercholesterolaemia is tendon xanthomata. These are localized infiltrates of lipid-containing macrophages that resemble atherosclerotic plaques; they develop from the third decade onwards. The commonest sites are the Achilles tendon and the extensor tendons of the hands, particularly over the knuckles (Fig. 18.35). Other sites include the tibial tuberosities, at the site of insertion of the patellar tendon (subperiosteal xanthomata) or at the triceps tendon at the elbow.

As the cholesterol deposition is deep within the tendon and the swelling is fibrous, tendon xanthomata are felt as hard nodules along the length of the tendon. They occasionally become inflamed, and a tenosynovitis develops. On the extensor surface of the hands, they may overlie the knuckle and be very hard and quite easy to miss.

Xanthelasmata are deposits of lipid in the skin of the eyelids, more commonly the upper rather than the lower (see Fig. 18.27). Although a dramatic sign, they are not present in the majority of patients with familial hypercholesterolaemia. More common is a corneal arcus, seen as a rim of lipid deposit around the iris (Fig. 18.27). This can be seen at any age, although it is more common in older people; only in the minority is this sign associated with hypercholesterolaemia.

The characteristic sign of hypertriglyceridaemia is eruptive xanthomata (Fig. 18.36). These are yellow nodules or papules that usually appear on the extensor surface of the elbows, knees, buttocks and back. Striate palmar xanthomas are yellowish discoloration of the skin creases, usually seen best in the hands, and are due to hypertriglyceridaemia. In severe forms of hypertriglyceridaemia, hepatosplenomegaly may be seen. Funduscopy in severe hypertriglyceridaemia may show lipaemia retinalis, characterized by optic pallor and the retinal vessels appearing white (Fig. 18.37).

A careful cardiovascular examination should be performed in all patients with significant hyperlipidaemia, including a search for carotid or femoral bruits and signs of peripheral vascular disease. Patients with homozygous familial hypercholesterolaemia may have signs of aortic stenosis.

Investigation

All patients with lipid disorders should undergo a fasting lipid profile, comprising total cholesterol, LDL cholesterol, HDL cholesterol and triglycerides. In severe hypertriglyceridaemia, the serum may become turbid and take on the appearance

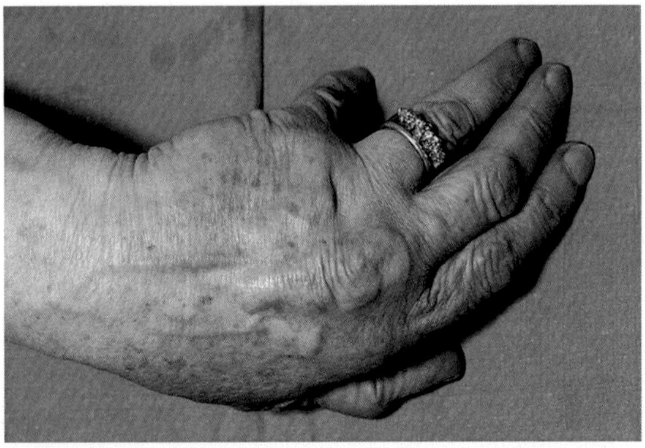

Figure 18.35 Tendon xanthoma of the hands. (Courtesy of Dr David Peterson.)

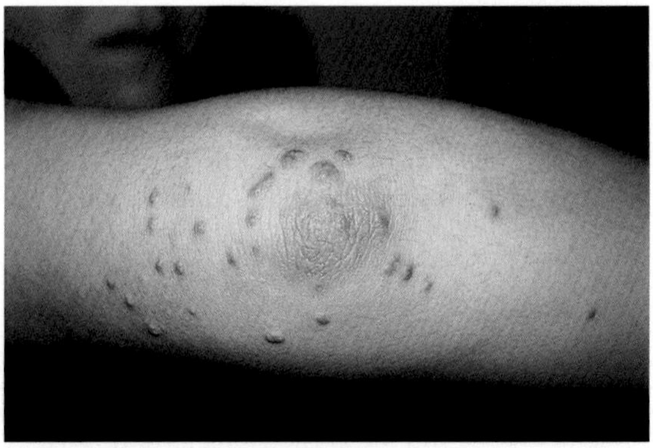

Figure 18.36 Eruptive xanthomata in severe hypertriglyceridaemia. (Courtesy of Dr David Peterson.)

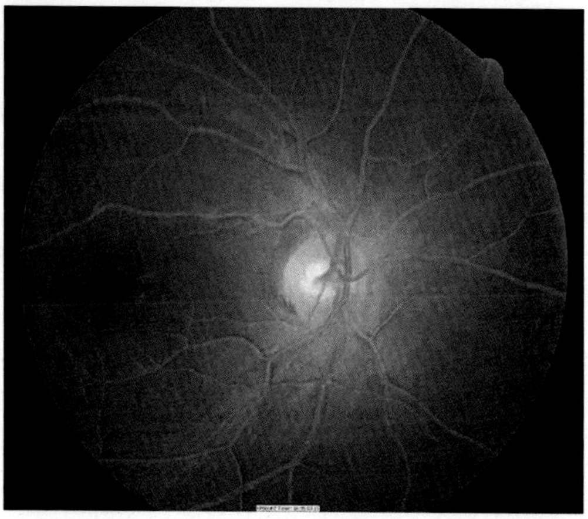

Figure 18.37 Lipaemia retinalis. (Courtesy of Dr Paul Dodson.)

of milk. Investigations to exclude secondary causes should include thyroid, liver and renal function and fasting glucose. Resting or exercise ECG may be checked to look for signs of ischaemic heart disease. Genotyping to determine the type of familial lipid abnormality may be required, especially for familial hypercholesterolaemia, although this is usually only available in specialist centres.

Acute pancreatitis can be diagnosed using serum amylase, which is frequently very elevated in the condition. In severe hypertriglyceridaemia, however, falsely low serum amylase can lead to diagnostic confusion, as triglycerides interfere with the amylase assay. Severe hypertriglyceridaemia can lead to a pseudohyponatraemia, and care should be exercised when interpreting serum sodium levels in the condition.

Skin, nails and hair 19

Rino Cerio

Introduction

The skin is the largest organ in the human body. Forming a major interface between man and his environment, it covers an area of approximately 2 m and weighs about 4 kg. The structure of human skin is complex (Figs 19.1 and 19.2), consisting of four distinct layers and tissue components with many important functions (Box 19.1). Reactions may occur in any of the components of human skin and their clinical manifestations reflect, among other factors, the skin level in which they occur, and sometimes they act as a 'window' of systemic changes elsewhere in the body, e.g. medical conditions discussed later in the chapter, such as those associated with pruritus (Box 19.9), systemic causes of erythema nodosum (Box 19.10) or paraneoplastic skin conditions (Box 19.2).

The accurate diagnosis of most skin lesions requires an adequate history, careful examination of the patient and, occasionally, laboratory investigation, but dermatology is predominantly a visual specialty.

History

Detailed information should be sought concerning the present skin condition. This should include the site of onset, mode of spread and duration of the disorder. Any personal history or family history of skin disease, including skin cancer and atopy (an allergic skin reaction becoming apparent more or less immediately on contact), is important. Previous medical conditions should be noted and a full drug history obtained, including use of over-the-counter and other preparations. The social and occupational history and, in some circumstances, details of recent travel, environmental exposure, especially sunshine and artificial ultraviolet light, and sexual activity are often important (see Box 19.3).

Examination

The whole skin, including hair, nails and assessable mucosae, should be fully inspected (preferably in natural light), but the patient's modesty should be protected. Sometimes a magnifying lens or dermatoscope is useful.

Colour and pigmentation

Before inspecting any rash or lesion, note the colour of the skin. Normal skin colour varies, depending on lifestyle and light exposure as well as constitutional and ethnic factors.

Pallor can have many causes. It may be:

- temporary, due to shock, haemorrhage or intense emotion
- persistent, due to anaemia or peripheral vasoconstriction.

Vasoconstriction is seen in patients with severe atopy – an inherited susceptibility to asthma, eczema and hay fever. Pallor is a feature of anaemia, but not all pale persons are anaemic; conjunctival and mucosal colour is a better indication of anaemia than skin colour. A pale skin resulting from diminished pigment occurs with hypopituitarism and hypogonadism.

Normal skin contains varying amounts of brown melanin pigment. Brown pigmentation due to deposited haemosiderin is always pathological. Albinism is an inherited generalized absence of pigment in the skin; a localized form is known as piebaldism. Patches of white and darkly pigmented skin (vitiligo) (Fig. 19.3) are due to a local and complete absence of melanocytes. Several autoimmune endocrine disorders are associated with vitiligo.

Abnormal redness of the skin (erythema) is seen after overheating, extreme exertion, sunburn and in febrile, exanthematous and inflammatory skin diseases. Flushing is a striking redness, usually of the face and neck, which may be transient or persistent. Local redness may be due to telangiectasia, especially on the face. Cyanosis is a blue or purple-blue tint due to the presence of excessive reduced haemoglobin, either locally, as in impaired peripheral circulation, or generally, when oxygenation of the blood is defective. The skin colour in methaemoglobinaemia is more leaden than in ordinary cyanosis; it is caused by drugs, such as dapsone, and certain poisons.

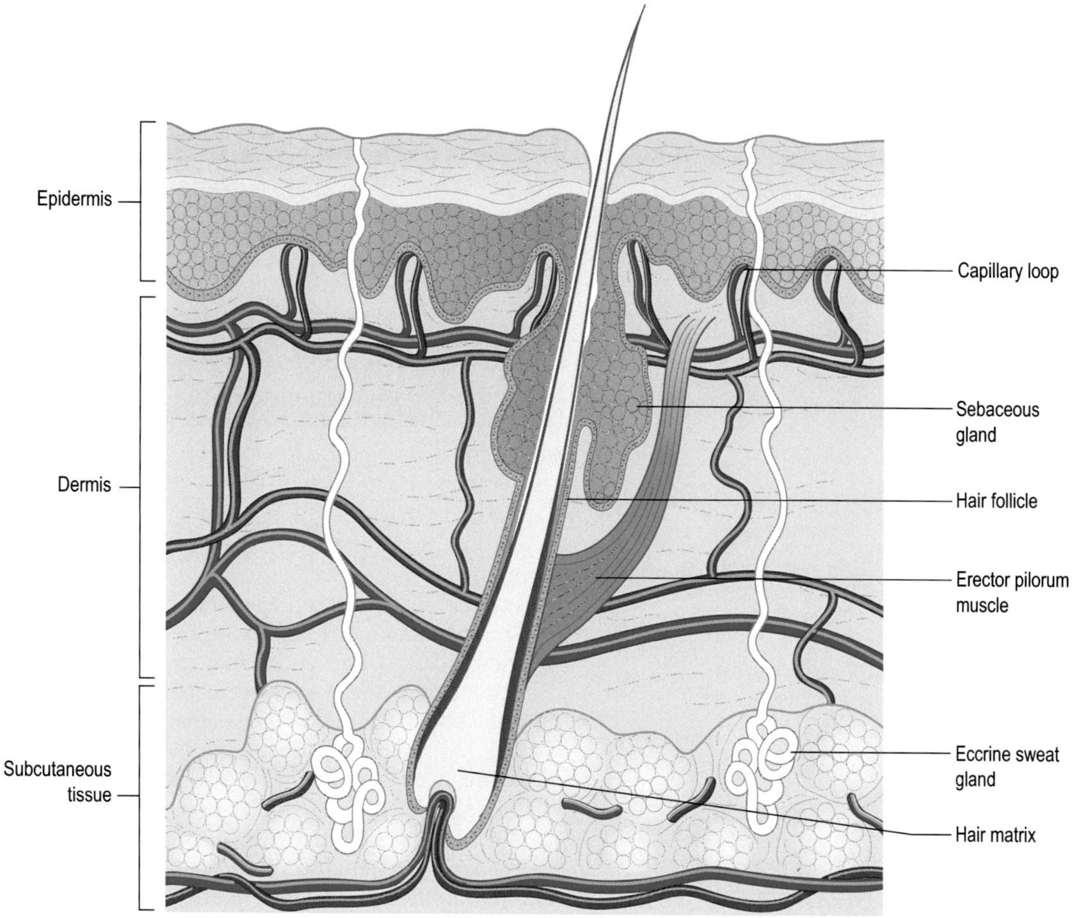

Figure 19.1 The anatomy of the full thickness of the skin in section.

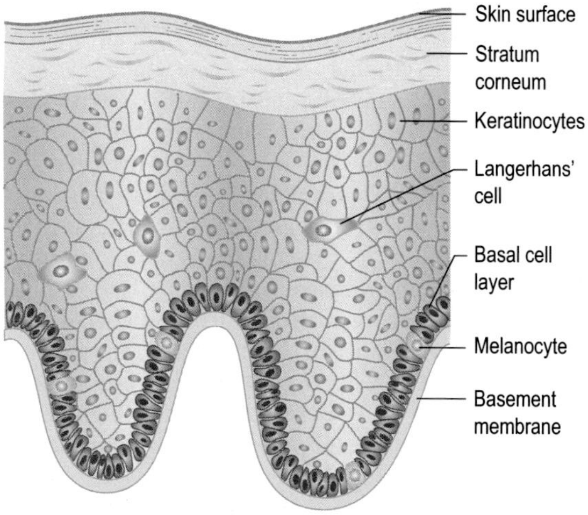

Figure 19.2 The anatomy of the epidermis.

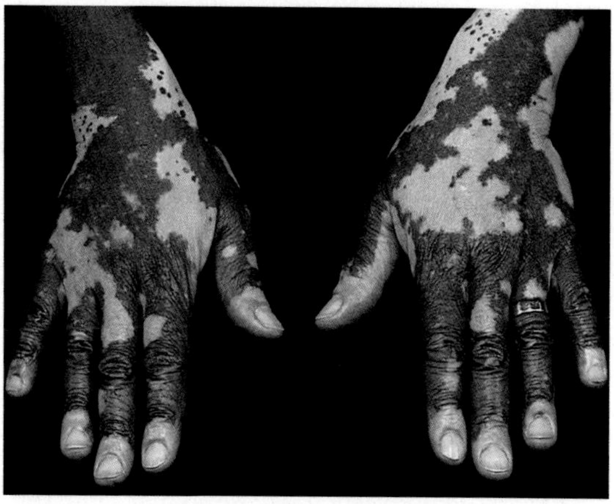

Figure 19.3 Vitiligo, a disorder of cutaneous pigmentation that is often autoimmune in origin and associated with other autoimmune disorders.

Jaundice varies from the subicteric lemon-yellow tints seen in pernicious anaemia and acholuric jaundice to various shades of yellow, orange or dark olive-green in obstructive jaundice. Jaundice, which stains the conjunctivae, must be distinguished from the rare orange-yellow of carotenaemia, which does not. Slight degrees of jaundice cannot be seen in artificial light.

Increased pigmentation may be racial, due to sunburn or connected with various diseases. In Addison's disease, there is a brown or dark-brown

Box 19.1 Functions of the human skin

- Protection: physical, chemical, infection – immune and innate
- Physiological: homoeostasis of electrolytes, water and protein
- Thermoregulation
- Sensation: specialized nerve endings – pain, touch and temperature
- Lubrication and waterproofing: sebum
- Immunological reactions: Langerhans' cells, lymphocytes, macrophages
- Wound healing
- Ultra violet-induced vitamin D synthesis
- Body odour: apocrine glands
- Psychosocial: cosmetic

Box 19.2 Paraneoplastic skin disorders

Dermatosis	Associated tumour
Dermatomyositis	Lung, GI tract, GU tract
Acanthosis nigricans	GI tract, lung, liver
Paget's disease of the nipple/ Extra-mammary Paget's disease of the perineum	Adenocarcinoma
Erythroderma	Haematological
Tylosis-thickening of palms and soles	Oesophageal carcinoma
Ichthyosis	Lymphoma
Erythema gyratum repens	Lung, breast
Necrolytic migratory erythema	Glucagonoma

Box 19.3 Approach to dermatological patient history

Time course of skin eruption
Distribution of lesions including initially
Symptoms – pruritus
Family history – atopy and psoriasis
Drug/allergy history
Past medical history
Contacts – family and partners
Provocating factors – sunlight and foods
Previous and current treatments

pigmentation affecting exposed parts and parts not normally pigmented, such as the axillae and the palmar creases; the lips and mouth may exhibit dark bluish-black areas. Note, however, that mucosal pigmentation is a normal finding in a substantial proportion of black patients.

More or less generalized pigmentation may also be seen in the following:

- Haemochromatosis, in which the skin has a peculiar greyish-bronze colour with a metallic sheen, due to excessive melanin and iron pigment

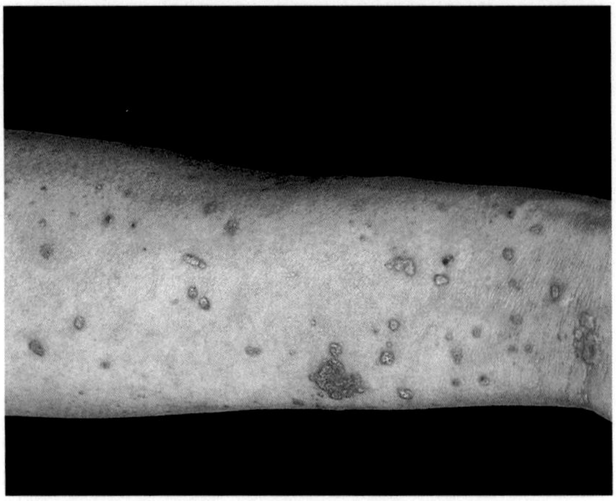

Figure 19.4 Flat-topped papules of lichen planus.

- Chronic arsenic poisoning, in which the skin is finely dappled affecting covered more than exposed parts
- Argyria, in which the deposition of silver in the skin produces a diffuse slate-grey hue
- The cachexia of advanced malignant disease

In pregnancy, there may be pigmentation of the nipples and areolae, of the linea alba and sometimes a mask-like pigmentation of the face (chloasma). Chloasma may also be induced by oral contraceptives containing oestrogen. A similar condition, melasma, may be seen in Asian and Afro-Caribbean males.

Localized pigmentation may be seen in pellagra and in scars of various kinds, particularly those due to X-irradiation therapy. Venous hypertension in the legs is often associated with chronic purpura, leading to haemosiderin pigmentation. The mixture of punctate and fresh purpura and haemosiderin may produce a golden hue on the lower calves and shins. Pigmentation may also occur with chronic infestation by body lice. Erythema ab igne, a reticular pattern of pigmentation, can be seen in patients who use local heat to relieve chronic pain or on the shins of people who habitually sit too near a fire. Livedo reticularis, a web-like pattern of reddish-blue discoloration mostly involving the legs, occurs in autoimmune vasculitis, especially in systemic lupus erythematosus (SLE) and antiphospholipid syndrome, when it is associated with cerebral infarction. The violet-coloured lesions of lichen planus are slightly raised, flat-topped papules (Fig. 19.4). Psoriasis usually presents as a symmetrical plaque on extensor surfaces (Fig. 19.5). Keloid consists of raised and inflamed, overgrown tender scar tissue (Fig. 19.6).

Skin lesions and eruptions

Skin eruptions and lesions should be examined with special reference to their morphology, distribution and arrangement. The terminology of skin lesions is summarized in Boxes 19.4 and 19.5. Colour, size, consistency, configuration, margination and surface characteristics should be noted.

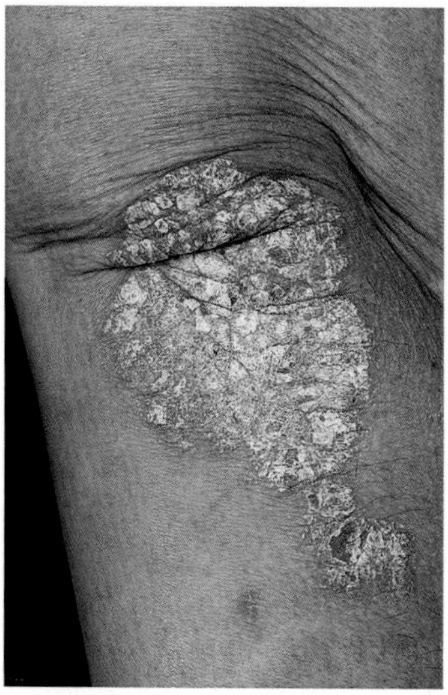

Figure 19.5 Salmon-pink plaque of psoriasis on elbow covered in characteristic silver scale.

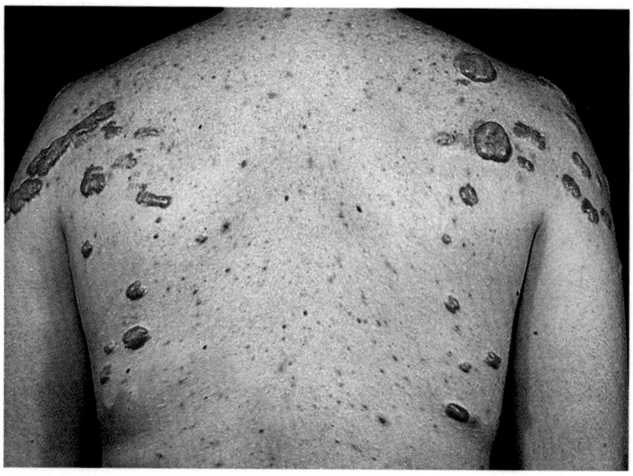

Figure 19.6 Multiple keloid scarring of the back due to acne vulgaris. There is a genetic predisposition to the formation of keloid in scar tissue.

Box 19.4 Primary skin lesions: a glossary of dermatological terms

Macule	Non-palpable area of altered colour
Papule	Palpable elevated small area of skin (<0.5 cm)
Plaque	Palpable flat-topped discoid lesion (>2 cm)
Nodule	Solid palpable lesion within the skin (>0.5 cm)
Papilloma	Pedunculated lesion projecting from the skin
Vesicle	Small fluid-filled blister (<0.5 cm)
Bulla	Large fluid-filled blister (>0.5 cm)
Pustule	Blister containing pus
Wheal	Elevated lesion, often white with red margin due to dermal oedema
Telangiectasia	Dilatation of superficial blood vessel
Petechiae	Pinhead-sized macules of blood
Purpura	Larger petechiae which do not blanch on pressure
Ecchymosis	Large extravasation of blood in skin (bruise)
Haematoma	Swelling due to gross bleeding
Poikiloderma	Atrophy, reticulate hyperpigmentation and telangiectasia
Erythema	Redness of the skin
Burrow	Linear or curved elevations of the superficial skin due to infestation by female scabies mite
Comedo	Dark horny keratin and sebaceous plugs within pilosebaceous openings

Morphology of skin lesions

Inspection and palpation

Assessment of morphology requires visual and tactile examination. Do not be afraid to feel the lesions. You will rarely be exposed to any infection risk, with the exception of herpes simplex, herpes zoster, syphilis, Hepatitis B and human immunodeficiency virus (HIV) disease. If these infections are suspected, it is wise to wear disposable plastic gloves when examining open or bleeding cutaneous lesions. Begin with palpation of the skin. Pass the hand gently over it, pinching it up between the forefinger and thumb, and note the following points:

- Is it smooth or rough, thin or thick?
- Is it dry or moist?
- Is there any visible sweating, either general or local?

The elasticity of the skin should be investigated. If a fold of healthy skin is pinched up, it immediately flattens itself out again when released. Sometimes, however, it only does so very slowly, remaining creased for a considerable time. This is found frequently in healthy old people but may be an important sign of dehydration, for example after severe vomiting and diarrhoea, or in uncontrolled diabetes mellitus.

Subcutaneous oedema

When oedema is present, firm pressure on the skin with a finger produces a shallow pit that persists for some time. In some cases, especially when the oedema is very long standing, pitting is not found. The best place to look for slight degrees of oedema in cardiac disease is behind the malleoli at the ankles in patients who are ambulant and over the sacrum in those who are confined to bed. The finger pressure should be maintained for 20-30 seconds or slight degrees of oedema will be overlooked. Pitting is minimal or absent in oedema due to lymphatic obstruction, where the skin is usually thickened and tough.

Box 19.5 Secondary skin lesions that evolve from primary lesions

Scale	Loose excess normal and abnormal horny layer
Crust	Dried exudate
Excoriation	A scratch
Lichenification	Thickening of the epidermis with exaggerated skin margin
Fissure	Slit in the skin
Erosion	Partial loss of epidermis which heals without scarring
Ulcer	At least the full thickness of the epidermis is lost. Healing occurs with scarring
Sinus	A cavity or channel that allows the escape of fluid or pus
Scar	Healing by replacement with fibrous tissue
Keloid scar	Excessive scar formation (see Fig. 19.6)
Atrophy	Thinning of the skin due to shrinkage of epidermis, dermis or subcutaneous fat
Stria	Atrophic pink or white linear lesion due to changes in connective tissue

Subcutaneous emphysema

Air trapped under the skin gives rise to a characteristic crackling sensation on palpation. It starts in, and is usually confined to, the neighbourhood of the air passages. On rare occasions, it may result from the clostridial infection of soft tissues after injury (gas gangrene).

Distribution of skin lesions

Consider the distribution of an eruption by looking at the whole skin surface:

- Is it symmetrical or asymmetrical? Symmetry often implies an internal causation, whereas asymmetry may imply external factors.
- Is the eruption centrifugal (radiating from the centre) or centripetal (radiating to the centre)? Certain common diseases such as chickenpox and pityriasis rosea are characteristically centripetal, whereas erythema multiforme and erythema nodosum are centrifugal. Smallpox, now eradicated, was also centrifugal.
- A disease may exhibit a flexor or an extensor bias in its distribution: atopic eczema in childhood is characteristically flexor, whereas psoriasis in adults tends to be extensor.
- Are only exposed areas affected, implicating sunlight or some other external causative factor?
- If sunlight is suspected, are areas normally in shadow involved?
- Are the genitalia involved?
- Localized distributions may point immediately to an external contact as the cause, for example contact dermatitis from nickel earrings, lipstick dermatitis, etc.

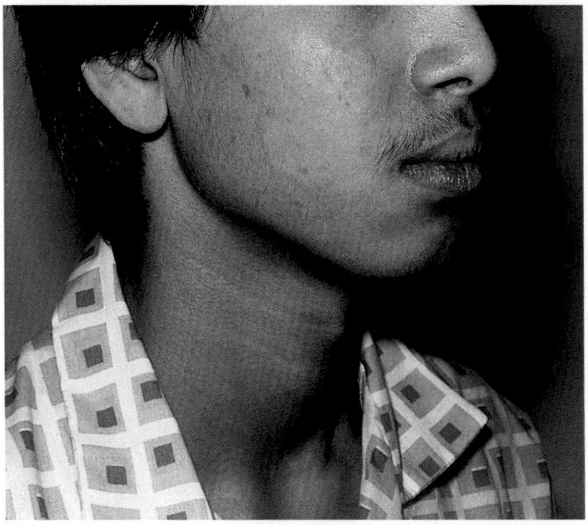

Figure 19.7 Hansen's disease. There is a depigmented area of anaesthetic and slightly pink skin on the exposed cheek. In this lepromatous lesion, acid-fast bacilli were found in scrapings.

Swelling of the eyelids is an important sign. Without redness and scaling, bilateral periorbital oedema may indicate acute nephritis, nephrosis or trichinosis. If there is irritation, contact dermatitis is the probable diagnosis. Dermatomyositis often produces swelling and heliotrope-coloured erythema of the eyelids without scaling of the skin. In Hansen's disease (leprosy), the skin lesions may be depigmented or reddened, with a slightly raised edge; they are also anaesthetic to pinprick testing (Fig. 19.7) and mainly located in skin that is normally cooler than core body temperature.

Configuration of skin lesions

Once the morphology of individual lesions and their distribution has been established, it is useful to describe their configuration on the skin (Box 19.6).

The hair

Hair colour and texture are racial characteristics that are genetically determined. The yellow-brown Mongol race has black straight hair, negroid people have black curly hair and Caucasians have fair, brown, red or black hair. Secondary sexual hair begins to appear at puberty and has characteristic male and female patterns. Androgenic male pattern baldness is genetically determined but requires adequate levels of circulating androgens for its expression. It occurs in women only in old age.

Growth of hair

Unlike other epithelial mitotic activity that is continuous throughout life, the growth of hair is cyclic (Fig. 19.8), the hair follicle going through alternating phases of growth (anagen) and rest (telogen). Anagen

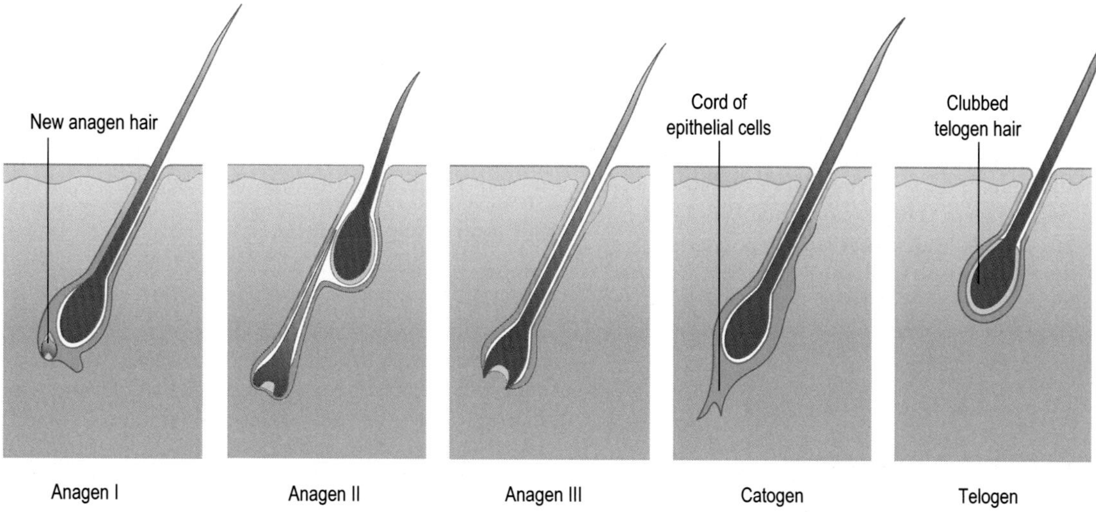

Figure 19.8 Hair follicle growth stages.

Box 19.6 Configuration of individual lesions

- Nummular/discoid
- Round or coin-like
- Annular
- Ring-like
- Circinate
- Circular
- Arcuate
- Curved
- Gyrate/serpiginous
- Wave-like
- Linear
- In a line
- Grouped
- Clustered
- Reticulate
- Net-like

Box 19.7 Causes of alopecia

Non-scarring

- Alopecia areata
- Trichotillomania (self-induced hair pulling)
- Traction alopecia
- Scalp ringworm (human)
- Metabolic iron deficiency, hypothyroidism)
- Drugs, e.g. heparin, retinoids, chemotherapy
- Sarcoidosis

Scarring

- Burns, trauma
- Aplasia cutis
- Discoid lupus erythematosus, lichen planopilaris
- Dissecting folliculitis
- Pseudopelade
- Kerion (see Fig. 19.30)
- X-irradiation
- Necrobiosis

in the scalp lasts 3-5 years; telogen is much shorter, about 3 months. Catagen is the conversion stage from active to resting and usually lasts a few days. The duration of the anagen phase determines the length to which hair in different body areas can grow. On the scalp, there are on average about 100 000 hairs. The normal scalp may shed as many as 100 hairs every day as a normal consequence of growth cycling. These proportions can be estimated by looking at plucked hairs (trichogram); the 'root' of a telogen hair is non-pigmented and visible as a white, club-like swelling. Normally 85% of scalp hairs are in anagen and 15% in telogen.

Alopecia

Hair loss (alopecia) has many causes. It is convenient to subdivide alopecia into localized and diffuse types. In addition, the clinician should determine whether the alopecia results in scarring and hence, permanent hair loss (Box 19.7).

Any inflammatory or destructive disease of the scalp skin may destroy hair follicles in its wake. Thus, burns, heavy X-ray irradiation or herpes zoster infection in the first division of the trigeminal nerve may cause scarring and alopecia. Alopecia in the presence of normal scalp skin may be patchy and localized, as in traction alopecia in nervous children, ringworm infections (tinea capitis) or autoimmune alopecia areata. Secondary syphilis is a rare cause of a patchy alopecia with a 'moth-eaten' appearance.

Scalp hair loss at the temples and crown, with the growth of male-type body hair, is characteristic of women with virilizing disorders. Metabolic causes of diffuse hair loss in women include hypothyroidism and severe iron deficiency anaemia. Antimitotic drugs may affect the growing hair follicles, producing a diffuse loss of anagen hairs, which are pigmented throughout their length. Dramatic metabolic upsets, such as childbirth, starvation and severe toxic illnesses, may precipitate follicles into the resting phase, producing an effluvium of telogen hairs 3 months later, when anagen begins again. This is called telogen alopecia. In the autoimmune disorder alopecia totalis (Fig. 19.9), there is complete loss of hair. Self-inflicted traction alopecia (Fig. 19.10) may indicate psychological problems.

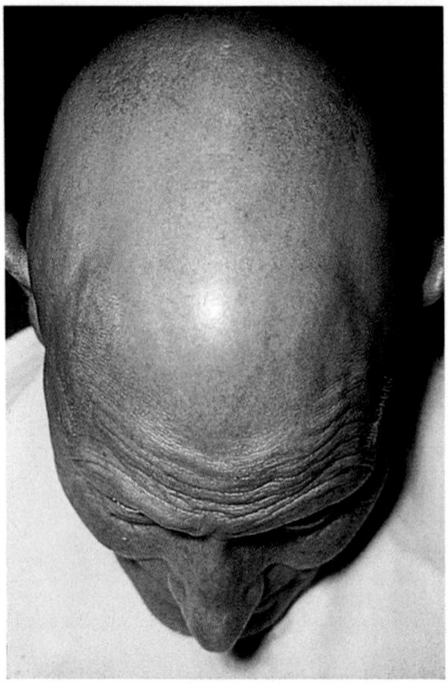

Figure 19.9 Alopecia totalis.

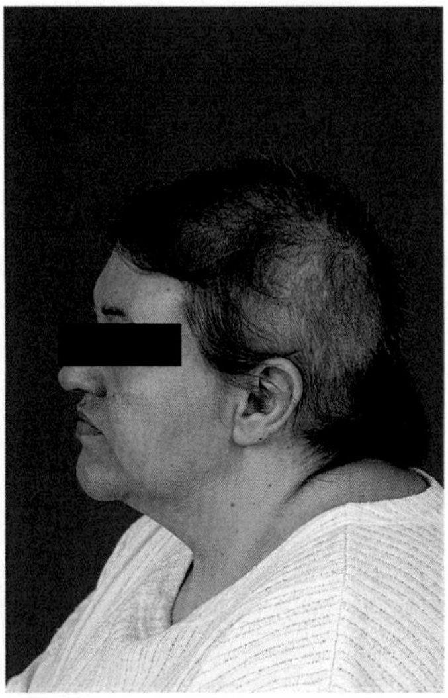

Figure 19.10 Traction alopecia in a psychologically troubled patient.

The nails

The nails should be examined carefully. The structure of the nail and nail bed is shown in Figs 19.11 and 19.12. The nail consists of a strong, relatively inflexible keratinous nail plate over the dorsal surface of the end of each digit, protecting the fingertip.

Nail matrix abnormalities

Thimble pitting of the nails is characteristic of psoriasis (Fig. 19.13), but eczema and alopecia areata may also produce pitting. A severe illness may temporarily arrest nail growth; when growth starts again, transverse ridges develop. These are called Beau's lines and can be used to date the time of onset of an illness. Inflammation of the cuticle or nail fold (chronic paronychia)

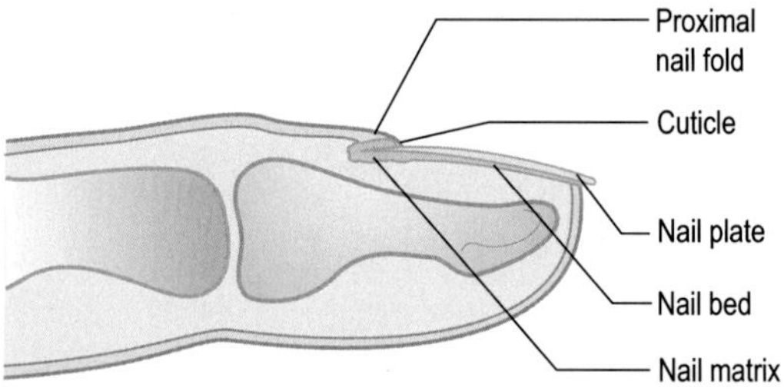

Figure 19.11 Structure of the nail (lateral view).

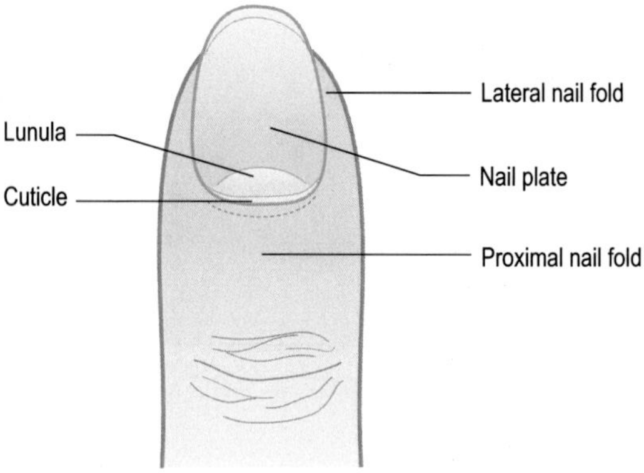

Figure 19.12 Structure of the nail (dorsal view).

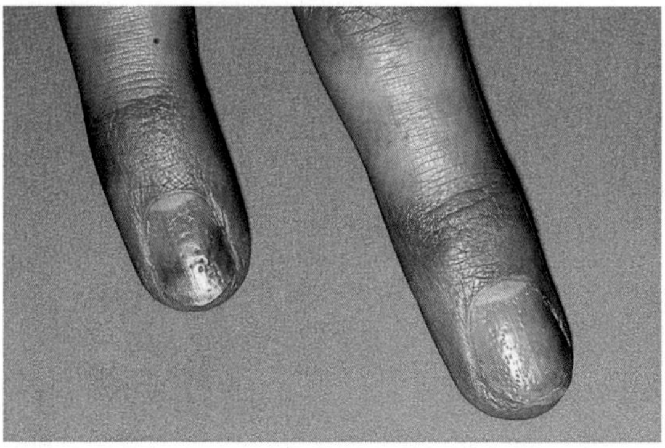

Figure 19.13 Psoriasis of the nail beds.

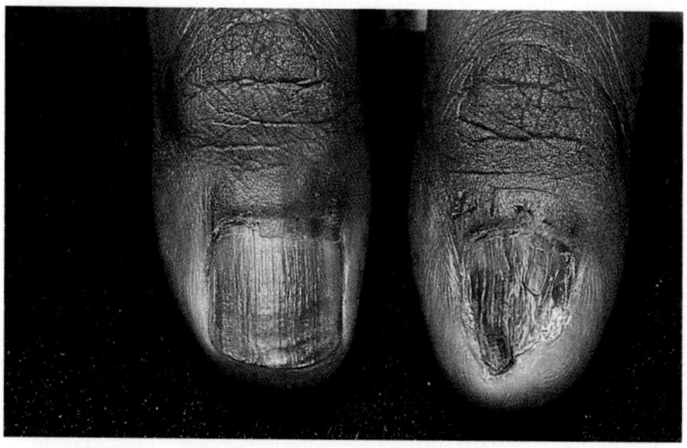

Figure 19.14 Lichen planus, showing longitudinal ridging of the nails and overgrowth of the cuticle on the nail plate (pterygium).

may produce similar changes. The changes described above arise from disturbance of the nail matrix.

Nail and nail-bed abnormalities

Disturbance of the nail bed may produce thick nails (pachyonychia) or separation of the nail from the bed (onycholysis). This occurs in psoriasis but may be idiopathic. Long-term tetracyclines may induce separation when the fingers are exposed to strong sunlight (photo-onycholysis). The nail may be destroyed in severe lichen planus (Fig. 19.14) or epidermolysis bullosa (a genetic abnormality in which the skin blisters in response to minor trauma). Nails are missing in the inherited nail-patella syndrome. Splinter haemorrhages under the nails may result from trauma, psoriasis, rheumatoid arthritis or other 'collagen vascular' diseases, bacterial endocarditis and trichinosis.

The nails in systemic disease

In long-lasting iron-deficiency states, the fingernails and toenails become soft, thin, brittle and spoon-shaped. They lose their normal transverse convex curvature, becoming flattened or concave (koilonychia). The 'half and half nail', with a white proximal and red or brown distal half, is seen in some patients with chronic renal failure. Whitening of the nail plates may be related to hypoalbuminaemia, as in cirrhosis of the liver (leuconychia). Some drugs, notably antimalarials, antibiotics and phenothiazines, may discolour the nail. Nail-fold telangiectasia or erythema is a useful physical sign in dermatomyositis (Fig. 19.15), systemic sclerosis and systemic lupus erythematosus. In dermatomyositis, the cuticle becomes ragged. In systemic sclerosis, loss of finger pads may lead to curvature of the nail plates. An impaired peripheral circulation, as in Raynaud's phenomenon, can lead to thinning and longitudinal ridging of the nail plate, sometimes with partial onycholysis. In bronchiectasis, the nails may take on a curved, yellow appearance (Fig. 19.16).

Clubbing

Clubbing is probably caused by hypervascularity and the opening of anastomotic channels in the nail bed.

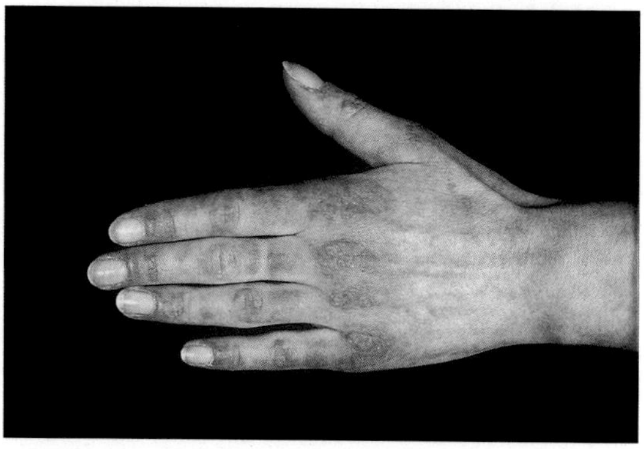

Figure 19.15 Typical heliotrope-coloured erythema seen in dermatomyositis (periungual and Gottron's papules over the knuckles).

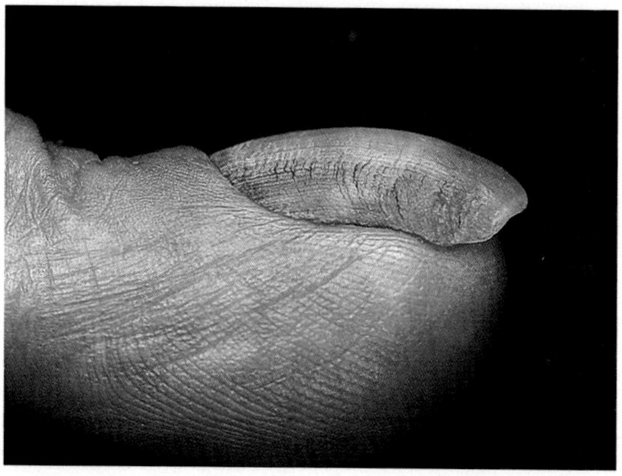

Figure 19.16 Yellow nail syndrome in bronchiectasis.

Rarely, clubbing may be congenital. The distal end of the digit becomes expanded, with the nail curved excessively in both longitudinal and transverse planes. Viewed from the side, the angle at the nail plate is lost and may exceed 180°. In normal nails, when both thumbnails are placed in apposition, there is a lozenge-shaped gap whereas, in clubbing, there is a reduction in this gap (Schamroth's window test, Fig. 19.17). In hypertrophic pulmonary osteoarthropathy, there is clubbing of the fingers and thickening of the periosteum of the radius, ulna, tibia and fibula, which can be tender. (The causes of clubbing are listed in Box 19.8.)

Cutaneous manifestations of internal disease

Genodermatoses (lesions of inherited origin)

White macules shaped like small ash leaves and present at birth may be the first sign of tuberous sclerosis. Sometimes they are difficult to see by natural

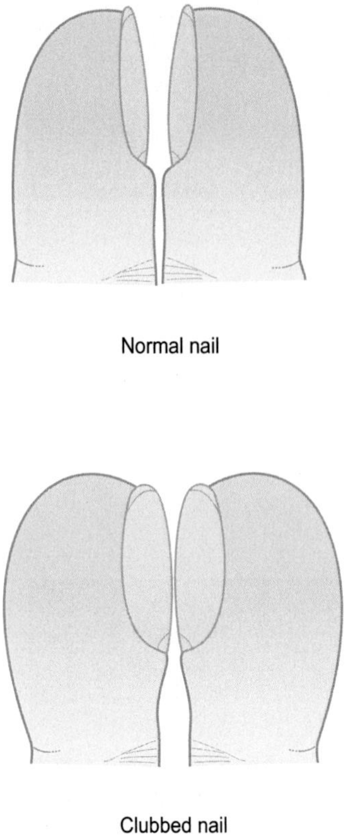

Figure 19.17 Schamroth's window test.

Box 19.8 Causes of clubbing of the fingers

Cardiopulmonary disorders

- Severe chronic cyanosis
- Cyanotic congenital heart disease
- Chronic fibrosing alveolitis
- Chronic suppuration in the lungs:
  - bronchiectasis
  - empyema
  - lung abscess
- Carcinoma of the bronchus
- Bacterial endocarditis

Chronic abdominal disorders

- Crohn's disease
- Ulcerative colitis
- Cirrhosis of the liver

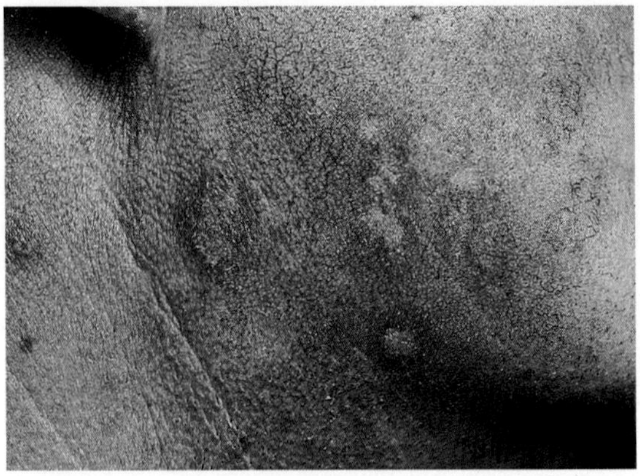

Figure 19.18 Discoid lupus erythematosus, showing atrophic scars.

light but show up under ultraviolet light (Wood's light). They should be looked for in infants with seizures. Pigmentation of the lips is a feature of the genetically determined Peutz-Jeghers syndrome, in which multiple polyps of the stomach or colon appear that may later undergo malignant transformation. Café au lait type macules, sometimes multiple, are a common sign of neurofibromatosis (NF). Another valuable sign in von Recklinghausen's neurofibromatosis is bilateral freckling of the axillary skin. The characteristic soft neurofibromata may be solitary or a few or hundreds may be scattered over the body. Ichthyosis (scaly fish skin) is usually present from childhood and is genetic, but if ichthyosis is acquired in adult life, a search should be made for malignancy or other underlying disease.

Non-organ-specific autoimmune disorders

Several of the so-called collagen vascular diseases show characteristic cutaneous eruptions. Systemic lupus erythematosus, seen in women between puberty and the menopause, may show a symmetrical 'butterfly' erythema of the nose and cheeks. In discoid lupus, the cutaneous lesion is localized (Fig. 19.18). In polyarteritis nodosa, reticular livedo of the limbs with purpura, vasculitic papules and ulceration occurs. In scleroderma (systemic sclerosis), acrosclerosis of the fingertips with scarring, ulceration and calcinosis follows a Raynaud's phenomenon of increasing severity. Dermatomyositis often presents with a heliotrope-coloured discoloration and oedema of the eyelids and with fixed erythema over the dorsa of the knuckles and fingers (see Fig. 19.15) and over the bony points of the shoulders, elbows and legs. There is usually weakness of the proximal limb muscles. Dermatomyositis in the middle aged is associated with internal malignancy in about 10% of cases.

Skin pigmentation

Acanthosis nigricans is a brownish velvety thickening of the axillae, groins and sides of the neck. Sometimes there is thickening of the palms and soles, and warty excrescences may develop on the skin, eyelids and oral mucosa. In the middle-aged, acanthosis nigricans is strongly associated with internal malignancy, but benign minor forms are seen in obese young women, especially in Arab people, and in children with endocrinopathies characterized by insulin resistance. Patchy depigmented macules which are hypoanaesthetic and associated with enlargement of the peripheral nerves are a feature of certain types of leprosy (Hansen's disease).

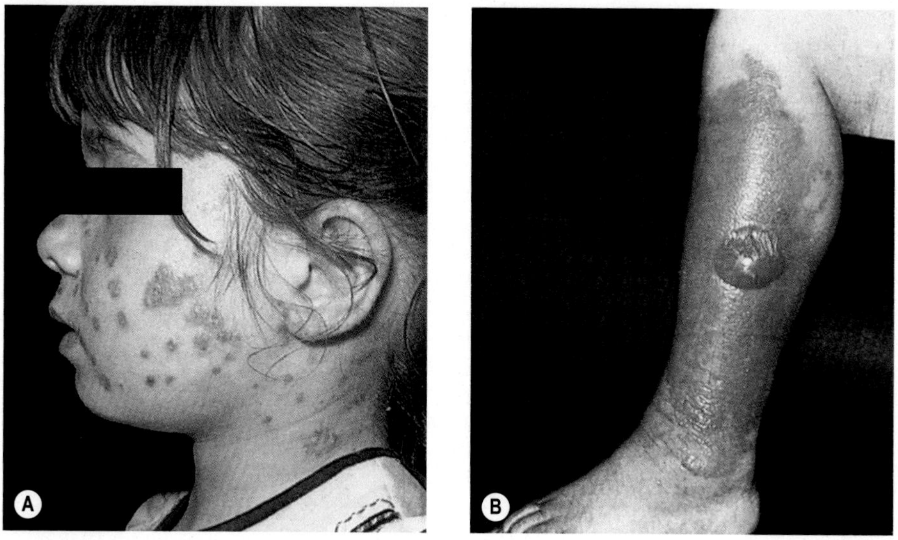

Figure 19.19 **(A)** Impetigo. **(B)** Erysipelas.

Box 19.9 Causes of pruritus in systemic disease

- Iron deficiency anaemia
- Diabetes mellitus
- Thyrotoxicosis or hypothyroidism
- Chronic renal failure
- Chronic hepatic failure
- Biliary obstruction including primary biliary cholangitis
- Lymphoma and other internal malignancies
- Drugs, e.g. cocaine, morphine
- HIV infection
- Polycythemia vera
- Parasites, e.g. onchocerciasis
- Psychogenic

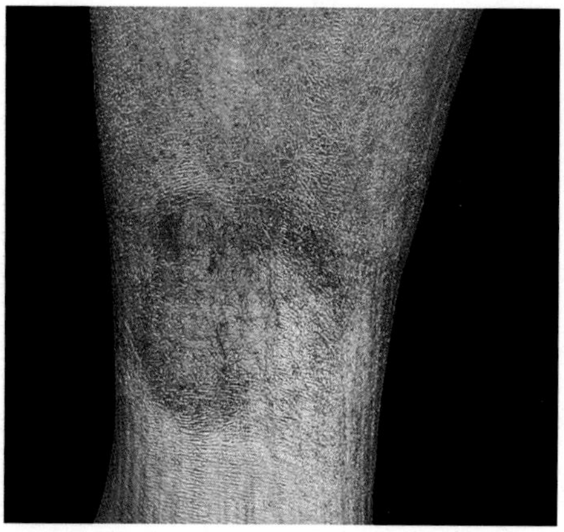

Figure 19.20 Necrobiosis lipoidica diabeticorum.

Generalized, severe persistent pruritus in the absence of obvious skin disease may be due to systemic disease (Box 19.9). However, in older people with dry skin, it is common and of no systemic significance. Diabetes mellitus has a number of skin manifestations; of these, pruritus vulvae, pruritus ani, balanoposthitis and angular stomatitis are due to *Candida* overgrowth. Boils, follicular pustules or ecthyma are staphylococcal in origin. Impetigo and erysipelas, both streptococcal infections, are uncommon (Fig. 19.19). Eruptive xanthomata are a rare feature of uncontrolled diabetes mellitus. Necrobiosis lipoidica diabeticorum (Fig. 19.20) produces reddish-brown plaques, usually on the shins, with central atrophy of the skin. It has to be distinguished from peritibial myxoedema (which is hypertrophic, not atrophic), the dermatoliposclerosis of chronic venous disease in the legs and the epidermal hypertrophy of chronic lymphatic obstruction.

Neuropathic ('perforating') ulcers are found on pressure points of the heel, ball of the foot or toes and are characteristically painless. Arteriopathic ulceration resulting from large vessel disease is seen on the foot and on the calves in small vessel disease. Spider naevi consist of a central arteriole feeding a cluster of surrounding vessels. Many young people have up to seven naevi on the face, shoulders or arms. In others, pregnancy, the administration of oestrogens (as in oral contraceptives) and liver disease may cause multiple lesions. Pregnancy and liver disease may also produce a blotchy erythema of the thenar and hypothenar eminences ('liver palms'). Leuconychia are seen in liver disease.

Erythema nodosum is a condition in which tender, painful, red nodules appear, typically on the shins. They fade slowly over several weeks, leaving bruising, but never ulcerate. Sarcoidosis and drug sensitivity are the commonest causes, but other systemic disorders should be considered (Box 19.10).

Xanthomata are yellow or orange papules or nodules in the skin caused by dermal aggregations of lipid-loaded cells. Different patterns of hyperlipoproteinaemia may induce varying patterns of xanthomatosis. Thus, the type Ia (hypercholesterolaemia) pattern

Box 19.10 Causes of erythema nodosum

- Sarcoidosis
- Drugs, e.g. sulfonamides
- Streptococcal infection
- Tuberculosis
- Inflammatory bowel disease
- Behçet's disease
- Other infections, e.g. leprosy, systemic mycoses, toxoplasmosis, lymphogranuloma venereum

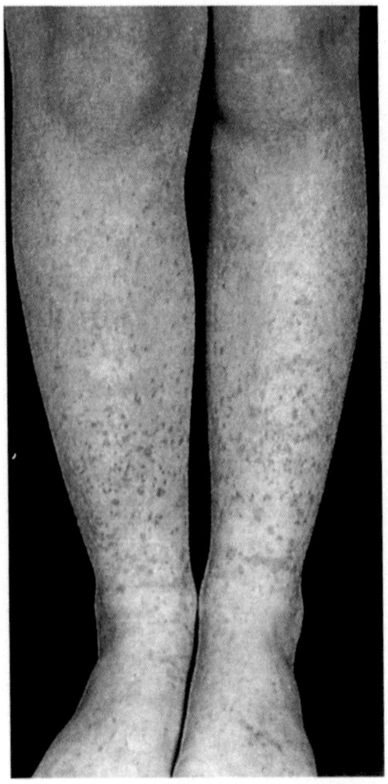

Figure 19.21 Purpura in Henoch-Schönlein disease.

typically causes tuberous xanthomata on the extensor aspects of the knees and elbows and on the buttocks, sometimes associated with tendon xanthomata. Widespread eruptive xanthomata are more characteristic of hypertriglyceridaemia. White deposits of lipid (arcus senilis) in the cornea may have a similar explanation but may be a normal feature in those over 60. Flat lipid deposits around the eyes (xanthelasma) may be due to hyperlipidaemia but are also seen in the middle-aged and elderly without any general metabolic upset.

Carotenaemia produces an orange-yellow colour to the skin, especially of the palms and soles. It occurs in those who eat great quantities of carrots and other vegetables, in hypothyroidism, in diabetic patients and also in those taking β-carotene for the treatment of porphyria.

Haemorrhage in the skin

Aggregations of extravasated red blood cells in the skin cause purpura (Fig. 19.21). Purpura may be punctate from capillary haemorrhage or may form larger macules, depending on the extent of haemorrhage and the size of vessels involved. Palpable purpura should raise suspicion of leucocytoclastic vasculitis. The Hess test for capillary fragility involves deliberately inducing punctate purpura on the forearm by inflating a cuff above the elbow at 100 mmHg for 3 minutes. Sensitivity to drugs such as aspirin may cause widespread 'capillaritis'.

The term ecchymosis implies a bruise, usually with cutaneous and subcutaneous haemorrhage causing a palpable lump. A frank fluctuant collection of blood is a haematoma. Unlike erythema and telangiectasia, purpura cannot be blanched by pressure. It must not be confused with senile haemangioma (cherry angioma or Campbell de Morgan spot), which is common in later life on the trunk and has no pathological significance. Haemorrhage into the thick epidermis of the palm or sole due to trauma (e.g. 'jogger's heel') may induce brown or almost black macules that take weeks to disappear, inviting confusion with melanoma.

The skin in sexually transmitted diseases

The skin is involved in various sexually transmitted diseases. The primary chancre of syphilis may occur on the genitalia of either sex, at or near the anus, on the lip or, rarely, elsewhere. The rash of secondary syphilis is brownish-red and maculopapular and is one of the few rashes involving the palms and soles. It does not itch. Other manifestations of the secondary stage are condylomata lata around the anogenital area and snail-track ulceration and 'mucous patches' in the mouth. There may be low-grade fever, lymphadenopathy and splenomegaly.

Septicaemia is a rare complication of gonorrhoea that occurs particularly in pregnant women presenting with pustular skin lesions. Recurrent type II herpes simplex is common on the penis; it occurs less often on the buttocks, where relapses may be heralded by a radiating neuralgia. Genital viral warts are common in both sexes. They are particularly important in females because there is evidence that certain viral subtypes are responsible for chronic cervical dysplasia with malignant potential.

HIV-related syndromes have many cutaneous manifestations, including disseminated Kaposi's sarcoma, candidiasis, molluscum contagiosum, seborrhoeic dermatitis, folliculitis and oral hairy leukoplakia (Fig. 19.22).

Viral infection of the skin

Several of the most common viral infections and illnesses of childhood are characterized by fever and a distinctive rash (exanthem), including measles, varicella and rubella. In measles, upper respiratory symptoms are quickly followed by a characteristic maculopapular and erythematous rash. In rubella (German measles), the rash is more transient, with small papules, and associated with occipital lymphadenopathy and only slight malaise. The exanthem of varicella (chickenpox)

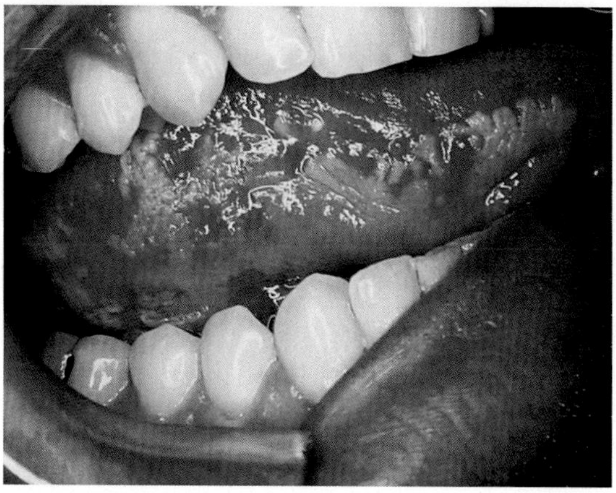

Figure 19.22 Hairy leukoplakia.

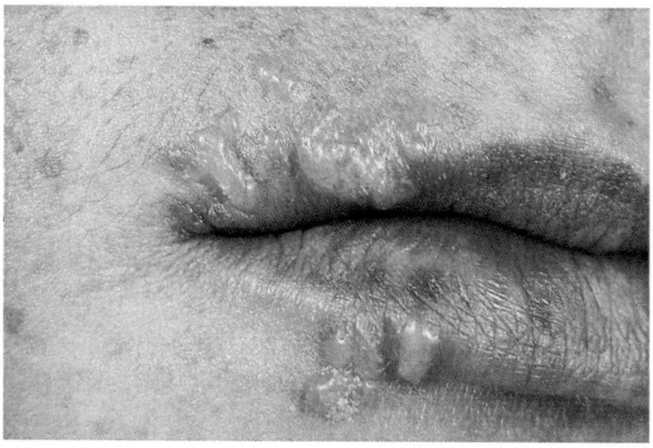

Figure 19.23 Herpes simplex (type I).

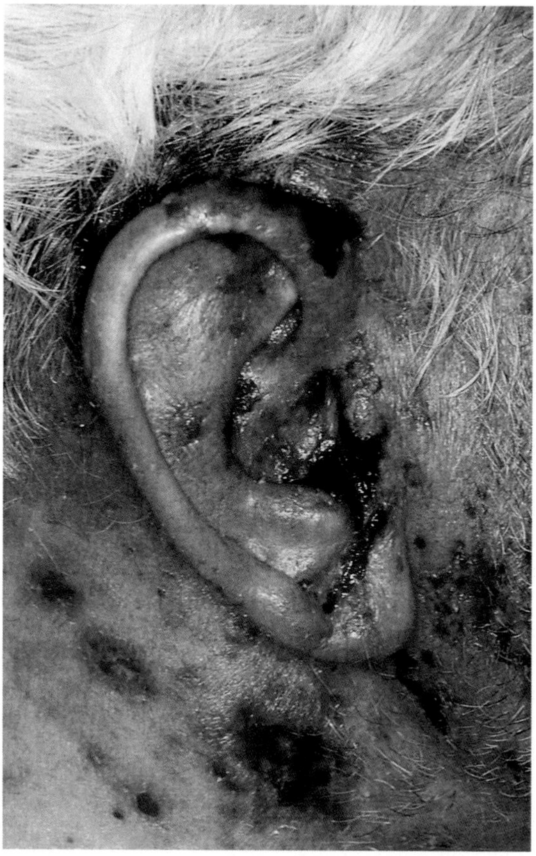

Figure 19.24 Herpes zoster vesicles on the ear lobe involving the C2 dermatome.

is papulovesicular and centripetal, and there may be lesions in the mouth. In herpes zoster and herpes simplex infections (Fig. 19.23), there is a non-follicular papulovesicular rash in which the vesicles are planted in an inflamed base. The rash is painful. In herpes zoster, the rash follows a segmental distribution, corresponding with skin of a dermatome. The vesicular lesion becomes encrusted (Fig. 19.24) and later, secondary infection may occur.

Other less common viral infections associated with a rash include erythema infectiosum, due to a parvovirus, in which the exanthem on the face gives a 'slapped-cheek' appearance, and roseola infantum, a disease of toddlers which mimics rubella.

Drug eruptions

In the last 40 years, eruptions caused by drugs have become common. Most such rashes are due to allergic hypersensitivity. Drug rashes can mimic almost every pattern of skin disease. Thus, urticaria may be caused by penicillin or opiates; a measles-like (morbilliform) rash may be induced by ampicillin, especially when given to patients with infectious mononucleosis; eczema-like rashes are seen with methyldopa and phenylbutazone therapy; and gold and chloroquine rashes mimic lichen planus. A palpable rash looking like Henoch-Schönlein purpura indicates leucocytoclastic vasculitis. Generalized exfoliative dermatitis may be induced by sulfonylureas, indomethacin and allopurinol. Increasing use of biologics in clinical medicine has identified unusual skin eruptions.

Drugs that may sensitize the skin to sunlight (phototoxic reaction) include tetracyclines, sulfonamides and nalidixic acid. Acne-like rashes may follow high-dose prednisolone therapy and are common with phenytoin therapy. Certain cytotoxic drugs and sodium valproate cause hair loss. Both erythema nodosum and erythema multiforme may be induced by sulfonamides, including co-trimoxazole. Laboratory tests are of little value in the diagnosis of drug eruptions. A carefully taken history and knowledge of the common patterns of drug reactions usually allow accurate diagnosis (Box 19.11).

Tumours in the skin

Exposure to the sun may, after many years, result in the development of many common skin tumours, for example squamous or basal cell carcinoma or melanoma. These tumours are especially common in fair-skinned people. Basal cell carcinoma arises

Box 19.11 Common drug eruptions

Morphological type	Drug
Maculopapular	Penicillin/amoxicillin
Urticaria	Penicillin, non-steroidal drugs
Vasculitis	Hydralazine
Fixed drug eruption	Tetracyclines, phenolphthalein
Pigmentation	Amiodarone, minocycline
Photosensitivity	Thiazides, sulfonamides
Lupus erythematosus	Isoniazid, penicillamine
Erythema nodosum	Oral contraceptive pill, sulfonamides
Erythema multiforme	Barbiturates
Acneform	Steroids
Pustular	Carbamazepine
Lichenoid	Thiazides, antimalarials, allopurinol
Psoriasiform	Beta-blockers, lithium, antimalarials
Toxic epidermal necrolysis / Stevens-Johnson syndrome / erythema multiforme	Carbamazepine, non-steroidal drugs, co-trimoxazole
Pemphigus	ACE inhibitors
Linear IgA disease	Vancomycin
Erythroderma	Sulfonylureas, ACE inhibitors, allopurinol

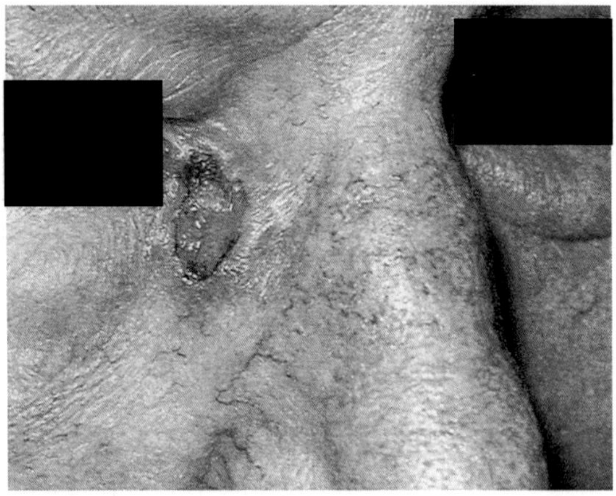

Figure 19.25 Basal cell carcinoma.

especially on the face, near the nose or on the forehead (Fig. 19.25). The lesion may be ulcerated with a firm, rounded edge, or papular. Melanomas may develop on the torso in men and legs in females. They may be pigmented or amelanotic and may in about a third of cases develop rapidly in a pre-existing benign mole (Fig. 19.26). Staging by assessing draining regional sentinel lymph nodes is becoming increasingly routine in cutaneous oncology. Seborrhoeic keratoses are familial, resulting in a raised warty pigmented lesions

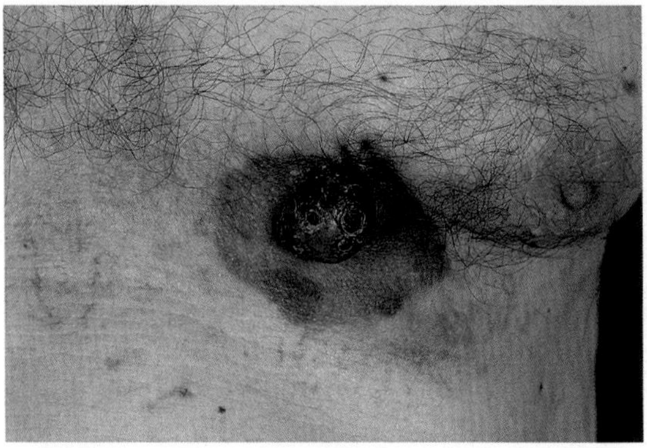

Figure 19.26 Malignant melanoma on a male chest. The nodule is invasive.

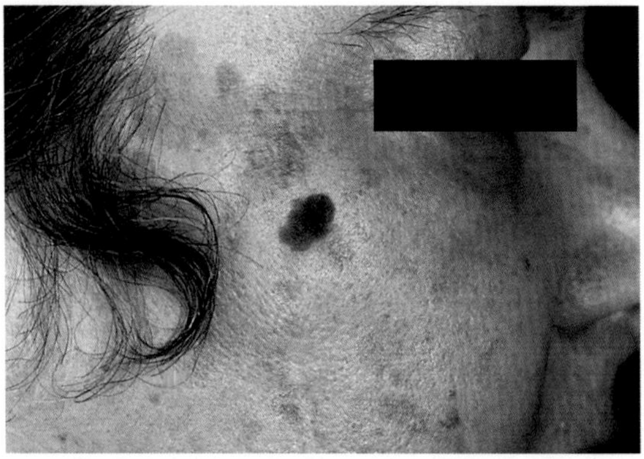

Figure 19.27 A pigmented basal cell papilloma (seborrhoeic keratosis) on the face. This is a benign lesion.

found in the sun-exposed elderly, especially on the dorsa of hands as 'liver spots' (Fig. 19.27). A symptomatic pigmented skin lesion having an asymmetric, ragged border, three or more colours and diameter of >7 mm, particularly if it is increasing in size or bleeding and found on sun-damaged freckled skin, should be regarded as suspicious of malignant melanoma.

Special techniques in examination of the skin

The skin is uniquely available to the examining physician. There are a number of diagnostic procedures and blood tests (Box 19.12).

Tzanck preparation

Tzanck preparation, an often forgotten old but valuable technique, is useful for emergency diagnosis of vesicular infections or blistering eruptions such as pemphigus. The intact blister is opened and the base gently scraped. The material obtained is smeared onto the microscope slide, allowed to air dry and then stained. Viral lesions will show typical multinucleated giant cells, and pemphigus will show acantholytic cells.

Box 19.12 Dermatology blood investigations

Blood test	Clinical example
FBC	Pruritus
Ferritin and iron studies	Hail and nail
Biochemistry renal and liver function	Pruritus
Streptococcal serology	Cellulitis
Autoantibodies	Autoimmune disorders
Hepatitis screen	Lichen planus
HSV 1 & 2 serology	Erythema multiforme
Syphilis serology	Secondary syphilis
HIV	Persistent infections
HLA typing	Dermatitis herpetiformis
DNA analysis	Epidermolysis bullosa

Microscopic examination – Dermatoscopy (direct assessment of skin lesions)

Dermatoscopic and/or microscopic examination is useful in the diagnosis of scabies, pediculosis (lice) and fungal infection (tinea and candidiasis). The established routine use of the dermatoscope has become essential in the assessment of pigmented skin lesions and aids in diagnosis of skin malignancy, especially malignant melanoma.

Scabies

Scabies is caused by the mite *Acarus (Sarcoptes) scabei*. The female is larger than the male and burrows in the epidermis, depositing eggs. These burrows should be looked for between the fingers, on the hands or wrists and on the sides of the feet. They can be recognized with the naked eye as short dark lines terminating in a shining spot of skin. The eggs lie in the dark line, the mite in the shining spot. It may be picked out by means of a flat surgical needle and placed on a microscope slide for more detailed examination.

Pediculosis

Three forms of pediculosis or louse infestation occur: *Pediculus capitis* on the head, *Pediculus corporis* on the trunk, and *Pediculus pubis* on the pubic and axillary hairs. The eggs or nits of *P. pubis* and *P. capitis* adhere to the hairs. From their position on the hairs, one can judge roughly the duration of the condition, as they are fixed at first near the root of the hair and are carried up as the hair grows, so the higher the nits are, the longer the pediculi have been present. *P. corporis* should be looked for in the seams of the clothes, especially where the clothes come into contact with the skin, for example over the shoulders. The bites of the parasite produce haemorrhagic spots, each with a dark centre and a paler areola. Marks of scratching should be looked for on parts accessible to the patient's nails. *P. pubis* is venereally acquired and causes intense pubic itching. The nits are laid on the pubic hair and the lice themselves are easily visible. *P. corporis* is seen only in the grossly deprived, living in rough conditions of war or social upheaval. In contrast, *P. capitis* is common in school children, however clean they and their families may be, and is endemic in many schools.

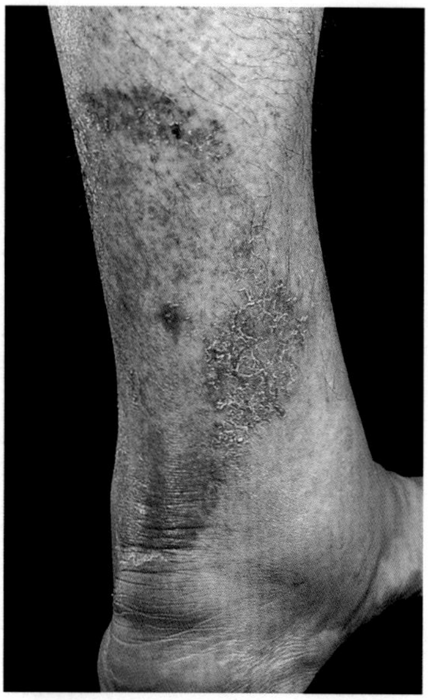

Figure 19.28 Tinea rubrum (ringworm infection).

Fungal infections

Fungus may grow in the skin, nails or hair and can cause disease (ringworm or tinea), for example athlete's foot (tinea pedis).

The most common sites of fungal infection are the skin between the toes (tinea pedis) and the soles of the feet and the groin (tinea cruris). The lesions may be scaly or vesicular, tending to spread in a ring form with central healing (Fig. 19.28); macerated, dead, white, offensive-smelling epithelium is found in the intertriginous areas, such as the toe clefts.

Nail discoloration, deformity, hypertrophy and abnormal brittleness may result from fungus infection (tinea unguium).

Ringworm of the scalp (tinea capitis) is most common in children. It presents as round or oval areas of baldness covered with short, lustreless broken-off hair stumps. These hair stumps may fluoresce bright green under Wood's light. Some fungi do not fluoresce with Wood's light, however, and these can be detected only by microscopy and culture (Figs 19.29 and 19.30).

Microscopic examination for fungus infection

Scales from the active edge of a lesion are scraped off lightly with a scalpel or the roofs of vesicles are snipped off with scissors. The material is placed in a drop of 10% to 20% aqueous potassium hydroxide solution on a microscope slide, covered with a coverslip and left for 30 minutes to clear. It is then examined under the light microscope with the 8-mm or 4-mm objective using low illumination. The mycelia are recognized as branching, refractile threads that boldly transgress

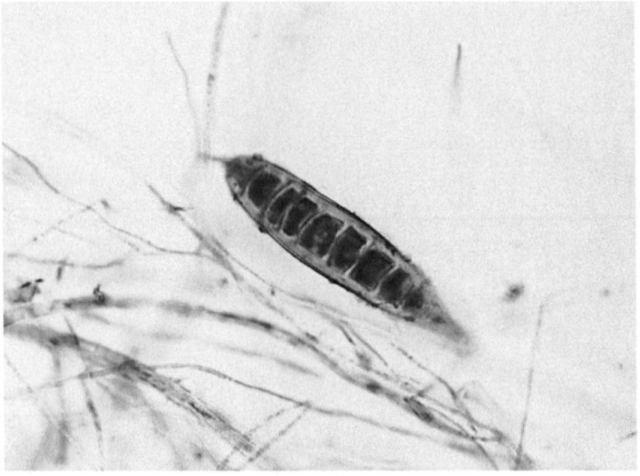

Figure 19.29 Lactophenol blue preparation showing macronidia of Microsporum species, isolated from skin scrapings from a patient with ringworm.

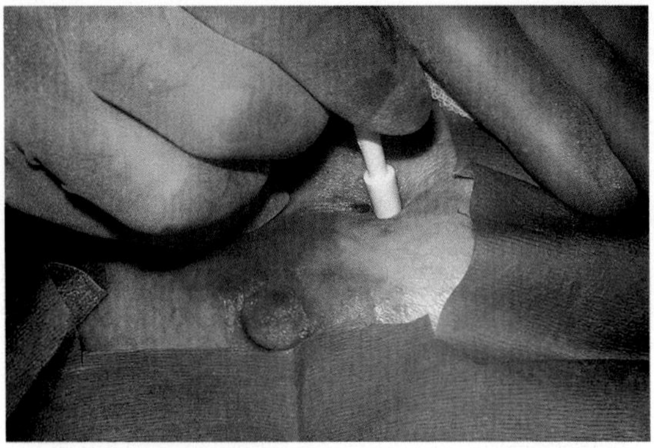

Figure 19.31 Disposable punch skin biopsy, especially useful where minimal scarring is desirable.

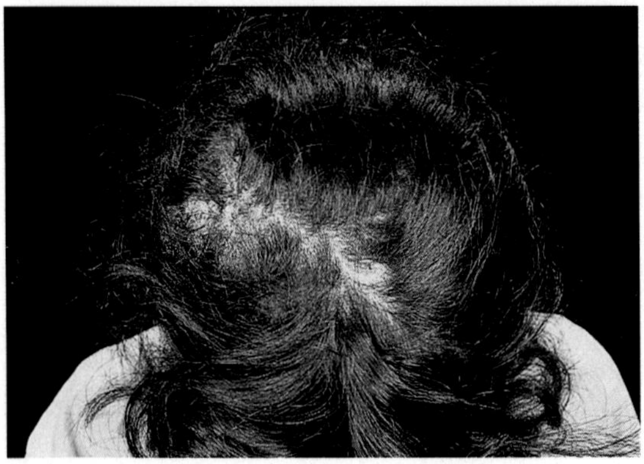

Figure 19.30 Kerion due to localized deep dermatophyte infection in the scalp.

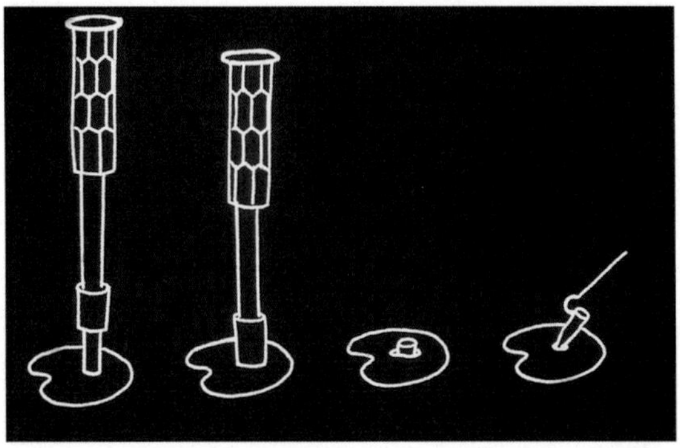

Figure 19.32 A 4-mm punch diagnostic biopsy.

the outlines of the squamous cells. Nails are examined in much the same way, but it is necessary to break up the snippings and shavings into small fragments. These are either heated in potassium hydroxide or are left to clear in it overnight before being examined.

A scalp lesion is cleaned with 70% alcohol or with 1% cetrimide; infected stumps and scales are removed by scraping with a scalpel. The hairs are cleaned in potassium hydroxide in the same way as skin scales. Examination under the microscope reveals spores on the outside of the hair roots and mycelia inside the hair substance. The species of fungus responsible may be established by culture on Sabouraud's glucose-agar.

Wood's light

A Wood's light lamp emits long-wave ultraviolet light at a peak of 360 nm. Wood's light examination is performed in a darkened room and is useful to identify the fluorescence of fungi and corynebacterial infection (erythrasma), elevated porphyrins in urine or in the localization of pigmentary abnormalities.

Contact allergy patch testing

Contact allergy patch testing is an important and valuable tool for the diagnosis of suspected allergic dermatitis due to contact (contact dermatitis). The formulation of the allergens is critical, and various standard contact allergen test batteries have been developed in different countries and clinics to include the commonest culprits. Patch testing is simple, but the results are not always easy to interpret. Allergens are placed in shallow aluminium 1-cm^2 wells and applied in strips to the patient's back for 48 hours for initial reading and a second reading at 96 hours. This ensures that any delayed-type hypersensitivity (e.g. Coomb's type IV reaction to an allergen) can be identified.

Skin biopsy

Biopsy of the skin is used not only for the excision of benign and malignant tumours but also to identify the nature of reactive and/or inflammatory lesions. Punch biopsy (Figs 19.31 and 19.32) is popular because of its convenience and its minimal scarring. The biopsy can be studied by conventional histology, often supplemented by immunofluorescence and sometimes immunohistochemistry or molecular biology, to identify specific proteins or genetic abnormalities. Skin biopsy of fresh tissue can be sent for the microbiology of unusual infections and is increasingly used in diagnosis and in assessing the progress of skin diseases.

Eyes 20

Andrew Coombes

Introduction

Although proportionally a greater contribution towards the diagnosis of ophthalmic disorders is made by the examination compared to the history, it is important to obtain a detailed account of the presenting complaint and associated visual symptoms from the patient with an ocular problem.

History

Disturbance of vision, the most important ocular symptom, may be sudden or gradual, unilateral or bilateral, and lead to loss of central vision or partial field loss. Simultaneous, bilateral visual symptoms are usually due to disease in optic pathways at or posterior to the optic chiasm. Sudden visual disturbance should be assessed urgently. Visual hallucinations may be formed or unformed. Some visual symptoms have particular significance (Table 20.1). For example, haloes around lights occur in acute angle-closure glaucoma due to corneal oedema. 'Floaters' and flashes (photopsia) are indicative of vitreous or retinal disorders, respectively. The latter may also cause objects to appear smaller (micropsia), larger (macropsia) or distorted (metamorphopsia). Disorders of ocular movement may cause double vision (diplopia) or visual blurring. Are the visual symptoms binocular or monocular? Are they related to eye movements?

Other common presentations include a red eye, abnormal lid position, protrusion of the globe and pupillary or eyelid abnormality. Ocular pain is often associated with a red eye (Table 20.2). Ocular pain due to a foreign body may be described as 'a gritty sensation' in the eye, often worsened by blinking. It may be associated with sensitivity to light (photophobia) but this, particularly in conjunction with ocular aching, usually indicates serious corneal or intraocular disease. Severe ocular pain with vomiting may indicate acute glaucoma. Migraine often presents with bilateral visual symptoms and headache. Raised intracranial pressure and giant cell arteritis should also be considered when headache is associated with visual symptoms. Pain may be referred to the eye because of neighbouring disease, for example sinusitis. Excessive tear production (lacrimation) associated with discomfort may indicate ocular surface disease. There may be abnormal secretions from the eye, such as mucus or pus. With insufficient tears, the eye typically feels dry, whereas a painless overflow of tears (epiphora) typically indicates blockage of the lacrimal drainage system.

Note any previous ophthalmic history, such as a squint in childhood, and any pre-existing poor vision or previous ocular injury or surgery. Note what type of glasses or contact lenses are worn: extended-wear soft contact lenses are associated with an increased risk of corneal infection. The family history may reveal glaucoma, decreased visual acuity, colour blindness, squint or neurological disease associated with visual loss. In addition to the ocular history, the medical, drug and social histories are important.

Examination

Eye examination is part of the cranial nerve examination. It includes ocular movements (cranial nerves III, IV and VI), corneal sensation (ophthalmic division of the trigeminal nerve) and eye closure (VII). Assess the optic (II) nerve by testing visual acuity, colour vision, the visual fields and the pupillary light reaction. Inspect the optic nerve head (the optic disc and cup) with the ophthalmoscope. Detailed examination of the anterior segment of the eye requires use of the slit lamp which, with additional equipment, can also be used to test the intraocular pressure (IOP) and examine the retina.

Visual acuity

Visual acuity is most reliably tested at 6 m (20 ft) using a standard chart such as the Snellen (Fig. 20.1a) or Log MAR chart (Fig. 20.1b). Tests of acuity in near vision are portable but limited by age-related loss of accommodation (presbyopia), which necessitates refractive correction in older patients. These use test types of varying sizes, based on the point system of the printers (Fig. 20.2), and the smallest type that can be read comfortably at a distance of 33 cm is recorded (normally N4.5 or N5 type).

Table 20.1 Sudden visual disturbance

Diagnosis		**History: visual symptoms**	
Vascular	Ocular	Amaurosis fugax	Transient (minutes), unilateral
		Retinal artery/vein occlusion	Permanent, unilateral, often associated with systemic vascular disease, e.g. ischaemic heart disease, hypertension, diabetes
		Non-arteritic ischaemic optic neuropathy (NAION)	Permanent, unilateral, often associated with systemic vascular disease, e.g. ischaemic heart disease, hypertension, diabetes
		Arteritic ischaemic optic neuropathy (AAION)	Permanent, unilateral, typically associated with symptoms of giant cell arteritis, e.g. temporal headache/tenderness, jaw claudication, features of polymyalgia rheumatica
		Papilloedema/optic disc swelling	Transient (seconds), bilateral visual obscurations, often precipitated by coughing or bending
	Cortical	Transient ischaemic attack (TIA)	Transient (minutes), bilateral, associated with systemic vascular disease, e.g. ischaemic heart disease, hypertension, diabetes, etc.
		Migraine	Transient, bilateral, typically followed by nausea and headache
		Cerebrovascular accident (CVA)	Permanent homonymous field defect, may be preceded by TIA symptoms; note central acuity usually preserved except in bilateral occipital lobe infarction
Non-vascular	Vitreous	Posterior vitreous detachment (PVD)	Transient (weeks), unilateral, floaters, occasional photopsia, central vision normal
		Vitreous haemorrhage	Transient (weeks), unilateral, multiple floaters, central vision typically reduced
	Retina	Wet age-related macular degeneration (AMD)	Progressive, unilateral central visual distortion (metamorphopsia) This condition is also known as exudative or neovascular AMD
		Retinal detachment	Progressive, unilateral field loss, central vision reduced if macula involved, often associated with symptoms of PVD
	Optic nerve	Optic neuritis	Transient (months), unilateral, may be associated with features of multiple sclerosis
		Acute compression	Progressive, unilateral, bilateral if chiasm involved, e.g. pituitary apoplexy (infarction of a pituitary tumour)
Pseudo		Suddenly noticed	Unilateral gradual visual loss from, e.g. dry AMD or cataract
		Functional	Bilateral or unilateral; diagnosis of exclusion

Snellen distance vision

On the Snellen chart, each line of letters is designated by a number that corresponds to the distance at which those letters can be read by someone with 'normal' distance vision. For example, the largest letter, at the top of the chart – designated 60 – would be read at 60 m by a person with 'normal' vision.

Technique

The patient sits or stands 6 m (20 ft) from the chart. Where space is limited, a mirror may be used 3 m from both patient and chart, with the patient facing away from the chart and reading the letters in the mirror, giving a total of 6 m. However, increasingly, electronic computer screens are being used and the letter size can be adjusted to allow test distance to be varied between 3 and 6 m. Distance glasses should be worn if necessary and each eye tested separately. The patient should read line by line from the top of the chart. If a patient cannot see the largest letter, designated 60, then the test distance should be reduced. If at 1 m the 60 letter cannot be seen, assess the following:

- Counting fingers held up at about 1 m (CFs)
- Hand movements (HMs)
- Perception of light (PL)

When testing low vision, ensure that the eye not being tested is completely covered. If a patient cannot read 6/6 or better in either eye, check the vision again using a pinhole occluder (Fig. 20.3). This test distinguishes patients with poor vision due to refractive error from those who have ocular or neurological conditions. In a myopic (short-sighted) eye, the rays of light are focused in front of the retina. In hypermetropia (long-sightedness), light is focused behind the eye, because the eye is abnormally short. In astigmatism, the cornea is not uniformly curved and light is not focused evenly on the retina. When using a pinhole, only the central rays of light pass through to the retina and refractive errors are significantly reduced.

Table 20.2 Red eye

Diagnosis	History	Examination
Subconjunctival haemorrhage	Typically asymptomatic, spontaneous May be associated with trauma	Unilateral (except some trauma), contiguous red area
Viral conjunctivitis	FB sensation, watering, no visual loss or photophobia Recent contact with person with red eye or URTI?	Bilateral, prominent inflamed conjunctival vessels and follicles, enlarged tender preauricular lymph node
Bacterial conjunctivitis	FB sensation, discharge, no visual loss or photophobia	Bilateral, prominent inflamed conjunctival vessels, mucopus
Allergic conjunctivitis	Itch, watering, no visual loss or photophobia, history of atopy	Bilateral, prominent inflamed conjunctival vessels and follicles
Iritis (anterior uveitis)	Reduced vision, aching sensation, photophobia PMH or systemic enquiry may elicit underlying disease	Unilateral, prominent pericorneal vessels, small pupil, aqueous cells and flare (protein) (at slit lamp), hypopyon
Acute angle-closure glaucoma	Severe pain, haloes/rainbows around lights, reduced vision, hypermetropic, elderly	Unilateral, pericorneal prominent vessels, semidilated (oval) pupil, corneal oedema, shallow anterior chamber (slit lamp)
Episcleritis	Mild discomfort, tenderness, no visual loss or photophobia, young adult, otherwise fit and well	Unilateral, typically sectorial prominent inflamed subconjunctival vessels (may also be nodular or diffuse)
Scleritis	Significant aching pain, tender, photophobia, occasionally reduced vision, systemic enquiry may elicit underlying disease	Unilateral, typically sectorial prominent inflamed deep scleral vessels (may also be nodular or diffuse)
Bacterial keratitis	FB sensation, watering/discharge, visual loss, photophobia Pre-existing ocular surface disease, recent trauma or contact lens wear?	Unilateral, opacity in cornea (slit lamp) stains with fluorescein
Herpetic viral keratitis	FB sensation, watering/discharge, visual loss, photophobia Cold sores or ophthalmic shingles?	Unilateral, branching linear dendrite(s) on cornea (slit lamp) stains with fluorescein

FB, foreign body; PMH, past medical history; URTI, upper respiratory tract infection.

Recording visual acuity

The top figure, the numerator, records the distance of the subject from the test chart – usually 6 m. The bottom figure records the line read by the patient. The normal person can read the line designated 6 at 6 m (i.e. 6/6 (20/20) vision).

Record a mistake of one letter in a line as '–1' and a single letter read from the next smaller line as '+1'. Thus, if all except one of the letters on the line designated 6 are read correctly, the visual acuity is recorded 6/6 –1. If only one letter on that line is read correctly, the visual acuity is recorded 6/9 +1. Like all ophthalmic findings except visual fields, right eye visual acuity is traditionally written on the left side of the page (as the patient's eye appears to you) and vice versa. Whether the patient was using glasses, pinhole (ph) or was unaided (ua) is recorded in the middle (Fig. 20.4).

Log MAR charts

Increasingly, Snellen acuity tests are being replaced by use of a Log MAR chart, which superficially appears similar to a Snellen chart but addresses its problems, namely different number of letters per line, irregular spacing between letters/lines and unequal graduation from one line to the other. On a LogMar chart each letter has a score value of 0.02 log units with 5 letters per line (each line therefore scores 0.1 log units). 6/6 is equivalent to LogMar score 0.00 and 6/60 is 1.00. Each letter read contributes to the score; for example, 6/6-1 would be recorded as 0.02. The digital output is also helpful for research and audit purposes.

Colour vision

Tests of colour vision are important because colour perception, especially for red, is affected in optic nerve disease before changes in visual acuity can be detected. Show the patient a red target one eye at a time (any bright red target can be used) and ask if there is a difference between the eyes. In the affected eye, red appears 'washed out' (desaturated). Acquired defects of colour vision may also occur in macular disease. The Ishihara test (Fig. 20.5) was devised to test for congenital colour anomalies (colour blindness) but is often used to assess acquired visual disorders. Most inherited colour blindness occurs in males (sex-linked recessive inheritance). It ranges from total colour blindness (monochromatopsia) to subtle confusion between colours, typically between red

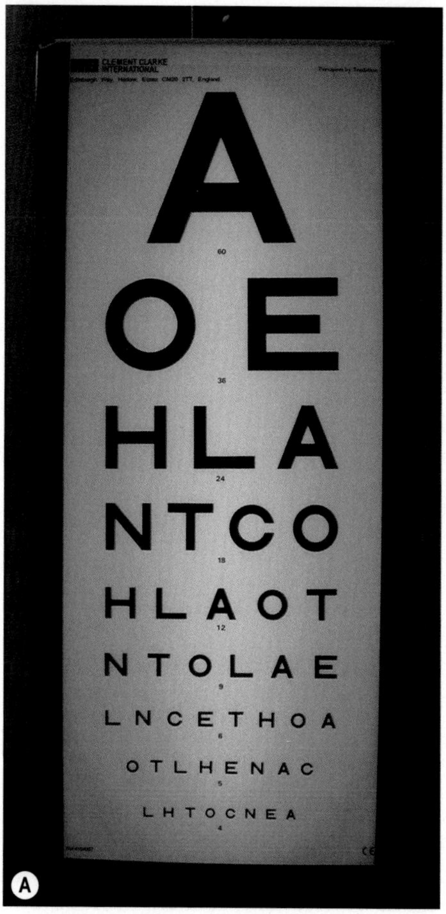

Figure 20.1a Snellen chart for testing distance vision.

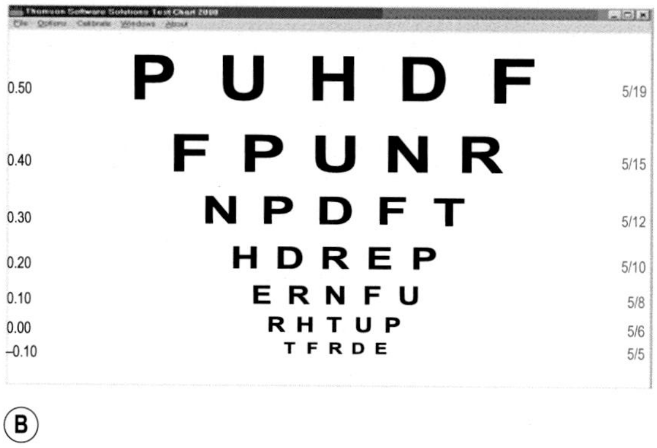

Figure 20.1b Log MAR chart for testing distance vision.

and green. About 8% of men and 0.5% of women in the UK have congenital colour perception defects. Blue/yellow deficiencies and total colour blindness are uncommon.

Visual field testing

Visual field testing is described in Chapter 16. Field defects may affect one or both eyes. Symmetric bilateral (homonymous) field defects are characteristic of lesions posterior to the optic chiasm, and asymmetric field defects are usually due to lesions anterior to the chiasm (i.e. in the optic nerves or retinae). Characteristic field defects (scotoma) occur in glaucoma, when damage to nerve fibres occurs at the optic disc, typically at the inferior or superior aspect of the optic cup. Fundoscopy shows an increase in vertical length of the optic cup (see later in the chapter for details about how to examine the fundi) and field loss is arc-shaped (arcuate scotoma). If both the inferior and superior fields are involved, a ring-shaped scotoma develops. Untreated glaucoma results in loss of the peripheral field so that only a small central island of vision remains (tunnel vision). Computerized perimetry is useful in identifying early visual field loss. The Humphrey field test analyser (Carl Zeiss), for example, provides statistical information indicating the reliability of the test in comparison with a group of age-matched controls (Fig. 20.6).

Pupils

Examination of the pupils in neurology is discussed in Chapter 16. In ophthalmic practice, there are three key aspects to pupil examination: size, shape and reactions.

Pupil size: anisocoria

In 12% of normal individuals, the pupils are slightly unequal, particularly in bright light (anisocoria), but in these subjects they react normally. Abnormal pupils dilate and constrict abnormally, and the degree of anisocoria varies with the ambient illumination. However, it is often difficult to decide which pupil is abnormal. In the absence of local eye disease, a small pupil may be due to paralysis of the dilator pupillae muscle (sympathetic innervated), part of Horner's syndrome (Fig. 20.7), in which anisocoria is more pronounced in low ambient light. An enlarged pupil suggests a parasympathetic lesion, which may be preganglionic in oculomotor lesions or postganglionic as in the tonic pupil of Adie's syndrome. Adie's tonic pupil tends to be dilated in bright light and is very slow to react. A feature of both parasympathetic and sympathetic lesions is denervation hypersensitivity caused by upregulation of receptors at the neuromuscular junction (adrenergic in sympathetic and cholinergic in parasympathetic). This is the basis of pharmacological pupil testing. In both pre- and postganglionic parasympathetic blockade, the pupil is supersensitive to weak cholinergic drops (e.g. pilocarpine 0.1%). In sympathetic block, dilute adrenergic agonists such as phenylephrine 1% are unreliable, so the uptake blocker, cocaine 4%, is used. This dilates normal pupils but has no effect in pre- or postganglionic lesions. Hydroxyamfetamine 1% causes noradrenaline (norepinephrine) release from normal or intact postganglionic neurons and allows pre- and postganglionic lesions to be distinguished (the synapse is located in the superior cervical ganglion). In complex pupil abnormalities, for example bilateral

READING TEST TYPES
as approved by
THE FACULTY OF OPHTHALMOLOGISTS,
LONDON, ENGLAND

N. 5

He moved forward a few steps: the house was so dark behind him, the world so dim and uncertain in front of him, that for a moment his heart failed him. He might have to search the whole garden for the dog.
Then he heard a sniff, felt something wet against his leg — he had almost stepped upon the animal. He bent down and stroked its wet coat. The dog stood quite still, then moved forward towards the house, sniffed at the steps, at last walked calmly through the open door as though the house belonged to him. Jeremy followed, closed the door behind them; then there they were in the little dark passage with the boy's heart beating like a drum, his teeth chattering, and a terrible temptation to sneeze hovering around him. Let him reach the nursery and .establish the animal there and all might be well, but let them be discovered, cold and shivering, in the passage, and out the dog would be flung. He knew so exactly what would happen.

(From "Jeremy" by Hugh Walpole).

wire sons vain error unwise cream remove

N. 6

The camp stood where, until quite lately, has been pasture and ploughland; the farm house still stood in a fold of the hill and had served us for battalion offices; ivy still supported part of what had once been the walls of a fruit garden; half an acre of mutilated old trees behind the wash-houses survived of an orchard. The place had been marked for destruction before the army came to it. Had there been another year of peace, there would have been no farmhouse, no wall, no apple trees. Already half a mile of concrete road lay between bare clay banks, and on either side a chequer of open ditches showed where the municipal contractors had designed a system of drainage. Another year of peace would have made the place part of the neighbouring suburb. Now the huts where we had wintered waited their turn for destruction.

(From "Brideshead Revisited" by Evelyn Waugh)

nervous manner immune over unanimous wear

N. 8

And another image came to me, of an arctic hut and a trapper alone with his furs and oil lamp and log fire; the remains of supper on the table, a few books, skis in the corner; everything dry and neat and warm inside and outside the last blizzard of winter raging and the snow piling up against the door. Quite silently a great weight forming against the timber; the bolt straining in its socket; minute by minute in the darkness outside the white heap sealing the door, until quite soon when the wind dropped and the sun came out on the ice slopes and the thaw set in a block would move, slide and tumble high above, gather way, gather weight, till the whole hillside seemed to be falling, and the little lighted place would crash open and splinter and disappear, rolling with the avalanche into the ravine.

(From "Brideshead Revisited" by Evelyn Waugh)

immense snow came near arrow use.

Figure 20.2 Near vision chart based on the point system of the printer.

Horner's syndrome, infrared pupil imaging can be valuable. Causes of anisocoria are highlighted in Box 20.1. In congenital Horner's syndrome, the affected iris is depigmented and appears blue.

Pupil reactions: afferent and central defects

The swinging light test is used to detect a relative afferent pupillary defect (RAPD) resulting from retinal or optic nerve disease. The test loses sensitivity in symmetrical bilateral optic nerve disease, but this is rare, and in most bilateral cases the defect will be detected on the more abnormal side. RAPD is often associated with reduced vision, but if central vision is retained, the acuity will be normal, although severe peripheral field damage may cause RAPD. In neurosyphilis, the pupils are small and irregular and show the Argyll Robertson phenomenon (normal pupil constriction to a near target but reduced reaction to light) owing to a midbrain defect. In Parinaud's syndrome, the pupils are typically large and poorly reactive to light, with abnormal vertical gaze, convergence retraction nystagmus and lid retraction on attempted upgaze (Collier's sign). The causes of light-near dissociation are given in Box 20.2.

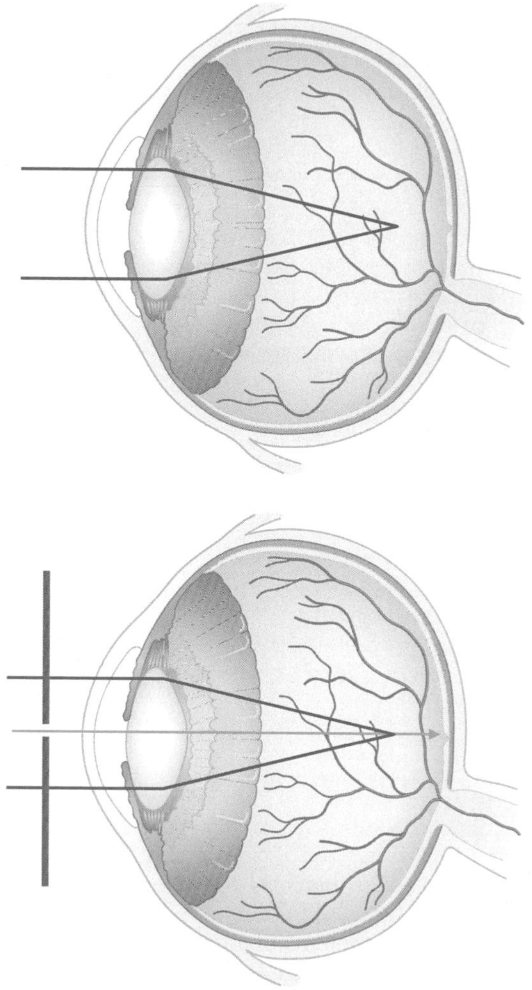

Figure 20.3 Testing vision with a pinhole. Top: light is not focused on the retina owing to refractive error (in this case in front of the retina, as in myopia, or short-sightedness). Bottom: the use of a pinhole selects rays of light not needing to be focused, giving a better indication of a patient's true best corrected visual acuity despite refractive error.

Box 20.1 Causes of anisocoria

- Idiopathic (12% population)
- Parasympathetic:
  - third nerve palsy (external ophthalmoplegia)
  - tonic pupil (internal ophthalmoplegia, e.g. Holmes-Adie)
- Sympathetic:
  - Horner's syndrome
- Argyll Robertson
- Pharmacological
- Ocular:
  - iris inflammation, e.g. iritis
  - iris ischaemia
  - trauma
  - iatrogenic

Box 20.2 Light-near dissociation

- Argyll Robertson pupil
- Holmes-Adie pupil
- Parinaud's syndrome
- Aberrant third nerve regeneration
- Myotonic dystrophy
- Diabetes mellitus

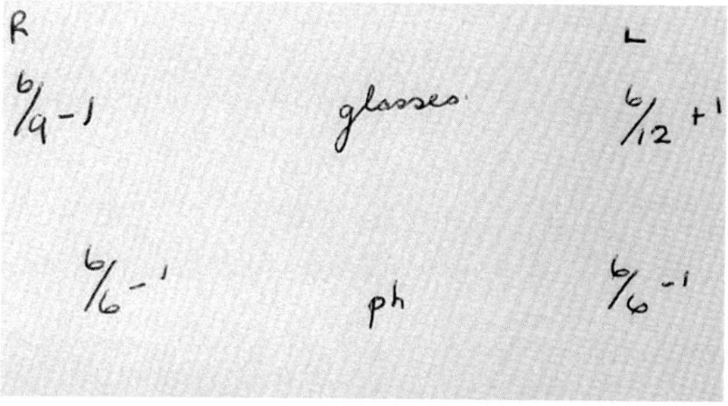

Figure 20.4 Recording visual acuity: the numerator is the test distance. ph, pinhole.

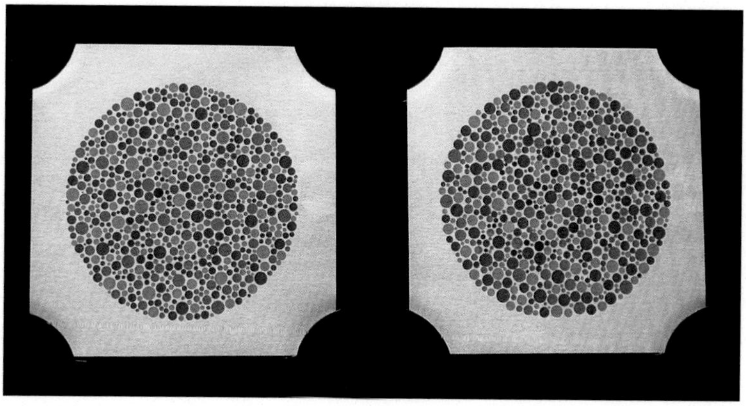

Figure 20.5 Ishihara colour vision test.

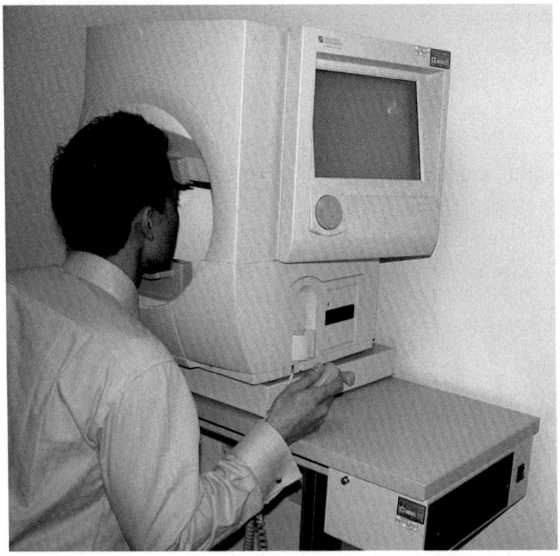

Figure 20.6 Automated static perimetry: the Humphrey field test analyser.

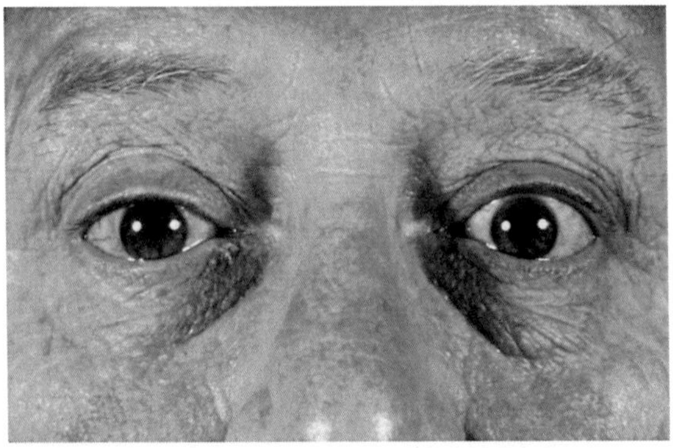

Figure 20.7 Horner's syndrome. On the affected side there is ptosis, which may be very slight, and a small pupil (miosis) that reacts to both light and accommodation. (Reproduced with permission from Mir, 2003 Atlas of Clinical Diagnosis, 2nd edn, Saunders, Edinburgh.)

Pupil shape

Slit-lamp examination is the best technique to assess intrinsic ocular disease that may affect the shape and position of the pupil (Box 20.3).

Box 20.3 Causes of abnormal pupil shape

- Congenital: Rieger's anomaly (anterior segment cleavage anomalies)
- Trauma
- Iatrogenic (sphincterotomies, iridectomy, cataract surgery)
- Inflammatory (posterior synechiae in iritis)
- Tumour (ectropion uveae in ciliary body malignancies)
- Ischaemic: herpes zoster, angle-closure glaucoma
- Idiopathic: iridocorneal endotheliopathy (ICE) syndrome (which also features multiple pupils (polycoria) and misplaced pupils (correctopia))

Box 20.4 Risk factors for acute angle-closure glaucoma: *dilate pupils cautiously*

- Intermittent symptoms of angle-closure attack (see symptoms in Table 20.2)
- High hypermetropia
- Old age
- Narrow anterior chamber angles (detected on slit-lamp gonioscopy)
- Family history of acute angle-closure glaucoma

Direct ophthalmoscopy

The direct ophthalmoscope is an indispensable clinical instrument that allows direct visualization of the retina – which is part of the CNS – and its circulation. It consists of a bright, focused light source that illuminates the retina to allow the observer to see the image, magnified about 15 times.

Preparation

1 Decide the objective of the examination.
2 Consider dilating the pupils with 1% cyclopentolate (Mydrilate) (0.5% in children under 6 months) or 1% tropicamide (Mydriacyl). This blurs the vision for at least 2 hours, so patients should be forewarned and instructed not to drive. Some patients have a predisposition to closed-angle glaucoma (Box 20.4) and dilation may precipitate an attack. At-risk individuals must be warned to return if symptoms of acute angle closure occur.
3 Briefly explain the examination so that the patient can cooperate fully. Ask the patient to fixate on a distant target – the patient should continue to look in this direction even if the examiner's head obscures the target.
4 Dim the room lights.
5 Set the ophthalmoscope lens wheel to zero dioptres (D), unless correcting for your own short- or long-sightedness.
6 Ensure that the ophthalmoscope light is bright. Unless the pupil is small, select a large light spot size (Box 20.5, Fig. 20.8).

Examining the fundi

Look carefully at the optic disc/cup, the retinal vessels and the retina and macula (Fig. 20.9).

Optic disc

This marks the point where the retinal axons exit the back of the eye to form the optic nerve. It corresponds to the physiological blind spot. The normal disc is round or slightly oval. If there is astigmatism, the disc may appear more oval than normal. There

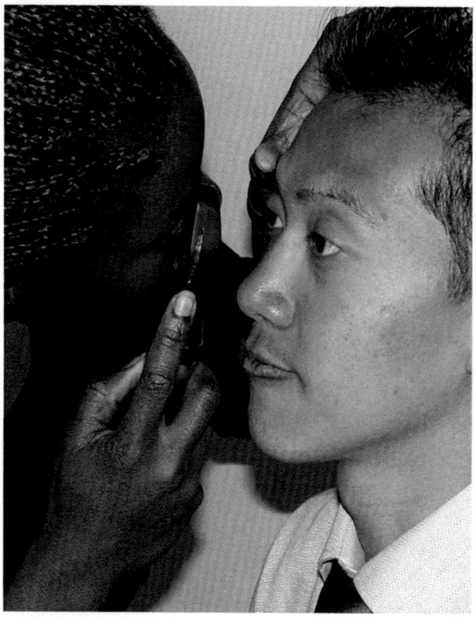

Figure 20.8 Examining the right eye with the direct ophthalmoscope.

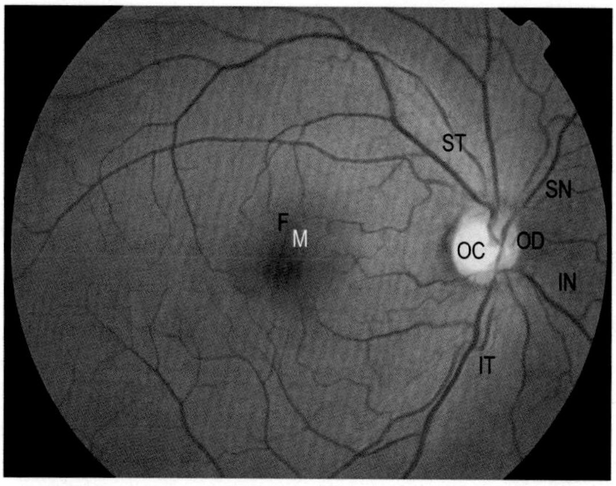

Figure 20.9 Normal fundus anatomy. OC, optic cup; OD, optic disc. Retinal vascular arcades: F, fovea; IN, inferonasal; IT, inferotemporal; M, macula; SN, superonasal; ST, superotemporal.

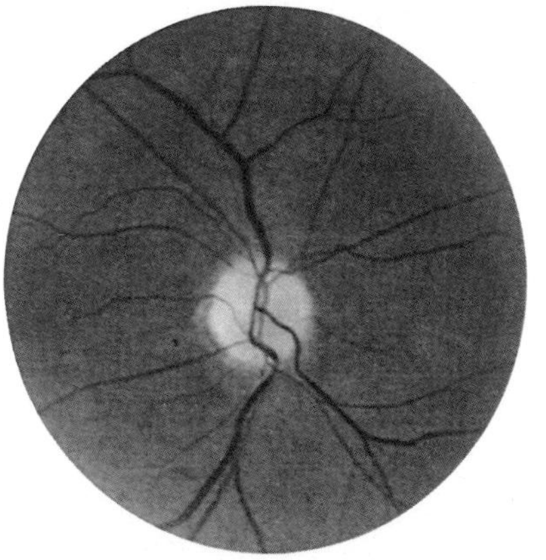

Figure 20.10 Primary optic atrophy. The disc is pale and whiter than normal, and its edges are unusually sharply demarcated from the retina. The retinal vessels are slightly attenuated.

Box 20.5 Technique of ophthalmoscopy

- Use your LEFT eye for the patient's LEFT eye, holding the ophthalmoscope with your LEFT hand and using your RIGHT hand with thumb over the LEFT brow to steady the patient's head (the opposite approach is used for the right eye) (Fig. 20.8).
- First, at arm's length, look for and examine the red reflex (like that in flash photographs). The red reflex is dimmed in elderly people with cataracts, and these may obscure the retina. In a child, congenital cataract and retinoblastoma may abolish the red reflex.
- Looking at the red reflex through the ophthalmoscope, gradually close in on the eye to examine the anterior ocular structures. Use the +20 D lens to view the cornea and the +15 D lens for the iris. Some ophthalmoscopes have a lever to switch to these lenses.
- Then, with a zero lens setting, locate the optic disc. If it is difficult to find, locate any blood vessel and follow it towards the optic disc. Fine-tune the focus with 1-2 D lens steps; if the focus worsens, reverse the other way. If your eye is emmetropic and your accommodation is relaxed, the strength of the lens necessary to bring the fundus into focus gives an indication of the refractive error of the patient's eye (plus or red lenses indicate hypermetropia and minus or black lenses myopia).
- Compare the two eyes. There is a broad range of normal appearances, so if an unusual appearance is symmetrical, it could be a variant of normal.

Box 20.6 Causes of optic atrophy

- Congenital:
  - dominant and recessive
- Optic neuritis
- Chronic papilloedema
- Toxic:
  - tobacco, lead, alcohol
- Optic nerve compression:
  - thyroid
  - tumour
- Post-traumatic (direct optic nerve or indirect vascular damage)

are four key questions to consider when viewing the optic disc:

1 Is the colour normal? The normal disc is yellow-pink and its temporal side is paler. An abnormally pale disc is a sign of optic atrophy (Fig. 20.10). In addition, in optic atrophy there is a reduction in the number of capillaries crossing the edge of the disc, from the normal 10 to 7 or fewer (Kestenbaum's sign). The causes of optic atrophy are listed in Box 20.6. In primary optic atrophy due to optic nerve lesions, the disc is flat and white, with clear-cut

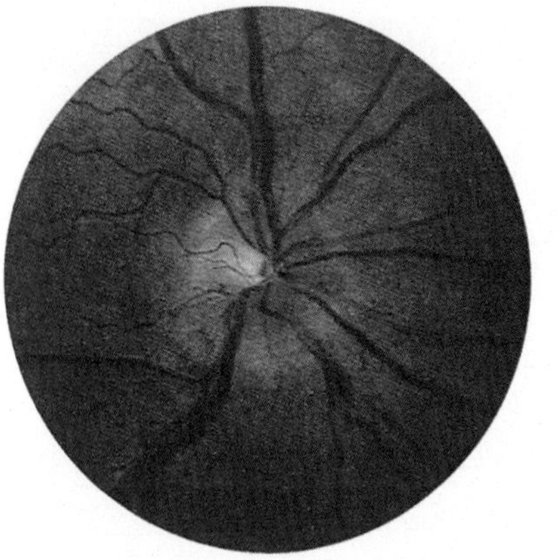

Figure 20.11 Papilloedema: optic disc swelling due to raised intracranial pressure.

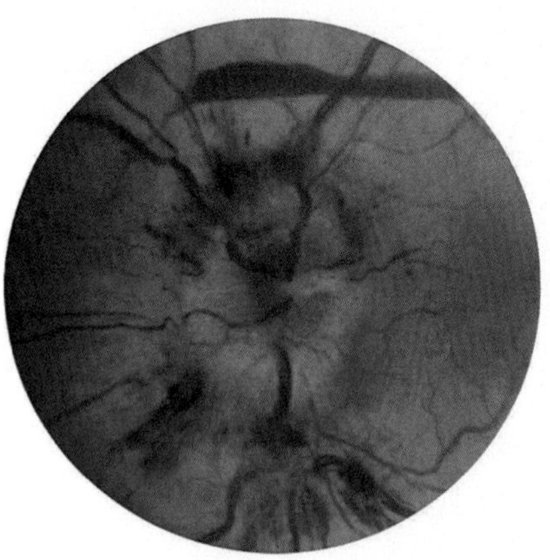

Figure 20.12 Severe papilloedema with retinal haemorrhages.

Box 20.7 Causes of the appearance of optic disc swelling

- Raised intracranial pressure (papilloedema)
- Infiltration:
  - lymphoma
  - sarcoid
- Vascular:
  - hypertension (grade 4)
  - central retinal vein occlusion
  - anterior ischaemic optic neuropathy
- Pseudopapilloedema:
  - congenital small discs
  - high hypermetropia
- Optic disc drusen

edges. Secondary optic atrophy follows swelling of the optic disc due to papilloedema: the disc is greyish-white, with indistinct edges.

2 Are the margins distinct? The disc margin should be sharply defined. In optic disc swelling, this clear edge is obscured (Fig. 20.11) and venous pulsations are abolished. However, venous pulsations may be difficult to see in some normal subjects. Some important causes of disc swelling are listed in Box 20.7. In papilloedema, caused by raised intracranial pressure, the disc is abnormally red and its margins are blurred, especially at the upper and lower margins, and particularly in the upper nasal quadrant. The physiological cup becomes obliterated and the retinal veins are slightly distended. As the condition progresses, the disc becomes more definitely swollen (Fig. 20.12). In order to measure the degree of swelling, start with a high plus lens in the ophthalmoscope and reduce the power until the centre of the disc is just in focus. The retina, a short distance from the disc, is then brought into focus by further reduction of the lens power. This further reduction indicates the degree of swelling of the disc (3 D is equivalent to 1 mm of swelling). If papilloedema develops rapidly, there will be marked engorgement of the retinal veins with haemorrhages and exudates on and around the disc, but with papilloedema of slow onset there may be little or no vascular change, even though the disc may become very swollen. The retinal vessels will, however, bend sharply as they dip down from the swollen disc to the surrounding retina. The oedema may extend to the adjacent retina, producing greyish-white striations near the disc (Paton's lines), and a macular fan of hard exudates temporal to the fovea may develop in some cases.

3 Is the central cup enlarged? The cup is a physiological central depression formed at the optic disc as nerve fibres leave the retina to form the optic nerve. It marks the point where the retinal vessels enter and leave the eye. It is paler than the surrounding rim of the disc. The optic cup : disc ratio is estimated by comparing their ratios vertically. In chronic open-angle glaucoma, the ratio is increased (>0.3) – optic disc cupping. When the cup is deep, in advanced glaucoma, retinal vessels disappear as they climb from the floor to the rim, and reappear as they bend sharply over the edge of the rim (bayonetting); in less advanced cases, the cup appears as a vertical oval extending to the edge of the disc (Fig. 20.13). In myopic individuals, the disc and cup appear large, and mimic glaucoma. Myopes often have a partial ring of pigmentation or white sclera surrounding the disc, which is easily mistaken for the edge of the cup. In severe myopia, degenerative chorioretinal changes may occur in the fundus, which can involve the macula and impair central vision.

4 Are there any other abnormal features? In proliferative diabetic retinopathy, new blood vessels (neovascularization) develop at the optic disc. Myelinated nerve fibres have a dramatic

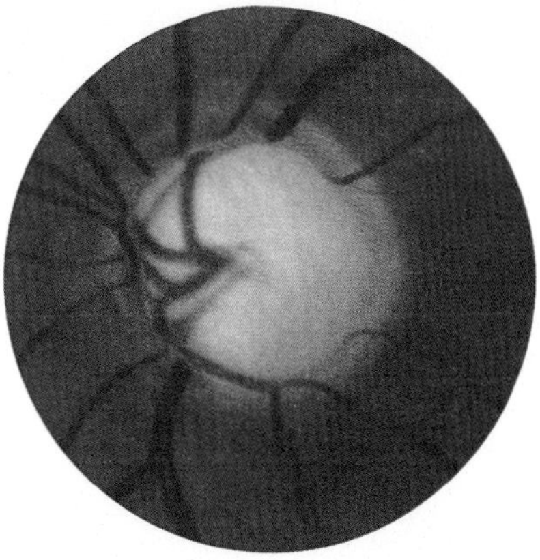

Figure 20.13 Glaucomatous disc cupping. The cup is oval in the vertical plane and appears pale. The retinal vessels are displaced nasally.

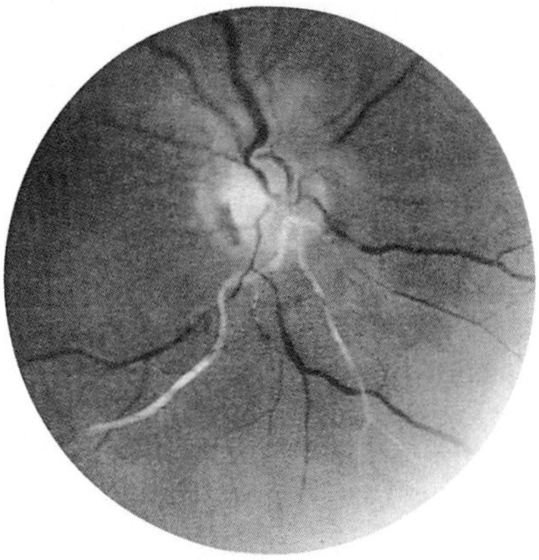

Figure 20.15 Retinal arteriolar emboli. Cholesterol emboli in the retinal arteries of a patient with atheromatous disease of the internal carotid artery in the neck.

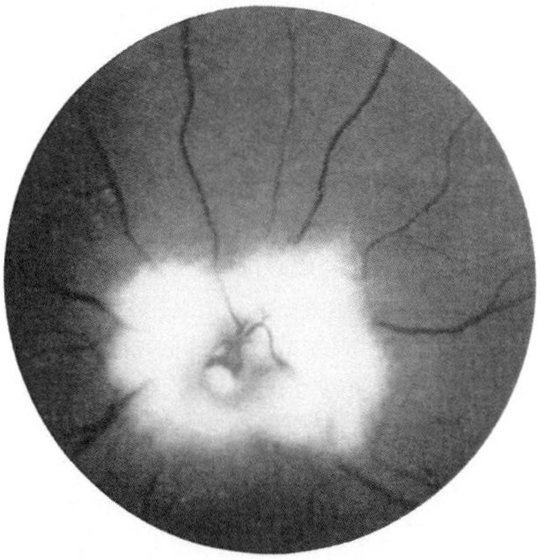

Figure 20.14 Myelinated nerve fibres: the white area obscures the disc; this is a normal variant.

white appearance, but they are a unilateral, harmless and non-progressive congenital anomaly (Fig. 20.14). They have a characteristic feathered edge that may obscure the retinal vessels.

Blood vessels

There are four pairs of arterioles and venules, which form the main retinal vascular arcades that emerge from the optic disc: superotemporal (above the macula), inferotemporal (below the macula), superonasal, and inferonasal. Study each in turn. Arterioles are thin, bright red in colour and with a longitudinal streak of light reflection. In branch arteriolar occlusion, a bright yellow (cholesterol) embolus may occasionally be seen (Fig. 20.15). In diabetes or venous occlusion, the venules are larger, darker and often dilated or tortuous. Look carefully at arteriolar/venous crossings: compression and localized dilatation of venules (arteriovenous (AV) nipping) with arteriolar narrowing (attenuation) is a sign of hypertension (Box 20.8, Fig. 20.16). Spontaneous arteriolar pulsation is an

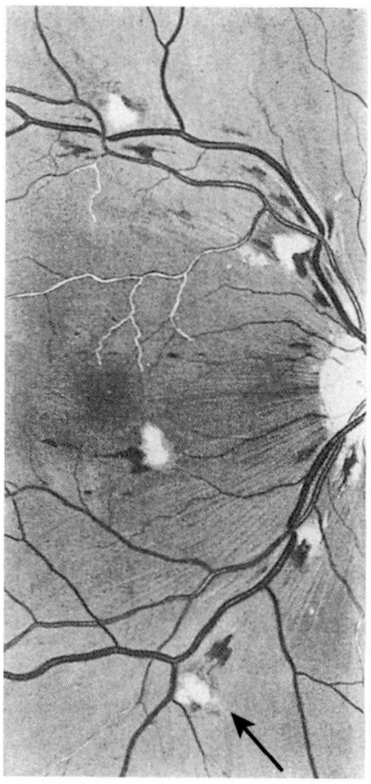

Figure 20.16 Hypertensive retinopathy. The arteries are irregular in calibre and show 'silver wiring'. Arteriovenous nipping is present. Characteristic 'flame-shaped' haemorrhages and 'cotton wool' spots (arrow) can be seen.

Box 20.8 Appearance and classification of hypertensive retinopathy

- Grade 1: arteriolar narrowing (attenuation) and vein concealment
- Grade 2: profound arteriolar attenuation and venous deflections at crossings (AV nipping)
- Grade 3: severe attenuation 'arteriolar copper wiring', haemorrhages, cotton wool spots and hard exudates
- Grade 4: all of the above, plus very severe attenuation 'arteriolar silver wiring' and optic disc swelling

abnormal finding that may occur if the IOP is very high or the central retinal artery pressure very low. Spontaneous venous pulsation is frequently seen in normal eyes, but is reduced in papilloedema.

Retina and macula

As each main vascular arcade is followed and examined, the adjacent and peripheral retina can be systematically assessed. The macula is the central retinal area bounded by temporal vascular arcades. It measures approximately five disc diameters across. The fovea at its centre is one disc diameter in size. The fovea, with its high density of cone photoreceptors, is responsible for fine discriminatory vision. To find the fovea, locate the optic disc and move the ophthalmoscope beam temporally (move yourself toward the nose). Alternatively, ask the patient to look directly into the light. However, if the pupil is undilated, it tends to constrict at this point, and the patient may recoil because of dazzle (you can dim the light beam to make it more comfortable). In young patients, the retina is very reflective and there is often a small yellow dot in the middle of the fovea (macula lutea or fovea centralis). Box 20.9 and Figs 20.17 and 20.18 identify common retinal abnormalities by their colour and appearance.

Slit lamp and intraocular pressure

The slit lamp (Fig. 20.19) provides a stereoscopic, magnified view of the eye and is the key examination tool for ophthalmologists. Many accident and

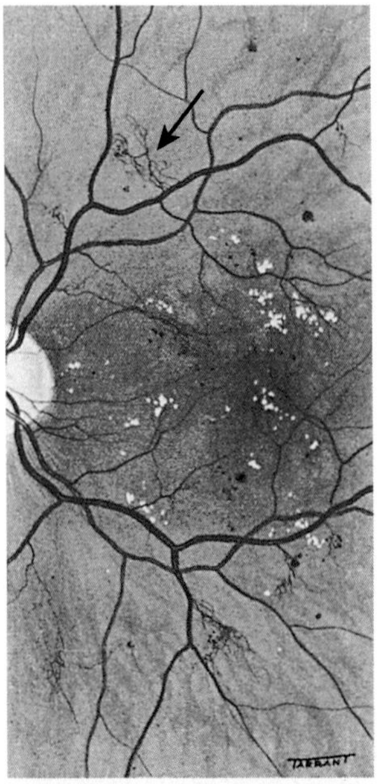

Figure 20.17 Diabetic retinopathy. Microaneurysms (tiny red dots), blot haemorrhages, hard exudates and areas of new vessel formation (arrow) are characteristic of this condition. In many patients, hypertensive retinopathy is also present.

Box 20.9 Common retinal abnormalities

White

- Cotton wool spots: white, fluffy, indistinct areas indicative of retinal ischaemia. This is the accumulation of axonal proteins in the nerve fibre layer. Causes include severe hypertension, diabetes and retinal vein occlusion
- Chorioretinal atrophy: well-defined 'punched-out' lesions (the white is the sclera). May occur in conjunction with retinal pigment hypertrophy. Associated with previous retinal inflammation or injury (including retinal laser)

Yellow

- Hard exudates: bright yellow with well-demarcated edges consisting of lipid deposits that have leaked out of abnormal blood vessels. Most commonly associated with microaneurysms in diabetes (Fig. 20.17)
- Drusen: small multifocal round yellow features, usually located in the central macula. Generally smaller and less bright yellow than hard exudates. Typically bilateral and relatively symmetrical. Common in elderly people associated with 'dry' age-related macular degeneration

Red

- Microaneurysms: the dots that typify diabetic retinopathy. They may leak to cause exudates or bleed to cause blot haemorrhages (Fig. 20.17)
- Blot haemorrhages: rounded localized intraretinal blood, typically due to diabetic retinopathy, but other causes include severe hypertension and retinal vein occlusion
- Deep large haemorrhages: associated with retinal ischaemia when numerous
- Flame haemorrhages: have a characteristic feathery shape as the blood is in the nerve fibre layer; may be present in retinal vein occlusion (Fig. 20.18). Not typically associated with ischaemia

Black

- Retinal pigment hypertrophy: well-defined black lesions, often in conjunction with chorioretinal atrophy. May occur with previous retinal inflammation or injury (including retinal laser therapy).

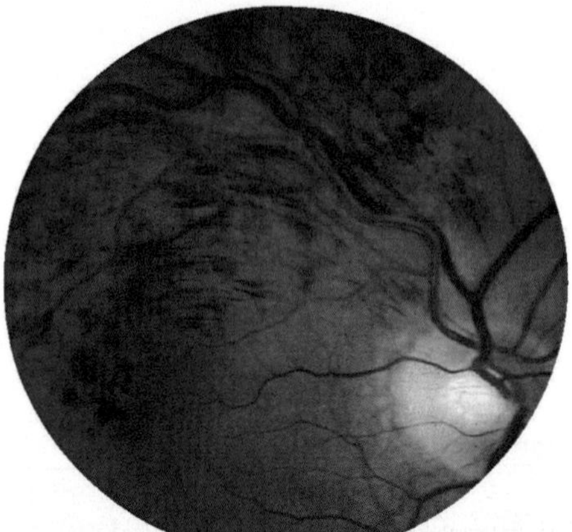

Figure 20.18 Branch retinal vein occlusion. There are flame-shaped retinal haemorrhages, but the disc is normal.

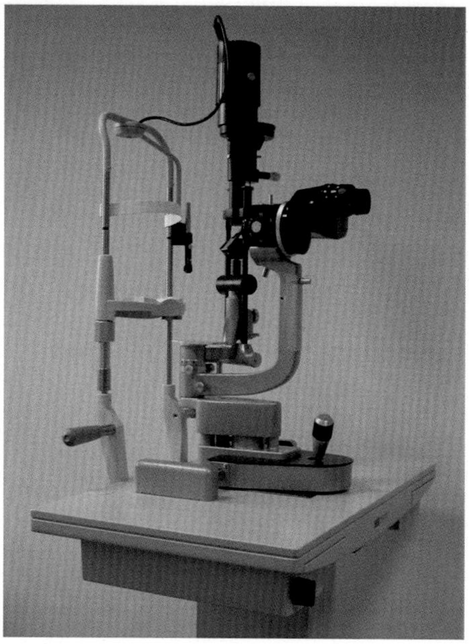

Figure 20.19 Slit lamp.

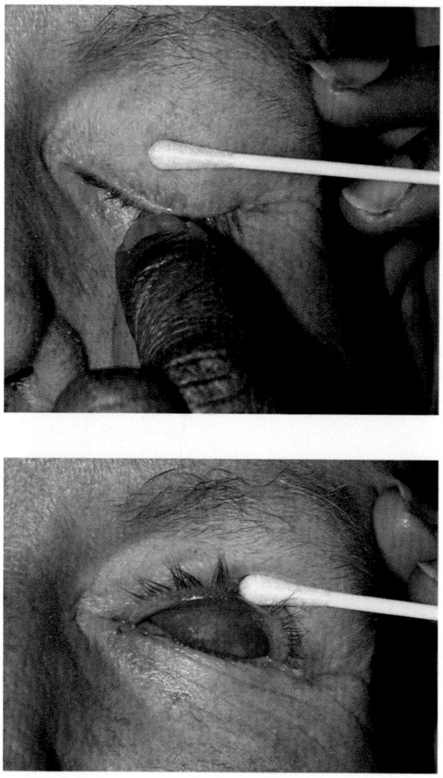

Figure 20.20 Everting the upper eyelid to expose the tarsal conjunctiva.

emergency departments have a slit lamp, and it can be invaluable for assessing suspected foreign bodies and corneal abrasions. Some direct ophthalmoscopes are equipped with a slit-lamp beam, which can be useful. Alternatively, the anterior orbital structures and globe can be examined with a bright torch and basic magnification, and the same principles of systematic examination apply. The slit lamp comprises a table-mounted binocular microscope column with an adjustable illumination source that produces a narrow, slit beam of light.

The patient is seated with forehead and chin supported. The slit beam illumination and microscope have a common axis of rotation and coincident focal lengths, allowing the angle of illumination to be varied along with its width, length and intensity. Projected onto the globe, the slit beam illuminates an optical cross-section of the eye's transparent structures, and this can be viewed with magnification varying from 10× to 40× power. An attachment allows the IOP to be measured (tonometry). The drainage angle can be seen with a special contact lens (gonioscopy) and, with the aid of a hand-held lens or a contact lens, the retina can also be viewed.

The following structures can be examined:

- Lid margins, meibomian gland orifices and lashes. Inflammation of the lid margins (blepharitis) is one of the commonest ophthalmic conditions. It is related to chalazia, blocked meibomian glands and infected lash follicles (styes). The puncta, on the medial aspect of the lids, drain tears into the canalicular tear drainage pathway. Misdirected lashes (trichiasis) causing foreign body sensations occur with chronic lid disease.
- Conjunctival surfaces (tarsal, forniceal and bulbar). This mucous membrane lines the eyeball (bulbar conjunctiva) and the inner surface of the eyelids (tarsal conjunctiva). The conjunctiva may be pale in anaemia, yellow in jaundice or red (injected) in conjunctivitis and other inflammatory eye disorders. Directing the patient's gaze up, down, left and right ensures that all the bulbar conjunctiva is viewed. To examine the inferior tarsal conjunctiva of the lower lid, the lower lid should be gently everted and the patient asked to look upwards. To examine the superior tarsal conjunctiva – for example if a foreign body is suspected – ask the patient to look downwards (Fig. 20.20). Grasp the lashes between the forefinger and thumb, gently pull down on them and rotate the eyelid upwards over either the other thumb or a cotton bud.
- Cornea and tear film. The transparent cornea can be viewed in cross-section. The addition of a drop of 2% fluorescein reveals defects or foreign bodies in the corneal epithelium and the tear film can be assessed (Fig. 20.21). The tear meniscus on the lower eyelid should be symmetrical and less than 1 mm thick, and the tear break-up time should be more than 10 seconds. Fluorescein also aids the identification of aqueous leakage in a penetrating corneal

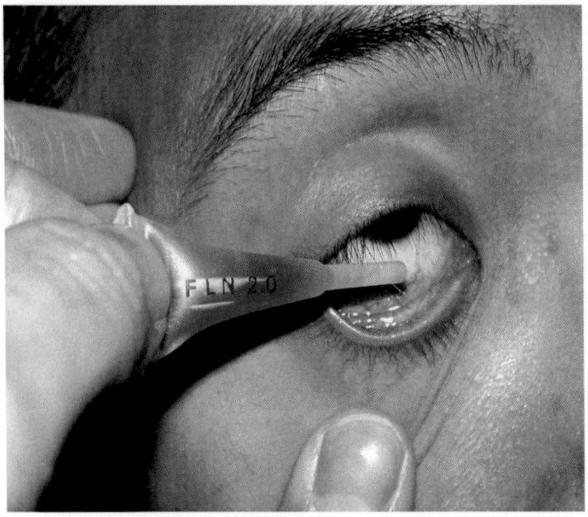

Figure 20.21 Fluorescein used to stain the cornea and tear film.

injury (Seidel's test). Arcus senilis is a common crescentic opacity near the periphery of the cornea. It usually starts at the lower part of the cornea, extending to form a complete circle. It is common in old people but may occur in the young (arcus juvenilis) in association with type IV hyperlipoproteinaemia. Corneal sensation should be tested.

- Anterior chamber (filled with aqueous). In iritis, a cause of red eye, there is inflammation in the aqueous, with flare (protein) and cells (typically leukocytes). In severe iritis, the inflammatory exudate settles inferiorly to create a white fluid level in the anterior chamber (hypopyon). Hyphaema has a similar but red appearance caused by bleeding into the anterior chamber, usually due to trauma.
- Iris. Note any difference in the colour of the two eyes (heterochromia), abnormality in the shape or size of the pupils or signs of iritis. In iritis, the pupil may be constricted (miosis) or irregular owing to the formation of adhesions (posterior synechiae) between the edge of the pupil and the anterior surface of the lens. Blunt trauma can cause a dilated (mydriasis) unreactive pupil with radial ruptures in the iris. An irregular or teardrop-shaped pupil and a history of a high-velocity foreign body is highly suspicious of a penetrating eye injury where the iris has plugged the leaking wound. Other abnormalities of the pupils are described in Chapter 16.
- Lens. Cataracts are usually due to ageing (central nuclear sclerosis) but also occur in diabetes mellitus, after injury and in certain hereditary diseases, for example myotonic dystrophy. Posterior subcapsular cataract is a common side effect of corticosteroid therapy. Blunt eye injury may cause partial dislocation of the lens (subluxation) or complete dislocation into the vitreous cavity.

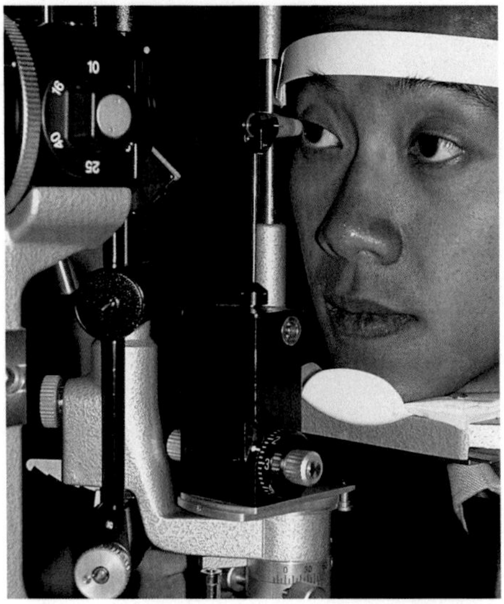

Figure 20.22 Goldman tonometry.

- Anterior vitreous. This is best examined when the pupil is dilated. Opacities may be observed, most easily using a green light. Cells in the vitreous may be associated with ocular inflammation (vitritis), trauma (vitreous haemorrhage) or retinal holes/detachment (retinal pigment).

Measuring intraocular pressure: applanation tonometry

Intraocular pressures between 10 and 21 mmHg are considered normal. An increased IOP is a characteristic feature of glaucoma. A diminished IOP occurs in diabetic coma and in severe dehydration from any cause. The IOP may be assessed by palpating the eyeball, although only gross variations from normal can be appreciated. More accurate is applanation tonometry, in which the force required to flatten (applanate) an area of a sphere (the cornea) is proportional to the pressure within the sphere (Fig. 20.22). Topical anaesthetic and fluorescein are applied to the cornea and a bright cobalt blue filter is used to illuminate the sterile tonometer head. Contact between tonometer head and cornea creates a thin green circular outline of fluorescein, and a prism in the head splits this into two semicircles. The tonometer force is adjusted manually until the semicircles just overlap, and is read in millimeters of mercury (mmHg; Fig. 20.23).

Eyelid, lacrimal and orbital assessment

Eyelids

People of Asian origin have a long, narrow palpebral aperture with an upward and outward obliquity and a characteristic fold of skin along the upper lid. The

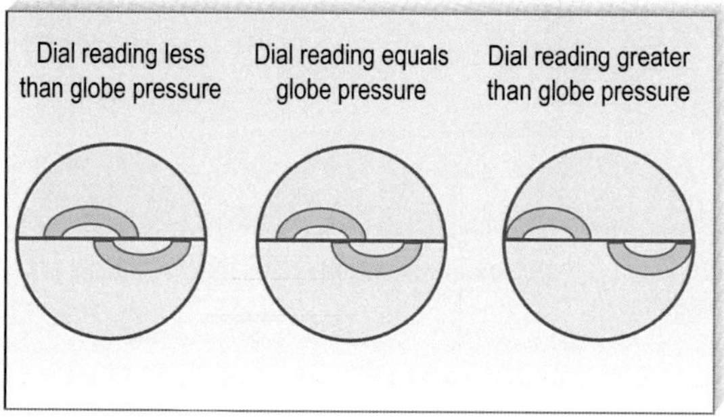

Figure 20.23 Diagrammatic representation of tonometry.

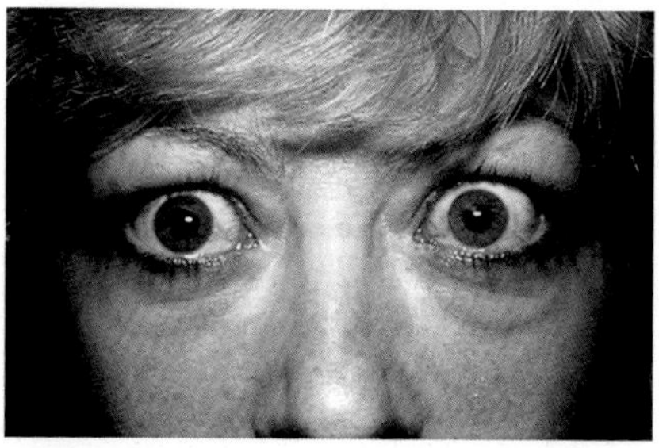

Figure 20.24 Thyroid eye disease with upper eyelid retraction and mild exophthalmos (bilateral proptosis).

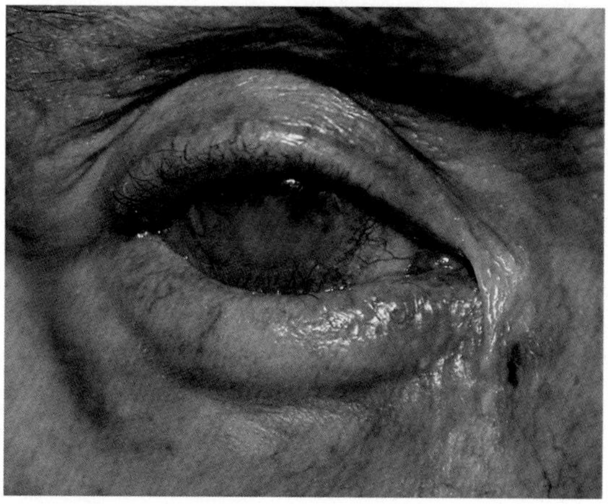

Figure 20.25 Lower eyelid entropion causing infective keratitis and corneal opacification.

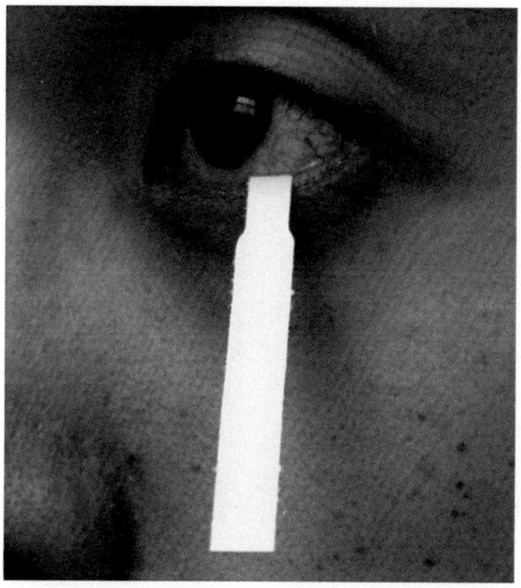

Figure 20.26 Schirmer's test for dry eyes.

highest point of the aperture is typically at the junction of its middle and inner thirds. In Down's syndrome, the palpebral fissure is also oblique. However, it is also short and wide, with its highest point at the centre of the lid.

Normally no sclera is visible above the limbus (the corneoscleral junction). The commonest cause of scleral show is eyelid retraction (Fig. 20.24) due to dysthyroid eye disease, accompanied by other signs such as lid lag, in which movement of the upper lid seems to lag behind that of the eyeball when the patient looks downwards. In parkinsonism, there may be reduced blink frequency. Look for reduced eyelid closure (lagophthalmos) and levator muscle function. Ptosis (drooping of the upper lid) may be congenital or acquired (check old photographs). In age-related ptosis, owing to levator disinsertion, levator function is retained and there is a high upper eyelid skin crease. In ptosis due to myogenic or neurogenic lesions, there is reduced levator function (see Ch. 16). In entropion, there is inversion of the lid margin with associated malpositioning of the lashes, which may rub on the cornea (Fig. 20.25); and in ectropion, eversion of the eyelid is often associated with watering. The lower lid is prone to skin tumours, particularly basal cell and squamous cell carcinomas (see Fig. 19.25). Xanthelasmas are fatty deposits that develop in the upper and lower eyelids in patients with long-standing hypercholesterolaemia.

Lacrimal

Examine the lacrimal gland by pulling up the outer part of the upper lid while the patient looks downwards and inwards. Acute inflammation (dacryoadenitis) causes a tender swollen gland, with oedema of the upper lid and localized conjunctival injection. Chronic dacryoadenitis, a painless enlargement of the lacrimal gland which is frequently bilateral, occurs in sarcoidosis and lymphoproliferative disorders. Tumours of the lacrimal gland produce a hard swelling of the gland associated with displacement of the globe. Involvement of the lacrimal gland by any disease process may cause a dry eye.

Assess the position and size of the puncta (see above). Painless watering is a feature of obstruction of the tear drainage pathway, but exclude reflex tearing and overflow from, for example, a dry eye. Schirmer's test uses a standardized strip of filter paper to detect dry eyes by assessing the extent of wetting at 5 minutes (Fig. 20.26). Overt nasolacrimal duct blockage can be excluded if the patient reports fluid at the back of the throat on probing and syringing with normal saline (Fig. 20.27).

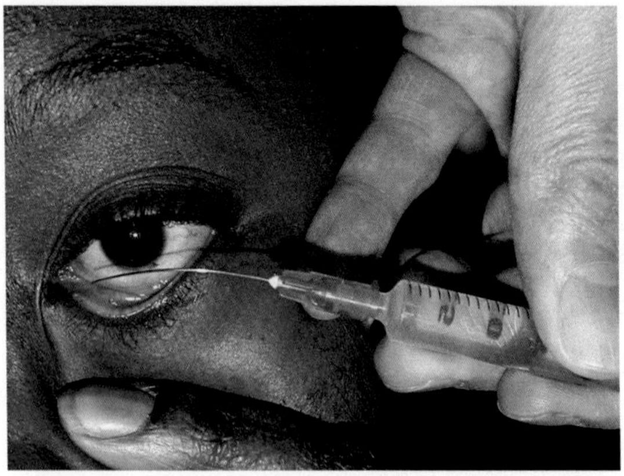

Figure 20.27 Syringe and probing to assess nasolacrimal duct function.

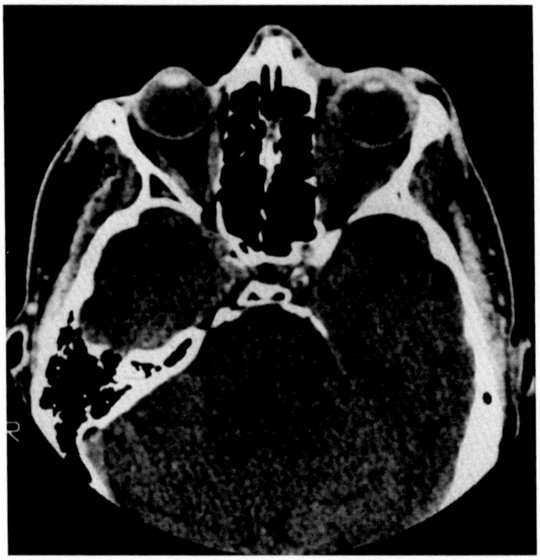

Figure 20.28 Axial CT orbits in TED. Left-sided thyroid eye disease with exophthalmos and marked hypertrophy (inflammation) of the medial and lateral rectus muscles on that side. These muscles in the other eye are also slightly enlarged. The optic nerve can clearly be seen between the enlarged muscles on the left side.

Orbit

The most common cause of forward displacement of the eyeball – proptosis when unilateral, or exophthalmos when bilateral – is thyroid eye disease (TED) (see Fig. 18.13). This can cause corneal exposure and ulceration. Optic nerve damage may occur despite minimal proptosis. Axial proptosis, in the primary direction of the eye in forward gaze, is typical of TED and of tumours in the extraocular muscle cone behind the eye (intraconal mass lesions) (Fig. 20.28). Non-axial proptosis occurs in association with space-occupying orbital lesions outside the muscle cone, for example lacrimal gland tumours; these displace the globe forward and inferomedially. Apparent ('pseudo') proptosis causes diagnostic confusion: for example in ipsilateral eyelid retraction or myopia (where the eye is longer than normal) or when there is contralateral ptosis or enophthalmos.

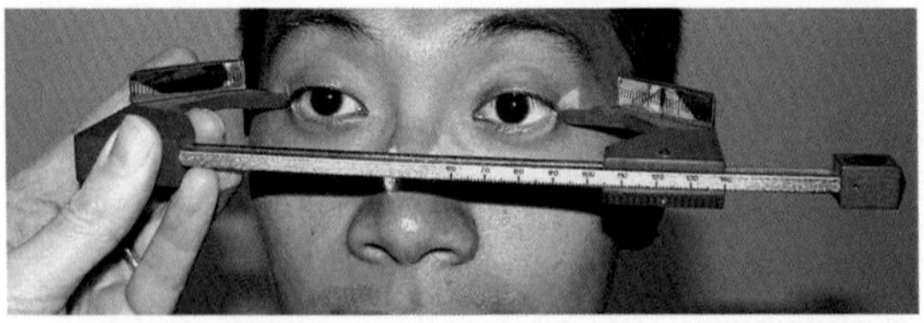

Figure 20.29 Hertel exophthalmometry to quantify proptosis or exophthalmos.

Proptosis and enophthalmos can be measured with the Hertel exophthalmometer (Fig. 20.29). A difference of >2 mm between sides is abnormal. A proptosis that increases while the patient performs a Valsalva manoeuvre is suggestive of a venous abnormality. Pulsatile proptosis with an orbital bruit is a feature of carotid cavernous fistula.

Blunt trauma to the orbit may cause a blowout fracture of the thin orbital floor. Orbital contents may prolapse through the fracture, restricting the movement of the inferior rectus muscle and limiting upgaze. A full orbital examination should include palpation, eye movement examination, optic nerve assessment and testing of the trigeminal nerve for altered sensation.

Examination of the eye in children

The advice given in Chapter 6 on the examination of children in general is also important when examining children's eyes. Children may object strongly to lights and instruments, particularly when they are wielded by white-coated strangers. Allow the child to get used to the surroundings while taking a history from the parent, but do not ignore the child. Constantly observe the child, noting visual behaviour, the position and movements of the eyes and the general appearance of each eye.

Visual maturation continues after birth and without a focused retinal image, the visual pathways fail to develop properly, a condition known as amblyopia. Untreated, sight loss from amblyopia becomes irreversible. It is therefore important to assess visual acuity in preverbal and young children. Babies should rapidly fix a large object – for example the examiner's face – and follow it. After 6 months, 'continuous' and 'steady' fixation that is 'maintained' ('CSM') during a blink should be demonstrable. If an infant strongly objects to your covering an eye for even a short time, consider whether the non-covered eye may not be seeing well. A more sophisticated assessment can be made using 'preferential looking'. Cards are presented to the child with a grating drawn at one end and none at the other. The child will prefer to look at the image rather than nothing. Successively smaller

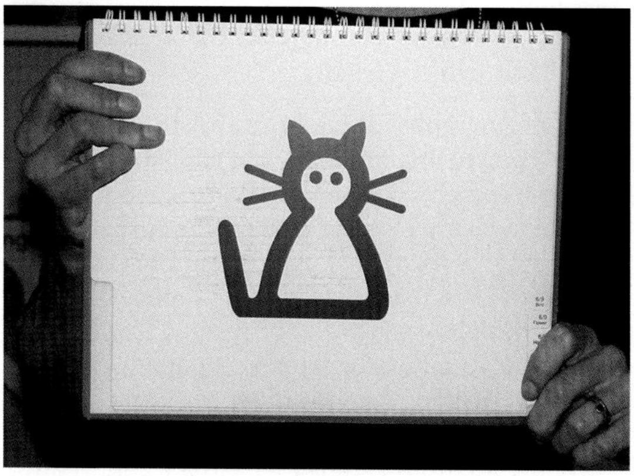

Figure 20.30 Kay picture-matching test to assess the visual acuity of children 2 years and older.

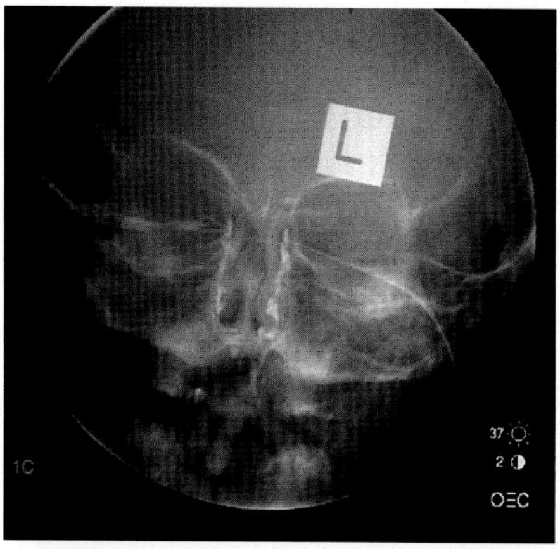

Figure 20.31 Dacryocystogram showing restricted flow of radiopaque dye in the right nasolacrimal duct.

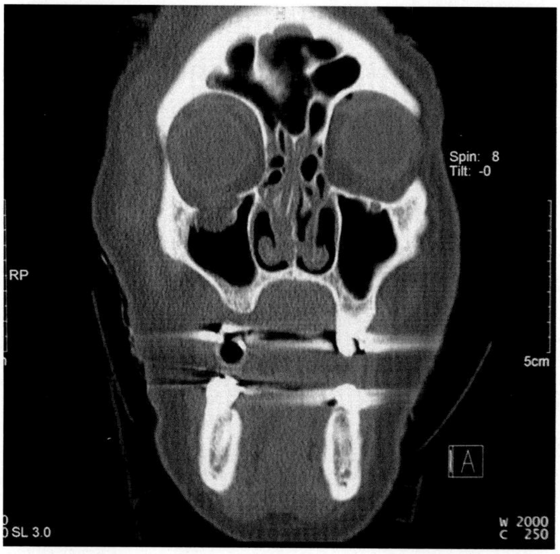

Figure 20.32 Coronal CT orbits in blowout fracture. The right bony orbital floor is fractured and the orbital contents prolapsed.

spatial gratings are shown until the child does not see them. The grating seen can be converted to an approximate Snellen acuity (the vision of a 1-year-old equates to approximately 6/12), although testing each eye independently in this age group is difficult. From the age of 2 years, a more accurate estimate of acuity can be made using the Kay picture-matching test (Fig. 20.30), and from 3 years the Sheridan-Gardiner letter-matching test. In these tests, the child, or the child's parent, holds a card with a number of pictures or numbers on it. The examiner holds up an image and asks the child to match this target to one on the card – the targets vary in size.

Next, the position and movements of the eyes should be assessed. The least disturbing method is to observe the corneal light reflex: a light held at about 1 m should produce a reflection in the centre of each pupil. If the reflection in one eye is at a different location from that in the other, there may be a squint (although a wide intercanthal distance may give this appearance). If a squint is suspected, a cover and alternate cover test should be performed. Assess the ocular movements and the pupillary responses to light and accommodation. Examine the media and fundi with the ophthalmoscope through the dilated pupil. Because of limited cooperation, refraction testing may be limited to the retinoscopy assessment. In general, only children with refractive errors so severe that there is a risk of amblyopia require treatment.

Imaging

Plain X-rays

Plain X-rays have a limited role in the detection of foreign bodies, but have been largely superseded by computed tomography (CT) or magnetic resonance imaging (MRI). Ultrasound is used to assess the globe. A dacryocystogram uses a radiopaque dye introduced into the lacrimal drainage system to identify sites of lacrimal duct obstruction (Fig. 20.31). It is particularly useful in the watering eye, when carcinoma is suspected, when repeat surgery is planned or when trauma has occurred.

Computed tomography and magnetic resonance imaging

CT and MRI are used extensively in the diagnosis of orbital disease. CT is often considered superior because it defines the bony orbit, but the X-ray dose to the eye and lens is not inconsiderable. CT is the investigation of choice in blunt orbital trauma and blowout fractures (see above), where fine-cut coronal spiral images are desirable (Fig. 20.32).

A- and B-mode ultrasound

The A-mode scan is a one-dimensional time-amplitude study commonly used to assess axial length, which is an essential measurement for lens implant calculation prior to cataract surgery. The B-mode scan gives a two-dimensional cross-sectional view of the eye for the diagnosis of both intraocular and orbital tumours, retinal detachments and intraocular disorders when the fundal view is impaired (e.g. with vitreous haemorrhage; Fig. 20.33).

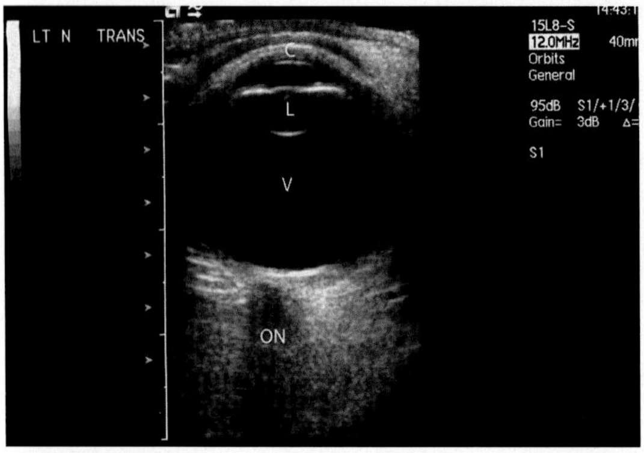

Figure 20.33 B-mode ultrasound scan showing lens opacity and vitreous opacities but no retinal detachment following penetrating trauma. C, cornea; L, lens; ON, optic nerve; V, vitreous.

Retinal photography and fundus fluorescein angiography

Retinal photography alone is useful to document posterior segment abnormalities and allow monitoring, for example of a choroidal naevus. In conjunction with the intravenous injection of sodium fluorescein photography it gives a detailed assessment of the retinal and choroidal vasculature (Figs 20.34 and 20.35). A blue filtered light excites fluorescence (530 nm) as the dye circulates. Fundus fluorescein angiography is useful in investigating diabetic retinopathy, age-related macular degeneration and retinal ischaemia. Minor side effects, including transient nausea and yellow discoloration of the skin and urine, are common. Severe anaphylaxis is, fortunately, very rare.

Retinal and optic disc tomography

Optical coherence tomography (OCT) and optic disc tomography

Becoming increasingly widely used clinically, optical coherence tomography (OCT) is based on interferometry, typically using near infrared light, to obtain

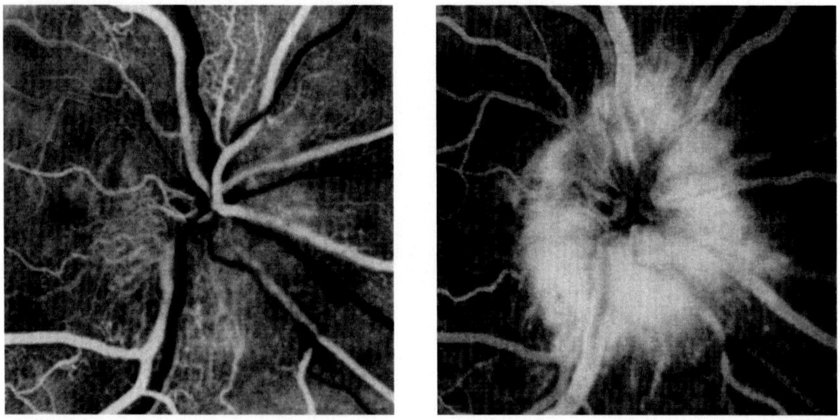

Figure 20.34 Fluorescein retinal angiogram of fundus in papilloedema. Note the late-phase leakage of the dye.

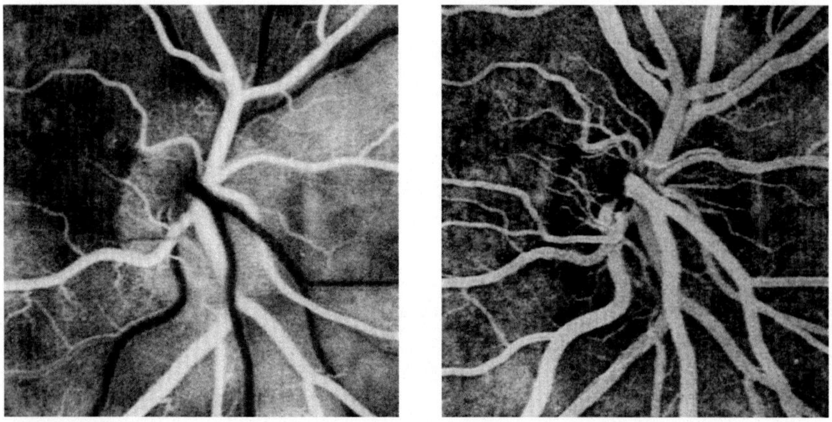

Figure 20.35 Fluorescein retinal angiogram of fundus in pseudopapilloedema.

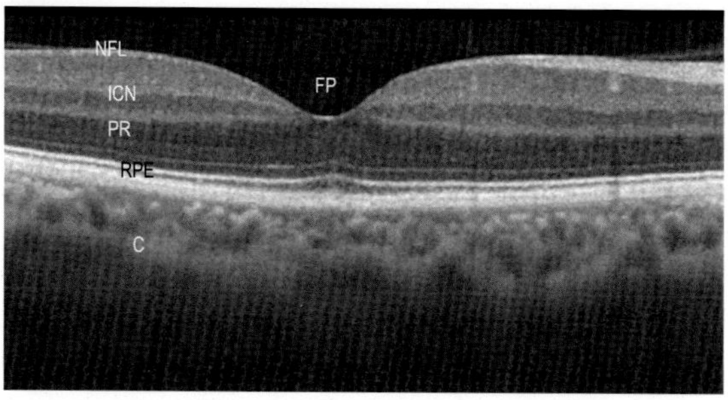

Figure 20.36 Ocular coherence tomography image of a normal macula. C, choroid; RPE, retinal pigment epithelium; PR, photoreceptor layer; ICN, inter-connecting neurone layer; NFL, nerve fibre layer; FD, foveal depression.

high-resolution (2-20 μm) cross-sectional images of the retina (Fig. 20.36) and optic disc. Optical coherence tomography angiography (OCTA) is a newer development that compares motion contrast imaging to high-resolution volumetric blood flow information to generate non-invasive retinal angiography images without injection of fluorescein. OCT has also been developed to generate images of the anterior segment (ACOCT), for example showing the angle structures in high resolution. In addition to OCT, a variety of techniques have been developed to image and assess the shape of the optic disc that are particularly useful in the management of glaucoma. These include scanning laser polarimetry (SLP) and the scanning laser ophthalmoscope (SLO) which assesses nerve fibre thickness indirectly.

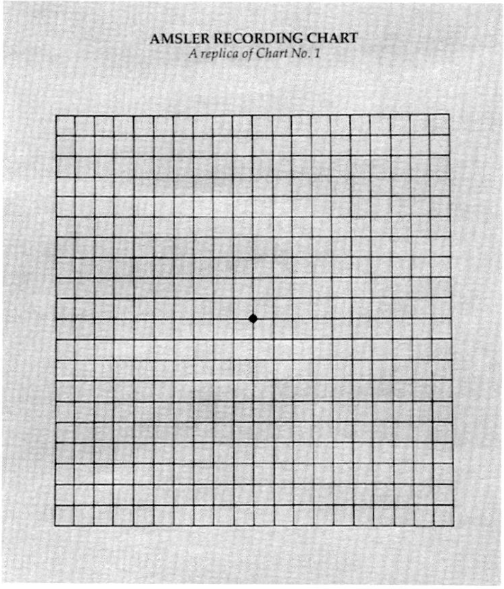

Figure 20.37 Amsler grid for testing macular function.

Special examination techniques

Refraction and refractive assessment

A refraction test will ascertain the optical power of an eye, with a view to prescribing glasses or contact lenses. An objective refraction is performed using neutralizing lenses in conjunction with a retinoscope. In adults and cooperative children, this is then refined subjectively by placing neutralizing lenses in front of the eye and simultaneously assessing visual acuity. Increasingly, the retinoscope is being replaced by an automated technique (the autorefractor).

Amsler grid

The Amsler grid is a sensitive test of macular function. It comprises a series of vertical and horizontal lines with a central spot for fixation (Fig. 20.37). The patient is asked to look at this spot and describe any distortions or missing areas in the grid.

Indirect ophthalmoscopy

Binocular indirect ophthalmoscopy, using a light source supported on the examiner's head and a hand-held lens in front of the patient's eye, allows a much greater area of the fundus to be visualized (Fig. 20.38). The retinal periphery is more readily seen.

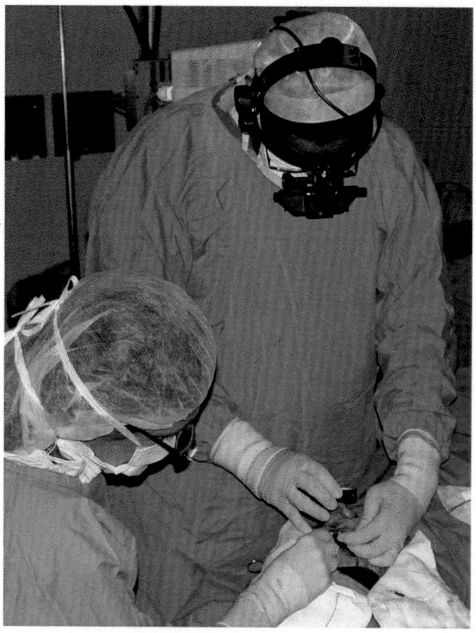

Figure 20.38 Indirect ophthalmoscopy, here used intraoperatively. Note the head light and hand-held 20 D lens.

Electrophysiological tests

Visual evoked potentials (VEP), recorded from the occipital cortex using scalp electrodes while the patient views an alternating black-and-white chequerboard stimulus, have a role in the diagnosis of disease of the visual pathway. The principal waveform recorded from the scalp is a positive deflection occurring about 100 ms after the stimulus (the P100 wave).

This is attenuated in amplitude and increased in latency in disease of the optic nerve, for example optic neuritis or optic nerve compression. Electroretinograms (ERG) measure the electrical potential across the eye, recorded with a corneal electrode, with a reference electrode placed on the forehead. Flash, flicker or pattern stimuli are used to generate electrical responses from retinal activation. This is useful in assessing hereditary or acquired retinal degeneration.

Ear, nose and throat 21

Michael J. Wareing

Introduction

This chapter describes the assessment of potential diseases of the ear, nose and throat. The formal title of the specialty is otorhinolaryngology, which has many interactions with oral and maxillofacial surgery, although more details of the latter are too specialized for an undergraduate textbook.

There is a close functional and anatomical relationship between the ear, the nose and the throat. Disease in one area may have manifestations in another area. Symptoms in one area may likewise refer to another area, so an accurate assessment requires a thorough history and examination of the entire area to elucidate a cause. Ear, nose and throat (ENT) is a highly clinical subject because much is visible, especially with modern examination techniques. Therefore, myriad modern imaging and other investigations are often unnecessary.

The ear

Anatomy

The ear (Fig. 21.1) consists of the external, middle and inner ears. The external ear consists of the pinna and external auditory canal (meatus). The cartilaginous pinna is covered with perichondrium and skin, forming the helix and antihelix. The meatus has an outer cartilaginous and an inner bony component. The skin overlying the external auditory meatus contains hair cells and modified sebaceous glands which produce wax (cerumen). Desquamated skin debris, mixed with cerumen, migrates outward from the drum and deep canal and makes the external ear a self-cleaning system.

The opaque or semitranslucent eardrum (tympanic membrane) separates the middle and external ears (Fig. 21.2). The pars tensa, the lower part of the drum, is formed from an outer layer of skin, a middle layer of fibrous tissue and an inner layer of middle ear mucosa. It is attached to the annulus, a fibrous ring that stabilizes the drum to the surrounding bone. The pars flaccida, the upper part of the drum, may retract if there is prolonged negative middle ear pressure secondary to Eustachian tube dysfunction. The malleus, incus and stapes are three small connecting bones (ossicles) (Fig. 21.3) that transmit sound across the middle ear from the drum to the cochlea. The handle of the malleus lies within the fibrous layer of the pars tensa. Within the middle ear, the head of the malleus articulates with the incus in the attic, the upper portion of the middle ear space. The long process of the incus articulates with the stapes. This articulation (the incudostapedial joint) is liable to disruption from trauma or chronic infection. The stapes footplate sits in the oval window, and transmits and amplifies sound to the fluid-filled inner ear.

The inner ear has two portions. The cochlea (Fig. 21.4), the spiral organ of hearing, is a transducer that converts sound energy into digital nerve impulses that are transmitted by the eighth cranial nerve (cochlear) to the brainstem and thence to the auditory cortex. The organ of Corti (Fig. 21.5) within the cochlea contains hair cells that detect frequency-specific sound energy; low-frequency sounds are detected in the apical region and high-frequency sounds are detected in the basal region. The inner ear is also concerned with balance. The semicircular canals and the vestibule contain receptors that detect angular and linear motion in the three cardinal x, y and z planes. The inner ears are only one component of the balance system; visual input and proprioception from joints and muscles are also important.

The facial (seventh cranial) nerve (Fig. 21.6) is important in otological practice. It runs from the brainstem through the cerebellopontine angle to the internal auditory meatus (IAM) with the cochlear and vestibular (eighth) nerves. The facial nerve passes through the temporal bone and leaves the skull through the stylomastoid foramen near the mastoid process. It may be damaged when there is suppurative middle ear disease or trauma. The chorda tympani leaves the descending portion of the facial nerve in the temporal bone to provide taste fibre innervation to the anterior two-thirds of the tongue. The facial nerve supplies the facial muscles through upper and lower divisions that arise as it passes through the parotid gland.

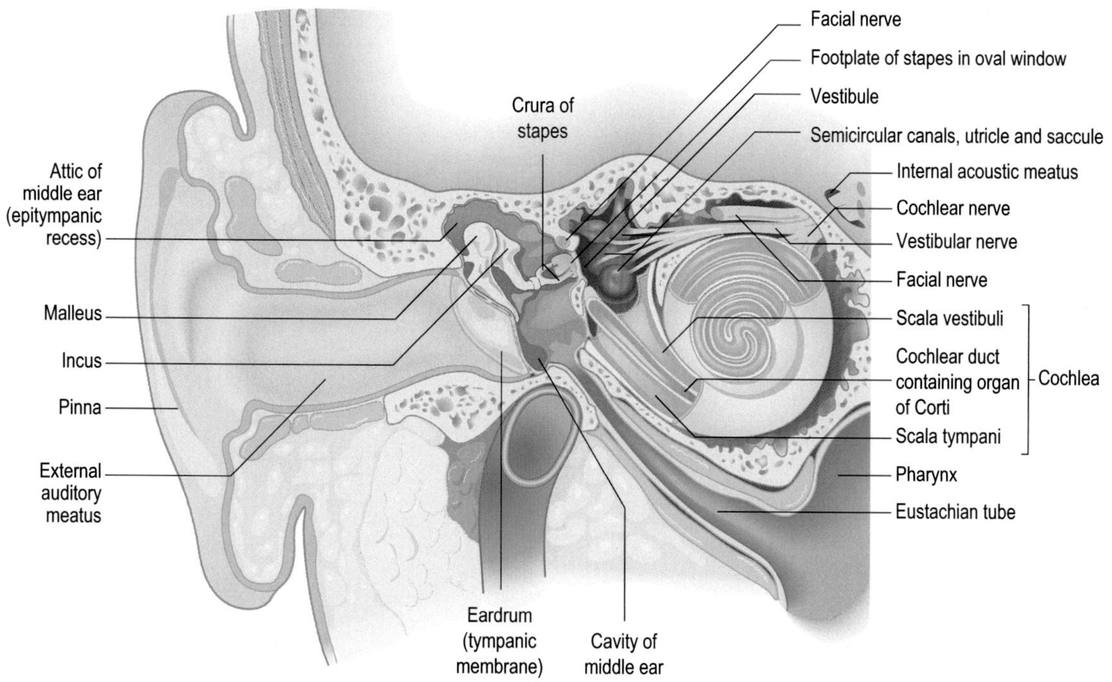

Figure 21.1 Anatomy of the ear.

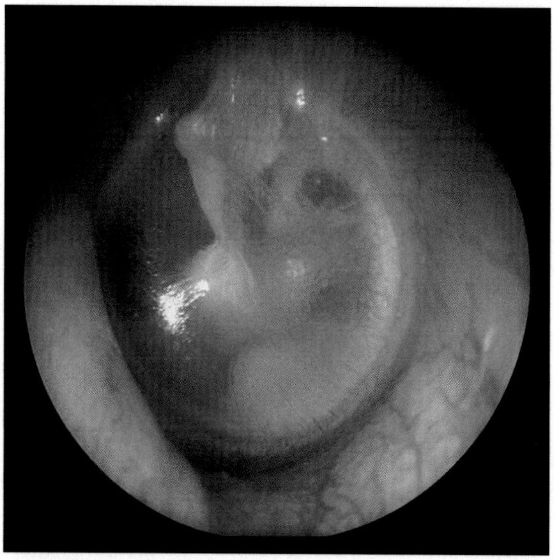

Figure 21.2 A normal left tympanic membrane.

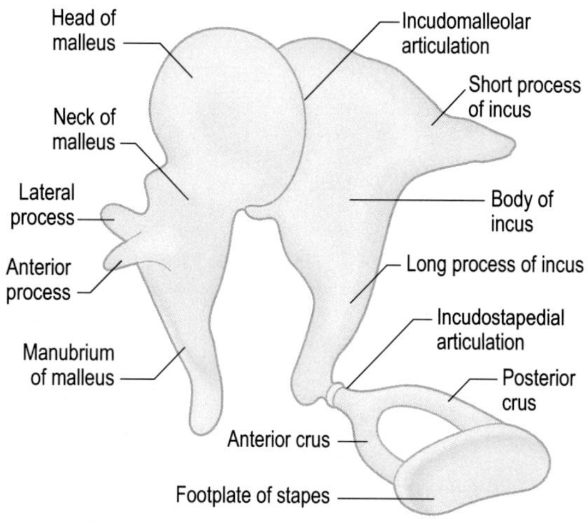

Figure 21.3 The ossicles.

Symptoms of ear disease

The five main symptoms of ear disease are:

1 otalgia: earache or pain.
2 otorrhoea: discharge.
3 hearing loss.
4 tinnitus: a perception of sound in the absence of an appropriate auditory stimulus.
5 vertigo: an illusion of movement.

Otalgia

Pain from disease of the external ear, tympanic membrane and middle ear reaches the brain by branches of the fifth, ninth and tenth cranial nerves, together with nerves from C2 and C3 roots. Because branches of these nerves also supply the larynx and pharynx, as well as the temporomandibular joint and teeth, disease of these structures may give rise to referred pain in the ear. Therefore, if otoscopic examination is normal, examination of these other sites should be considered. In half of affected patients, the ear pain is referred.

The main causes of otalgia are listed in Box 21.1. Of the otological causes, acute infection of the cartilage of the pinna (perichondritis) can be very painful. Malignant otitis externa is not neoplastic. It is due to infection (usually *Pseudomonas*) and can spread to the skull base, especially in diabetic or immunocompromised individuals.

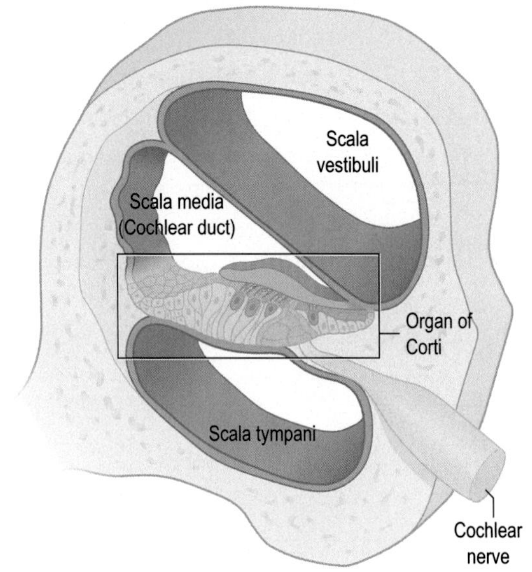

Figure 21.4 Section through the cochlea.

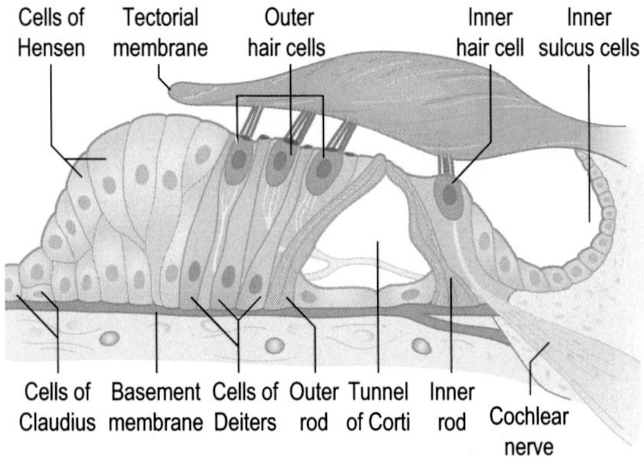

Figure 21.5 The organ of Corti.

Box 21.1 Causes of otalgia

Otological

- Acute suppurative otitis media, mastoiditis
- Acute otitis externa
- Barotrauma
- Furunculosis
- Perichondritis
- Herpes zoster (Ramsay Hunt syndrome – shingles of the facial nerve)
- Myringitis bullosa – viral myringitis
- Necrotizing external otitis (malignant otitis externa)
- Neoplasia

Non-otological

- Tonsillitis or quinsy
- Dental disease
- Temporomandibular joint pathology
- Cervical spine disease
- Carcinoma in the upper air and food passages

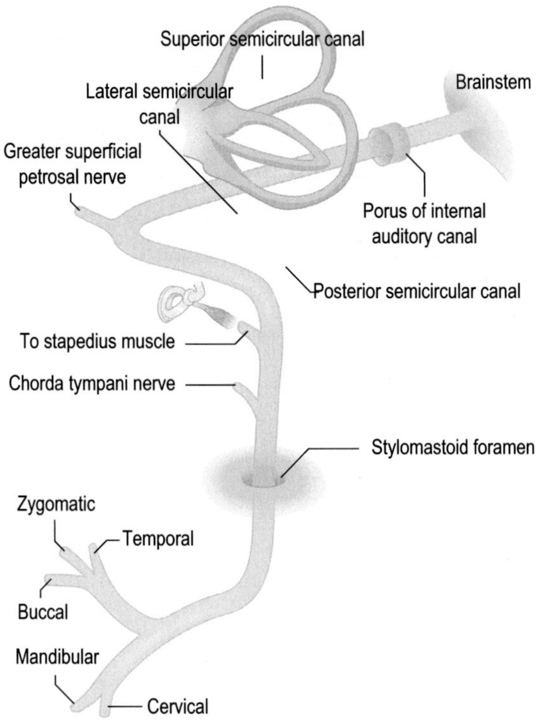

Figure 21.6 The course of the peripheral facial nerve.

Otorrhoea

Pus draining from the ear varies in character depending on its origin (Table 21.1). A profuse mucoid discharge with pulsation suggests a tympanic membrane perforation. The length of history is important. Persistent discharge suggests chronic otitis media with perforation (Table 21.2). Cholesteatoma usually begins with tympanic membrane retraction and blockage of migrating desquamated skin from the drum and external meatus. The retraction deepens and infection leads to destruction of middle ear structures, sometimes causing damage to the facial nerve or inner ear. The infection may spread outside the temporal bone, even causing meningitis or intracranial abscess. Bleeding from a chronically discharging ear is usually due to infection but may rarely indicate malignant change. Cranial trauma followed by bleeding and leakage of cerebrospinal fluid (CSF) indicates fracture of the base of the skull.

Hearing loss

Deafness may be gradual or sudden, bilateral or unilateral. There may be an obvious precipitating cause, such as trauma or noise exposure. There are two characteristics of hearing loss: to use the analogy of a radio, a decrease in volume or a change in the tuning corresponding to impaired speech discrimination so that words are not clear even with a hearing aid. Hearing loss may be conductive, sensorineural or mixed, with both conductive and sensorineural components (Box 21.2). Conductive deafness is due

Table 21.1 Characteristics of otorrhoea in relation to site and aetiology

Diagnosis	Purulent	Mucopurulent	Mucoid	Serous	Watery
Acute otitis externa (OE)	✓✓	✓		✓	
Chronic OE	✓✓	✓		✓✓	
Acute suppurative otitis media (SOM)	✓	✓✓	✓		
Chronic SOM	✓	✓✓	✓✓		
Cerebrospinal fluid leak				✓	✓✓

Table 21.2 Classification of chronic otitis media (COM)

COM classification (synonym)	Otoscopic abnormalities
Healed COM (healed perforation with or without tympanosclerosis)	Thinning and/or local or generalized opacification of the pars tensa without perforation or retraction
Inactive mucosal COM (dry perforation)	Permanent perforation of the pars tensa but the middle ear mucosa is not inflamed
Active mucosal COM (discharging perforation)	Permanent defect of the pars tensa with an inflamed middle ear mucosa that produces mucopus which may discharge
Inactive squamous epithelial COM (retraction)	Retraction of the pars flaccida or pars tensa (usually posterosuperior) which has the potential to become active with retained debris
Active squamous epithelial (cholesteatoma)	Retraction of the pars flaccida or tensa that has retained squamous epithelial debris and is associated with inflammation and the production of pus, often from the adjacent mucosa

Box 21.2 Causes of deafness

Conductive

- Occluding wax in the external meatus
- Middle ear effusion
- Acute suppurative otitis media
- Chronic otitis media: perforation, ossicular erosion, cholesteatoma
- Otosclerosis
- Trauma to the drum or ossicular chain
- Otitis externa
- Congenital atresia of the external meatus or congenital ossicular fixation
- Carcinoma of the middle ear

Sensorineural

- Age-associated hearing loss: presbycusis
- Noise-induced hearing loss
- Genetic: syndromal or non-syndromal
- Ménière's disease
- Infective: meningitis, measles, mumps, syphilis
- Sudden sensorineural hearing loss (idiopathic)
- Perinatal: hypoxia, jaundice
- Prenatal: rubella
- Trauma: head injury, surgery
- Ototoxicity: aminoglycosides, diuretics, cytotoxics
- Neoplastic: vestibular schwannoma, other cerebellopontine angle lesions

to disease in the external ear canal, tympanic membrane or middle ear. Characteristically, the patient retains normal speech discrimination. Sensory deafness implies pathology in the cochlea, and neural deafness implies pathology in the cochlear nerve or the central connections of hearing, but in practice this distinction is difficult to make and rarely useful, and the term sensorineural deafness is used instead. Sensorineural deafness causes impairment of speech discrimination with recruitment; the latter is an abnormal perception of the increase of intensity of sound with increasing signal volume that results from damage to the hair cells in the cochlea. This leads to a decreased functional dynamic range, so that a small increase in sound intensity is uncomfortable. The patient may also notice an apparent difference in the pitch or frequency of a tone between the two ears (diplacusis). Most hearing loss is gradually progressive and related to ageing. Deafness is often secondary to occupational or social noise exposure and is often inherited. Many drugs are ototoxic, and there are associations between hereditary hearing loss and neurological and renal disorders. Occasionally, sensorineural hearing loss occurs suddenly. A cause is only rarely identifiable.

Tinnitus

Tinnitus is a ringing, rushing or hissing sound in the absence of an appropriate auditory stimulus. It can be caused by almost any pathology in the auditory pathways. It is strongly associated with hearing loss, although it occasionally occurs with normal hearing. It is common, affecting up to 18% of the population of industrialized countries. In a small proportion

(0.5%), daily life is affected. Correction of coexisting depressive illness may be of value. Management of tinnitus includes the use of hearing aids or masking devices. It usually improves with time, but in most cases there is no specific treatment.

Vertigo

Vertigo is an illusion of movement such that the patient either feels the world moving or has a sensation of moving in the world. Patients frequently have difficulty describing the symptom. Higher centre dysfunction, as in anxiety states or drug effects, may also cause dizziness. There are therefore many causes for symptomatic 'dizziness' (Box 21.3). A feeling of the room spinning associated with nausea or vomiting suggests an acute labyrinthine cause, especially if there are changes in hearing or tinnitus. Fortunately, most acute vestibular events are self-limiting, because even if one vestibular system is abnormal, the central connections can 'reset' the system over a period of a few days. The elderly are less able to compensate. In all age groups, vertigo may cause residual vague imbalance, particularly in association with movement or after alcohol ingestion. It is important to test for positional changes, as the commonest cause of vestibular vertigo is benign paroxysmal positional vertigo (BPPV), secondary to loose debris floating in the posterior semicircular canal.

Box 21.3 Causes of vertigo

Of sudden onset

- Acute viral labyrinthitis
- Vestibular neuritis

With focal features

- Brainstem ischaemia (transient ischaemic attack)
- Multiple sclerosis
- Migraine
- Temporal lobe epilepsy

With deafness and tinnitus

- Ménière's disease
- Vestibular schwannoma

With positional change

- Benign paroxysmal positional vertigo (BPPV)
- Cervical vertigo

After trauma

- BPPV
- Perilymph fistula

With motion

- Motion sickness

Drug induced

- Vestibulotoxic drugs, e.g. gentamicin, salicylate, quinine, antihypertensives

With aural discharge

- Middle ear disease

With systemic disorders

- Postural hypotension
- Syncope
- Cardiac dysrhythmia
- Carotid sinus hypersensitivity
- Anxiety and panic attacks
- Hyperventilation syndrome

Clinical examination of the ear and hearing

Pinna and postauricular area

First, inspect the pinna and the surrounding skin. Congenital abnormalities may be associated with accessory skin tags, abnormal cartilaginous fragments in the skin surrounding the ear or small pits and sinuses. Look also for any lymphadenopathy (associated with otis externa or scalp cellulitis) and for surgical scars. A hot, tender postaural swelling, pushing the pinna forward, suggests mastoid infection (Fig. 21.7). Incomplete development of the ear

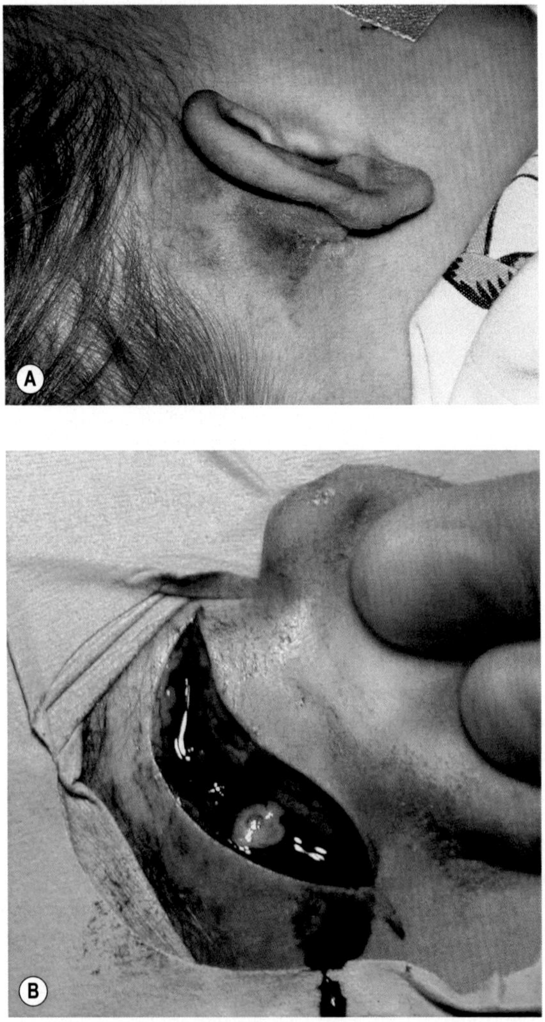

Figure 21.7 Acute mastoiditis **(A)** before and **(B)** after incision.

(microtia) occurs with narrowing (atresia) of the external meatus, but the auricle can also be displaced from its normal position (melotia) or pathologically enlarged (macrotia). These abnormalities may be associated with cysts or infection in a preauricular sinus.

External ear canal

Inspect the external auditory canal using a hand-held otoscope (Fig. 21.8). To bring the cartilaginous meatus into line with the bony canal, retract the pinna backwards and upwards. Always use the largest speculum that will comfortably fit the ear canal. Hold the otoscope like a pen between thumb and index finger, with the ulnar border of your hand resting gently against the side of the patient's head. In this way, any movement of the patient's head during the examination causes synchronous movement of the speculum, limiting any risk of accidental injury to the ear canal. With a young child, sit him on his parent's lap with the head and shoulder held (Fig. 21.9).

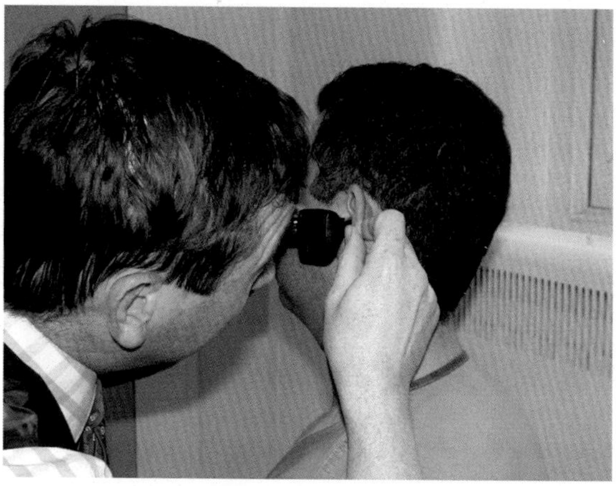

Figure 21.8 Examining the ear in an adult.

Wax may be removed with a Jobson Horne probe or wax hook or by syringing with water. Never syringe if there is a history of previous perforation or discharge. It is important to use water at 37°C lest vertigo be induced by caloric stimulation of the labyrinth. Keratin debris, pus or mucopus in the meatus can be removed and can be sent for microbiology. Foreign bodies in the ear canal are sometimes found in children; they may be difficult to remove without a general anaesthetic.

The tympanic membrane

The hand-held otoscope is satisfactory for most examinations, but the outpatient microscope offers the best view. Be familiar with the variability in appearance of the normal drum. The most common abnormality is tympanosclerosis (Fig. 21.10), which consists of white chalky patches in the drum caused by hyaline degeneration of the fibrous layer due to previous infection. Prolonged negative middle ear pressure may cause the drum to become thinned and atelectatic (Fig. 21.11), either diffusely or with a retraction pocket. Eustachian tube dysfunction and/or acute otitis media may cause a middle ear effusion (Fig. 21.12). Fluid behind the drum is often obvious, but when the drum is opaque, increased vascularity or retraction are useful clues. Perforations of the pars tensa are either central or marginal (Fig. 21.13). Marginal perforations extend to the annulus and may be associated with cholesteatoma (Fig. 21.14), whereas with central perforations there is a rim of retained membrane between the defect and the annulus. Both are described by their position in relation to the handle of the malleus (anterior, posterior or inferior) and by their size (Fig. 21.15).

The fistula test is indicated if the patient is dizzy with middle ear pathology. Press on the tragus to occlude the meatus and then apply more pressure. If the labyrinth is open, this pressure change will be applied to the inner ear. The patient will be dizzy and nystagmus may be induced.

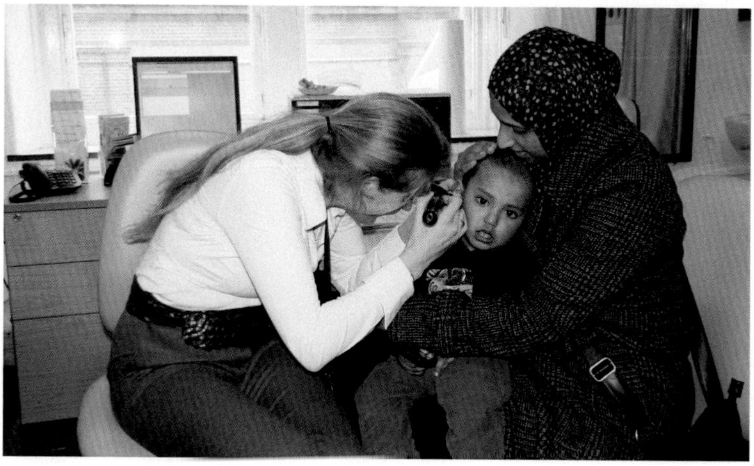

Figure 21.9 Examining the ear in a child.

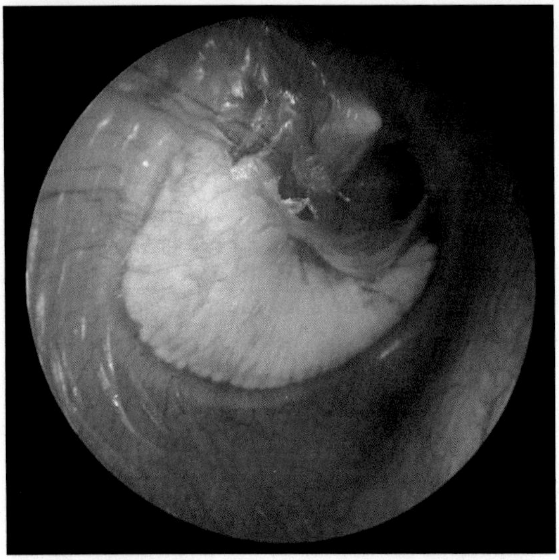

Figure 21.10 A right tympanic membrane showing marked posterior tympanosclerosis and a small anterior perforation.

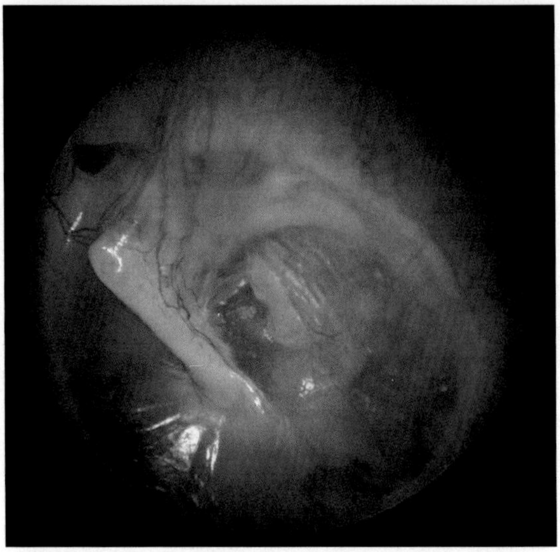

Figure 21.11 A left tympanic membrane showing atelectasis and posterior retraction on to the long process of the incus.

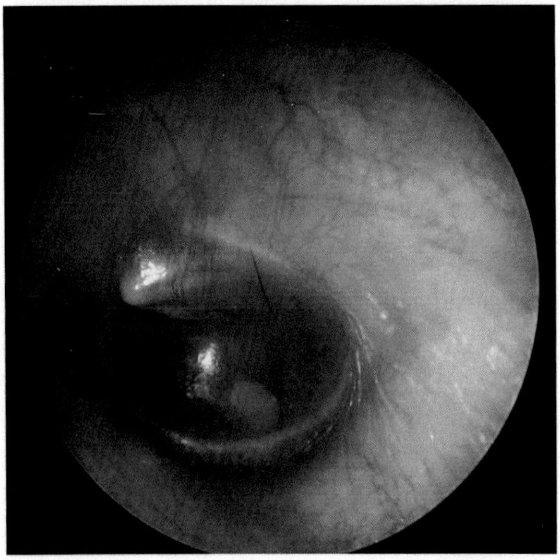

Figure 21.12 A left tympanic membrane with a middle ear effusion.

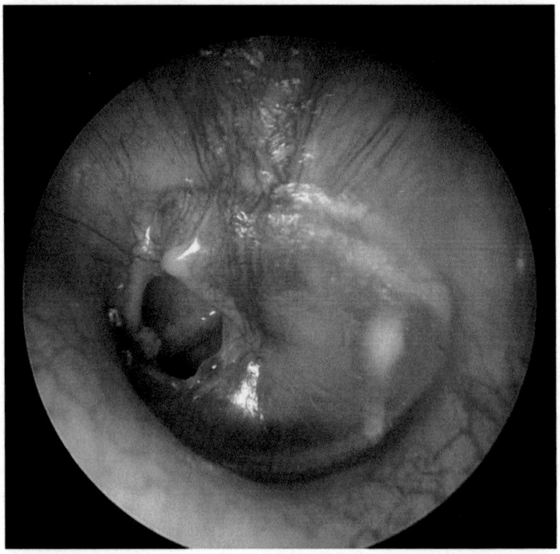

Figure 21.13 A left tympanic membrane with an anterior central perforation.

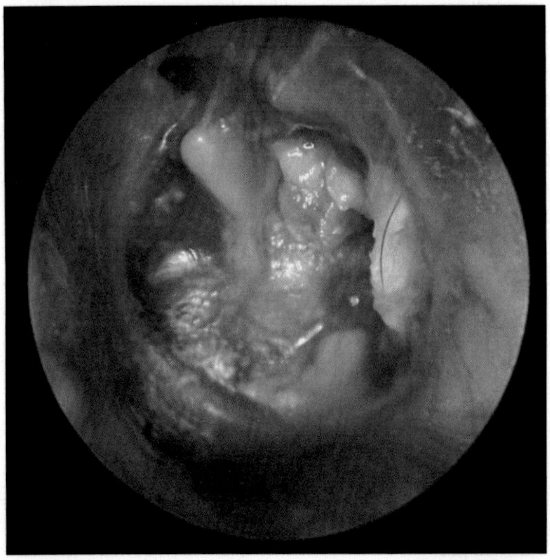

Figure 21.14 A left tympanic membrane with cholesteatoma in the posterosuperior quadrant.

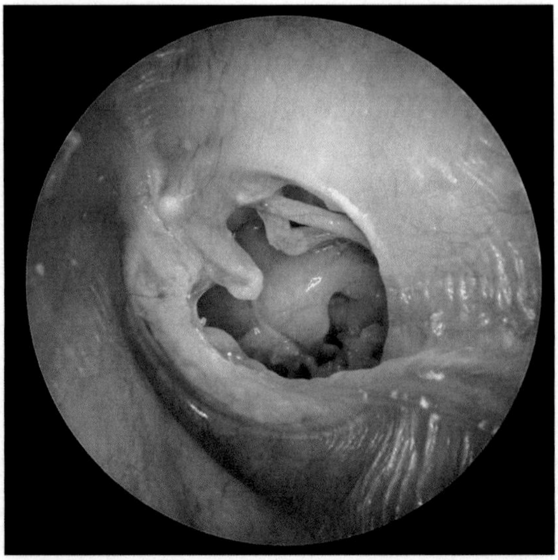

Figure 21.15 A left tympanic membrane with a subtotal perforation. The chorda tympani and long process of the incus can clearly be seen, as can the round window niche.

Table 21.3 The House-Brackmann facial nerve grading scale

Grade	Function
I	Normal
II	Normal at rest Slight weakness on close inspection Complete eye closure with minimal effort Slight asymmetry of mouth with movement Good to moderate forehead movement
III	Normal at rest Obvious asymmetry on movement Synkinesis ± hemifacial spasm Complete eye closure with effort Slight to moderate forehead movement Slight weakness of mouth with maximal effort
IV	Normal at rest Asymmetry on movement is disfiguring Incomplete eye closure No perceptible forehead movement Asymmetrical mouth motion with maximal effort
V	Asymmetric at rest Barely noticeable movement No forehead movement Incomplete eye closure Slight mouth movement with effort
VI	No facial function perceptible

The facial nerve

Test the facial movements. Unilateral weakness is much easier to identify than bilateral weakness. A peripheral facial palsy can be graded using the House-Brackmann scale (Table 21.3). Function of the greater superficial petrosal nerve can be tested with Schirmer's test: absorbent paper strips are applied to the inferior margin of the eye to detect tear formation (Ch. 20). Chorda tympani function can be tested by the sense of taste and by electrogustometry.

Clinical assessment of hearing

Conversational hearing will indicate any possible deafness. The television may be too loud or varying amounts of background noise make conversation unexpectedly difficult. Establish which is the patient's better-hearing ear. Test using words or numbers. Stand to the side of the ear to be tested and mask the non-test ear by gently rubbing the tragus. The test starts with a whispered voice at 60 cm (approximate intensity 15 dB) and proceeds with a whispered voice at 15 cm (35 dB). If there is no response, try a conversational voice at 60 cm (50 dB); this is then repeated, if necessary, at 15 cm (55-60 dB) from the test ear. With experience, a surprisingly accurate assessment can be made. It is valuable in correlating the history and results of more formal audiometry.

The Rinne test (Fig. 21.16) compares hearing by air and bone conduction using a 512- or 256-Hz tuning fork. Strike the tuning fork and hold it near the external ear canal with the prongs vibrating towards the meatus (air conduction) and then against the mastoid process (bone conduction). Ask the patient which sound was louder. In subjects with normal hearing and those with sensorineural loss, air conduction is better than bone conduction (Rinne positive.) In conductive deafness, bone conduction is louder (Rinne negative), although patients with a small conductive loss (up to 30 dB) may remain Rinne positive; it is only when the difference between air and bone conduction exceeds 40 dB that the Rinne test is consistently negative. Moreover, patients with a profound unilateral sensorineural hearing loss will report a Rinne-negative response if the contralateral ear has normal or reasonable hearing. This is because although the vibrating tuning fork held adjacent to the test ear will only be heard in that ear, the same tuning fork placed on the mastoid process will also be heard in the non-test ear. For these reasons, masking (by rubbing) the non-test ear should always validate a negative response. If there is doubt, a Barany box should be used to mask the contralateral ear.

In the Weber test, the base of the vibrating tuning fork is placed firmly on the vertex or forehead in the midline. With eyes shut, ask the patient whether the sound is heard in the midline or whether it is lateralized. With normal response or with hearing symmetrically reduced, the sound is heard in the midline. However, when one ear is normal, the noise will be louder on the side opposite to an ear with pure sensorineural loss and on the same side as an ear with purely conductive hearing loss. The Weber test is simple and quick, but there is a high test-retest variability. Because all clinical tests of hearing have limited reliability, accurate formal audiometry in the ENT clinic is essential.

Clinical assessment of balance

The unsteady patient requires a full neuro-otological examination. It is also necessary to examine the cardiovascular system (see Ch. 13). The aim is to localize the site of any potential lesion and possibly confirm a diagnosis, although sometimes all that is possible is to differentiate between central (brainstem) and peripheral (labyrinthine) lesions.

- Examine the cranial nerves (see Ch. 16), particularly testing the eyes and for nystagmus.
- Nystagmus (see Ch. 20). The characteristic saw-toothed nystagmus of vestibular disease has a slow (labyrinthine) and a fast (central) component and is enhanced by movement of the eyes in the direction of the fast phase. Eye movements can also be assessed using Frenzel's glasses (Fig. 21.17). These are illuminated and have 20-dioptre lenses that abolish visual fixation for the patient, thereby possibly unmasking nystagmus.

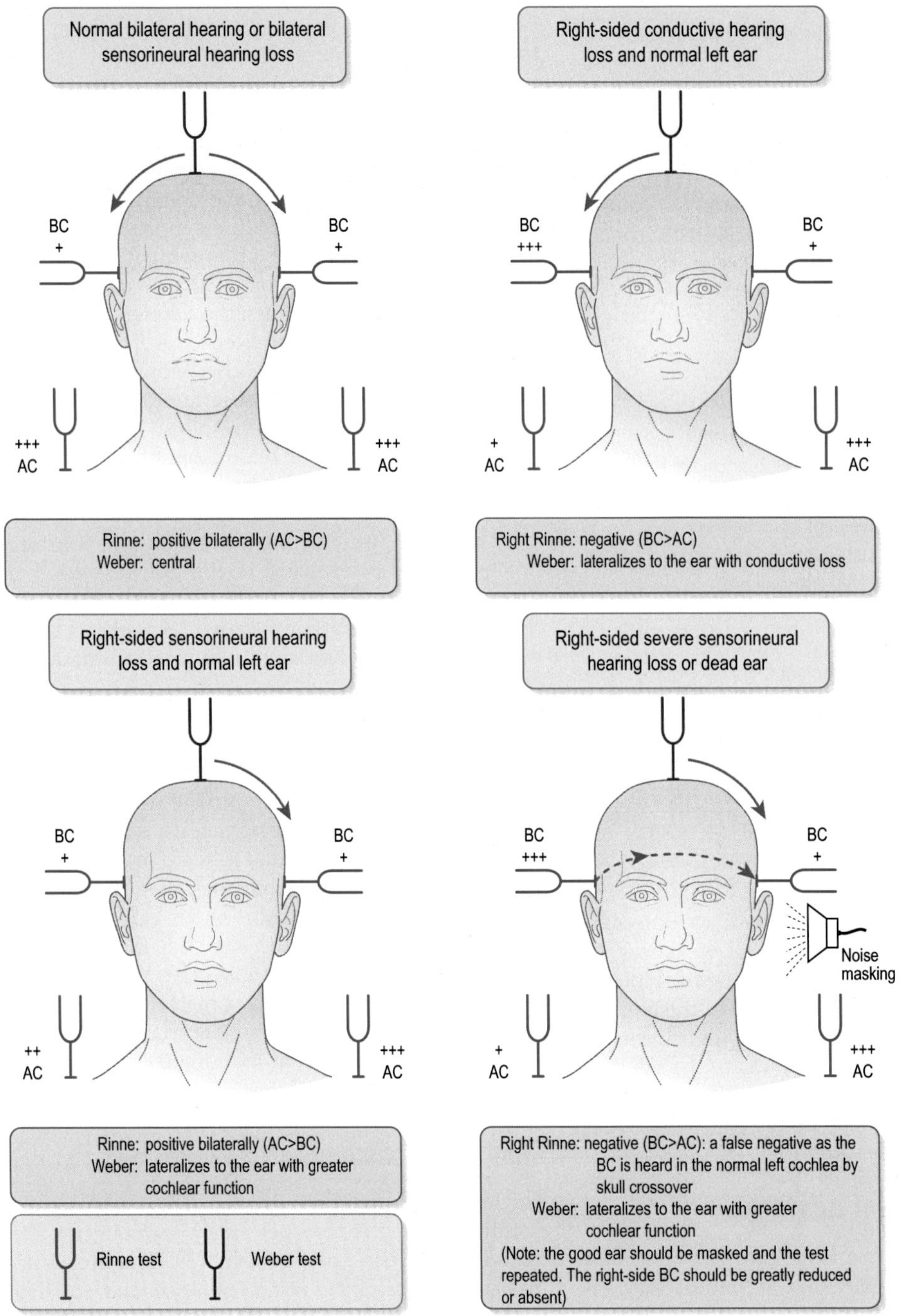

Figure 21.16 Interpretation of tuning fork tests.

- Pursuit (slow) movements, which depend on the fovea and the occipital cortex of the brain, are seen when the patient tracks an object moved slowly horizontally and vertically across the visual field about 35 cm away.
- Saccadic movements are driven by the frontal lobes and the pontine gaze centres are seen when the patient alternates the gaze rapidly between two objects held approximately 30° apart.
- Romberg's test. The patient stands with the feet together, initially with the eyes open and then closed. Patients with disorders of the spinal posterior columns (impaired position sense) will sway or fall with closed eyes but will stand normally if eyes are open. Patients with uncompensated unilateral labyrinthine dysfunction are unstable, tending to fall to the side of the lesion. Patients with central

dysfunction sway to both sides, whether the eyes are open or shut.

- Unterberger's stepping test has the patient standing with arms outstretched and eyes closed and taking steps on the spot. Unilateral vestibular hypofunction leads to rotation to the affected side.
- Gait assessment. The patient walks heel to toe with eyes first open and then closed. The patient with a cerebellar lesion is unable to do either. The patient with a peripheral vestibular lesion will struggle, particularly with the eyes closed.
- The Dix-Hallpike test assesses the effect of positional change. The patient sits on an examination couch. First test neck movements, to make sure they are free and painless. The head is then turned 45° to the side of test. The patient is laid back rapidly with his head extended over the end of the bed (Fig. 21.18). The classic response in BPPV involves a variable latent period when nothing happens. There is then a torsional nystagmus beating to the lower ear, with a variable feeling of vertigo. This lasts perhaps 5-30 seconds. With repetition, the response becomes less or absent. The condition is caused by debris in the posterior semicircular canal. It is frequently self-limiting, but if it persists it may be cured by the Epley particle repositioning manoeuvre. Other positive results are possible. Persistent immediate positional nystagmus without vertigo implies central pathology.

Special investigations of hearing

Pure tone audiometry

A single-frequency tone is presented at standardized levels into each ear in turn. This is done in noise-free surroundings, usually in a soundproofed booth (Fig. 21.19). Air conduction is tested first through

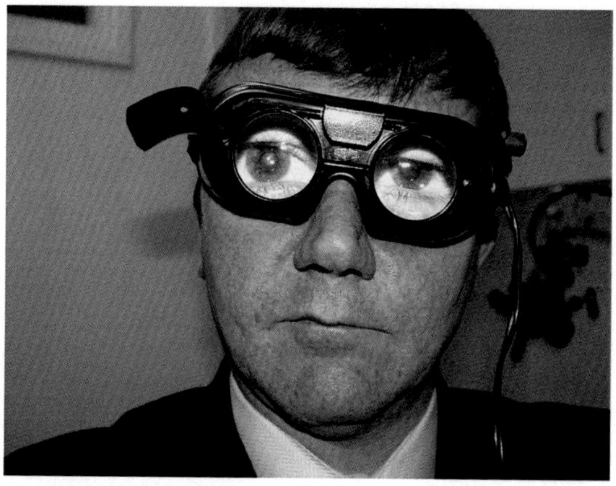

Figure 21.17 Frenzel's glasses.

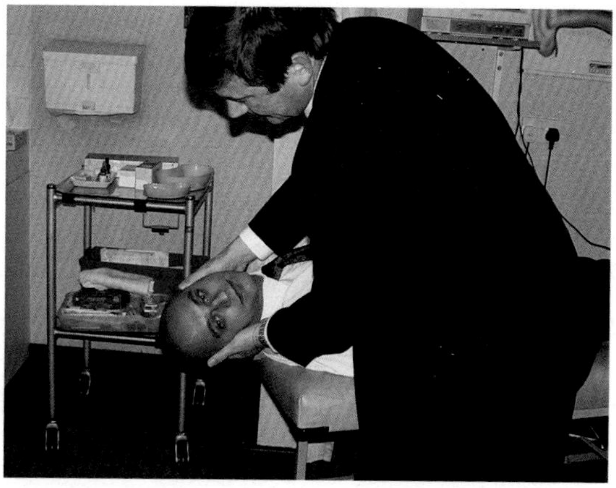

Figure 21.18 The Dix-Hallpike test position.

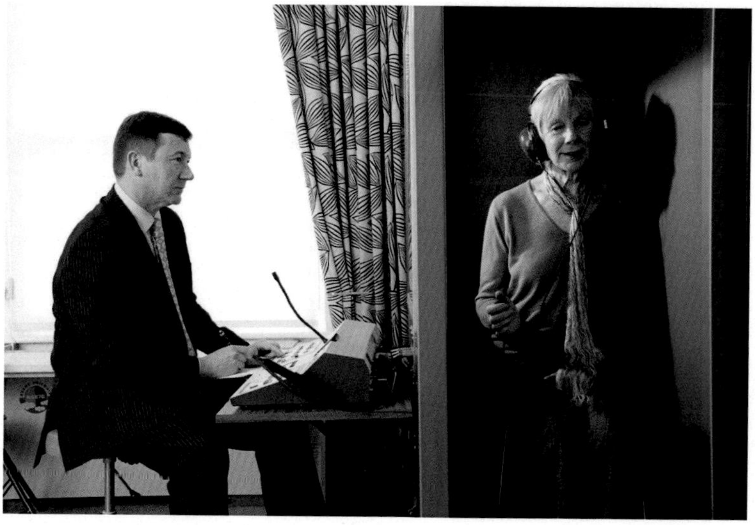

Figure 21.19 Pure tone audiometry.

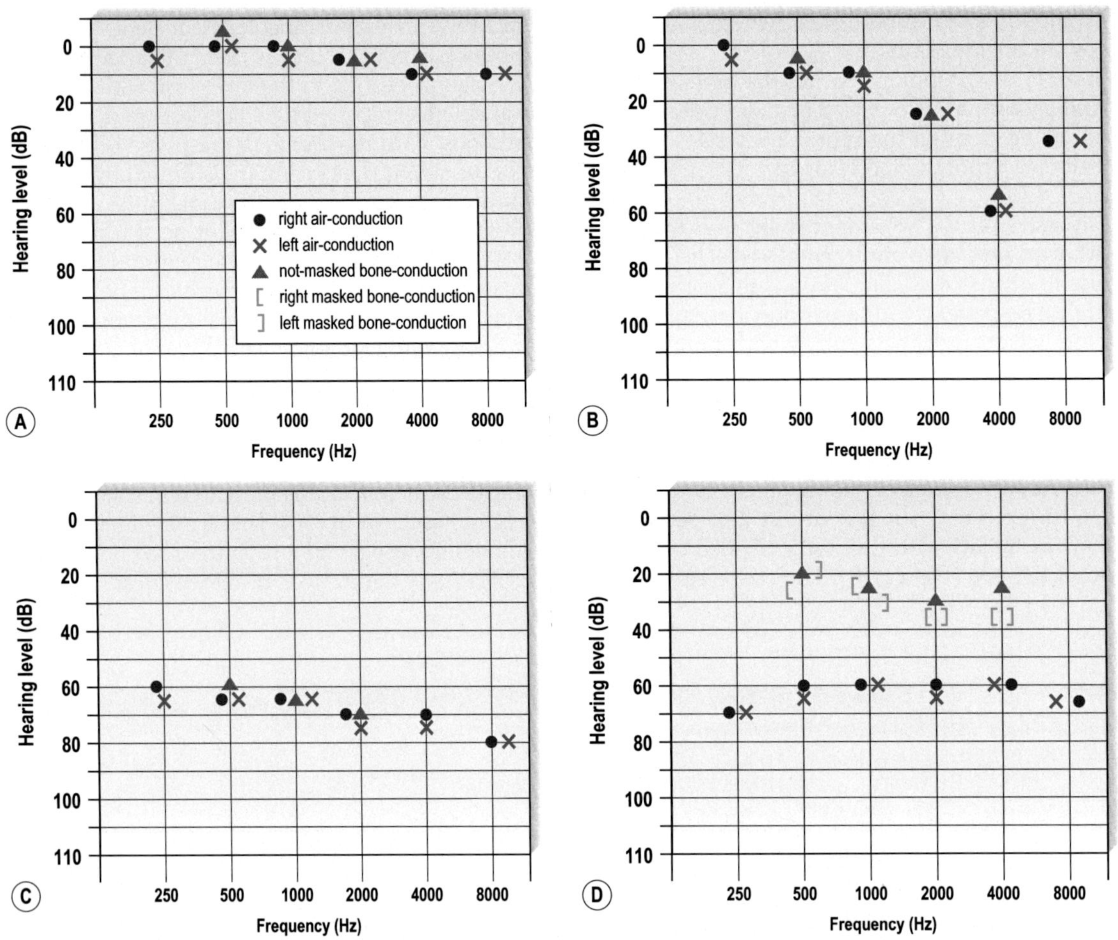

Figure 21.20 Pure tone audiograms: **(A)** normal; **(B)** noise-induced hearing loss; **(C)** presbycusis; **(D)** bilateral conductive hearing loss.

headphones. A level well above threshold, as predicted by free field testing, is chosen and the patient responds when he hears the sound. The intensity is then reduced in 10-dB steps until the patient cannot hear it. It is then increased in 5-dB steps to establish the quietest sound that can be heard – the threshold. The better ear is tested first at 1, 2, 4 and 8 kHz, then at 250 and 500 Hz (Fig. 21.20). Bone conduction tests are performed using a vibrating headset applied to the mastoid. In conductive loss, the difference is called the air-bone gap. This may be correctible by surgery to the middle ear and tympanic membrane.

Speech audiometry

A pure tone audiogram does not test discrimination. A speech audiogram measures the patient's ability to recognize words from phonetically balanced lists delivered at different sound levels to the test ear from a tape recording. The percentage of words correctly repeated by the subject is noted at each level. With normal hearing, all words are heard (100% optimal speech discrimination – ODS) at a sound intensity of 40 dB. Patients with sensorineural deafness are often unable to achieve 100% ODS and, in particular, patients with neural/retrocochlear loss have poor ODS (Fig. 21.21).

Tympanometry

An earpiece is inserted into the external meatus through which pass three channels. The first delivers a continuous tone into the ear canal during the test (probe tone); the second has a microphone to record the sound intensity level within the ear canal; the third channel connects to a manometer so that the pressure within the canal can be altered (Fig. 21.22).

The external meatus is a rigid tube with a compliant end (the drum). Normally the middle ear and ear canal pressures are equal, and most of the sound introduced into the meatus is transmitted into the ear; only a minimum of sound energy is reflected back and measured by the microphone. Changing the pressure difference between the external and the middle ear causes the tympanic membrane to become less compliant. This increases the sound energy reflected back to the probe. These changes are plotted graphically on a tympanogram (Fig. 21.23). The test

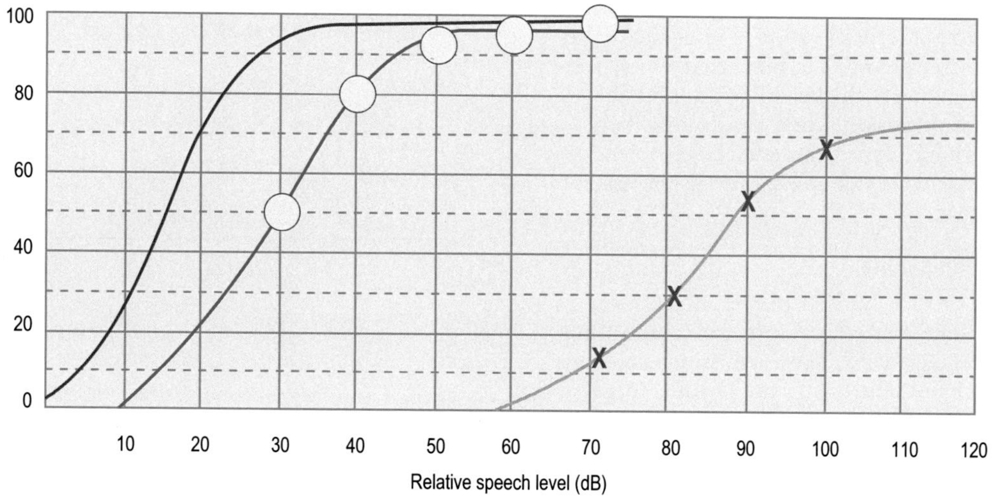

SPEECH MATERIAL

FREE FIELD / EARPHONE

SCORING: PHONEME / WORD / SENTENCE

SPEECH LEVEL	RIGHT %	LEFT %
30	50	
40	80	
50	93	
60	97	
70	100	17
80		30
90		53
100		67

COMMENTS:

100% at 70 dB in the right ear
67% at 100 dB in the left ear
(maximum level of the audiometer reached with appropriate masking)

Figure 21.21 Speech audiogram.

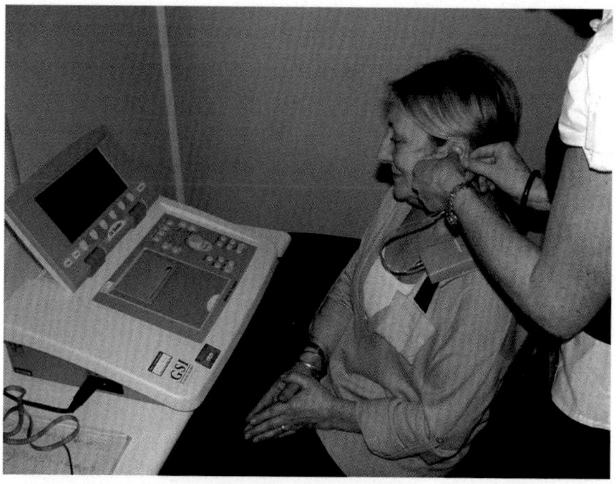

Figure 21.22 A tympanogram being performed.

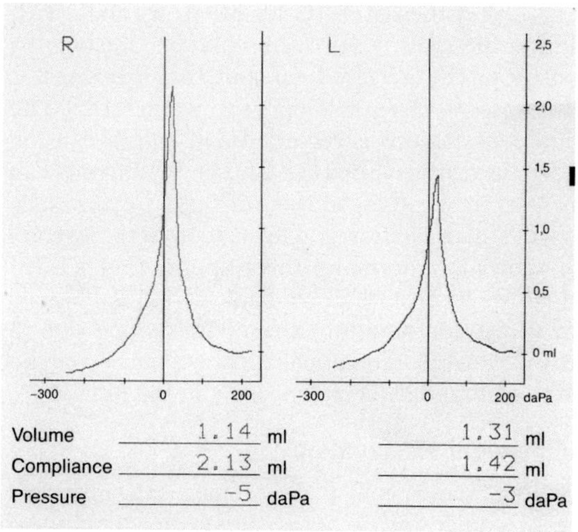

Figure 21.23 A tympanogram.

also measures the volume of the canal: a large volume indicates a tympanic perforation. Impedance (the reciprocal of compliance) is increased when the tympanic membrane is thickened or the middle ear has fluid and is decreased when the drum is hypermobile or atrophic. Tympanometry is an objective test. It has particular value in children in the assessment of glue ear.

Otoacoustic emissions

When a click or tone-burst is played into the ear, a very small noise is emitted in return, probably arising from the outer hair cells. These emissions are particularly prominent in neonates but become increasingly difficult to elicit with age. Testing does not require cooperation. When there is hearing loss there is no response. The technique is valuable in the screening of neonates and forms the backbone of the Universal Neonatal Hearing Screen programme.

Evoked-response audiometry

A click presented to the ear causes a nerve impulse to be sent to the auditory cortex via the brainstem. If a large number (>2000) of responses are averaged, then evoked responses in brainstem and cortex can be seen and amplitudes and latencies measured. The auditory brainstem response is not affected by sedation and the main indication is in the establishment of hearing thresholds, especially in infants. Cortical-evoked responses are less widely used. They require an awake and alert patient.

Special tests of balance

Caloric testing is the most commonly performed routine test of the vestibular end-organ. The patient lies on a couch with the head up 30° in order to bring the lateral semicircular canals into the vertical plane. With the patient fixing on a point in central gaze, each external ear canal is irrigated with water at 30°C, and then at 44°C for 30-40 seconds, with suitable intervals. Cold water induces nystagmus away from the irrigated ear and the opposite for warm water (COWS: cold opposite, warm same). The induced nystagmus is recorded and analysed using electronystagmography (Fig. 21.24). Nystagmus can be enhanced by the abolition of optic fixation (see Frenzel's glasses above). The videonystagmoscope also allows monitoring of this response (Fig. 21.25) and allows recordings to be made. Peripheral lesions tend to cause a diminished response on one side (a canal paresis). A directional preponderance may be due to central disorders, especially in the brainstem.

Radiological examination

Computed tomography (CT) scanning is the investigation of choice but is not a substitute for clinical assessment of chronic ear disease. It is not specifically diagnostic of cholesteatoma (Fig. 21.26) but is useful in cranial trauma (Fig. 21.27) and in the evaluation

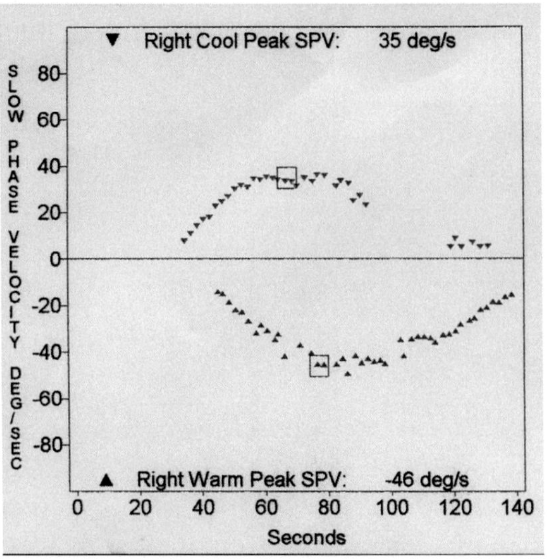

Figure 21.24 A computerized caloric test result.

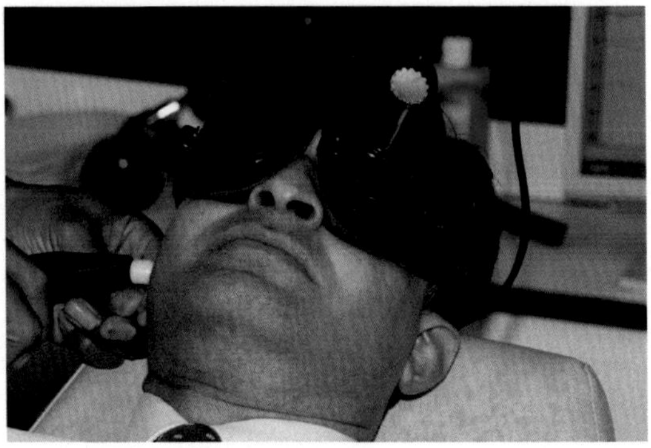

Figure 21.25 Videonystagmography.

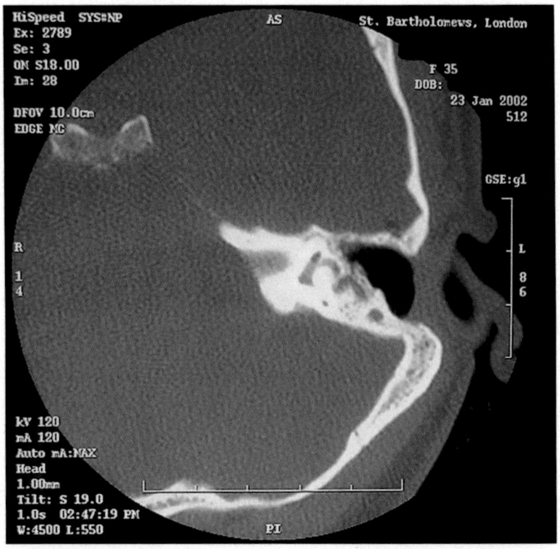

Figure 21.26 CT scan of left ear showing a fistula of the lateral semicircular canal in a patient who had previously undergone a mastoidectomy.

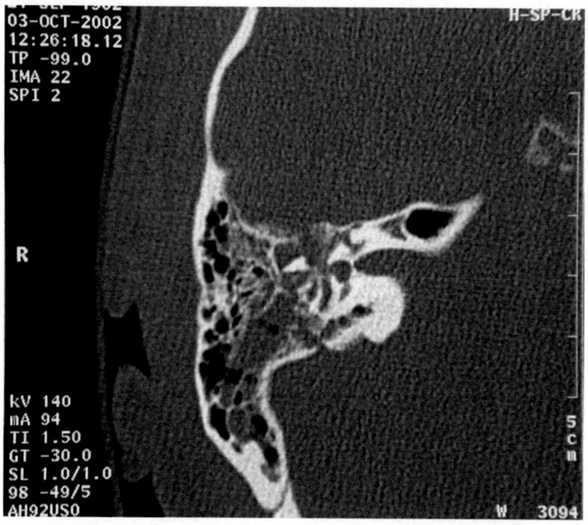

Figure 21.27 CT scan of a right ear showing a fracture across the middle ear. The incus is seen and is lying in a displaced position.

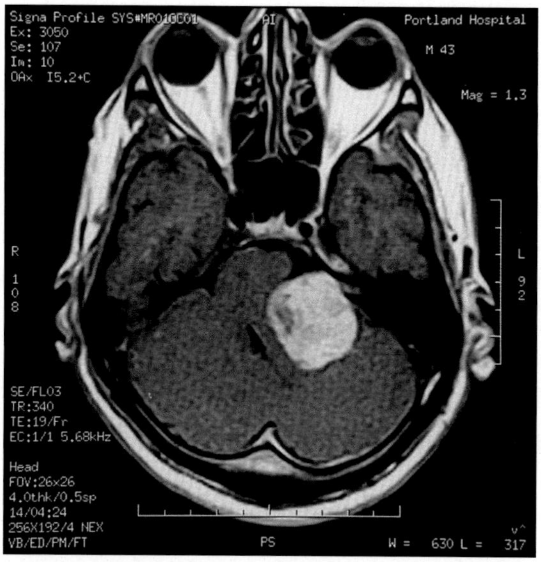

Figure 21.28 MRI scan demonstrating a large left vestibular schwannoma with brainstem compression.

Box 21.4 Functions of the nose

- Respiration
- Filtration
- Heating
- Humidification
- Smell

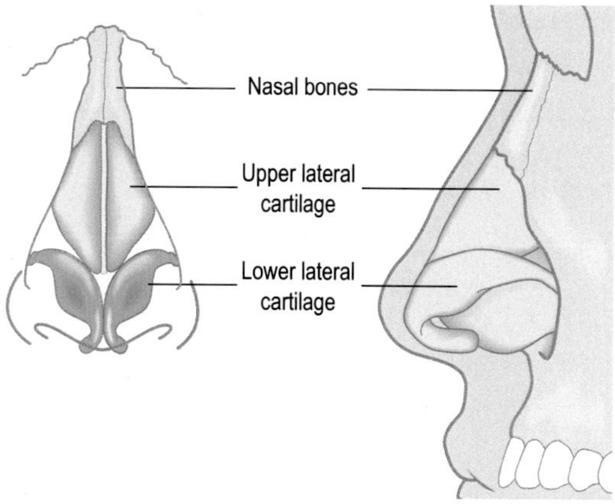

Figure 21.29 The external nose.

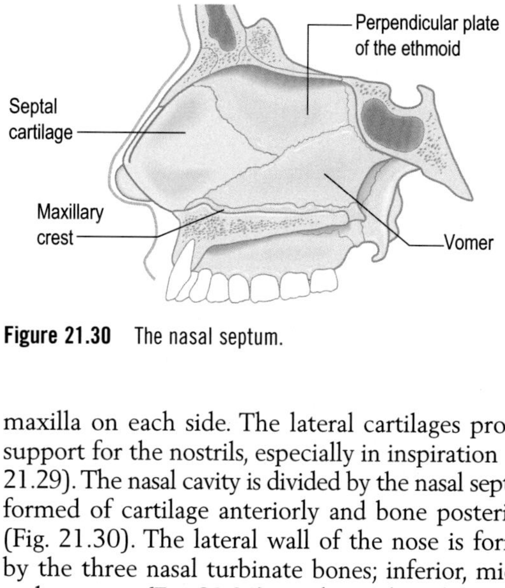

Figure 21.30 The nasal septum.

of temporal bone neoplasia. Magnetic resonance imaging (MRI) is more useful in identifying soft tissue abnormalities in the cerebellopontine angle, especially vestibular schwannoma (Fig. 21.28). These present with asymmetric sensorineural hearing loss. MRI also helps assess tumour spread outside the temporal bone. MR angiography helps in assessment of pulsatile tinnitus and vascular lesions. Formal angiography is useful for embolization of vascular tumours.

The nose and paranasal sinuses

Anatomy

The nose (Box 21.4) is formed by the two nasal bones which articulate with the nasal process of the maxilla on each side. The lateral cartilages provide support for the nostrils, especially in inspiration (Fig. 21.29). The nasal cavity is divided by the nasal septum, formed of cartilage anteriorly and bone posteriorly (Fig. 21.30). The lateral wall of the nose is formed by the three nasal turbinate bones; inferior, middle and superior (Fig. 21.31). Under each turbinate is a corresponding meatus. The nose constantly produces mucus – a pint a day – which is constantly propelled backwards by the cilia to the posterior choanae, whence it is swallowed, usually unnoticed.

The paranasal sinuses are air-filled spaces in the bones of the facial skeleton (Figs 21.31 and 21.32). They comprise the paired maxillary, frontal and ethmoid sinuses and the unpaired but bisected sphenoid sinus, and form the structure of the adult

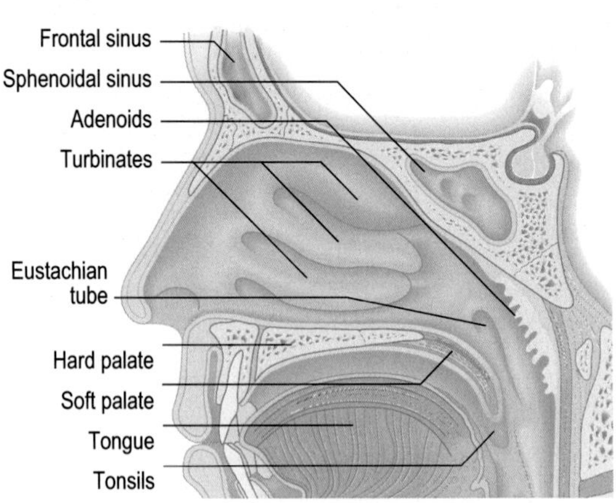

Figure 21.31 The lateral wall of the nose.

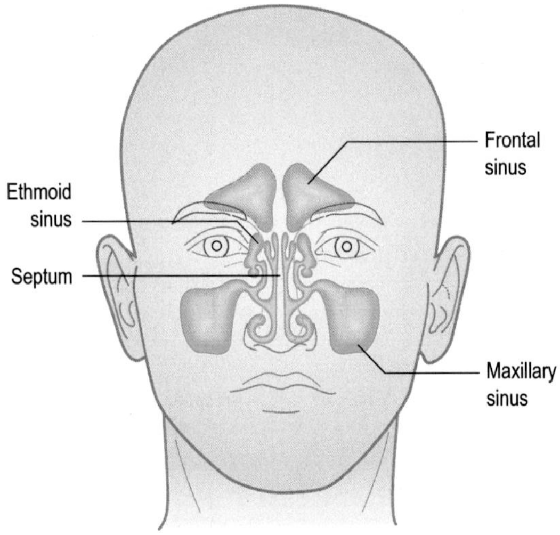

Figure 21.32 Cross-section through the sinuses (semischematic).

face. The ethmoidal cells or labyrinth comprises a number of small bony cells. The sinuses open into the nose via small drainage channels (ostia). Their mucus is swept by cilia through the ostia to be mixed with mucus secreted by the nose. The middle meatus is the common pathway for drainage from the maxillary, the anterior ethmoid and the frontal sinuses. The anterior ethmoids are important because disease in these areas will compromise maxillary and frontal sinus drainage. Blockage of the ostia due to inflammation in the nose, with retention of mucus and secondary infection, is the presumed mechanism for sinus infection (rhinosinusitis). The upper teeth are closely related to the floor of the maxillary sinus; infection here may lead to sinus problems.

The olfactory neuroepithelium of the nose is located in the roof of the nasal cavity. Neurons run through the cribriform plate to the olfactory bulb lying on the floor of the anterior cranial fossa. The postnasal space contains the adenoids, which are lymphoid tissue, part of Waldeyer's ring, which includes the palatine tonsils. These are largest in childhood and regress from the age of about 8 years onwards, although rarely they may persist into adult life. The inferior opening of the Eustachian tube is on the lateral wall of the postnasal space.

Symptoms of nasal disease

The important symptoms of nasal and sinus disease are:

- nasal blockage
- rhinorrhoea – nasal discharge
- epistaxis (nasal bleeding)
- sneezing and itching
- disturbances of smell
- facial pain.

General features

Orbital and facial pain, proptosis, diplopia, periorbital swelling and conjunctival chemosis may develop if infection or neoplasia spread outside the sinuses. Pathology in the postnasal space may lead to otological symptoms secondary to Eustachian tube involvement.

Nasal blockage

Unilateral or bilateral blockage of the nose is common. Maximum resistance to airflow occurs at the front of the nose near the inferior turbinate. In the nasal cycle (2-6 hours long), one side is congested and one side decongested at any one time. The commonest cause of nasal blockage is allergic rhinitis. A constant blockage suggests a structural abnormality (deviated nasal septum, nasal polyposis, adenoidal hypertrophy (children)).

Rhinorrhoea

Nasal discharge may be mucoid, purulent or watery. It may contain blood. A purulent discharge suggests infection, either in the nose or in the sinus. In a child, unilateral discharge may be due to a foreign body retained in the nose. Mucoid discharge is more suggestive of allergic rhinitis. Watery discharge is indicative of vasomotor rhinitis. CSF leak is a rare but important cause; the discharge is clear, watery and salty tasting. Epistaxis (a nose bleed) varies in severity from a minor intermittent problem to a life-threatening major haemorrhage that may require cautery. It tends to occur in children and the elderly. The arterial supply of the nose is from branches of the sphenopalatine artery (external carotid), and from the anterior and posterior ethmoidal arteries (internal carotid). These vessels anastomose in the anterior nasal septum, the site of most epistaxes. Epistaxis is associated with hypertension, trauma (including nose-picking), rhinitis and bleeding disorders.

Itching and sneezing

Sneezing is a protective expulsive reflex that helps clear the nasal airway of irritants. Paroxysmal sneezing, associated with rhinorrhoea, nasal obstruction and palatal and conjunctival itching, occurs with allergic rhinitis.

Disturbances of smell

Loss of smell (anosmia) or impaired sense of smell is most often due to nasal obstruction, for example with nasal polyposis or allergic rhinitis. It also follows damage to nerve fibres passing through the cribriform plate after craniofacial trauma. Rarely, viral infection may cause permanent anosmia. Cacosmia is an unpleasant smell, usually unnoticed by the patient, caused by chronic anaerobic sepsis in the nose.

Facial pain

Pain in the face is very common, but pain limited to the nose is rare. Pain centred over a sinus may indicate infection or, rarely, a malignancy. There are many causes of facial pain. Some, such as cluster headache (causing transient nasal blockage and rhinorrhoea) and trigeminal neuralgia, are functional disorders, with well-defined features (see Ch. 16). Structural disorders, such as infection or tumour involving facial structures, may also present with facial pain. Investigation should usually include imaging by CT or MRI.

Other symptoms

Always enquire about any history of allergy. Most people are aware of hay fever but house dust mite allergy is also common.

Examination of the nose and face

Inspect the nose and face from the front, side and back in a good light. Note the colour of the skin and any asymmetry of facial contours. Observe for scars and pigmentary changes. With age, the tip of the nose tends to droop. Deformities of the nasal bone and cartilage, such as saddle deformity, often follow a nasal fracture or other destructive disorders of the bony or cartilaginous septum. Palpate the nose and facial skeleton, especially the orbital margins, noting tenderness and any swelling, expansion or depression of bone. Facial swelling is unusual in maxillary sinusitis, but occurs with dental root infections and in carcinoma of the maxillary antrum. Inspect and palpate the palate and alveoli from inside the mouth using a gloved finger.

Examine the nasal vestibule and intranasal contents by gently pushing the tip of the nose upwards with a finger, preferably using reflected illumination from a head mirror. The nasal vestibule is lined with skin and contains vibrissae (thicker hairs); these become prominent in older men. Inspect the anterior nasal cavity with Thudicum's nasal speculum or an otoscope (Fig. 21.33). The nasal septum is rarely completely straight but should not be so bent that it is not possible to see the anterior end of the inferior turbinate. The majority of nasal resistance to airflow occurs in the front of the nose. Look for any area of granulation

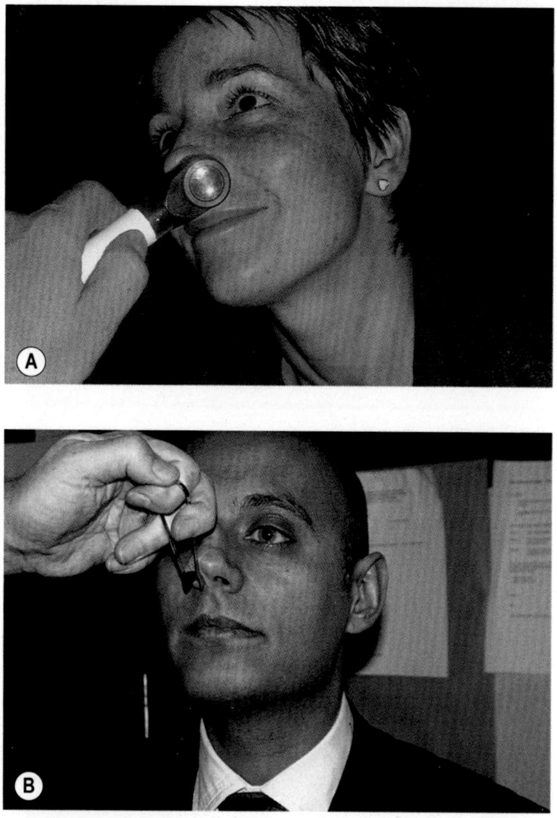

Figure 21.33 Examining the nose.

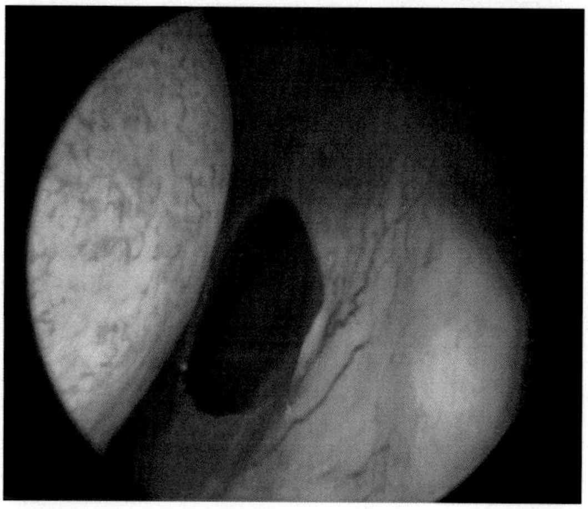

Figure 21.34 A septal perforation.

on the nasal septum and for any perforation (Fig. 21.34). Perforations may be secondary to cocaine snorting, digital trauma (nose-picking), surgical trauma, granulomatous conditions or inhalation of industrial dusts, notably nickel and chrome.

Nasal polyps are usually easily identifiable by their pale colour (Fig. 21.35) and their softness and lack of sensitivity to probing. In a child, an apparent polyp may be seen arising from the roof of the nose; this should not be probed as it may be the intranasal presentation of a meningocele. In children and adults, airflow through a patent nostril causes misting on a

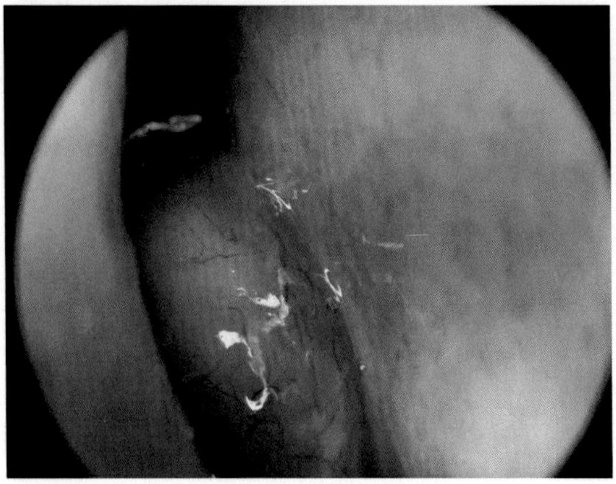

Figure 21.35 A large polyp in the right nasal cavity.

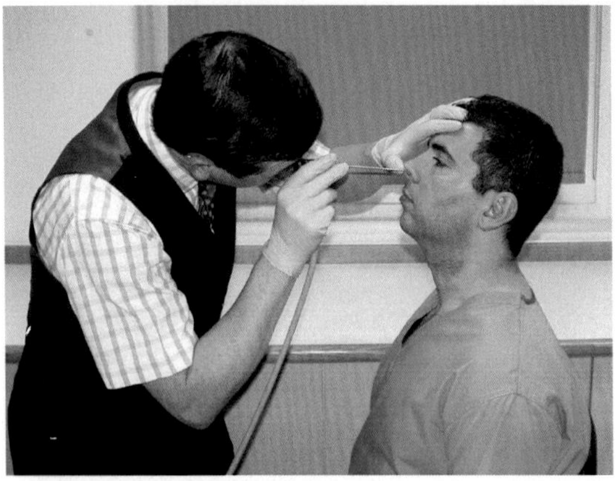

Figure 21.36 Rigid nasal endoscopy.

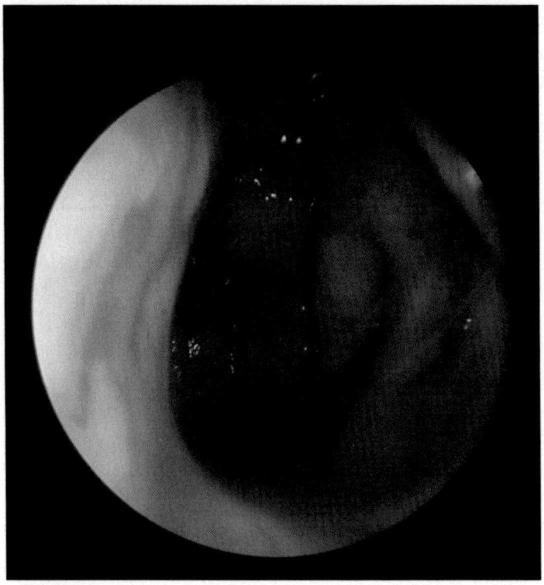

Figure 21.37 Endoscopic view of the Eustachian tube orifice and the postnasal space.

Box 21.5 Common inhalant allergens

- House dust and house dust mite
- Grass pollen
- Tree pollen
- Weed pollen
- Animal dander: cat, dog, rabbit
- Feathers
- Moulds

cold metal tongue depressor or mirror held at the nose. In a neonate, nasal patency is best estimated by observing any movement of a wisp of cotton wool held in front of each nostril after blocking each in turn with the thumb. Nasal endoscopy (Fig. 21.36), after applying a topical decongestant such as xylometazoline with topical lidocaine anaesthesia, allows inspection of the middle meatus for oedema, draining pus or polyps. The postnasal space and the opening of the Eustachian tube (Fig. 21.37) can be seen, with the fossa of Rosenmuller, the site of origin of postnasal space carcinomas, lying directly above and behind. In children and young adults, look for adenoidal swelling.

Special tests

Allergy testing

If allergic symptoms are severe, there is merit in confirming extrinsic allergy by skin-prick testing (see Ch. 19). An important component of treating allergy is allergen avoidance, and certainty of responsible allergens may encourage compliance. The common inhalant allergens (Box 21.5), together with any agents that have been suspected from the history, should be tested and compared to positive and negative controls (histamine and saline). Unfortunately, however, a negative response does not definitely exclude atopy. If clinical suspicion is strong, the radioallergosorbent test (RAST), which measures specific IgE in blood, may be considered, although it is expensive. Nasal provocation tests are time consuming, as only one allergen at a time can be tested.

Nasal patency

Objective assessment of nasal patency is difficult. Rhinomanometry, which measures nasal airflow and resistance, and acoustic rhinometry, which measures nasal volume and cross-sectional area, remain specialized research tools.

Mucociliary clearance

Mucociliary clearance is a test of impaired ciliary function used, for example, in Kartagener's syndrome of impaired ciliary motility. A strong, sweet taste such as saccharin placed on the anterior end of the inferior turbinate should be tasted in the mouth about 20 minutes later.

Radiological examination

Plain X-rays are unreliable in the management of sinus disease but may be helpful in the absence of more specialized tests. A lateral X-ray may be useful in estimating the degree of adenoidal hypertrophy in young children (Fig. 21.38). Endoscopic nasal examination and CT scanning are the investigations of choice for sinus disease (Fig. 21.39). CT is useful in the management of chronic infection, trauma and neoplasia. However, there is a radiation dosage to the eyes, and the investigation should be used only when the diagnosis is uncertain or to provide accurate anatomical information before surgery. MRI is less useful in sinus disease because of difficulties in interpretation. MRI is highly sensitive to changes in the mucosal lining of the sinuses. However, it tends to overdiagnose and interpretation requires caution. It does have value in assessing spread of sinus neoplasia.

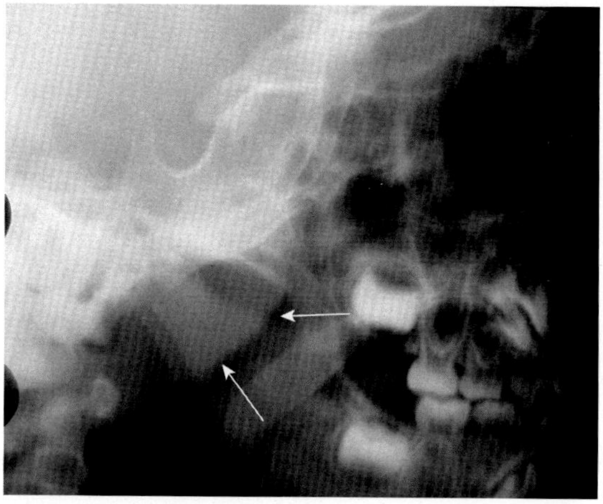

Figure 21.38 Lateral X-ray of the nasopharynx demonstrating adenoidal hypertrophy (arrow).

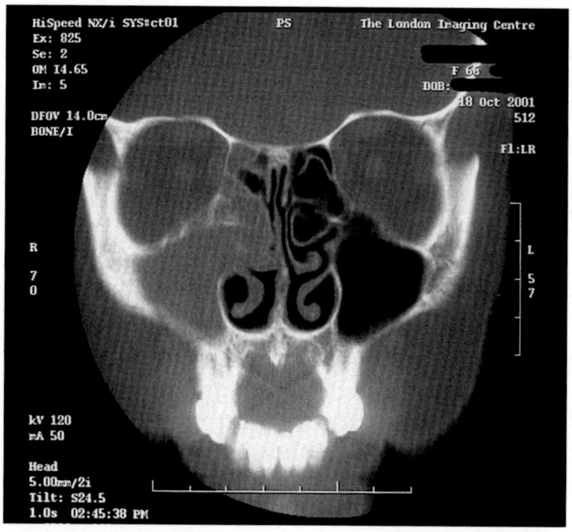

Figure 21.39 Coronal CT scan of the nose showing an opaque right maxillary antrum and anterior ethmoid cells.

The throat

Anatomy

The throat includes the oral cavity, the pharynx (oropharynx, nasopharynx and hypopharynx), the larynx and the major salivary glands. The oral cavity extends from the lips to the anterior faucial pillars. The oral cavity proper is bounded by the teeth laterally, the tongue and floor of the mouth inferiorly and the hard and soft palate superiorly. The pharynx extends from the base of the skull to the cricopharyngeal sphincter (Fig. 21.40). The oropharynx is bounded above by the soft palate and below by the upper surface of the epiglottis. Its anterior margin is defined laterally by the anterior faucial pillar, containing the palatoglossus muscle, and by the posterior third of the tongue. The posterior pharyngeal wall is its posterior boundary. The palatine tonsils are situated laterally between the anterior and posterior pillars of the fauces. The base of the tongue contains the lingual tonsils. This lymphoid tissue, together with the adenoids and the tubal tonsil (lymphoid tissue around the Eustachian tube opening), makes up Waldeyer's ring, an important line of immunological defence. The hypopharynx consists of the posterior pharyngeal wall, the piriform fossae and the postcricoid area. The piriform fossae, which comprise the lateral walls of the pharynx adjacent to the larynx, are the routes by which food is passed into the upper oesophagus. The larynx is a rigid structure consisting of cartilages, the most prominent of which are the paired thyroid cartilages, which articulate with the cricoid cartilage below. The epiglottis is attached to the inner surface of the thyroid cartilage and aids the separation of air and food passages during swallowing. The larynx consists of three compartments (Fig. 21.41): glottis, supraglottis and subglottis. The glottis is formed by the vocal folds. The glottis has poor lymphatic drainage, which may help to delay the spread of malignancy from this area. The epiglottis extends from the false cords below to the hyoid bone above. It has a rich lymphatic drainage, and therefore malignancy in this area is more frequently associated with metastatic disease. The subglottis is the narrowest part of the upper respiratory tract and extends from the glottis to the lower border of the cricoid.

The prime function of the larynx is to separate breathing and swallowing, thereby protecting the airway. Voice production is a secondary function that has arisen with evolution. Phonation occurs with movement of the vocal folds into the midline (Fig. 21.42). Changes in volume of the voice are caused by alterations in the subglottic pressure, whereas alterations in pitch are due to modification of the

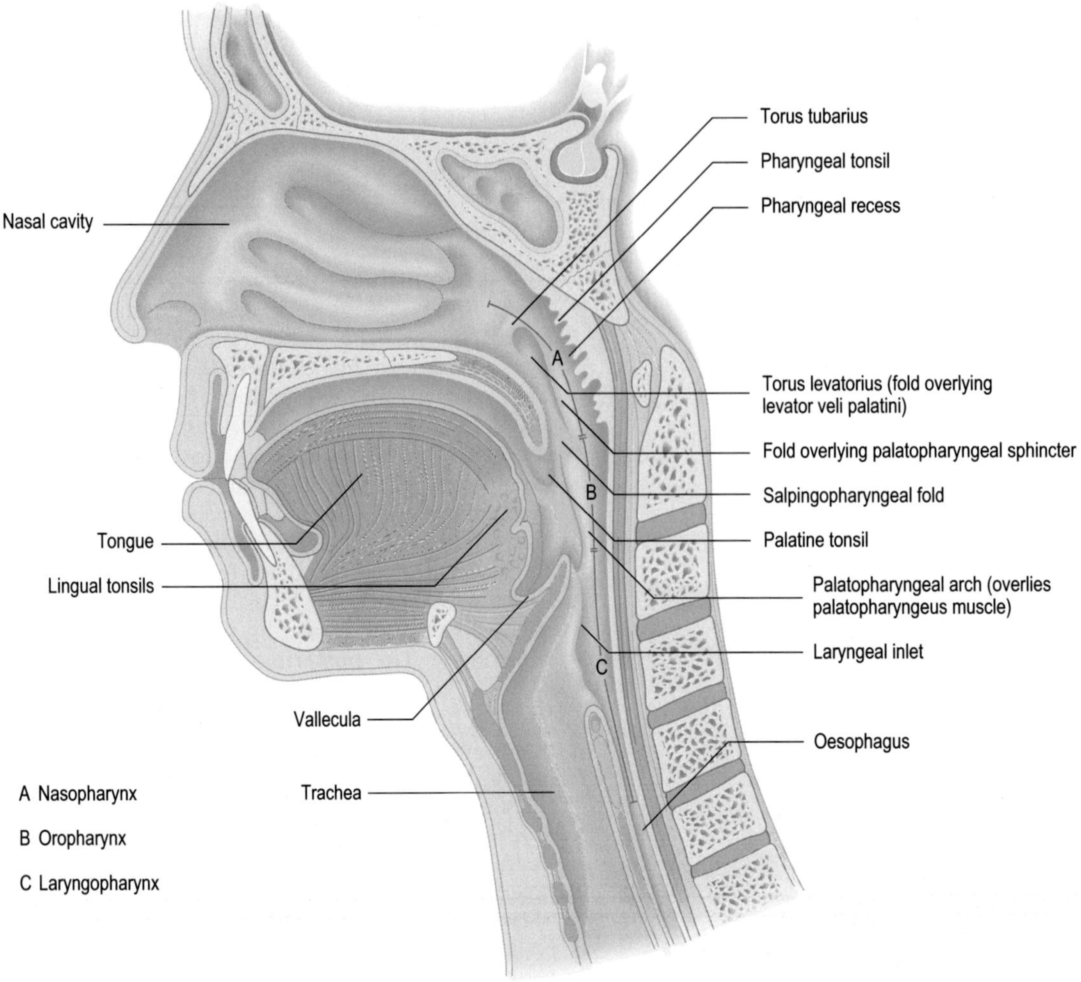

Figure 21.40 Midline sagittal section demonstrating the pharynx.

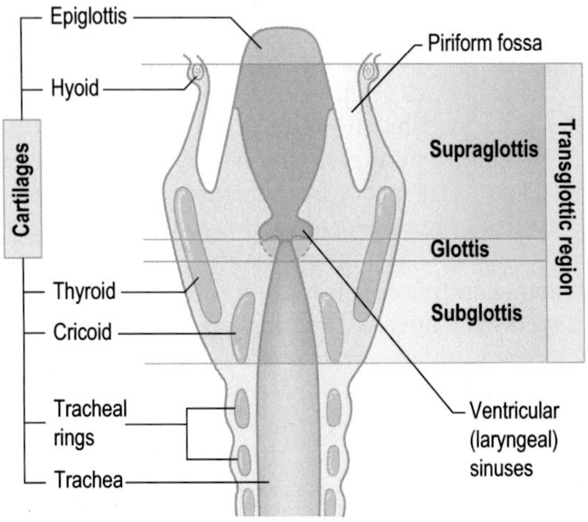

Figure 21.41 The divisions of the larynx.

length and tension of the vocal folds. The quality of this basic laryngeal sound is modulated by resonance in the pharynx, air sinuses, mouth and nose.

The pharynx is innervated from the pharyngeal plexus (cranial nerves IX, X and XI). Interruption of this nerve supply by lesions at the jugular foramen leads to swallowing problems and severe morbidity. All the muscles of the larynx except the cricothyroid are supplied by the recurrent laryngeal branch of the vagus (cranial nerve X). In the chest, this nerve loops around the arch of the aorta on the left and the subclavian artery on the right, before running up to enter the larynx. The long course of the left recurrent laryngeal nerve means it is more frequently affected by disease. The cricothyroid is supplied by the external branch of the superior laryngeal nerve (cranial nerve X).

There are three paired major salivary glands (Fig. 21.43). The parotid gland lies anterior to the ear. Its duct opens opposite the second upper molar tooth.

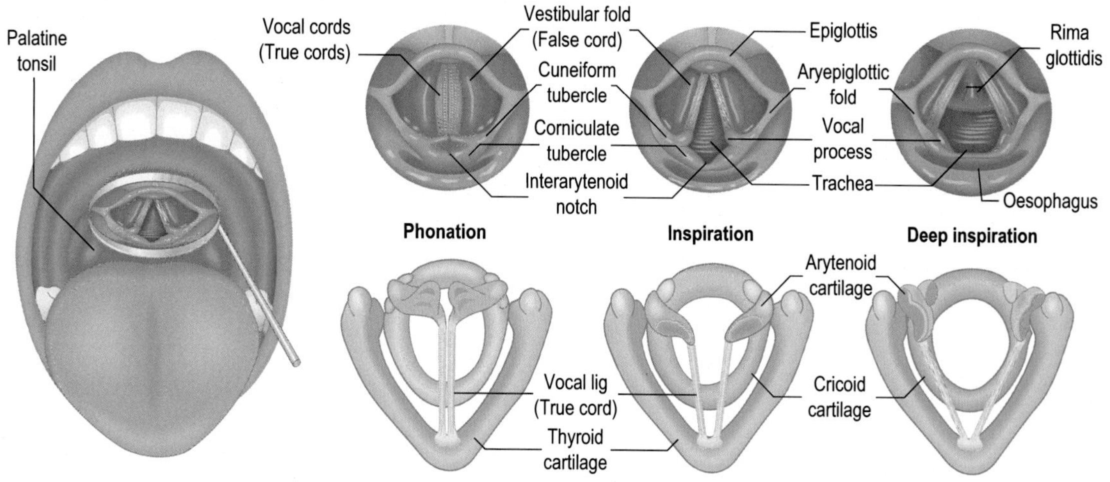

Figure 21.42 The mechanism of phonation.

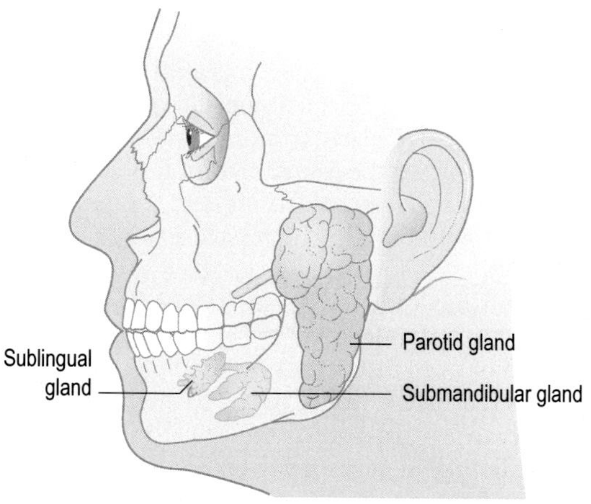

Figure 21.43 The major salivary glands.

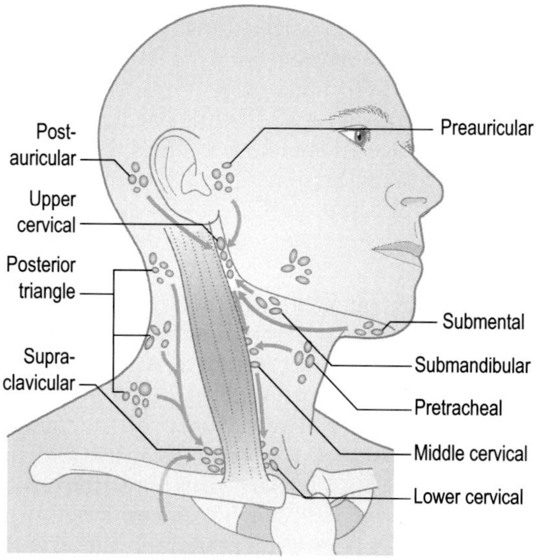

Figure 21.44 The cervical lymph node groupings.

The submandibular gland lies far posterior in the floor of the mouth and may be palpated in the neck, under the mandible. Its duct opens anteriorly in the floor of the mouth adjacent to the frenulum of the tongue. The smaller sublingual gland lies anteriorly in the floor of the mouth and its duct joins the submandibular duct.

The lymph nodes of the head and neck (Fig. 21.44) provide a barrier to the spread of disease, whether inflammatory or neoplastic. Enlargement implies that there is either primary disease within the nodes or that they have become involved secondary to pathology in the areas they drain. Occasionally they may become involved by pathology below the clavicle.

Symptoms of throat disease

Patients with throat disorders present with:

- pain
- ulceration
- stridor, or stertorous (noisy) breathing
- dysphonia (hoarseness)
- dysphagia (difficulty in swallowing)
- a mass in the neck.

Occasionally lesions in the upper airway may present with overspill of food and fluids into the upper trachea or nose or with weight loss. Malignant mouth, throat and airway disease is very strongly associated with smoking, with alcohol intake an important synergistic factor.

Oral ulceration and pain

An ulcer is the commonest oral lesion. Traumatic ulcers heal quickly although, if due to ill-fitting dentures or broken teeth, will rapidly recur, if not fail to heal. Aphthous ulcers are small, painful superficial ulcers of the tongue, buccal mucosa and

Box 21.6 Causes of a burning sensation in the mouth

- Deficiency states:
  - iron deficiency
  - vitamin B_{12} deficiency
  - folate deficiency
- Infection:
  - candidiasis
- Diabetes mellitus
- Erythema migrans
- Psychogenic:
  - anxiety
  - depression
  - cancer phobia

palate, of uncertain cause which are painful but generally heal quickly. There is a high incidence of recurrence. Oral carcinoma may present as an ulcer and is frequently painless. Sometimes there will be other symptoms such as bleeding, loose teeth or halitosis but suspicious non-resolving lesions need to be biopsied. Thrush (fungal infection with *Candida albicans*) is a frequent cause of white patches or pain. Rare causes of ulceration include Crohn's disease and Behçet's syndrome. The sensation of 'burning mouth' has a number of causes outlined in Box 21.6.

Sore throat

A sore throat is one of the commonest of all symptoms. Viral pharyngitis is the most common cause. Tonsillar inflammation is also common. Acute follicular tonsillitis begins with local redness, developing into a punctate or confluent yellow exudate on the tonsils, often due to group A *Streptococcus* infection. In glandular fever (Epstein-Barr virus infection), the tonsils are covered with a white membrane with palatal petechiae. A grey membrane is the classic feature of the now-rare infection with *Corynebacterium diphtheriae*. A throat swab for culture and sensitivity is a useful test. Find out the frequency and severity of attacks of tonsillitis, as estimated by the amount of time lost from school or work, and any antibiotic treatment; such considerations help to decide whether tonsillectomy is merited. Generally in children, at least four attacks a year for 2 years is the minimum indication for tonsillectomy.

An abscess adjacent to the tonsil (quinsy) is very painful, causing dysphagia and trismus (spasm in the lower jaw). Surgical drainage is usually required. Squamous cell carcinoma of the tonsil is also often painful. It presents as an exophytic mass or ulcer. In the early stages, diagnosis is difficult. Ulceration in the oropharynx also occurs in glandular fever, rubella and streptococcal tonsillitis.

Stridor and stertor

Stridor is noisy breathing associated with upper airway obstruction at the laryngeal level (Box 21.7). Stertor is noisy breathing at the oropharyngeal level and is nearly always caused by adenotonsillar hypertrophy. Epiglottitis is particularly important in infants and small children up to the age of 7 years. It is associated with infection by *Haemophilus influenzae* type B, and may present with rapidly progressive airway obstruction and dyspnoea, fever, pharyngeal pain and drooling. Vaccination has reduced its incidence. Immediate antibiotic therapy may need to be supplemented by intubation or even tracheostomy. In adults, laryngeal carcinoma may cause stridor owing to direct blockage of the airway, to fixation of the vocal fold or with recurrent laryngeal nerve involvement. Croup, acute laryngotracheobronchitis in young children, causes less severe airway obstruction. The thick tenacious secretions are relieved by air humidification.

Box 21.7 Causes of stridor

Neonatal

- Congenital tumours and cysts
- Laryngomalacia
- Subglottic stenosis

Children

- Supraglottitis (epiglottitis)
- Laryngotracheobronchitis
- Acute laryngitis
- Foreign body
- Retropharyngeal abscess
- Papillomatosis

Adults

- Acute laryngitis
- Laryngeal trauma
- Laryngeal carcinoma
- Supraglottitis (epiglottitis)

Dysphonia

Dysphonia or hoarseness covers a range of symptoms, from subtle changes noticed by professional voice users to aphonia, when there is no voice. It may be caused by structural problems affecting the vocal fold or by neurological disease (Box 21.8). Hoarseness followed by increasing airway obstruction is the typical presentation of a laryngeal neoplasm (Fig. 21.45). Damage to the recurrent laryngeal nerve anywhere along its course usually leads to hoarseness, although compensation from the unaffected side will limit symptoms. A lesion of the vagus above the exit of the superior laryngeal nerve produces a more breathy voice, as there is also loss of cricothyroid function. Acute vocal abuse and acute inflammation cause dysphonia, which is usually self-limiting. Long-term vocal abuse may lead to a number of changes of the vocal folds: singer's nodules, polyps (Fig. 21.46) or Reinke's oedema. These will often respond to speech therapy, although surgery may be necessary.

Box 21.8 Causes of dysphonia

Inflammatory

- Acute and chronic laryngitis
- Smoke inhalation

Neoplasia

- Carcinoma
- Laryngeal papillomatosis

Recurrent laryngeal nerve

- Post thyroidectomy
- Carcinoma of lung/breast

Neurological

- Myasthenia gravis
- Spasmodic dysphonia
- Systemic: hypothyroidism, rheumatoid arthritis

Habitual dysphonias

- Reinke's oedema
- Singer's nodules
- Vocal cord polyps
- Vocal process granuloma

Gastro-oesophageal/laryngopharyngeal reflux

Psychogenic

- Musculoskeletal tension
- Ventricular
- Dysphonia
- Conversion disorders
- Mutational falsetto (pubophonia)

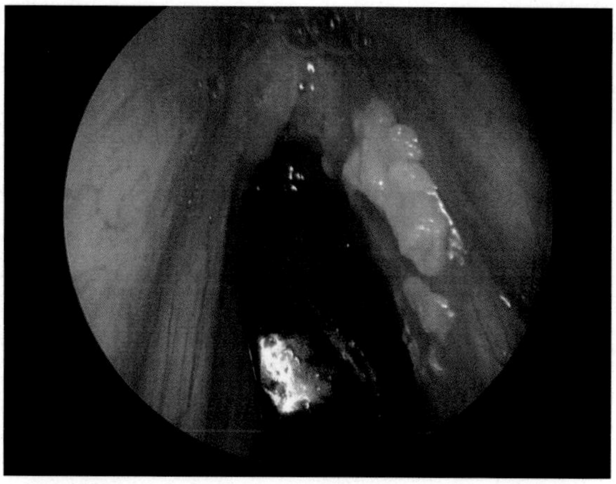

Figure 21.45 Laryngeal carcinoma at the anterior commissure with hyperkeratosis of the right vocal cord.

It is also worth considering whether gastro-oesophageal (laryngopharyngeal) reflux may be implicated. Malignancy should be considered in any patient with dysphonia of more than 4 weeks' duration.

Dysphagia

Any lesion that interrupts the normal sequence of coordinated muscular activity necessary for swallowing may cause dysphagia (Box 21.9). Dysphagia results from structural disease of the pharyngo-oesophagus or from neurological disorders. Persistent dysphagia, especially if associated with regurgitation of undigested food, weight loss, dysphonia, otalgia or a mass in the neck, requires urgent investigation. Pooling of saliva in the piriform fossa seen at laryngoscopy implies obstruction in the cervical oesophagus or in the postcricoid area (see Ch. 14 for discussion of dysphagia below the cricopharyngeus).

Box 21.9 Causes of dysphagia

- Neuromuscular: motor neuron disease, multiple sclerosis, myasthenia gravis
- Intrinsic lesions: oesophageal stricture, oesophageal web, achalasia, pharyngeal pouch, pharyngeal and oesophageal neoplasia
- Extrinsic lesions: thyroid enlargement, primary or secondary neoplasia, aortic aneurysm
- Systemic: scleroderma
- Psychosomatic: globus pharyngeus

Box 21.10 Salivary gland enlargement

- Bacterial infection: acute usually unilateral painful swelling (sialadenitis)
- Viral infection: mumps; painful bilateral swelling and rash
- Obstruction by stone: calculus; variable swelling and pain
- Salivary tumour: gradual increase in size

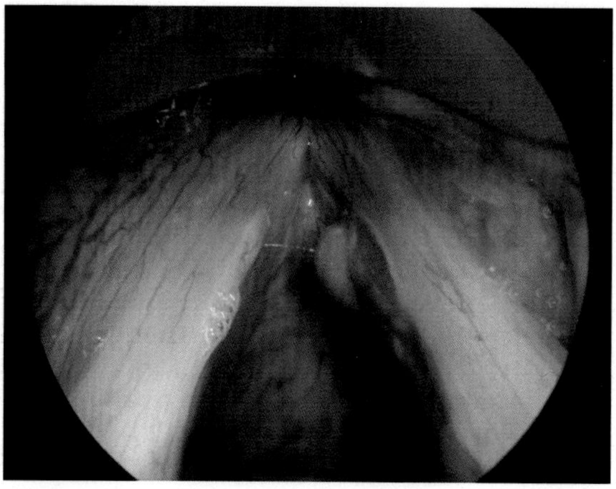

Figure 21.46 A traumatic right vocal cord polyp.

Lump in the neck

The causes of salivary gland swelling are outlined in Box 21.10.

The neck has a rich lymphatic system of nodes and channels that drain the head and neck (see Fig. 21.44).

Box 21.11 Causes of neck lumps by age (these groupings are not exclusive)

Less than 20 years

- Inflammatory/infective lymph nodes
- Thyroglossal and branchial cysts, midline dermoid, cystic hygroma
- Lymphoma

20-40 years

- Salivary gland pathology: calculus, infection, tumour
- Thyroid pathology: goitre, inflammatory thyroiditis, tumour
- Chronic infection: HIV, tuberculosis, actinomycosis
- Lymphoma

Over 40 years

- Secondary malignancy
- Primary malignancy: lymphoma
- Thyroid pathology: goitre, tumour

The deep cervical lymph nodes run in the carotid sheath. The most prominent of these is the jugulodigastric node, which can be palpated just posterior to the angle of the mandible and anterior to the anterior edge of sternomastoid. This is the most commonly enlarged node in upper respiratory tract infections, especially following tonsillitis. The commonest mass in the neck is a lymph node following infection, especially in children. Tuberculosis and atypical mycobacterial infection should always be considered with persistent cervical lymphadenopathy. The diagnosis of a neck lump is partly suggested by the age of the patient (Box 21.11). Features that suggest malignancy are progressive enlargement, hardness, lack of tenderness, fixation to deep structures and size (a node more than 1 cm in diameter is more likely to be malignant). Ultrasound is a valuable investigation, particularly combined with fine needle aspiration cytology.

Examination of the mouth and throat

With practice it is possible to inspect all of the oral cavity, the pharynx and the larynx. Use a headlight or a head mirror to ensure adequate illumination and keep both hands free for the manipulation of instruments. First check the lips, teeth and gums, the floor of the mouth and the openings of the submandibular and parotid ducts. Observe the corners of the mouth for cracks or fissures (angular stomatitis or cheilitis). In children, this is usually due to bacterial infection, but poor dentition in the elderly leads to cracks and candidiasis (thrush). This may also be seen in severe iron-deficiency anaemia and in vitamin B_2 (riboflavin) deficiency. Grouped vesicles on the lips on a red base with crusted lesions are seen in herpes simplex labialis. This viral infection is acute and the lack of induration and ulceration serves to distinguish it from malignancy.

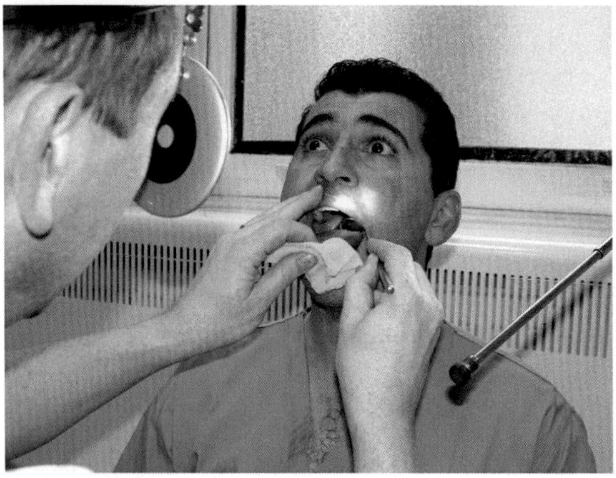

Figure 21.47 Indirect laryngoscopy.

If salivary gland pathology is suspected, bimanual palpation, with one gloved finger in the mouth and synchronous palpation of the gland, may help to define pathology. Palpation is also valuable for examining the cheeks, tongue and even the tonsils on occasion. Tongue mobility (cranial nerve XII) should be assessed by protrusion and side-to-side movement. Look for wasting or fasciculation. Depress the tongue to inspect the tonsillar pillars, the palatine tonsils, soft palate and uvula. The tonsils and soft palate should be nearly symmetrical. Check the gag reflex (cranial nerve IX). The more distant portions of the pharynx can be inspected only with a laryngeal mirror or fibreoptic laryngoscope. For indirect laryngoscopy (Fig. 21.47), remove any dentures; gently hold the protruded tongue and ask the patient to take slow deep breaths. With the mouth opened wide, a warmed or demisted laryngeal mirror is introduced gently but firmly to the soft palate. Displace the soft palate upwards and backwards with the mirror and instruct the patient to say 'ee' or 'ah'. The larynx elevates towards the examining mirror. The vallecula, epiglottis, supraglottis and glottis are examined in turn. The whole length of each vocal fold should be clearly visible and the mobility of each side noted. Vision can be helped in the gagging patient by using a 2% lidocaine anaesthetic spray. If an inadequate view is obtained (this depends upon the skill of the examiner), the flexible fibreoptic nasal endoscope (Fig. 21.48) allows a good view in almost every case. If available, the flexible endoscopic examination is mostly used due to its superior view and for recording the examination for clinical review. Videolaryngostroboscopy (Fig. 21.49) is a specialized endoscopic examination, useful for detailed visualization of the vocal folds. In this technique, stroboscopic light is used through the endoscope to visualize the mucosal wave of the vocal fold and heighten diagnostic capabilities.

Examination of the neck

Examination of the neck is part of the routine assessment of any patient with suspected or proven disease

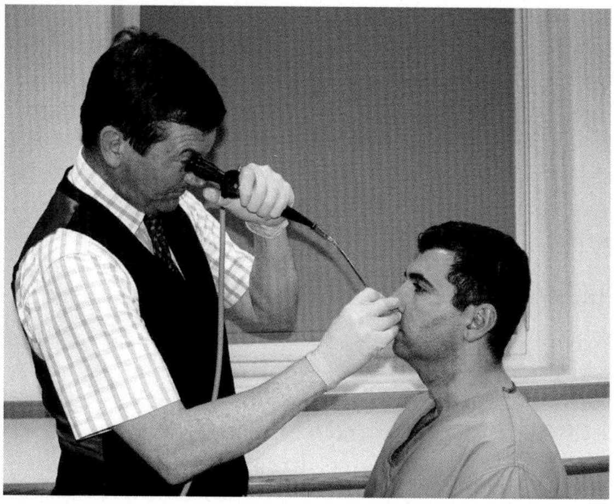

Figure 21.48 Flexible fibreoptic nasendoscopy.

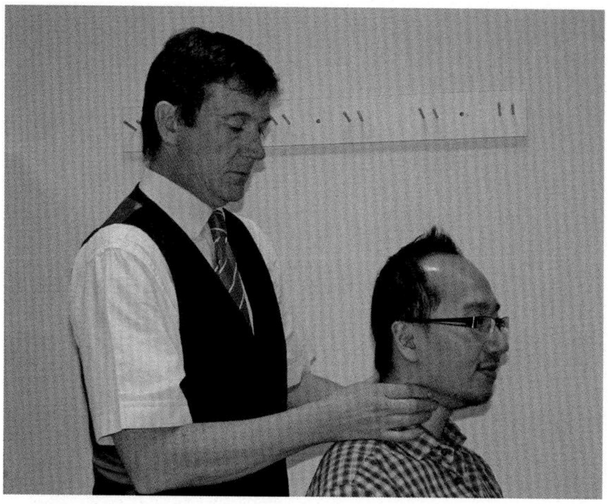

Figure 21.50 Examination of the neck.

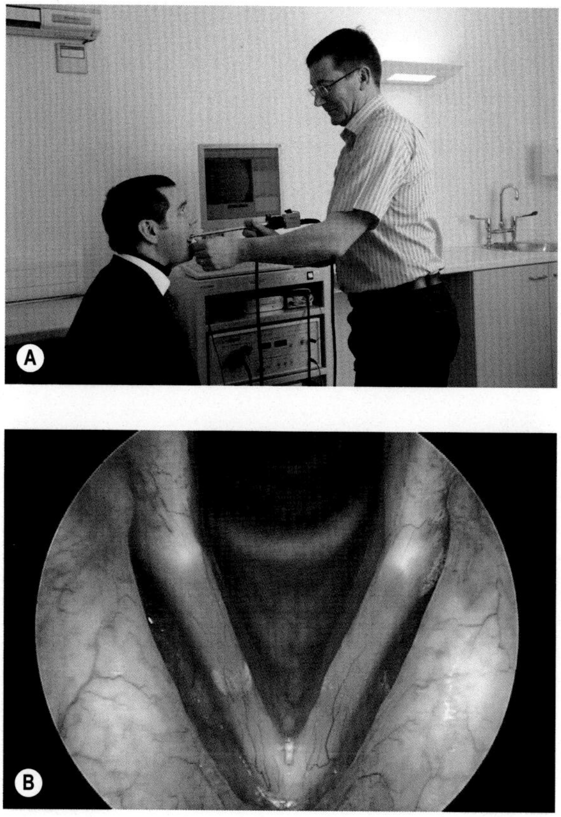

Figure 21.49 **(A)** Videolaryngostroboscopy and **(B)** the image.

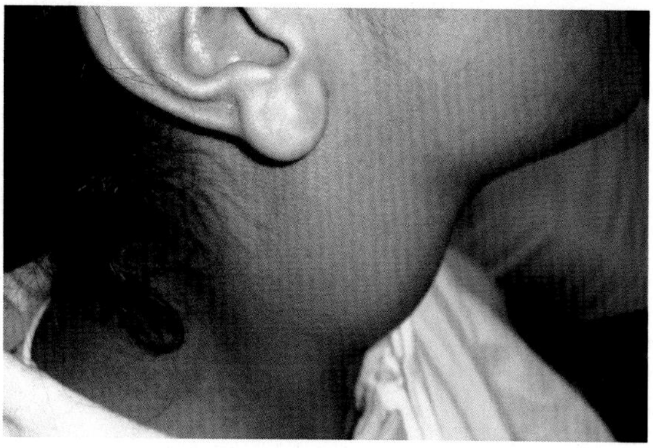

Figure 21.51 Thyroglossal cyst.

in the throat. The neck is exposed and inspected from the front and side before the examiner stands behind the patient (Fig. 21.50) and follows a well-rehearsed routine so that no area is missed. Start by palpating the nodes in the posterior auricular region and then progressively feel for the nodes on the anterior border of the trapezius muscle down to the supraclavicular fossa. The latter area is palpated forwards from behind. The examining fingers then pass up the jugular vein, where the most important groups of nodes in the head and neck are situated, towards the ear. The jugular, parotid and preauricular areas are then examined, followed by submandibular and submental nodes. Finally, the nodes associated with the anterior jugular chain are examined. This brings the fingers to the thyroid gland (details of thyroid examination are in Ch. 18). Midline lumps should also be assessed with the patient protruding the tongue. Movement suggests attachment to the base of the tongue and implies the presence of a thyroglossal cyst (Fig. 21.51). The larynx should be mobile from side to side, and if the thyroid cartilage is held between thumb and first finger and gently moved against the cervical spine, it should grate. This laryngeal crepitus is a normal phenomenon. It may be reduced or abolished by hypopharyngeal pathology or a mass in the prevertebral space displacing the larynx away from the cervical spine. Finally, auscultate the carotid arteries and the thyroid gland.

Tissue sampling

Fine needle aspiration cytology is useful in virtually all neck lumps. If correctly performed, this will

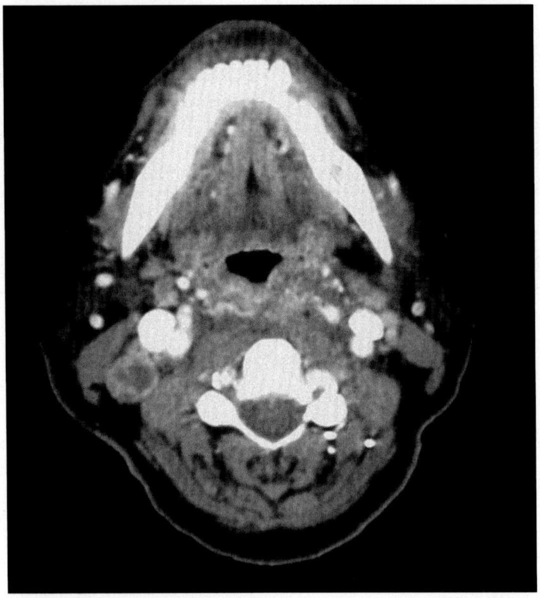

Figure 21.52 CT scan of neck demonstrating a large metastatic lymph node with central necrosis.

diagnose the vast majority of metastatic squamous carcinomas. It is less accurate in distinguishing lymphoma from reactive changes. If doubt remains, then core or excision biopsy should be performed. Accessible lesions in the oral cavity and oropharynx may be biopsied in the clinic with either topical anaesthesia or a local anaesthetic injection (usually with lidocaine).

Radiological examination

A soft-tissue lateral neck X-ray is not a sensitive investigation, even for detecting foreign bodies. A barium swallow is a dynamic investigation and can locate obstruction in the oesophagus or demonstrate incoordinate swallowing. It can be combined with video recording (videofluoroscopy). It is less helpful in evaluating the hypopharynx, where endoscopy under a general anaesthetic is the preferred investigation. Endoscopy is also helpful in taking biopsies in suspected malignancy. Ultrasound is useful for the evaluation of neck masses and the thyroid gland. Doppler ultrasound assesses the cervical vasculature. CT scanning helps to stage neoplastic disease and may demonstrate metastatic spread that has eluded palpation (Fig. 21.52). MRI complements CT as an imaging technique.

Index

Page numbers followed by '*f*' indicate figures, '*t*' indicate tables, and '*b*' indicate boxes.

A

B

D

E

F

G

I

J

K

N

Q

R

T

U

V

W

X

Y

Z

Printed in the United States
By Bookmasters